The Acute Leukemias

HEMATOLOGY

Series Editor

Kenneth M. Brinkhous, M.D.
Department of Pathology
University of North Carolina
School of Medicine
Chapel Hill, North Carolina

Other Volumes in Preparation

The Acute Leukemias

Biologic, Diagnostic, and Therapeutic Determinants

edited by

Sanford A. Stass
The University of Texas System Cancer Center
M. D. Anderson Hospital and Tumor Institute
Houston, Texas

Marcel Dekker, Inc. • New York and Basel

Library of Congress Cataloging-in-Publication Data

The Acute Leukemias.

(Hematology ; v. 6)
Includes index.
1. Acute leukemia. I. Stass, Sanford A.
II. Series: Hematology (New York, N.Y.) ; v. 6.
[DNLM: 1. Acute Disease. 2. Leukemia--diagnosis.
3. Leukemia--therapy. W1 HE873 v.6 / WH 250 A1892]
RC643.A318 1987 616.99'419 87-13468
ISBN 0-8247-7766-2

MARCEL DEKKER, INC.
270 Madison Avenue, New York, New York 10016

Current printing (last digit):
10 9 8 7 6 5 4 3 2 1

PRINTED IN THE UNITED STATES OF AMERICA

Series Introduction

For most of this century hematology has followed a pattern of major scientific discoveries, improved understanding of disease, and rapid application of new knowledge in the clinic. The rate of advance continues at an accelerating pace, so that all but the most zealous have difficulty in keeping up with the literature in even a limited area of specialized interest. As the explosive development of knowledge continues apace, it is a continuing challenge to keep abreast of significant new developments as they impact on clinical and laboratory hematology. The Marcel Dekker, Inc. Hematology series is designed to help in this respect, by providing up-to-date and expert presentations on important subject areas in our field. It is hoped that these works, both individually and collectively, will become important volumes for updating information and for reference for the clinician, investigator, teacher, and student, and in this manner contribute to the advancement of hematology.

This volume on the acute leukemias is the sixth in this Hematology series. Like its predecessors, it presents the current state of the art of the topic, bringing together the many facets of the subject during a stage of rapid advance in the field. In perspective, we are nearing the centennial of the publication in 1889 by Wilhelm Ebstein, the German physician, which clearly identified acute leukemia as an entity distinct from chronic leukemia. The subsequent slow and tortuous progress in subclassifying the acute leukemias by cell type was punctuated by the discovery in midcentury of chemotherapeutic agents causing remission of the disease by such pioneers as Sidney Farber and George Hitchings and their colleagues. This event, coupled with the advances in cell biology and pathology, provided the stimulus and the methods for better characterization of the cells of acute leukemia. The advent of the new immunology and molecular genetics and the application of these new technologies to the study of leukemic cells added still new dimensions for study. The results of this new focus and their applications to clinical management of the acute leukemias are expertly covered in this volume by a distinguished group of contributors under the able leadership of the editor, Sanford A. Stass.

Kenneth M. Brinkhous
Series Editor

Preface

The series to which this book belongs is intended to discuss the spectrum of current directions and knowledge in hematology. This particular volume is focused on one of the most dynamic areas of hematology: characterization of acute leukemia and its biologic, diagnostic, and therapeutic determinants.

In the past few years there has been a rapid expansion in our ability to characterize acute leukemia. This has resulted from the endeavors of scientists from multiple disciplines applying their expertise to the study of leukemic cells. Fields such as immunology, cytogenetics, biochemistry, and molecular biology have enabled detailed characterization of acute leukemia and opened new vistas of understanding never before imagined. In the last five years the biologic revolution in the study of acute leukemia has influenced clinical and basic scientists alike. Such knowledge has directly translated into better and more sensitive methods for the diagnosis of acute leukemia and a better understanding of the process of leukemogenesis. Furthermore, it is clear that the refinement of our ability to characterize and diagnose acute leukemia has resulted in the identification of nonrandom phenotypic and biologic features which have important clinical and prognostic implications. Information developed in the laboratory has rapidly become relevant at the bedside. Thus, in order for basic scientists, pathologists, hematopathologists and clinical and laboratory hematologists to keep pace with and understand future developments and applications in acute leukemia, a clear understanding of recent progress in the study of the characterization of acute leukemia is essential.

This book unifies the current complex and multifaceted approach to the characterization of acute leukemia and places in perspective the usefulness of the divergent studies that are currently available for evaluation of the leukemic cell. Subjects discussed by distinguished experts include specialized morphologic and cytochemical studies, flow cytometry, cytogenetics, immunologic phenotyping, biochemical markers, molecular biology, cytogenetics, and therapeutic implications of leukemic cell characterization. DNA technology, an explosive area of investigation, has provided one of the newest and most precise means for studying and classifying leukemic cells using oncogene and lineage-associated probes. The merging of molecular biology with the studies on nonrandom chromosomal findings, which are important for the classification and prognosis of acute leukemia, has greatly benefited our understanding of the leukemic cell. The insights from such investigations have excited both the basic scientist and the clinical physician. Therefore, several chapters address these subjects.

It is hoped that this book will not only serve as a resource for understanding the significance of biological studies of the leukemic cell but will also result in a better understanding of the clinical significance of leukemic cell characterization and diagnosis, and therefore be a practical guide for both the laboratorian and clinician. The concepts and studies in acute leukemia are changing so rapidly that our approach to this subject will very likely be different in the next decade. Given the present pace of discoveries, future volumes on acute leukemia will certainly include new concepts regarding past discoveries and will present novel studies to answer current questions. However, we hope that this book will be viewed as a timely resource for understanding the characterization of acute leukemia and the resultant biologic, diagnostic, and therapeutic determinants.

Sanford A. Stass

Contributors

Michael J. Ahearn, Ph.D. Associate Professor of Laboratory Medicine, Division of Laboratory Medicine, The University of Texas System Cancer Center, M. D. Anderson Hospital and Tumor Institute, Houston, Texas

Bart Barlogie, M.D. Professor of Medicine and Pathology, Department of Hematology, The University of Texas System Cancer Center, M. D. Anderson Hospital and Tumor Institute, Houston, Texas

Frederick G. Behm, M.D. Associate Member, Department of Pathology and Laboratory Medicine, St. Jude Children's Research Hospital, Memphis, Tennessee

Craig C. Childs, M.D. Assistant Professor of Laboratory Medicine, Hematopathology Program, Division of Laboratory Medicine, The University of Texas System Cancer Center, M. D. Anderson Hospital and Tumor Institute, Houston, Texas

Jeffrey Cossman, M.D. Senior Investigator, Laboratory of Pathology, National Cancer Institute, National Institutes of Health, Bethesda, Maryland

*Gary V. Dahl, M.D.** Associate Member, Leukemia and Lymphoma Service, St. Jude Children's Research Hospital, Memphis, Tennessee

Willard Dalton, Jr., M.D. Assistant Professor of Laboratory Medicine, Hematopathology Program, Division of Laboratory Medicine, The University of Texas System Cancer Center, M. D. Anderson Hospital and Tumor Institute, Houston, Texas

Dennis O. Dixon, Ph.D. Associate Professor of Biometrics, Department of Biomathematics, The University of Texas System Cancer Center, M. D. Anderson Hospital and Tumor Institute, Houston, Texas

---

**Current affiliation*: Associate Professor of Pediatrics, Department of Pediatrics, University of California–Davis Medical Center, Sacramento, California

Benjamin Drewinko, M.D. Professor of Laboratory Medicine and Chief, Section of Laboratory Hematology, Division of Laboratory Medicine, The University of Texas System Cancer Center, M. D. Anderson Hospital and Tumor Institute, Houston, Texas

Carolyn A. Felix, M.D. Medical Staff Fellow, Pediatric Branch, National Cancer Institute, National Institutes of Health, Bethesda, Maryland

Murray B. Gardner, M.D. Professor and Chairman, Department of Medical Pathology, School of Medicine, University of California–Davis, Davis, California

*Winfried B. Graninger, M.D.** Research Associate, Howard Hughes Medical Institute, Washington University School of Medicine, St. Louis, Missouri

Dennis A. Johnston, Ph.D. Associate Professor of Biomathematics, Department of Biomathematics, The University of Texas System Cancer Center, M. D. Anderson Hospital and Tumor Institute, Houston, Texas

David K. Kalwinsky, M.D. Associate Member, Department of Hematology-Oncology, St. Jude Children's Research Hospital; and the Division of Hematology-Oncology, Department of Pediatrics, University of Tennessee College of Medicine, Memphis, Tennessee

Michael J. Keating, M.D. Professor of Medicine, Department of Hematology, The University of Texas System Cancer Center, M. D. Anderson Hospital and Tumor Institute, Houston, Texas

Geoffrey R. Kitchingman, Ph.D. Associate Member, Department of Virology and Molecular Biology, St. Jude Children's Research Hospital, Memphis, Tennessee

Turid Knutsen, MT(ASCP), CLSp(CG) Cytogenetic Oncology Section, Medicine Branch, National Cancer Institute, National Institutes of Health, Bethesda, Maryland

Stanley J. Korsmeyer, M.D. Associate Professor, Division of Hematology-Oncology, Departments of Medicine and Microbiology-Immunology, Howard Hughes Medical Institute, Washington University School of Medicine, St. Louis, Missouri

Kenneth B. McCredie, M.B., Ch.B. Professor of Medicine, Department of Hematology; and Chief, Leukemia Service, The University of Texas System Cancer Center, M. D. Anderson Hospital and Tumor Institute, Houston, Texas

Joseph Mirro, Jr., M.D. Associate Member, Department of Hematology-Oncology, St. Jude Children's Research Hospital; and Associate Professor, Department of Pediatrics, University of Tennessee College of Medicine, Memphis, Tennessee

**Current affiliation*: Second Department of Medicine, University of Vienna, Vienna, Austria

*Arnon Nagler, M.D., M.Sc.** Department of Hematology, Rambam Medical Center; and Faculty of Medicine, Technion Israel Institute of Technology, Haifa, Israel

Stefania Pittaluga, M.D. Visiting Associate, Laboratory of Pathology, National Cancer Institute, National Institutes of Health, Bethesda, Maryland

Gary Spitzer, M.D. Professor of Medicine, Internist, Department of Hematology, The University of Texas System Cancer Center, M. D. Anderson Hospital and Tumor Institute, Houston, Texas

Sanford A. Stass, M.D. Director, Hematopathology Program, Division of Laboratory Medicine; and Professor of Laboratory Medicine and Pathology, The University of Texas System Cancer Center, M. D. Anderson Hospital and Tumor Institute, Houston, Texas

Jose M. Trujillo, M.D. Professor of Laboratory Medicine, The University of Texas System Cancer Center, M. D. Anderson Hospital and Tumor Institute, Houston, Texas

Ronald S. Walters, M.D. Assistant Professor of Medicine, Department of Hematology, The University of Texas System Cancer Center, M. D. Anderson Hospital and Tumor Institute, Houston, Texas

Jacqueline Whang-Peng, M.D. Chief, Cytogenetic Oncology Section, Medicine Branch, National Cancer Institute, National Institutes of Health, Bethesda, Maryland

John J. Wright, M.D., Ph.D. Medical Staff Fellow, Metabolism Branch, National Cancer Institute, National Institutes of Health, Bethesda, Maryland

---

Current affiliation:
*Research Associate, Department of Hematology, Stanford Medical Center, Stanford, California

Contents

The Acute Leukemias

1

Introduction

Characterization and Diagnosis of the Acute Leukemias

CRAIG C. CHILDS and SANFORD A. STASS *The University of Texas System Cancer Center, M. D. Anderson Hospital and Tumor Institute, Houston, Texas*

I. INTRODUCTION

The acute leukemias are a heterogeneous group of hematopoietic malignancies characterized by a clonal expansion of immature cells. Techniques for cellular characterization have demonstrated heterogeneity beyond the categories of acute lymphoblastic (ALL) and acute nonlymphoblastic leukemia (ANLL), and have led to the recognition of additional subtypes with therapeutic and prognostic significance. The variety of data that can be generated in the process of characterizing leukemic cells is apparent from a reading of the table of contents of this book; what may be less evident is the relative value of the various modalities when applied towards diagnosis, classification, and prognosis. The distinction is not always clear between those tools with practical and established roles in patient management and those of primarily research significance. Certain modalities of clinical value such as determination of the DNA index in childhood ALL (Look et al., 1985) may not be available in every clinical setting. Research techniques used in only a few institutions may prove to have important clinical relevance and eventually become a routine part of the acute leukemia workup. An example of this would be the application of molecular lineage probes in ALL (Korsmeyer et al., 1981, 1983; Arnold et al., 1983; Aisenberg and Wilkes, 1985; Kitchingham et al., 1986). The purpose of this introductory chapter is to place in perspective the characterization and diagnosis of acute leukemia by providing a general overview of some of the topics to be covered later in the book. The chapter will offer general guidelines for application and interpretation of data in acute leukemia.

II. DIAGNOSIS AND PROGNOSIS

A. FAB Classification

The diagnosis and classification of acute leukemia should be based on standard morphologic criteria, best represented at present by the French-American-British (FAB) cooperative group proposals (Bennett et al., 1976, 1981b, 1982, 1985a, 1985b) (see Chapter 2). The advantages of a standardized approach are compelling. The light microscopic examination of the bone marrow including Romanovsky and special cytochemical stains is the standard tool for the diagnosis of acute leukemia. Morphologists require a means to communicate to one another the specific morphologic features identified when rendering a diagnosis; in a larger sense, standardization is crucial to achieve the interinstitutional uniformity necessary to allow meaningful comparison of clinical trials. Most important, a classification system must identify subgroups which have common biologic and clinical features.

In order to be useful, a classification system must be reproducible and have biologic significance and clinical relevance. The reproducibility and prognostic significance of the FAB classification have varied among institutions (Foon et al., 1979; Viana, 1980; Mertelsmann et al., 1980; Miller et al., 1981, 1985; Sultan et al., 1981; Bennett, 1981a; Head et al., 1985; Kalwinsky et al., 1985; van Eys, 1986; Childs, Stass, and Bennett, 1986). Despite the conflicting reports in the literature, we feel the reproducibility is acceptable for routine use if the criteria are closely adhered to and interpreted in a logical fashion. The FAB group has recognized four areas of imprecision in the criteria for the subclassification of acute myelocytic leukemia (AML): the distinction between AML without maturation (FAB-M1) and with maturation (FAB-M2); between FAB-M2 and acute myelomonocytic leukemia (AMML; FAB-M4); between FAB-M4 and acute monocytic leukemia (AMOL; FAB-M5); and between erythroleukemia (FAB-M6) and myelodysplastic syndrome (Bennett, 1985b). The group has recently published revised criteria to address these problems in hopes of improving the performance of the FAB classification (Bennett, 1985b).

The FAB classification identifies subgroups which have common biologic and clinical features. For example, certain subtypes have characteristic cytogenetic abnormalities: t(8;14) in ALL, L3 (Zech, Haglund, and Nilsson, 1976); t(8;21) in FAB-M2 (Rowley, 1973); t(15;17) in acute promyelocytic leukemia (FAB-M3) (Rowley et al., 1977); inversion 16 in acute myelomonocytic leukemia with eosinophilia (FAB-M4 with eosinophilia) (Arthur and Bloomfield, 1983), and abnormalities of 11q in FAB-M5 (Berger et al., 1980). The ALL L3 subtype also has a characteristic B-cell phenotype with detectable surface immunoglobulin. Clinical relevance is demonstrated beyond the important distinction between lymphoid and nonlymphoid lineage, as illustrated by the association of FAB-M3 and FAB-M5 with disseminated intravascular coagulopathy, and extramedullary involvement in FAB-M5.

Despite the conflicting reports concerning prognostic significance, the FAB classification is an important tool in diagnosis and classification. Invariably institutions (and individuals) will tailor the criteria based on personal experience or in response to published exceptions to the rule (Mertelsmann et al., 1980; Head et al., 1985; Miller et al., 1985). This process is unavoidable, but does not necessarily detract from the importance of morphology. However, rational use of the FAB classification requires awareness of the limitations of the criteria in light of present knowledge. The FAB cooperative group has now formally recognized the contribution of cell characterization techniques in the diagnosis of acute megakaryoblastic leukemia (Bennett et al., 1985). We emphasize that the diagnosis and classification of acute leukemia in general is a cumulative effort in which light microscopic findings and cytochemical stains must often be integrated with other parameters such as the electron microscopy, cytogenetics, immunophenotype, flow cytometry, or clinical presentation. These correlates may be essential to arrive at a diagnosis and determine prognosis.

III. ACUTE MYELOCYTIC LEUKEMIA (AML)

A. Diagnosis and Subclassification

The FAB classification is based on the light microscopic appearance of the leukemic cells in the marrow in conjunction with cytochemical stains. We recommend as a minimum a myeloperoxidase (MPO) stain and a nonspecific esterase (NSE) either the α-napthyl butyrate esterase (ANB) or the α-napthyl acetate esterase stain with flouride inhibition (ANA-F). The MPO reaction is positive in myeloblastic leukemia, and is vital for making the distinction from acute lymphoblastic leukemia (ALL). Although Sudan black B has been considered an alternative stain, we feel this is not justified. Sudan black B is not specific for AML, as shown in a review of 350 patients with newly diagnosed ALL, in which six patients (1.6%) were found to have 5% or greater Sudan black positive blasts (Stass et al., 1984). In every newly diagnosed case of acute leukemia, MPO must be performed. As no cytochemical marker exists that is specific for lymphoid lineage commitment, the diagnosis of ALL requires demonstrated absence of myeloperoxidase activity. Some cases of acute leukemia can morphologically resemble lymphoblasts but will show strong MPO positivity and should be classified as AML. In addition, the presence of MPO negative azurophilic cytoplasmic granules has been described in ALL (Grogan et al., 1981; Stein et al., 1983). This emphasizes what we have already noted: cytochemistries should be done in conjunction with morphology prior to rendering a diagnosis. Stains other than MPO, although associated with myeloid lineage, are not as sensitive or specific. Sudan black positivity in ALL has been mentioned. The chloracetate esterase (CAE) generally parallels the MPO stain but may be weakly positive or negative in AML, and punctate positivity can occur in ALL (Keifer, Abromowitch, and Stass, 1985). It is extremely rare for AML to be MPO negative and CAE positive, although we have seen such a case with the diagnosis of AML confirmed by the demonstration of ultrastructural peroxidase. The PAS stain does not distinguish ALL from AML. As many as 43% of cases of ALL can be PAS negative (Flandrin and Daniel, 1973), and block positivity can occur in AML (Catovsky and Costello, 1979). The NSE stain is required for confirmation of monocytic differentiation in the diagnosis of acute myelomonocytic (FAB-M4) or monocytic (FAB-M5) leukemia (Bennett et al., 1976). Monocytes, promonocytes, and monoblasts (but not granulocytes are diffusely positive with the ANB reaction and the positive ANA stain is fluoride sensitive. Thus, the M4 leukemia shows MPO and NSE activity; the FAB-M5 subtype is either MPO negative or less than 20% positive, and NSE positive (Bennett et al., 1976). Our preference of NSE substrates is the butyrate reaction. In our experience the ANB stain is more specific for distinguishing monocyte cells from granulocytes, is simpler to interpret and perform, and fluoride inhibition is not necessary. It is imperative that the ANB be interpreted in the proper morphologic setting as focal positivity can be seen in as many as 25% of ALL (Stass, unpublished data). In summary, we consider the MPO and ANB reactions as essential in any diagnostic workup of acute leukemia.

Electron microscopy is a powerful tool in the classification of acute leukemia (Chapter 3), although ultrastructural criteria are in general not incorporated in the FAB classification. Often examples of acute leukemia that are undifferentiated or unclassifiable at the light microscope can be diagnosed as acute myelocytic leukemia based on the demonstration of ultrastructural myeloperoxidase (Glick et al., 1978; Youness, 1980). The electron microscope is essential for diagnosis in about 5% of cases (Glick et al., 1978). The ultrastructural platelet peroxidase reaction is usually positive in cases of acute megakaryoblastic leukemia (Chan et al., 1983; Koike, 1984; Sariban et al., 1984; Pui et al., 1985) and has been incorporated into the FAB criteria for the diagnosis of the M7 subtype (Bennett et al., 1985a).

B. Surface Immunophenotype

The application of monoclonal antibodies directed against surface membrane antigens has led to an immunophenotypic subclassification of ALL (Sallan et al., 1980; Bowman et al., 1981; Greaves, 1981; Greaves et al., 1981; Pullen et al., 1981; Kersey et al., 1982), although the value of immunophenotype as an independent prognostic parameter in ALL has been challenged (Greaves, 1981; Greaves et al., 1981; Kalwinsky et al., 1985). Immunophenotypic heterogeneity has been demonstrated for AML (Nadler et al., 1981; Griffin et al., 1981, 1983b; Van der Reijden et al., 1983; Pessano et al., 1984). However, the limitations of immunophenotype in the differential diagnosis, subclassification, and prognosis of acute lymphoid and myeloid leukemia are significant. Immunologists have not convincingly identified any leukemia-specific antigenic marker, and few if any surface antigens as defined by monoclonal antibodies are lineage specific. For example, coexpression of lymphoid and myeloid surface antigens occurs in acute leukemia (Smith et al., 1983; Stass and Mirro, 1985; Mirro et al., 1985b; Greaves et al., 1986). The value of lineage-associated monoclonals is not well established other than as confirmatory data, and should not be considered an independent diagnostic parameter. This caveat can be illustrated by the example of a case in which the leukemic cells are undifferentiated at the light and electron microscope and demonstrate one or more myeloid associated antigens. We do not feel at present that a diagnosis of acute myelocytic leukemia would be justified, and the diagnosis would remain as undifferentiated. The FAB group has incorporated immunophenotypic data in the diagnosis of acute leukemia of megakaryocytic lineage (FAB-M7), although correlation with cytochemistries, morphology, clinical presentation, and ultrastructural platelet peroxidase reaction is important in making the diagnosis (Bennett et al., 1985a). We would not base a diagnosis of FAB-M7 solely on the basis of platelet antibody reactivity, and require the demonstration of platelet peroxidase.

Immunophenotype as determined with a comprehensive panel including appropriate B and T cell, myeloid, and monocytic markers (see Chapters 7 and 8) can be important as confirmatory evidence of the morphologic diagnosis (Chan, Pegram, and Greaves, 1985). Immunologic data, if inconsistent with the morphologic impression, should certainly prompt reevaluation of the case. Although the immunophenotype should not be used as a sole criterion for the diagnosis, there is recent evidence that the immunophenotype in AML diagnosed by standard criteria may have prognostic significance. Griffin (1986) has recently presented data from a series of 196 patients with AML in which 82% of patients with the [$My4^-My7^-$] phenotype achieved clinical remission while all other cases showed a 54% clinical remission rate.

C. Cytogenetics

Clonal, nonrandom chromosomal abnormalities can be detected in a majority of patients with acute nonlymphocytic leukemia (Rowley, 1984). Chromosomal rearrangements appear to play a role in the malignant process, in light of the association between consistent translocation breakpoints and cellular oncogenes (Yunis, 1983; Rowley, 1984). As already mentioned, karyotype analysis has revealed a number of nonrandom translocations associated with subtypes of AML within the FAB classification. Cytogenetic abnormalities have been shown to have important prognostic significance in AML (see Chapter 5). For example, t(8;21), t(15;17), and inv 16 are associated with a favorable prognosis, whereas t(9,22), −5(or −5q), −7(or −7q), and t(4;11) are less favorable. Certain abnormalities have been described only in nonlymphoid leukemia (see Table 1), the presence of which would favor myeloid lineage. However, karyotype analysis is primarily performed for purposes of prognostication.

IV. ACUTE LYMPHOBLASTIC LEUKEMIA (ALL)

A. Morphologic Diagnosis and Subclassification

The criteria for the diagnosis of ALL demonstrates the concept that a cumulative interpretation of data rather than reliance on a single parameter is necessary in the diagnosis of acute leukemia. The role of cytochemistries in the distinction between ALL and AML is discussed above. No cytochemical marker exists that is specific for lymphoid lineage. The morphologic diagnosis is based on the light microscopic appearance and the demonstrated absence of myeloperoxidase, and in this sense is almost a diagnosis of exclusion. The morphologic appearance of ALL is distinctive and usually easily recognized; as mentioned, however, we have seen cases that look lymphoid but are shown to be AML on the basis of MPO positivity. The morphologic features which favor ALL include nuclear pleomorphism, indistinct or one or two nucleoli, coarse nuclear chromatin, and high nuclear-cytoplasmic ratio (except in the L2 subtype). The FAB group has proposed a scoring system for the subclassification of ALL into L1 and L2 subtypes to improve concordance amongst observers (Bennett et al., 1981b). The scoring system, if carefully adhered to, can achieve significant degrees of concordance (Bennett et al., 1981b; Miller et al., 1985; Childs, Stass, and Bennett, 1986), especially if supplemented by differential counts when scoring (Miller et al., 1985; Childs, Stass, and Bennett, 1986). The significance of L1 and L2 subtypes as an independent prognostic parameter has been questioned in some studies (Kalwinsky et al., 1985; van Eys et al., 1986) but not others, in which L2 morphology imparts a less favorable clinical course (Viana, Maurer, and Ferenc, 1980; Miller et al., 1981, 1985). It is important to remember that if morphologic subtyping is to be incorporated into treatment decisions, a high degree of concordance is vital.

B. Immunophenotype as a Diagnostic Parameter

Terminal deoxynucleotidyl transferase (TdT), the common acute lymphoblastic leukemia antigen (cALLa), and T11 are lymphoid associated markers that have gained widespread application and will be discussed in detail.

Terminal Deoxynucleotidyl Transferase (TdT)

TdT is a recognized marker of lymphoblasts that is *usually* associated with ALL (Bollum, 1979). TdT is a nuclear enzyme that catalyzes the polymerization of deoxynucleoside triphosphates without a requirement for template formation (Bollum, 1979). The enzyme is detected on air-dried blood and marrow smears with either indirect immunofluorescence (Stass et al., 1979) or immunoperoxidase (Stass et al., 1982; Lanham, Melvin, and Stass, 1985), and can be routinely included in a battery of cytochemistries. TdT is a valuable marker for hematopoietic malignancies in that it is found in more than 90% of cases of ALL in children and adults (Hutton et al., 1979), and in 3% to 10% of cases of AML, depending on the percentage of TdT-positive cells and the technique used (Jani et al., 1983). ALL classically will be TdT positive in greater than 40% of marrow cells (Stass et al., 1979). In a large series of patients with acute leukemia in which the incidence of TdT expression was studied with immunofluorescence techniques, approximately 10% of AML patients demonstrated increased numbers of TdT-positive cells (greater than 10%), but only 3% of the cases had greater than 50% positivity (Jani et al., 1983). Rarely AML can show as high as 90% TdT-positive cells (McGraw et al., 1981). If immunoperoxidase is used, 46% of cases of AML will show greater than 10% positivity (Lanham, Melvin, and Stass, 1985). B-cell ALL (L3 type) is usually TdT negative; only rare cases are reported as positive (Drexler et al., 1986). TdT is normally present in immature cortical thymocytes and a small population of bone marrow and circulating peripheral blood lymphocytes (Bollum, 1979; Froehlich et al., 1981; Bradstock, Kerr, and Bollum, 1985) that express the common ALL phenotype rather than T-cell surface markers (Janossy et al., 1979; Bradstock, Kerr, and Bollum, 1985).

Several explanations for TdT expression in AML are suggested. Some patients probably have 2 populations of cells: TdT-negative myeloblasts and TdT-positive lymphoblasts. Other cases on the basis of percentages have coexpression of myeloid characteristics and TdT by the same cell. This occurrence has been documented with a dual staining technique that demonstrated MPO and TdT in the same cell (Lanham et al., 1984). In either case, a common precursor with both myeloid and lymphoid developmental potential is postulated, either recapitulating normal hematopoietic differentiation (lineage fidelity) or occurring as a result of aberrant expression (lineage infidelity). However, presently we have no evidence for a normal cell which contains both MPO and TdT. In light of these findings, TdT, although a valuable tool for identifying ALL, is not lineage specific in the sense that MPO is still considered specific for AML, and TdT is not adequate as a sole parameter for the diagnosis of ALL. TdT does provide strong confirmatory evidence provided other parameters are met, including clinical presentation, morphology, cytochemistries, ultrastructure, immunophenotype, or appropriate results using lineage-associated molecular probes. As demonstration of this caveat, we recently encountered two cases that could not be classified by morphology and cytochemistries but were TdT positive in a majority of the cells. Electron microscopy demonstrated myeloperoxidase in both of these cases, documenting the myeloid origin of the leukemia.

TdT-positive cells can be increased in the marrow in the range of 20% in benign conditions such as idiopathic thrombocytopenic purpura (Nunnery et al., 1980). Low levels of TdT-positive cells in regenerating marrows (up to 11% of the cells) and remission marrows (2-7%) can occur without heralding relapse (Stass et al., 1981; van Dongen, 1986).

TdT determinations are presently performed utilizing polyclonal (heterologous) antibodies (Bollum, 1975). Monoclonal antibodies directed against human TdT have been developed (Bollum et al., 1984). In a comparative study of heterologous and monoclonal antibodies to TdT, the monoclonals were found less sensitive than the polyclonals in detecting ALL. However, while 2 of 5 cases of AML were positive for TdT with polyclonal antisera, none was reactive with the monoclonal. This suggested that the TdT of myeloid malignancy may not be identical to that in ALL (Lanham, Bollum, and Stass, 1986).

Common Acute Lymphoblastic Leukemia Antigen (cALLa)

The experience with cALLa as a hematopoietic surface marker is a classical demonstration of the inability to discover a leukemia-specific surface antigen. Originally defined in association with the prognostically favorable subset of non-T, non-B ALL, this surface antigen subsequently was shown to be neither leukemia, lineage, or hematopoietic specific (see Table 1). However, the distribution of cALLa within the setting of hematopoietic malignancy is well defined and has led (justifiably) to its widespread application as a marker of lymphoid lineage and in the immunologic subclassification of ALL. In our opinion, as with other surface antigens, the importance of cALLa as a diagnostic or prognostic variable depends on other parameters. For example, this surface antigen is expressed by approximately 25% of T-cell ALL (Roberts et al., 1978). The subgroup common ALL is immunologically defined by showing expression of cALLa with TdT and Ia, and the absence of T-cell surface antigens and cytoplasmic and surface immunoglobulin.

The expression of cALLa is relatively restricted within the setting of hematopoietic malignancy, and is useful in differential diagnosis as a marker of lymphoid differentiation, particularly in the distinction of ALL from AML or small round cell tumors in childhood (Greaves et al., 1983). The expression of cALLa in AML diagnosed by standard morphologic and cytochemical criteria is exceedingly rare. In a series of 573 cases of AML reported by Greaves in 1983, 14 expressed cALLa. On review 10 could not be confirmed as AML and were probably of lymphoid origin, one was a lymphoid relapse in a patient who originally had AML (lineage switch), and three were considered to have dual lymphoid-myeloid populations. Thus, expression of cALLa in acute leukemia with unequivocal myeloid differentiation was found in only 3 of 573 cases, or an incidence of approximately 0.5%. The incidence of cALLa expression in AML might seem unexpectedly low in light of the normal expression by mature granulocytes (Cossman et al., 1983). The biologic nature of cALLa in myeloid cells has been partially explored. The possibility exists that anti-cALLa monoclonal antibodies recognize the same epitope on molecules with distinct chemical characteristics (Pesando et al., 1981, 1986). As evidence of this, the glycoprotein identified with anti-cALLa monoclonal antibodies has a molecular weight of 100 kd in lymphoid cells and 110 kd in mature granulocytes (Pesando et al., 1986). Also, cALLa expression by neutrophils fails to undergo modulation when the cells are incubated with specific antibody, as occurs in cALLa positive lymphoid cells (Pesando et al., 1981, 1986). Whether

Table 1 Cellular Distribution of Common ALL Antigen (cALLa)

Cell type or condition	Reference
Normal hematopoietic cells	
Bone marrow	Greaves et al., 1983
Fetal thymus	Greaves et al., 1983
Peripheral blood	Bradstock et al., 1985
Mature granulocytes	Cossman et al., 1983
Normal nonhematopoietic cells	
Fetal small intestine	Metzgar et al., 1981
Breast myoepithelium	Metzgar et al., 1981
Renal tubules and glomeruli	Metzgar et al., 1981
Nonmalignant conditions	
Marrow transplant patients	Greaves et al., 1980b
Neonatal leukemoid reaction	Greaves et al., 1980b
Postchemotherapy lymphocytosis	Greaves et al., 1980a
Regenerating marrow	Greaves et al., 1980b
Hematopoietic malignancy	
Common ALL	Roberts et al., 1978
T-cell ALL	Roberts et al., 1978
B-cell ALL	Greaves et al., 1983
Pre B-cell ALL	Vogler et al., 1978; Greaves et al., 1979
Burkitt's lymphoma	Ritz et al., 1981
T-cell lymphoblastic lymphoma	Ritz et al., 1981
Follicular lymphoma	Ritz et al., 1981
CML-lymphoid or mixed blast crisis	Griffin et al., 1983a; Ha et al., 1985
Acute mixed lineage leukemia (AMLL)	Mirro et al., 1985b; Pui et al., 1984

or not this reflects distinct genetic mechanisms for the expression of cALLa in myeloid cells is uncertain, though this may be a possibility. As evidence that cALLa expression in myeloid malignancy does not necessarily imply B-cell lineage commitment, cases of chronic myelocytic leukemia in mixed blast crisis have been shown to express cALLa in the absence of heavy-chain immunoglobulin gene rearrangement (Bakhshi et al., 1983; Ha et al., 1985), although it has been shown that cALLa expression during B-cell differentiation is preceded by immunoglobulin gene rearrangement and B-cell lineage commitment (Korsmeyer et al., 1983). A single case of cALLa-positive AML in the series from St. Jude Children's Research Hospital demonstrated coexpression of cALLa and myeloperoxidase (but not TdT and myeloperoxidase) in individual leukemic cells (Mirro et al., 1985b). Although the heavy-chain gene was rearranged in this case, cell-sorting experiments were not performed in order to establish that the cALLa-positive/MPO-positive blasts were responsible for the rearranged band. Thus it was not established that cALLa expression by myeloperoxidase-positive blasts indicated simultaneous B-cell and myeloid lineage commitment.

Whereas the expression of cALLa by myeloperoxidase-positive acute leukemia is exceedingly rare, the coexpression of cALLa and myeloid-associated surface antigens in cases of ALL diagnosed with standard morphologic and cytochemical criteria is not uncommon. In the St. Jude Children's Research Hospital series cited above, 13 of 95 cases of childhood ALL demonstrated coexpression of cALLa and myeloid surface antigens (Mirro et al., 1985b). Similar findings are found for adult ALL. In a series reported from M. D. Anderson Hospital and Tumor Institute (Reuben et al., 1985), 2 of 28 cases demonstrated cALLa and My-9, a surface antigen reported to be found on early myeloid progenitor cells (Griffin, 1983b). Whether these patients represent an important clinical subgroup requires additional study (Mirro et al., 1985b; Stass and Mirro, 1985; Kitchingham et al., 1986). The diagnostic issue presented by these cases is distinct from that of cALLa positive AML in that it involves the diagnostic specificity of myeloid-monoclonal antibodies rather than the lineage specificity of cALLa. This demonstrates the importnace of interpretation of immunologic data in conjunction with other parameters.

T-11 Reactivity

The formation of spontaneous rosettes with sheep erythrocytes is the classic biologic marker for identifying T lymphocytes, and establishing T-cell lineage commitment in T-cell ALL. T-11 is a monoclonal antibody directed against a component of the E-rosette receptor that has met widespread application as a pan-T reagent. Although the lineage specificity of the E-rosette assay has not been challenged, the use of specific monoclonal antibody as a substitute is not recommended except when included in a panel with several other T-cell reagents. T-11 reactivity is not specific for lymphoid lineage since it has been reported in AML (Mirro et al., 1985a). A significant percentage of T-cell ALL will not form E-rosettes or show T-11 reactivity, but will react with other T-cell reagents.

C. Immunophentoype as a Prognostic Parameter

Immunophenotypic analysis of childhood ALL has proven useful in investigating the biological and clinical heterogeneity seen in this disease, and has identified subsets with prognostic significance and distinct clinical presentations (Sallan et al., 1980; Bowman et al., 1981; Greaves, 1981; Greaves et al., 1981; Pullen et al., 1981; Kersey et al., 1982). In general those patients with surface immunoglobulin (sIg) (B-cell ALL); cytoplasmic immunoglobulin (cIg) (pre-B-cell-ALL) (Vogler et al., 1978; Brouet et al., 1979); and T-cell phenotype (T-cell ALL) tend to have a worse prognosis. With multivariate analysis, however, the prognostic distinction between T-cell and common ALL disappears when adjustments are made for clinical features such as white blood cell count (Greaves, 1981; Greaves et al., 1981; Kalwinsky et al., 1985). The recent series from St. Jude Children's Research Hospital (Kalwinsky et al., 1985) found no difference in clinical outcome between T-cell ALL and common ALL with a high WBC count. The conclusion was made that clinical parameters (age, WBC count) and cytogenetic findings are more important than other variables such as cytochemistries, morphology, or surface immunophenotype in assigning risk in childhood ALL. The application of an immunophenotypic classification to adult ALL has not been as extensively investigated, but may be helpful in delineating similar biologically or prognostically significant categories (Sobol et al., 1985).

D. Cytogenetics

Cytogenetics has important prognostic implications in childhood ALL. Karyotypic studies have clearly shown that modal chromosome number (ploidy) has independent prognostic significance. Patients that are hyperdiploid with more than 50 chromosomes have the most favorable treatment responses, whereas patients with pseudodiploid karyotypes have the poorest responses. Patients with apparently normal, hypodiploid, or 47-49 chromosomes had intermediate responses (Williams et al., 1982). Additional analysis has shown that the frequency of chromosomal translocations accounts for the variability in prognosis in the different ploidy groups. Furthermore, when analyzed with other clinical and laboratory features, the presence of a translocation was the best single predictor of treatment failure. Statistical analysis showed that the presence of a translocation in childhood ALL increases the risk of treatment failure six times (Williams et al., 1986).

Certain cytogenetic abnormalities in ALL such as t(9;22) and t(4;11) are associated with a poor prognosis. Phenotype-specific translocations in ALL include t(8;14) in B-cell leukemia (Zech, Haglund, and Nilsson, 1976); t(11;14) in T-cell leukemia; and t(1;19) in pre-B-cell ALL (Williams et al., 1984).

V. Acute Mixed Lineage Leukemia

A. Definition

The term *acute mixed lineage leukemia* (AMLL) has been proposed for acute leukemia in which the malignant cells simultaneously express differentiation-associated characteristics of more than one cell lineage (Mirro et al., 1985b). Such lineage heterogeneity has important biologic and practical implications. The incidence of apparent mixed lineage expression is greater than previously realized (Mirro et al., 1985a, 1985b; Stass and Mirro, 1985; Reuben et al., 1985). Such cases demonstrate concurrent expression of both lymphoid and meyloid phenotypic markers, which precludes a clear assignment to a lymphoid or myeloid subtype. Such a distinction is obviously of extreme therapeutic importance. As these cases are not rare, an appreciation of this phenomenon is necessary in developing a rational approach to the diagnosis of acute leukemia. Since this chapter is directed towards the practical application of cell characterization techniques in acute leukemia, our discussion will focus on the diagnostic implications of AMLL. An important theme of this chapter has been the relative diagnostic value (or lineage specificity) of various studies employed in the diagnosis of leukemia. In the majority of cases, the FAB criteria supplemented with appropriate cytochemistries will be sufficient to make a diagnosis upon which appropriate treatment can be based. Additional phenotypic data (usually consisting of surface markers) will usually confirm the diagnosis or, if in conflict, prompt reevaluation of the case and perhaps reinterpretation. In a significant percentage of patients, however, the data will indicate mixed expression of lineage-associated characteristics and the diagnostician may be at a loss at how to proceed in terms of classification and appropriate therapy.

The following sections will briefly discuss the biological implications of AMLL, the more common patterns that have been described, and an approach to diagnosis.

B. Biologic Implications of AMLL

The ongoing theoretical debate concerning lineage fidelity, lineage infidelity, and even lineage promiscuity (Greaves et al., 1986) has been examined in detail in Chapter 12. What follows is a synopsis of the biological issues relevant to developing a rationale diagnostic approach.

The theory of hematopoietic leukemogenesis by Greaves (Greaves and Janossy, 1978; Greaves, 1982) proposes expansion of a malignant clone with adherence to lineage fidelity. According to this theory, the leukemic cell phenotype reflects that of a normal cell frozen or arrested at some stage of maturation or differentiation (Greaves and Janossy, 1978; Greaves, 1982). Thus within any leukemic population the phenotype is representative of normal gene expression with maintenance of lineage fidelity, rather than the product of abnormal gene expression. As a corollary, malignant phenotypes will not occur, nor will a leukemia-specific antigen be found. An opposing model of leukemogenesis involves aberrant gene expression in which abnormal assembly of "differentiation" programs occur from components that properly belong to normal programs (McCulloch et al., 1982; Smith et al., 1983; Stass and Mirro, 1985). The existence of individual leukemic cells with multiple lineage characteristics not normally coexpressed would challenge the former model and support the latter. Various examples of lineage infidelity have been forthcoming. The significance of such cases from a biological standpoint is dependent upon the lineage specifity of the particular parameters involved, and whether coexpression of these characteristics can occur in normal cells. What is important to understand for this discussion is that the term AMLL is not synonymous with lineage infidelity. The term, as defined, is used in recognition that many cases demonstrate conflicting phenotypic data, that recurrent patterns of AMLL occur (some of which may have clinical significance), and that the concept of lineage fidelity versus infidelity is not a settled issue. Although we favor the concept that lineage infidelity may be one explanation (Mirro, 1985b), we recognize that AMLL only raises the question (Stass and Mirro, 1985). In fact, mixed phenotypes identified in the context of AMLL, if found to have normal counterparts, would be consistent with lineage fidelity.

C. Diagnosis of AMLL

At first glance, the variety of reported cases of purported lineage infidelity seems hopelessly confusing. Many of the reports are isolated cases or short series, and utilize a wide variety of phenotypic and genotypic probes. Many if not most have been challenged on the basis of insufficient lineage specificity of the probes utilized. Greaves et al. (1986) have recently reviewed the literature on this subject. Relatively few prospective studies have been attempted with extensive panels of reagents that have been well characterized, and therefore the incidence of mixed lineage has been difficult to assess. For the purpose of this discussion, we would prefer to put aside the issue of lineage fidelity and concentrate on what is known about the incidence and clinical significance of AMLL. Tables 2 and 3 illustrate the degree of lineage specificity that can be expected from the various cell characterization techniques discussed in this book. If we limit the discussion (and the

Table 2 Lineage-Specific Cell Markers

Myeloid leukemia	*Lymphoid leukemia*
Auer rods (MPO+)	E rosettes (37°C)*
MPO (light or EM)	Surface immunoglobulin**
t(8;21)	Cytoplasmic immunoglobulin**
t(15;17)	t(8;14)
inv 16	Heavy *and* light chain immunoglobulin gene rearrangement
Platelet peroxidase (megakaryocytic)	

MPO = myeloperoxidase; EM = electron microscopy.
*Determination of E-rosette receptor associated antigen with monoclonal antibody (T11) is not specific for lymphoid lineage (see text).
**Monoclonal as determined by light chain restriction. Polyclonal surface immunoglobulin is not lineage specific.

Table 3 Lineage-Associated Cell Markers

Myeloid leukemia	*Lymphoid leukemia*
Morphology	Morphology
Sudan B black	cALLa
Chloracetate esterase	anti- T4, T-11, T-101 (Leu 1), B4, B1*
α-napthyl butyrate esterase	TdT
Myeloid surface markers	Heavy chain immunoglobulin gene rearrangement with light chains germ line
High RNA index	$T\beta$ cell receptor gene rearrangement
Heavy chain immunoglobulin and $T\beta$ cell receptor gene in germ line configuration	

cALLa = common ALL antigen; TdT = terminal deoxynucleotidyl transferase
*This is not meant to be an exhaustive list, but merely some of the more commonly used monoclonal antibodies.

entity of AMLL) to cases in which lineage infidelity can be proven, we would be confined to a small subset that would underestimate the frequency and significance of AMLL as a diagnostic and clinical problem.

AMLL represents a heterogeneous group of leukemias, the incidence and nature of which will depend upon the extent that patient's cells are routinely evaluated. The contention has been made, based on prospective studies, that AMLL is not rare, and that certain subsets may have clinical significance. The following data are primarily from the experience with pediatric and adult leukemia at 2 institutions: St. Jude Children's Research Hospital (Mirro et al., 1985b; Pui et al., 1984) and M. D. Anderson Hospital and Tumor Institute (Reuben et al., 1985) (see Chapter 12). In these studies, several patterns of mixed phenotypic expression emerged. The analytical approach involved classifying the cases according to standard criteria utilizing the FAB system, noting the phenotypic inconsistency, and where possible, the clinical significance. We prefer this approach as a general rule. The crucial clinical question for each patient is whether conflicting phenotypic data carried beyond morphology justifies a departure from the light microscopic diagnosis that may alter treatment. By adhering to standard criteria, rational analysis of otherwise potentially confusing data is possible.

D. Subtypes of AMLL

ALL with myeloid surface antigens. These are cases which meet standard morphologic and cytochemical criteria for ALL, usually including TdT positivity, with expression of one or more myeloid-associated surface antigens. The incidence may vary according to age group: 25% in childhood ALL (Mirro et al., 1985b) and 7% of adult ALL (Reuben et al., 1985). The incidence will vary as well according to the extent of the immunophenotypic panel. For example, the Pediatric Oncology Group reported a much lower incidence of 4.5% utilizing 2 myeloid monoclonals MY1 and DU-HL60 (Weiner et al., 1985). In that series the cases of non-T ALL with myeloid antigen expression had a significantly poorer clinical response rate. One study in adults has suggested that this group has a lower chance of achieving complete remission (Sobol et al., 1986); however, our preliminary experience at M. D. Anderson has not confirmed this finding (unpublished data). Future studies will be necessary to determine the clinical significance of myeloid antigen expression in ALL.

AML with lymphoid surface antigens. The incidence of AML diagnosed with standard criteria with expression of lymphoid surface antigens can be as high as 25% in childhood acute leukemia and 34% in adult cases of acute and chronic leukemia (Mirro et al., 1985b; Reuben et al., 1985). In children cALLa-positive AML occurs rarely (Pui et al., 1984); a more frequent pattern is seen in which a low percentage of MPO-positive blasts (less than 15%) were found with expression of the E-rosette-associated antigen or other T-cell markers. The formation of E rosettes was not observed in these cases (Mirro et al., 1985b). Other T-cell markers expressed included T-3 in children, and in adults T-11 was often concurrently expressed with the T-4 antigen, a marker of helper T cells. Pediatric patients who meet the standard criteria for AML and express T-11 may represent an important clinical subgroup of AMLL. These patients have a poorer response to induction therapy; those who fail AMLL-directed therapy may enter remission with ALL-directed treatment. Other reports of ALL with coexpression of markers of more than one lineage have suggested a poor response to therapy (Smith et al., 1983). Overall, the numbers are too few and followup insufficient to establish this group as a distinct therapeutic subset.

E. Summary

Although the incidence of AMLL is apparently greater than previously expected, there are only preliminary data suggesting clinical significance. The marked heterogeneity of mixed phenotypes further inhibits all-inclusive statements as to the appropriate treatment. The prudent course at the present time would be to adhere to the standard FAB criteria, although recognizing that some subsets of AMLL may prove to be clinically important.

VI. MINIMAL RESIDUAL DISEASE

This section is concerned with continued evaluation of the patient after the initial diagnosis is made and treatment begun. Protocols will vary as to the frequency and timing of the followup marrow examinations and the influence subsequent marrow findings will have on treatment decisions. In general, marrow examination should document the initial period of aplasia, regeneration, recovery, and the establishment of remission status. After remission is achieved, periodic marrows are required to monitor maintenance and to detect early relapse. In each case, the pathologist will be expected to assess the presence of blasts and evaluate the likelihood of residual (during aplasia), persistent (during the expected recovery phase or later) or relapsed acute leukemia (following a period of remission). In some cases, the pathologist may elect to repeat additional studies to detect or confirm low numbers of malignant cells (minimal residual disease). Knowledge of the sensitivity and specificity of cell characterization techniques is crucial when evaluating a marrow that is equivocal or suspicious for malignancy.

A. Remission Marrow: Definition

Complete remission is said to exist when a diagnosis of leukemia cannot be made except by history, and when certain hematologic parameters such as platelet count, hemoglobin, and granulocytes have returned to normal. In the marrow this usually implies less than 3-5% blasts and normal trilineage maturation. The conventional criterion of less than 5% is partly based on the fact that blasts are usually indistinguishable from normal precursors at this level. However, adherence to an arbitrary percentage ignores the increase in blast counts that can occur in regeneration and underestimates the limits of light microscopy. We feel a remission marrow is better defined as a marrow showing the absence of identifiably malignant blasts, regardless of the percentage, along with normal trilineage maturation. Not infrequently, malignant blasts can be identified at below the 3% to 5% level on the basis of distinctive or characteristic features: Auer rods in AML; vacuoles in ALL, L3; or unusual cytoplasmic granularity such as in granular ALL or promyelocytic leukemia. Such a marrow should not be designated as remission. Comparison with the diagnostic marrow can aid in the identification of malignant blasts in some cases. Increased blasts in the range of 5-10% or rarely as high as 30% can be seen in regenerating marrow (albeit transiently). This emphasizes the importance of interpreting the findings in conjunction with knowledge of the treatment stage and the expected findings. In some instances the distinction from residual leukemia may be impossible. In these circumstances, close followup with repeat marrows at frequent intervals is indicated. Certain morphologic abnormalities may be present that do not warrant a diagnosis of leukemia. The presence of myeloid or erythroid dysplasia in a patient undergoing chemotherapy should not be taken as evidence of residual acute leukemia. Such changes may be indistinguishable from chemotherapeutic effect and do not necessarily imply the presence of a malignant clone. Persistent monocytosis in a patient treated for acute myelomonocytic or monocytic leukemia could be confused with residual leukemia. Again, the important parameter is the number and appearance of the blasts. In these circumstances, karyotypic analysis may be of value to identify a malignant clone.

B. Detection of Minimal Residual Disease

Remission corresponds to a reduction of tumor burden beyond clearly detectable limits at which point normal function can return (Henderson, 1983). This corresponds to a tumor burden of 10^{10} or 10^9 cells, which from a biologic standpoint is still a considerable population (Henderson, 1983). Cell characterization techniques have been used to detect minimal disease in an effort to go beyond the sensitivity of the light microscope. If successful, relapse could be detected at an earlier stage or treatment strategies evaluated in terms of complete eradication of the malignant clone. Unfortunately, most techniques have not gone beyond the 1% detection limit set by light microscopy.

The hematologist when following a patient during treatment and relapse may be tempted to repeat certain diagnostic techniques such as immunophenotype or cytogenetics to follow the course of the disease. A brief discussion of those techniques that can be expected to yield useful information is in order. The detection of minimal residual disease should be considered in two levels. The first involves the study of marrows with increased blasts in which the light microscopic diagnosis is suspicious or equivocal for malignancy. The second involves detection of malignant cells when the marrow is in remission by standard criteria.

Immunophenotype. The role of surface markers is limited for detection of minimal disease for the same reasons as discussed in the section related to diagnosis. The surface antigenic phenotypes in most cases reflect normal differentiation stages, and thus cannot distinguish malignant cells from normal precursors. The elevated levels of cALLa and TdT in regenerating marrows has been mentioned. Although the sensitivity of flow cytometry in detecting small percentages of cells approximates the light microscope in many cases, the lack of leukemia-specific antigens or malignant phenotypes is a severe hindrance. Certain configurations can be useful, for example, the kappa/lambda ratio can detect monoclonal proliferation and is applicable to B-cell ALL. Certain markers can be utilized in extramedullary sites, such as detection of TdT-positive cells in the cerebral spinal fluid.

Cytogenetics. The sensitivity of karyotype analysis only rarely exceeds the light microscope, as in the reported finding of a t(8;14) in a remission marrow (Richardson and Dickerman, 1986). The advantage is that a marker diagnostic of malignancy is detected, and can be helpful in the evaluation of the suspicious or equivocal marrow.

Molecular lineage probes. DNA technology has produced tremendous advances in recent years. Molecular techniques may have important practical application. Detection of molecular rearrangements in lymphoid neoplasms has the advantage of sensitivity beyond the 1% level as shown with mixing experiments (Zehnbauer et al., 1986), and detects a clonal population. The detection of immunoglobulin gene rearrangement in "remission" marrows from patients treated for ALL has been reported and has heralded relapse (Arnold et al., 1983; Wright et al., 1986; Zehnbauer et al., 1986).

VII. FUTURE DIRECTIONS

A. Practical Applications

Although morphology at the light microscopic level remains the standard for diagnosis in most cases, cellular characterization techniques are increasing the refinement of subclassification and identifying subsets of patients—such as B-cell ALL or acute leukemia with t(4;11)—with specific biologic characteristics, which has important therapeutic significance. This is an important theme to be developed in later chapters. Further refinements in immunopathology may lead to the development of monoclonal antibodies that recognize leukemia-specific antigens or malignant phenotypes. Additional lineage-specific probes, particularly for myeloid differentiation, need to be developed. Progress in this area will most likely be made at the molecular level, with cloning of myeloid-specific genes such as myeloperoxidase (Chang et al., 1986). The BCR/abl transcript specific for the translocation in t(9;22) is indicative of future developments that will have enormous effect in diagnosis and treatment. The cloning of nonrandom chromosomal translocation sites and identification of their associated gene products in acute leukemia will provide a sensitive means for identifying leukemic clones and thus further the detection of minimal residual disease and the definition of biologically relevant leukemic subsets.

B. Future Classification

Heterogeneity has been found at the molecular level when probes are used to detect molecular gene rearrangements in lymphoid leukemia. It is becoming evident that the classic distinction of lymphoid and myeloid leukemia is less relevant than a classification based on specific biologic parameters. Since the purpose of a classification scheme is to provide insight into etiology, therapy and prognosis, future classifications will most likely be based on biologic parameters. Biologic classification schemes would be based on parameters such as cytogenetics, molecular characteristics, factors involved in the transformation of the leukemic cell, and cellular products resulting from genetic rearrangement in leukemic cells; they will most likely offer more insight and relevance to our approach to leukemia than morphology alone. This is the challenge of the future, and the approach that ultimately will best serve the basic researcher, diagnostician, and clinician.

REFERENCES

Aisenberg, A. C., and Wilkes, B. M. (1985). The genotype and phenotype of T-cell and non-T, non-B acute lymphoblastic leukemia. *Blood* 66:1215-1218.

Arnold, A., Cossman, J. C., Bakhshi, A., Jaffe, E. S., Waldman, T. A., and Korsmeyer, S. J. (1983). Immunoglobulin-gene rearrangements as unique clonal markers in human lymphoid neoplasms. *N. Engl. J. Med.* 309:1593-1599.

Arthur, P. C., and Bloomfield, C. D. (1983). Partial deletion of the long arm of chromosome 16 and bone marrow eosinophilia in acute nonlymphocytic leukemia: a new association. *Blood* 61:994-998.

Bakhshi, A., Minowada, J., Arnold, A., Cossman, J., Jensen, J. P., Whang-Peng, J., Waldman, T. A., and Korsmeyer, S. J. (1983). Lymphoid blast crisis of chronic myelogenous leukemia represents stages in the development of B cell precursors. *N. Engl. J. Med.* 309:826-831.

Bennett, J. M., and Begg, C. B. for the Eastern Cooperative Oncology Group (1981a). Eastern cooperative oncology group study of the cytochemistry of adult myeloid leukemia by correlation of subtypes with response and survival. *Cancer Res.* 41:4833-4837.

Bennett, J. M., Catovsky, D., Daniel, M. T., Flandrin, G., Galton, D. A. G., Gralnick, H. R., and Sultan, C. (1976). Proposals for the classification of the acute leukemias (FAB co-operative group). (1976). *Brit. J. Haem.* 33:451-458.

Bennett, J. M., Catovsky, D., Daniel, M. T., Flandrin, G., Galton, D. A. G., Gralnick, H. R., and Sultan, C. (FAB co-operative group) (1981b). The morphological classification of acute lymphoblastic leukemia: concordance among observors and clinical correlations. *Brit. J. Haem.* 47:553-561.

Bennett, J. M., Catovsky, D., Daniel, M. T., Flandrin, G., Galton, D. A. G., Gralnick, H. R., and Sultan, C. (The FAB co-operative group). (1982). Proposals for the classification of the myelodysplastic syndromes. *Brit. J. Haem.* 51: 189-199.

Bennett, J. M., Catovsky, D., Daniel, M. T., Flandrin, G., Galton, D. A. G., Gralnick, H. R., and Sultan, C. (1985a). Criteria for the diagnosis of acute leukemia of megakaryocyte lineage (M7). *Ann. Int. Med.* 103:460-462.

Bennett, J. M., Catovsky, D., Daniel, M. T., Flandrin, G., Galton, D. A. G., Gralnick, H. R., and Sultan, C. (1985b). Proposed revised criteria for the classification of acute myeloid leukemia. *Ann. Int. Med.* 103:626-629.

Berger, R., Berheim, A., Weh, H. J., Daniel, M. T., and Flandrin, G. (1980). Cytogenetic studies on acute monocytic leukemia. *Leuk. Res. 4*:119-127.

Bollum, F. J. (1975). Antibody to terminal deoxynucleotidyl transferase. *Proc. Natl. Acad. Sci. (USA)* 72:4119-4122.

Bollum, F. J. (1979). Terminal deoxynucleotidyl transferase as a hematopoietic cell marker. *Blood* 54:1203-1215.

Bollum, F. J., Augl, C., and Chang, L. M. S. (1984). Monoclonal antibodies to human terminal transferase. *J. Biol. Chem.* 259:5848-5850.

Bowman, W. P., Melvin, S. L., Aur, R. J. A., and Mauer, A. M. (1981). A clinical perspective on cell markers in acute lymphoblastic leukemia. *Cancer Res.* 41: 4794-4801.

Bradstock, K. F., Kerr, A., and Bollum, F. J. (1985). Antigenic phenotype of TdT-positive cells in human peripheral blood. *Cellular Immunol.* 90:590-598.

Brouet, J. C., Preud'homme, J. L., Periet, C., Valeusi, F., Rouget, P., and Seligmann, M. (1979). Acute lymphoblastic leukemia with Pre-B-cell characteristics. *Blood* 54:269-273.

Catovsky, D., and Costello, C. (1979). Cytochemistry of normal and leukaemic lymphocytes: a review. *Basic Appl. Histochem.* 23:255-270.

Chan, W. C., Brynes, R. K., Kim, T. H., Verras, A., Schick, C., Green, R. G., and Ragab, A. (1983). Acute megakaryoblastic leukemia in early childhood. *Blood* 62:92-98.

Chan, L. C., Pegram, S. M., and Greaves, M. F. (1985). Contribution of immunophenotype to the classification and differential diagnosis of acute leukaemia. *Lancet* i:475-479.

Chang, K. S., Trujillo, J. M., Cook, R. G., and Stass, S. A. (1986). Human myeloperoxidase gene: molecular cloning and expression in leukemic cells. *Blood* 68:1411-1414.

Childs, C. C., Stass, S. A., and Bennett, J. M. (1986). The morphological classification of acute lymphoblastic leukemia in childhood: observations on concordance utilizing a simple scoring system. *Am. J. Clin. Path.* 86:503-506.

Cossman, J., Neckers, L. M., Leonard, W. J., and Green, W. C. (1983). Polymorphonuclear neutrophils express the common acute lymphoblastic leukemia antigen. *J. Exp. Med.* 157:1064-1069.

Drexler, H. G., Messmore, H. L., Menon, M., and Minowada, J. (1986). A case of TdT-positive B-cell acute lymphoblastic leukemia. *Am. J. Clin. Path.* 85:735-738.

Flandrin, G., and Daniel, M. T. (1973). Practical value of cytochemical studies for the classification of acute leukemias. *Rec. Res. Cancer Res.* 43:43-56.

Foon, K. A., Naiem, F., Yale, C. Y., and Gale, R. P. (1979). Acute myelogenous leukemia: morphologic classification and response to therapy. *Leuk. Res.* 3: 171-173.

Froelich, T. W., Buchanan, G. R., Cornet, J. A. M., Sartain, P. A., and Smith, R. G. (1981). Terminal deoxynucleotidyl transferase-containing cells in peripheral blood: implications for the surveillance of patients with lymphoblastic leukemia or lymphoma in remission. *Blood* 58:214-220.

Glick, A. D., Paniker, K., Flexner, J. M., Graber, S. E., and Collins, R. D. (1978). Acute leukemia of adults. Ultrastructural, cytochemical, and histologic observations in 100 cases. *Am. J. Clin. Pathol.* 73:459-470.

Greaves, M., and Janossy, G. (1978). Patterns of gene expression and the cellular origins of human leukaemias. *Biochem. Biophys. Acta.* 516:193-230.

Greaves, M. F., Verbi, W., Vogler, L., Cooper, M., Ellis, R. Ganeshaguree, K., Hoffbrand, V., Janossy, G., and Bollum, F. J. (1979). Antigenic and enzymatic phenotypes of the pre-B subclass of acute lymphoblastic leukaemia. *Leuk. Res.* 3:353-362.

Greaves, M., Paxton, A., Janossy, G., Pain, C., Johnson, S., and Lister, T. A. (1980a). Acute lymphoblastic leukemia associated antigen III. Alterations in expression during treatment and in relapse. *Leuk. Res.* 4:1-14.

Greaves, M., Delia, D., Janossy, G., Rapson, N., Chessells, J., Woods, M., and Prentice, G. (1980b). Acute lymphoblastic leukaemia associated antigen: IV expression on non-leukaemic "lymphoid" cells. *Leuk. Res.* 4:15-32.

Greaves, M. F. (1981). Analysis of the clinical and biological significance of lymphoid phenotypes in acute leukemia. *Cancer Res.* 41:4752-4766.

Greaves, M. F., Janossy, G., Peto, J., and Humphrey, K. (1981). Immunologically defined subclasses of acute lymphoblastic leukemia in children: their relationship to presentation features and prognosis. *Brit. J. Haem.* 48:179-197.

Greaves, M. F. (1982). "Target" cells, cellular phenotypes and lineage fidelity in human leukaemia. *J. Cell. Physiol. Suppl.* 1:113-125.

Greaves, M. F., Hariri, G., Newman, R. A., Sutherland, D. R., Ritler, M. A., and Ritz, J. (1983). Selective expression of the common acute lymphoblastic leukemia (gp100) antigen on immature lymphoid cells and their malignant counterparts. *Blood* 61:628-639.

Greaves, M. F., Chan, L. C., Furley, A. J. W., Watt, S. M., and Molgaard, H. V. (1986). Lineage promiscuity in hemopoietic differentiation and leukemia. *Blood* 67:1-11.

Griffin, J. D., Ritz, J., Nadler, L. M., and Schlossman, S. F. (1981). Expression of myeloid differentiation antigens on normal and malignant myeloid cells. *J. Clin. Invest.* 68:932-941.

Griffin, J. D., Todd III, R. F., Ritz, J., Nadler, L. M., Canellas, G. P., Rosenthal, D., Gallivan, M., Beveridge, R. P., Weinstain, H., Karp, D., and Schlossman, S. F. (1983a). Differentiation patterns in the blastic phase of chronic myeloid leukemia. *Blood* 61:85-91.

Griffin, J. D., Mayer, R. J., Weinstein, H. J., Rosenthal, D. S., Coral, F. S., Beveridge, R. P., Schlossmann, S. F. (1983b). Surface marker analysis of acute myeloblastic leukemia: Identification of differentiation-associated phenotypes. *Blood* 62:557-563.

Griffin, J. D. (1986). Malignant phenotypes: AML. Leukemia Society Abstract. LSA Medical Conference Second National Symposium, March 20-22, 1986.

Grogan, T. M., Insalaco, S. J. Savage, R. A., and Vail, M. L. (1981). Acute lymphocytic leukemia with prominent azurophilic granulation and punctate acidic nonspecific esterase and phosphatase activity. *Am. J. Clin. Pathol.* 75:716-722.

Ha, K., Freedman, M. H., Hrincu, A., Petsche, D., Poon, A., and Gelfand, E. W. (1985). Separation of lymphoid and myeloid blasts in the mixed blast crisis of chronic myelogenous leukemia: No evidence of Ig gene rearrangement in cALLa-positive blasts. *Blood* 66:1404-1408.

Head, D. R., Cerezo, L., Savage, R. A., Craven, C. M., Bickers, J. N., Hartsock, R., Hasty, T. A., Saiki, J. H., Wilson, H. E., Morrison, F. S., Coltman, C. A., and Hutton, J. J. (1985). Institutional performance in application of the FAB classification of acute leukemia. The Southwest Oncology Group Experience. *Cancer* 55:1979-1986.

Henderson, E. S. (1983). Terminology and overview. In *Leukemia*, F. W. Guntz and E. S. Henderson (eds.). Grune and Stratton, New York, p. 490.

Hutton, J. J., Coleman, M. S., Keneklis, T. P., and Bollum, F. J. (1979). Terminal deoxynucleotidyl transferase as a tumor cell marker in leukaemia and lymphoma: results from 1000 patients. In *Advances in Oncology, Research and Education*, Vol. 4, M. Fox (ed.). Pergamon Press, Oxford and New York, p. 165.

Jani, P., Verbi, W., Greaves, M. F., Bevan, D., and Bollum, F. J. (1983). Terminal deoxynucleotidyl transferase in acute myeloid leukaemia. *Leukemia Res.* 7: 17-29.

Janossy, G., Bollum, F. J., Bradstock, K. F., McMichael, A., Rapson, N., and Greaves, M. F. (1979). Terminal transferase-positive human bone marrow cells exhibit the antigenic phenotype of common acute lymphoblastic leukemia. *J. Immunol.* 123:1525-1529.

Kalwinsky, K. D., Roberson, P., Dahl, G., Harber, J., Rivera, G., Bowman, W. P., Pui, C. H., Ochs, J., Abromowitch, M., Costlow, M. E., Melvin, S. L., Stass, S., Williams, D. L., and Murphy, S. B. (1985). Clinical relevance of lymphoblast biological features in children with acute lymphoblastic leukemia. *J. Clin. Oncol.* 3:477-484.

Keifer, J., Abromowitch, M., and Stass, S. (1985). Chloroacetate esterase positivity in acute lymphoblastic leukemia. *Am. J. Clin. Pathol.* 83:647-649.

Kersey, J., Abramson, C., Perry, G., Goldman, A., Nesbit, M., Gajl-Peczalska, K., and LeBien, T. (1982). Clinical usefulness of monoclonal antibody phenotyping in childhood acute lymphoblastic leukaemia. *Lancet* ii:1419-1423.

Kitchingham, G. R., Mirro, J., Stass, S., Rovigatti, U., Melvin, S. L., Williams, D. L., Raimondi, S. C., and Murphy, S. B. (1986). Biologic and prognostic significance of the presence of more than two μ heavy chain genes in childhood acute lymphoblastic leukemia of B precursor cell origin. *Blood* 67:698-703.

Koike, T. (1984). Megakaryoblastic leukemia: The characterization and identification of megakaryoblasts. *Blood* 64:683-692.

Korsmeyer, S. J., Hieter, P. E., Ravetch, J. V., Poplack, D. G., Waldman, T. A., and Leder, P. (1981). Developmental heirarchy of immunoglobulin gene rearrangements in human leukemic pre-B-cells. *Proc. Natl. Acad. Sci. USA* 78: 7096-7100.

Korsmeyer, S. J., Arnold, A., Bakhshi, A., Ravetch, J. V., Siebenlist, U., Hieter, P. A., Sharrow, S. O., LeBien, T. W., Kersey, J. H., Poplack, D. G., Leder, P., and Waldmann, T. A. (1983). Immunoglobulin gene rearrangement and cell surface antigen expression in acute lymphocytic leukemia of T cell and B cell precursor origins. *J. Clin. Invest.* 71:301-313.

Lanham, G. R., Bollum, F. J., Williams, P. L., and Stass, S. A. (1984). Simultaneous occurrence of terminal deoxynucleotidyl transferase and myeloperoxidase in individual leukemic blasts. *Blood* 64:318-320.

Lanham, G. R., Melvin, S. L., and Stass, S. A. (1985). Immunoperoxidase determination of terminal deoxynucleotidyl transferase in acute leukemia using PAP and ABC methods: experience in 102 cases. *Am. J. Clin. Pathol.* 83:366-370.

Lanham, G. R., Bollum, F. J., and Stass, S. (1986). Detection of terminal deoxynucleotidyl transferase in acute leukemias using monoclonal antibodies directed against native and denatured sites. *Am. J. Clin. Path.* 86:88-91.

Look, A. T., Roberson, P. K., Williams, D. L., Rivera, G., Bowman, W. P., Pui, C. H., Ochs, J., Abromowitch, M., Kalwinsky, D., Dahl, C. V., George, S., and Murphy, S. B. (1985). Prognostic importance of blast cell DNA content in childhood acute lymphoblastic leukemia. *Blood* 65:1079-1086.

McCulloch, E. A., Izaquiree, C. A., Chang, L. J.-A., and Smith L. J. (1982). Renewal and determination in leukemic blast populations. *J. Cell. Physiol. Suppl.* 1:103-111.

McGraw, T. P., Folds, J. D., Bollum, F. J., and Stass, S. A. (1981). Terminal deoxynucleotidyl transferase-positive acute myeloblastic leukemia. *Am. J. Hem.* 10:251-258.

Mertelsmann, R., Thaler, H. T., To, L., Gee, T. S., McKenzie, S., Schauer, P., Freidman, A., Arlin, Z., Cirrincione, C., and Clarkson, B. (1980). Morphological classification response to therapy and survival in 263 adult patients with acute nonlymphoblastic leukemia. *Blood* 56:773-781.

Metzgar, R. S., Borowitz, M. J., Jones, N. H., and Dowell, B. L. (1981). Distribution of common acute lymphoblastic leukemia antigen in nonhematopoietic tissues. *J. Exp. Med.* 154:1249-1254.

Miller, D. R., Liekin, S., Albo, U., Sather, H., and Hammond, D. (1981). Prognostic importance of morphology (FAB classification) in childhood acute lymphoblastic leukaemia (ALL). *Brit. J. Haem.* 48:199-206.

Miller, D. R., Krailo, M., Bayer, W. A., Lukens, J. N., Siegel, S. E., Coccia, P. R., Weiner, J., and Hammond, D. (1985). Prognostic implications of blast cell morphology in childhood acute lymphoblastic leukemia: a report from the Children's Cancer Study Group. *Cancer Treat. Rep.* 69:1211-1221.

Mirro, J., Antoun, G. R., Zipf, T. F., Melvin, S., and Stass, S. (1985a). The E Rosette-associated antigen of T cells can be identified on blasts from patients with acute myeloblastic leukemia. *Blood* 65:363-367.

Mirro, J., Zipf, T., Pui, C.-H., Kitchingman, G., Williams, D., Melvin, S., Murphy, S. B., and Stass, S. (1985b). Acute mixed lineage leukemia: clinicopathologic correlations and prognostic significance. *Blood* 66:1115-1123.

Nadler, L. M., Ritz, J., Griffin, J. D., Todd, R. F., Reinherz, E. L., Schlossman, S. F. (1981). Diagnosis and treatment of human leukemias and lymphomas utilizing monoclonal antibodies. *Prog. Hematol.* 12:187-225.

Nunnery, E. W., Stass, S. A., Stevens, R. C., Thomas, W., Schumacher, H. R., and Bollum, F. J. (1980). Terminal deoxynucleotidyl-transferase-positive cells in childhood idiopathic thrombocytopenic purpura. *Arch. Path. Lab. Med.* 104:493-494.

Pesando, J. M., Ritz, J., Lazarus, H., Tomaselli, K. J., and Schlossman, S. F. (1981). Fate of a common acute lymphoblastic leukemia antigen during modulation by monoclonal antibody. *J. Immunol.* 126:540-544.

Pesando, J. M., Hoffman, P., Martin, N., and Conrad, T. (1986). Anti-cALLa antibodies identify unique antigens on lymphoid cells and granulocytes. *Blood* 67:588-591.

Pessano, S., Palumbo, A., Ferrero, D., Pagliardi, G. L., Bottero, L., Lai, S. K., Meo, P., Carter, C., Hubbell, H., Lange, B., and Rovera, G. (1984). Subpopulation heterogeneity in human acute myeloid leukemia determined by monoclonal antibodies. *Blood* 64:275-281.

Pui, C.-H., Dahl, G. U., Melvin, S., Williams, D. L., Peiper, S., Mirro, J., Murphy, S. B., Stass, S. (1984). Acute leukemia with mixed lymphoid and myeloid phenotype. *Br. J. Haematol.* 56:121-130.

Pui, C.-H., Rivera, G., Mirro, J., Stass, S., Pieper, S., and Murphy, S. (1985). Acute megakaryoblastic leukemia. Blast cell aggregates simulating metastatic tumor. *Arch. Pathol. Lab. Med.* 109:1033-1035.

Pullen, D. J., Falleta, J. M., Crist, W. M., Vogler, L. B., Dowell, B., Humphrey, G. B., Blackstock, R., van Eys, J., Cooper, M. D., Metzger, R. S., and Meydrech, E. F. (1981). Southwest Oncology Group experience with immunological phenotyping in acute lymphocytic leukemia of childhood. *Cancer Res.* 41: 4802-4809.

Reuben, J., Dalton, W., Ahearn, M., Trujillo, J., Cork, A., McCredie, K., Keating, M., Freireich, E., and Stass, S. A. (1985). Mixed lineage leukemia (MLL): experience in adult acute and chronic leukemia. *Blood* 66:182a (suppl. 1).

Richardson, L. A., and Dickerman, J. P. (1986). 8;14 chromosome translocation in a negative bone marrow aspirate from a patient with Burkitt's lymphoma. *Cancer* 57:761-763.

Ritz, J., Nadler, L. M., Bhan, A. K., Notis-McConarty, J., Pesando, J. M., and Schlossman, S. F. (1981). Expression of common acute lymphoblastic leukemia antigen (CALLA) by lymphomas of B-cell and T-cell lineage. *Blood* 58:648-652.

Roberts, M., Greaves, M., Janossay, G., Sutherland, R., and Pain, C. (1978). Acute lymphoblastic leukemia (ALL) associated antigen-I. expression in different haemotopoietic malignancies. *Leuk. Res.* 2:105-114.

Rowley, J. D. (1973). Identification of a translocation with quinacrine fluorescence in a patient with acute leukemia. *Ann. Genet.* 16:109-112.

Rowley, J. D. (1984). Biological implications of consistent chromosome rearrangements in leukemia and lymphoma. *Cancer Res.* 44:3159-3168.

Rowley, J. D., Golomb, H. M., Vardiman, J., Fukuhara, S., Dougherty, C., and Potter, D. (1977). Further evidence for a non-random chromosomal abnormality in acute promyelocytic leukemia. *Int. J. Cancer* 20:869-872.

Sallan, S. E., Ritz, J., Pesando, J., Gelber, R., O'Brien, C., Hitchcock, S., Coral, F., and Schlossman, S. F. (1980). Cell surface antigens: Prognostic implications in childhood acute lymphoblastic leukemia. *Blood* 55:395-402.

Sariban, E., Oliver, C., Corash, L., Cossman, J., Whang-Peng, J., Jaffe, E. S., Gralnick, H. R., and Poplack, D. G. (1984). Acute megakaryoblastic leukemia in childhood. *Cancer* 54:1423-1428.

Smith, L. J., Curtis, J. E., Messner, H. A., Senn, J. S., Furthmayr, H., and McCulloch, E. A. (1983). Lineage infidelity in acute leukemia. *Blood* 61:1138-1145.

Sobol, R. E., Royston, I., LeBien, T. W., Minowada, J., Anderson, K., Davey, F., Cuttner, J., Schiffer, C., Ellison, R. R., and Bloomfield, C. D. (1985). Adult acute lymphoblastic leukemia phenotypes defined by monoclonal antibodies. *Blood* 65:730-735.

Sobol, R. E., Royston, I., Mick, R., Cuttner, J., Ellison, R. R., Dovey, F., Nelson, D., and Bloomfield, C. D. (1986). Clinical significance of mixed lymphoid and myeloid characteristics in adult acute lymphoblastic leukemia. *Proc. Amer. Soc. Clin. Oncol.* 5:C159.

Stass, S. A., Schumacher, H. R., Keneklis, T. P., and Bollum, F. J. (1979). Terminal deoxynucleotidyl transferase immuno-fluorescence of bone marrow smears. *Am. J. Clin. Pathol.* 72:898-903.

Stass, S. A., McGraw, T. P., Folds, J., and Bollum, F. J. (1981). Terminal transferase in acute lymphoblastic leukemia in remission. *Am. J. Clin. Pathol.* 75: 838-840.

Stass, S. A., Dean, L., Peiper, S. C., and Bollum, F. J. (1982). Determination of terminal deoxynucleotidyl transferase on bone marrow smears by immunoperoxidase. *Am. J. Clin. Pathol.* 77:174-176.

Stass, S. A., Pui, C.-H., Melvin, S., Rovigatti, U., Williams, D., Motroni, T., Kalwinsky, D., and Dahl, G. (1984). Sudan Black B positive acute lymphoblastic leukaemia. *Brit. J. Haem.* 57:413-421.

Stass, S. A., and Mirro, J. (1985). Unexpected heterogeneity in acute leukemia: mixed lineages and lineage switch. *Hum. Pathol.* 16:864-866.

Stein, P., Peiper, S., Butler, D., Melvin, S., Williams, D., and Stass, S. (1983). Granular acute lymphoblastic leukemia. *Am. J. Clin. Pathol.* 79:426-430.

Sultan, C., Deregnaucourt, J., Ko, Y. W., Imbert, M., D'Agay, M. F. R., Gouault-Heilman, M., and Brun, B. (1981). Distribution of 250 cases of acute myeloid leukemia (AML) according to the FAB classification and response to therapy. *Brit. J. Haem.* 47:545-551.

Van der Reijden, H. J., van Rhenen, D. J., Lansdorp, P. M., van't Veer, M. B., Langenhuijsen, M. M. A. C., Englefriet, C. P., and von dem Borne, A. E. G. K. (1983). A comparison of surface marker analysis and FAB classification in acute myeloid leukemia. *Blood* 61:443-448.

Van Dongen, J. J. M., Hooijkaas, H., Adriaansen, H. J., Hahlen, K., and Van Zanen, G. E. (1986). Detection of minimal residual acute lymphoblastic leukemia by immunological marker analysis: possibilities and limitations. In *Minimal Residual Disease in Acute Leukemia*, A. Hagenbeek and B. Lowenberg (eds.). Martinus Nijhoff Publishers, Dordrecht, Netherlands, pp. 113-133.

van Eys, J., Pullen, J., Head, D., Boyett, J., Crist, W., Falletta, J., Humphrey, G. B., Jackson, J., Riccardi, V., and Brock, B. (1986). The French-American-British (FAB) classification of leukemia. The Pediatric Oncology Group experience with lymphocytic leukemia. *Cancer* 57:1046-1051.

Viana, M. B., Maurer, H. S., and Ferenc, C. (1980). Subclassification of acute lymphoblastic leukemia in children: analysis of the reproducibility of morphological criteria and prognostic implications. *Brit. J. Haem.* 44:383-388.

Vogler, L. B., Crist, W. M., Bockman, D. E., Pearl, E. R., Lawton, A. R., and Cooper, M. D. (1978). Pre-B-cell leukemia: a new phenotype of childhood lymphoblastic leukemia. *New Engl. J. Med.* 298:872-878.

Weiner, M., Borowitz, M., Boyett, J., Civin, C., Metzger, R., McKolnis, J., Crist, W., Dowell, B., and Pullen, J. (1985). Clinical Pathologic aspects of myeloid antigen positivity in pediatric patients with acute lymphoblastic leukemia (ALL). *Proc. Am. Soc. Clin. Oncol.* 4:C671.

Williams, D. L., Tsiatis, A., Biodeur, G. M., Look, A. T., Melvin, S. L., Bowman, W. P., Kalwinsky, D. K., Rivera, G., and Dahl, G. V. (1982). Prognostic importance of chromosome number in 136 untreated children with acute lymphoblastic leukemia. *Blood* 60:864-871.

Williams, D. L., Look, T. A., Melvin, S. L., Roberson, P. K., Dahl, G., Flake, T., and Stass, S. (1984). New chromosomal translocations correlate with specific immunophenotypes of childhood acute lymphoblastic leukemia. *Cell* 36:101-109.

Williams, D. L., Harber, J., Murphy, S. B., Look, A. T., Kalwinsky, D., Rivera, G., Melvin, S., Stass, S., and Dahl, G. (1986). Chromosomal translocations play a unique role in influencing prognosis in childhood acute lymphoblastic leukemia. *Blood* 68:205-212.

Wright, J. J., Poplack, D. G., Bakhshi, M. B., and Korsmeyer, S. J. (1986). DNA rearrangements as unique markers of clonal evolution, recurrence, and translocation. In *Minimal Residual Disease in Acute Leukemia 1986*, A. Hagenbeek and B. Lowenberg (eds.). Martinus Nijhoff Publishers, Dordrecht, Netherlands, pp. 51-57.

Youness, E., Trujillo, J. M., Ahearn, M. J., McCredie, K. B., and Cork, A. (1980). Acute unclassified leukemia. A clinicopathologic study with diagnostic implications of electron microscopy. *Am. J. Hem.* 9:79-88.

Yunis, J. J. (1983). The chromosomal basis of human neoplasia. *Science* 221: 227-236.

Zech, L., Haglund, U., and Nilsson, K. (1976). Characteristic chromosomal abnormalities in biopsies and lymphoid-cell lines from patients with Burkitt and non-Burkitt lymphomas. *Int. J. Cancer* 17:47-56.

Zehnbauer, B. A., Pardoll, D. M., Burke, P. J., Graham, M. L., and Vogelstein, B. (1986). Immunoglobulin gene rearrangements in remission bone marrow specimens from patients with acute lymphoblastic leukemia. *Blood* 67:835-838.

2

A Morphologic and Cytochemical Approach to the Diagnosis of Acute Leukemia

WILLARD DALTON, JR. and SANFORD A. STASS *The University of Texas System Cancer Center, M. D. Anderson Hospital and Tumor Institute, Houston, Texas*

I. INTRODUCTION

The goal for classification systems in acute leukemia is to divide these heterogenous disorders into groups that are relatively homogeneous with respect to the feature of interest to an investigator, whether that be the etiology, the molecular pathways of leukemogenesis, the natural history, or the response to therapy. The most immediate concerns of a physician caring for a patient with acute leukemia are the selection of the therapeutic approach most likely to be effective and the ability to give prognostic information to the patient. Classification systems based on lineage as determined by morphology and cytochemistries have identified broad groups–acute lymphocytic leukemia (ALL) and acute nonlymphocytic leukemia (ANLL)–that have a useful degree of homogeneity for such therapeutic and prognostic purposes. The difference in clinical outcome between ALL and ANLL has long been apparent in children. Although these groups are also predictive of clinical outcome in adults, the difference is less striking in adults. Further morphologic subclassification of ALL and ANLL fails to improve clinical outcome prediction (Keating et al., 1980, 1982) except in those subtypes closely associated with several particular cytogenetic abnormalities. These subtypes include the Burkitt-cell type of ALL, associated with a reciprocal translocation usually involving chromosomes 8 and 14 [t(8;14)] ; acute myeloblastic leukemia (AML) with maturation, associated with t(8;21); acute promyelocytic leukemia, associated with t(15;17); and acute myelomonocytic leukemia with abnormal eosinophils, associated with abnormalities of chromosome 16, most commonly a pericentric inversion [inv(16)] (Trujillo et al., 1979; Kantarjian et al., 1986; Larson et al., 1986). The morphology of these subtypes is sufficiently distinctive to permit prediction of the associated cytogenetic abnormality in most cases. This fact certainly indicates that morphologic and cytochemical studies have some biological validity. Even where morphology correlates precisely with cytogenetics, the groups are not entirely homogeneous clinically, however. Better prediction of clinical outcome will require more than morphologic and cytochemical evaluation. Be that as it may, morphologic examination of Romanowsky-stained bone marrow smears and cytochemical stains has been and remains the benchmark for the diagnosis and classification of acute leukemias; initial validation of newer techniques still depends ultimately on careful comparison with these older, established morphologic evaluations.

Acute leukemias are a morphologically heterogenous group of disorders; with the exception of the above-mentioned leukemias associated with t(8;14), t(8;21), t(15;17) and inv(16), they do not fall easily into discrete morphological groups. This fact has led to variability and confusion in their classification. In 1976 a group of seven French, American, and British hematologists (the FAB group) proposed a set of guidelines for the classification of these disorders with the explicit intent of fostering uniformity and allowing meaningful comparison and analysis of data (Bennett et al., 1976). This initial proposal set forth criteria for determining subclasses of acute myelogenous leukemia based on the Wright-Giemsa (W-G) stain and selected cytochemistries. Based on morphological and cytochemical criteria, categories of ANLL (FAB, M1 through M6) were delineated using the type and extent of leukemic cell differentiation.

The FAB group also proposed criteria for the differentiation of acute leukemia from the dysmyelopoietic syndromes (DMPS). (A case was considered acute leukemia if there were 50% or more blasts plus promyelocytes present and DMPS if there were fewer than 50%.) They also devised categories of ALL based on W-G morphology including nuclear-cytoplasmic (N/C) ratio of the blasts; nuclear morphology, including nuclear outline and the presence, absence, and character of nucleoli; and heterogeneity of blast size (FAB-L1 through L3). In particular, they defined FAB-L2 and pointed out the importance of differentiating it from the FAB-M1 subtype of AML.

All of these morphologic subtypes of acute leukemia had been previously described. The FAB group merely devised a new, unambiguous nomenclature for the classes of acute leukemia and presented objective criteria for their diagnosis, including cytochemical parameters to define myeloid and monocytic differentiation.

Problems with the accurate discrimination between FAB-L1 and FAB-L2 soon became apparent, and in 1981 the FAB group introduced a scoring system to improve interobserver performance (Bennett et al., 1981). In 1982 the FAB group changed the criterion for acute leukemia to 30% or more blasts, refined the classification of the DMPS, and added the additional DMPS "refractory anemia with excess blasts in transformation" (RAEB-IT) (Bennett et al., 1982). Auer rods could be found in some cases of RAEB-IT; previously, some hematologists, including at least one member of the FAB group, felt that the presence of Auer rods per se established the diagnosis of acute leukemia (Gralnick et al., 1977). In September 1985, the group added another category, FAB-M7, to delineate acute leukemia of megakaryocytic lineage (Bennett et al., 1985a). Of note was the recommendation that surface immunophenotype (with regard to the presence of factor VIII or glycoprotein IB or IIB/IIIA) or ultrastructural demonstration of platelet peroxidase be used to establish the diagnosis of acute megakaryocytic leukemia. This was the first use of immunophenotype data by the FAB group. However, since antibody reactivity occasionally may not be specific for a given lineage, we have reserved the diagnosis of acute megakaryocytic leukemia for those cases that clearly demonstrate platelet peroxidase.

The FAB group proposed changes in the classification of the myeloid leukemias in October 1985, with major changes involving the diagnosis of erythroleukemia, FAB-M6 (Bennett et al., 1985b). These latest guidelines are precise, and the FAB group provides some evidence that they improve reproducibility. We find these proposed revisions rather complicated in lieu of any proof that they enhance the biological significance of the classification, however; we agree with others (Bloomfield and Brunning, 1985) that the revised system will have to be critically evaluated to determine how often changes in classification occur and whether these changes result in clinically or biologically more homogenous groups.

In the following descriptions of the morphologic subtypes of acute leukemia, we will adhere to the pre-October 1985 FAB guidelines, although we will also mention the impact of the newest FAB proposal under each specific type of myeloid leukemia. Since their publication in 1976 with revision in 1981-82, the FAB guidelines have been widely accepted and form the basis for the classification used in most studies on acute leukemia. They have also been demonstrated to be a useful framework for clinical, laboratory, and biological studies of acute leukemia and are especially important for interinstitutional comparison of results of clinical studies. However, as will be noted in subsequent chapters, future directions in the characterization and classification of acute leukemia will most likely include the use of biologic parameters that will more clearly identify relevant subgroups.

II. CRITERIA FOR DIAGNOSIS OF ACUTE LEUKEMIA IN ROMANOWSKY-STAINED BONE MARROW SMEARS

Examination of high-quality bone marrow smears stained with Wright-Giemsa (W-G) or other Romanowsky stains is generally the basis for the morphologic evaluation of acute leukemia. The smears should be evaluated in a well-spread area where the red cells are not touching in order to adequately appreciate cellular detail and accurately evaluate the N/C ratio. In our laboratory, trained technologists do a 500-cell differential count on all bone marrows. In difficult cases or where the blast percentage is borderline, a hematopathologist also does a formal differential count. The presence of 30% or more bone marrow blasts currently defines acute leukemia. This percentage is, of course, arbitrary but seems to be useful in practice. We also consider cases with at least 30% blasts in the peripheral blood as acute leukemia even if the bone marrow blast percentage is less than 30%. The FAB guidelines do not currently address this situation.

At this juncture we point out that occasional cases of round cell tumors such as neuroblastoma (Head, Kennedy, and Goyette, 1979; Abildgaard, 1980), rhabdomyosarcoma (Alamanaseen et al., 1984), Ewing's sarcoma and even medulloblastoma (Pollack, Miller, and Vye, 1981) can mimic acute leukemia on smears, with individual tumor cells spread rather evenly over the smears (Figure 1a). Therefore, it is extremely important that in every new case of suspected acute leukemia the slide be scanned for tumor cells. The presence of cohesive cells strongly suggests that one is dealing with a metastatic tumor rather than an acute leukemia (Figure 1b). Rarely, however, blasts in acute leukemia show a tendency to clump, especially those in acute megakaryocytic leukemia (Pui, Rivera, Mirro et al., 1985). Tumor simulating acute leukemia is most common in pediatric patients. In some instances (especially rhabdomyosarcoma), a primary lesion may never be found and a diagnosis may depend on ultrastructure or evaluation of the malignant cells in tissue culture.

Once the diagnosis of acute leukemia has been established, it is then classified as either lymphoid or myeloid. This first categorization is more important because of the differing therapy and prognosis of ALL and ANLL, especially in the pediatric age group. In many cases, classification of the acute leukemia into lymphoid or myeloid lineage may be apparent after examination of the W-G stained smears, but one must remember that the final diagnosis must rest on cytochemical stains. We have seen innumerable instances where the impression gained from the W-G stained smears did not match the cytochemical reactivity. Examination of the W-G stain is still useful, however, and clues to the lineage of the leukemia can be gleaned from assessment of the cell size, N/C ratio, the nuclear chromatin, nucleoli, and the presence or absence of cytoplasmic granules or rods.

As already mentioned, evaluation of the blasts' size and N/C ratio should be made in an area where the red cells are not touching. All cases will have a high N/C ratio if examined in thick areas of the smear! Large cells and a low N/C ratio are more in keeping with a myeloid leukemia, but it must be remembered that subgroups of ALL (FAB-L2 and L3) can have a low N/C ratio of 4:1 or less. The nuclear chromatin pattern in ALL is characterized by the presence of more heterochromatin (clumped chromatin) than in myeloid leukemias. We have noticed that the nuclear chromatin may become more finely granular at relapse in ALL compared to the initial presentation. Nucleoli tend to be more numerous (2 to 5) and prominent in myeloid leukemias than in lymphoid (1 to 2). Manual W-G stains seem to show nuclear detail and delineate nucleoli better than automated stains.

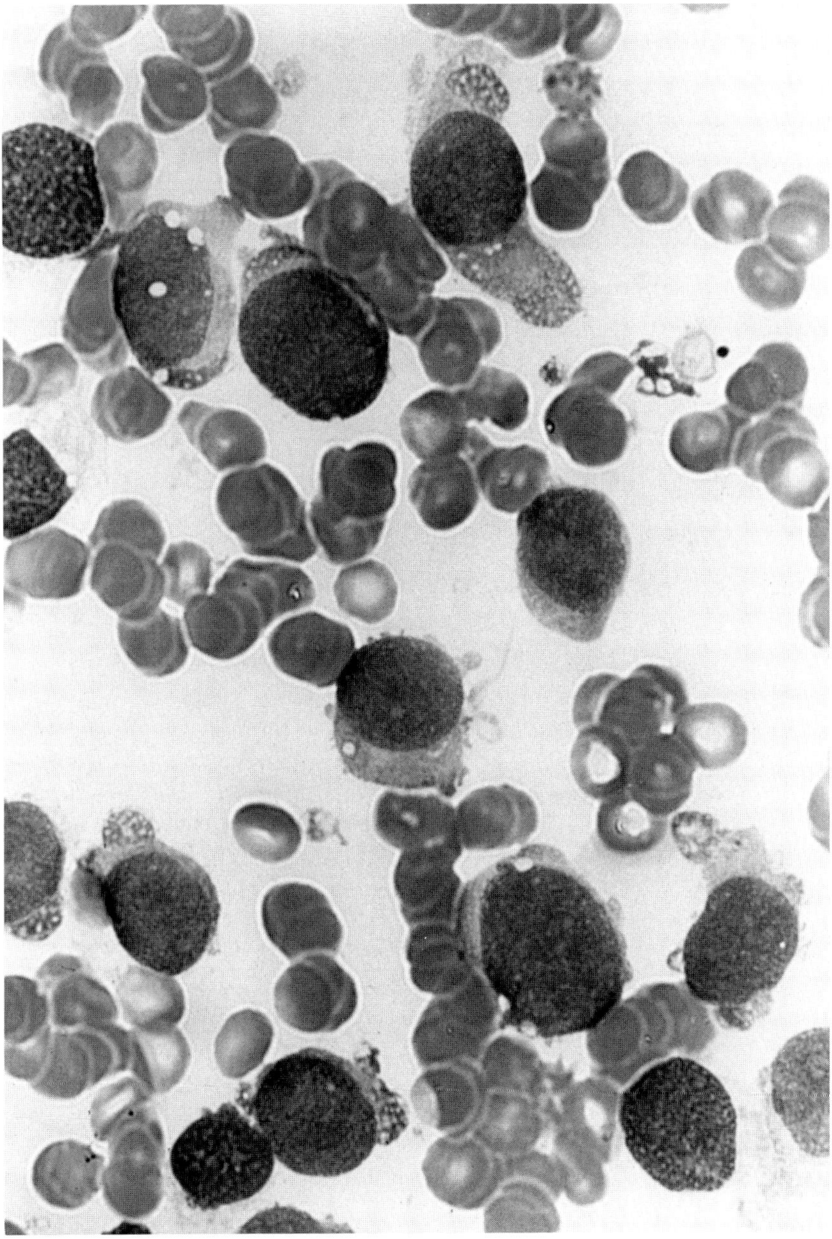

Figure 1a Metastatic tumor. Case of rhabdomyosarcoma simulating acute leukemia. (W-G, ×800)

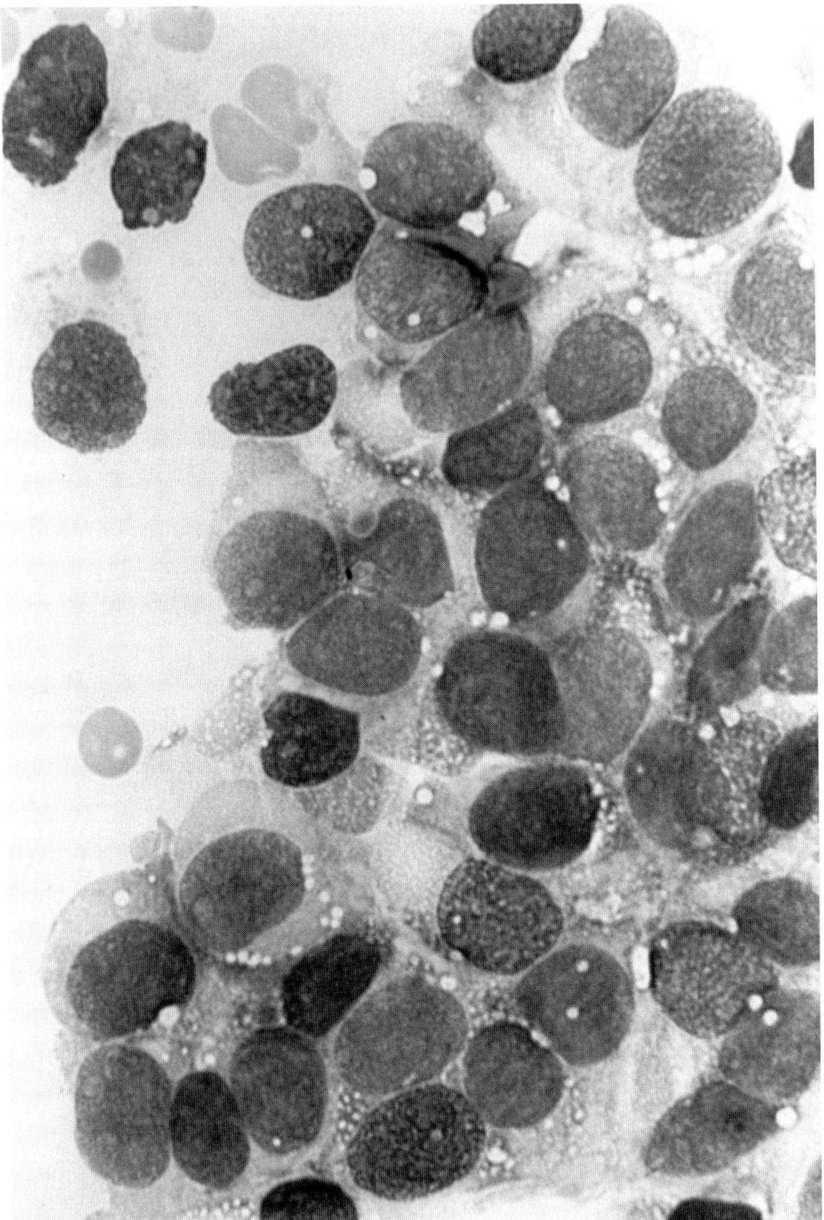

Figure 1b Metastatic tumor. Clusters of tumor cells establish the diagnosis of metastatic tumor in a case of rhabdomyosarcoma. (W-G, X800)

In practice we find that these nuclear and nucleolar features are of marginal value in the differential diagnosis of most cases of acute leukemia. It is the cytoplasma of the leukemic cells that offers the major clues for appraisal: lymphoid leukemias typically have a small amount of pale blue to dark blue cytoplasm, whereas myeloid leukemias have moderate to abundant amounts of gray to gray-blue cytoplasm. The color and intensity of bone marrow staining may vary from laboratory to laboratory or within the same laboratory from day to day depending upon the composition of the stains, length of incubation with the stain, pH, or the thickness of the smears. As a result the color of the cytoplasm is not always a reliable indicator of the lineage of leukemic cells. Lymphoid leukemias typically have agranular cytoplasm; myeloid leukemias may show either discrete "azurophilic" granules or a "dusting" of smaller granules. Cytoplasmic granules can also be seen in an occasional case of ALL (Grogan et al., 1981; Skoog, 1976; Stein et al., 1983; Yanagihara et al., 1980). These granules are usually large and distinct, standing in contrast to the surrounding translucent cytoplasm (Figure 2), and are always myeloperoxidase negative.

Auer rods may be identified in blasts and even in mature neutrophils (Stass, Lanham, Butler, et al., 1984) and provide strong evidence that the leukemia is myeloid, although it must be realized that similar red needlelike structures, which represent precipitated immunoglobulin, have been found in chronic lymphocytic leukemia (CLL) and multiple myeloma (Figure 3) (Raman and Van Slyck, 1983). In these cases, it is usually apparent that these needlelike structures are in lymphocytes (in CLL) or in plasma cells (in multiple myeloma) and not in myeloid cells, but cytochemical analysis can further insure against misinterpretation. Auer rods are usually myeloperoxidase positive whereas immunoglobulin is myeloperoxidase negative. Although we have seen a rare exception, it is also unusual to find genuine Auer rods unless most of the leukemic cells are myeloperoxidase positive, which of course would not be the case in CLL or multiple myeloma.

Cytoplasmic vacuoles are seen consistently in FAB-L3 and occasionally in FAB-L2 or even in FAB-L1. One study found vacuoles in 9.8% of cases of FAB-L1 in children and noted that the vacuoles were associated with a low initial leukocyte count and favorable age range, resulting in improved prognosis for this group (Potter et al., 1984). Vacuoles can also be seen in AML, especially during treatment or upon relapse. Phagocytosis of mature erythrocytes, platelets, or other formed elements has been associated with monocytic types of leukemia, but can also be seen in other acute myeloid leukemias, as well as in ALL (Figure 4), where it can occasionally be very striking (Colon-Otero et al., 1984). Round cell tumors involving the bone marrow, especially rhabdomyosarcoma, may show phagocytic activity (Figure 5) (Wheeler, Wilson, and Stass, 1981; Youness et al., 1980). Phagocytosis in ALL has been shown to correlate with the presence of particular myeloid-associated antigens on the surface of otherwise typical ALL blast cells (Pui, Mirro, Woodruff, et al., 1986). Cell fragments or "hyaline bodies"

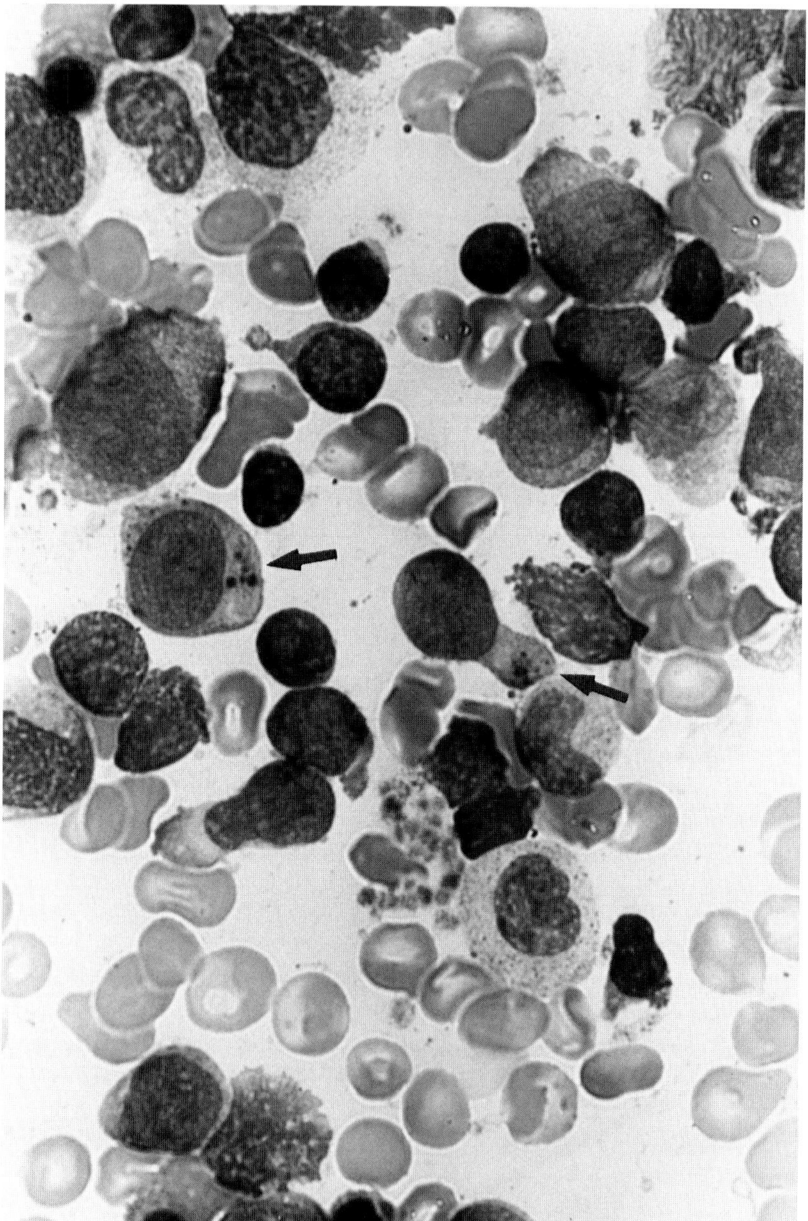

Figure 2 Acute lymphocytic leukemia, granular type. Two of the blasts contain large cytoplasmic granules (arrows), but the cytoplasm is otherwise translucent. (W-G, X800)

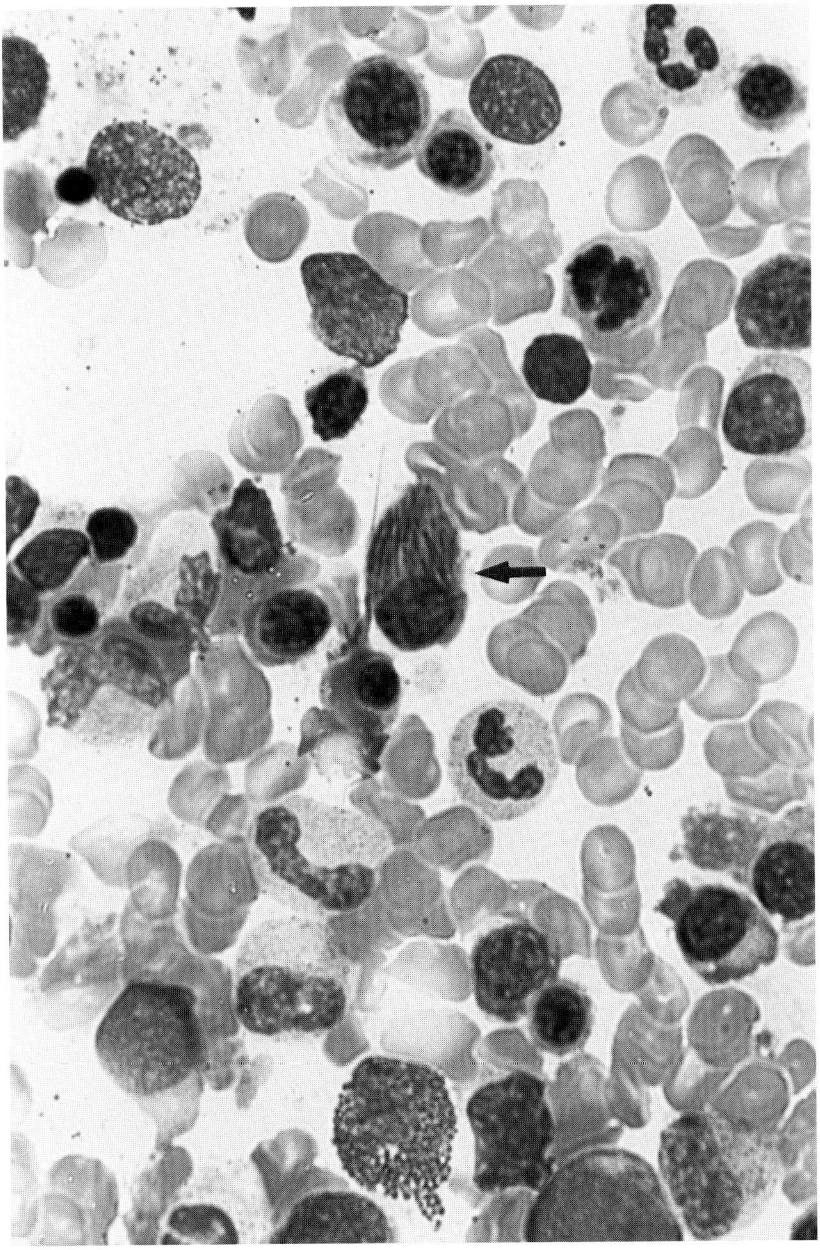

Figure 3 Plasma cell with inclusions. Plasma cell containing multiple needlelike inclusions resembling Auer rods (arrow). (W-G, ×800)

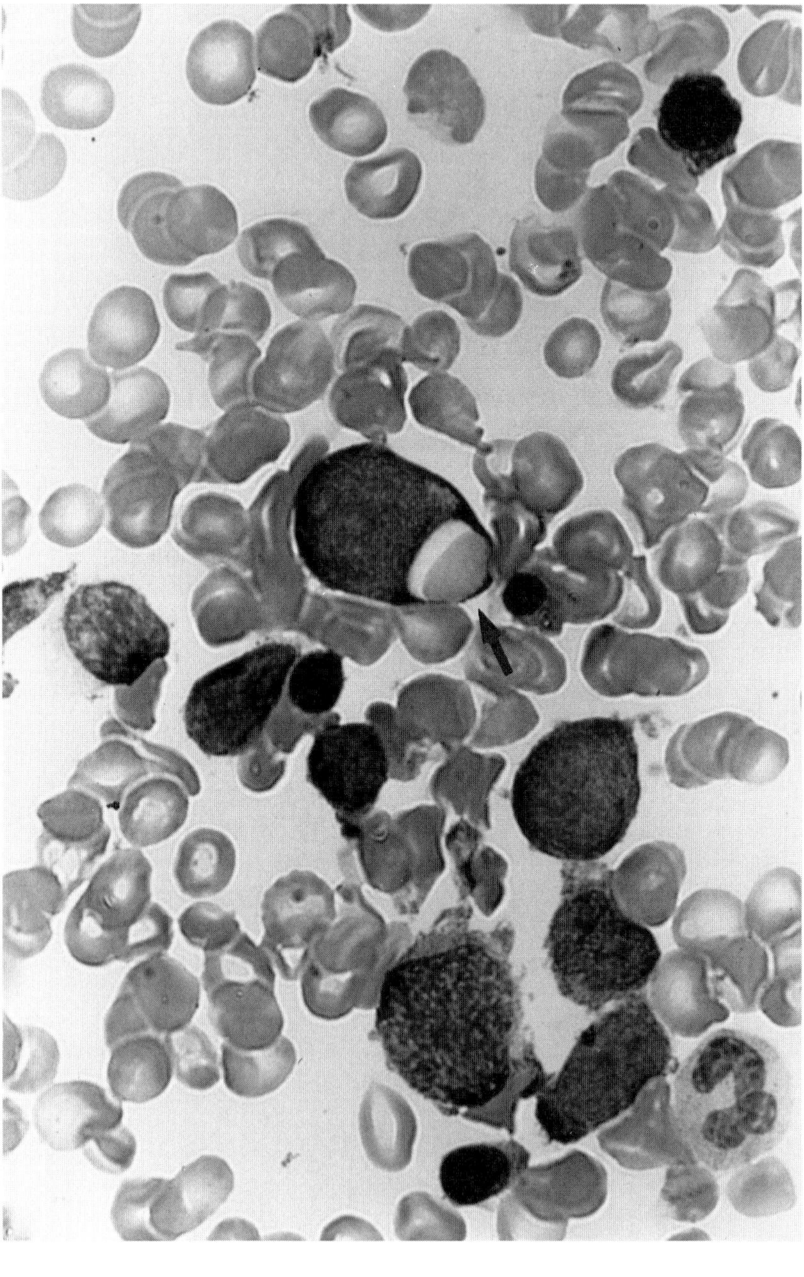

Figure 4a Acute lymphocytic leukemia. A blast has engulfed an erythrocyte (arrow). (W-G, ×800)

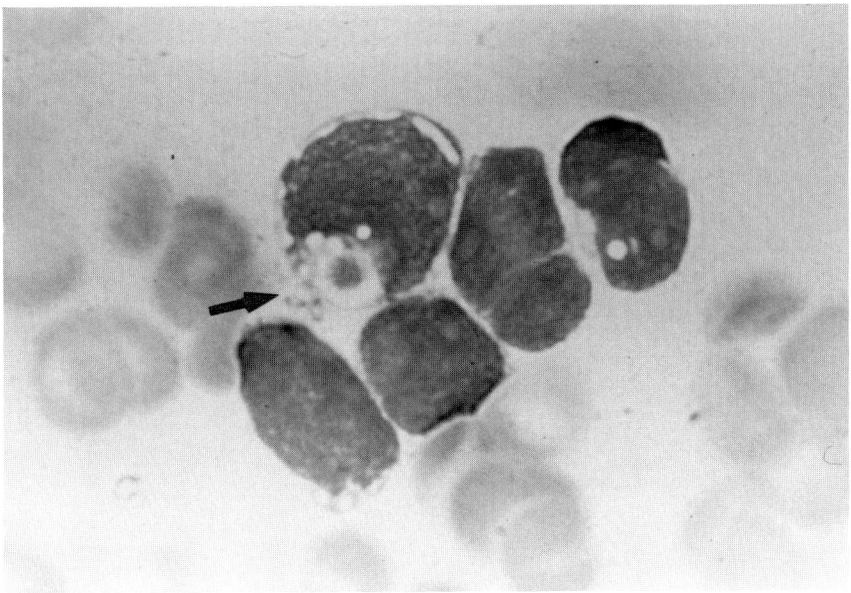

Figure 4b Acute lymphocytic leukemia. A blast has engulfed a platelet (arrow). (W-G, X800)

are seen somewhat more commonly in ALL, but can also be seen in AML. Smudge cells may be more common in ALL, but can be seen in AML. It is important to note that the presence of smudge cells cannot be used to support the diagnosis or classification of leukemia or any other malignancy! Normal cells may smudge depending on the pressure applied when smearing. Any diagnosis of leukemia or tumor must rest on the evaluation of intact cells.

A. Cytochemistries of Acute Leukemia

From a diagnostic point of view, the paramount feature of myeloid leukemic cells is the presence of myeloperoxidase in primary granules (see Table 1). We immediately do a myeloperoxidase stain (Kaplow, 1965) on a bone marrow smear of all patients being evaluated for possible acute leukemia. The stain is done as soon as the bone marrow aspirate arrives in the laboratory so that the W-G stain and the myeloperoxidase stains can be evaluated at the same time. This allows us to quickly relay accurate information on the lineage of the leukemia to the clinician, so that treatment planning can begin. An empirical definition is that when 3% or more of the *leukemic blasts* are myeloperoxidase positive by light microscopy, the leukemia is classified as myeloid. It should be noted that this is an

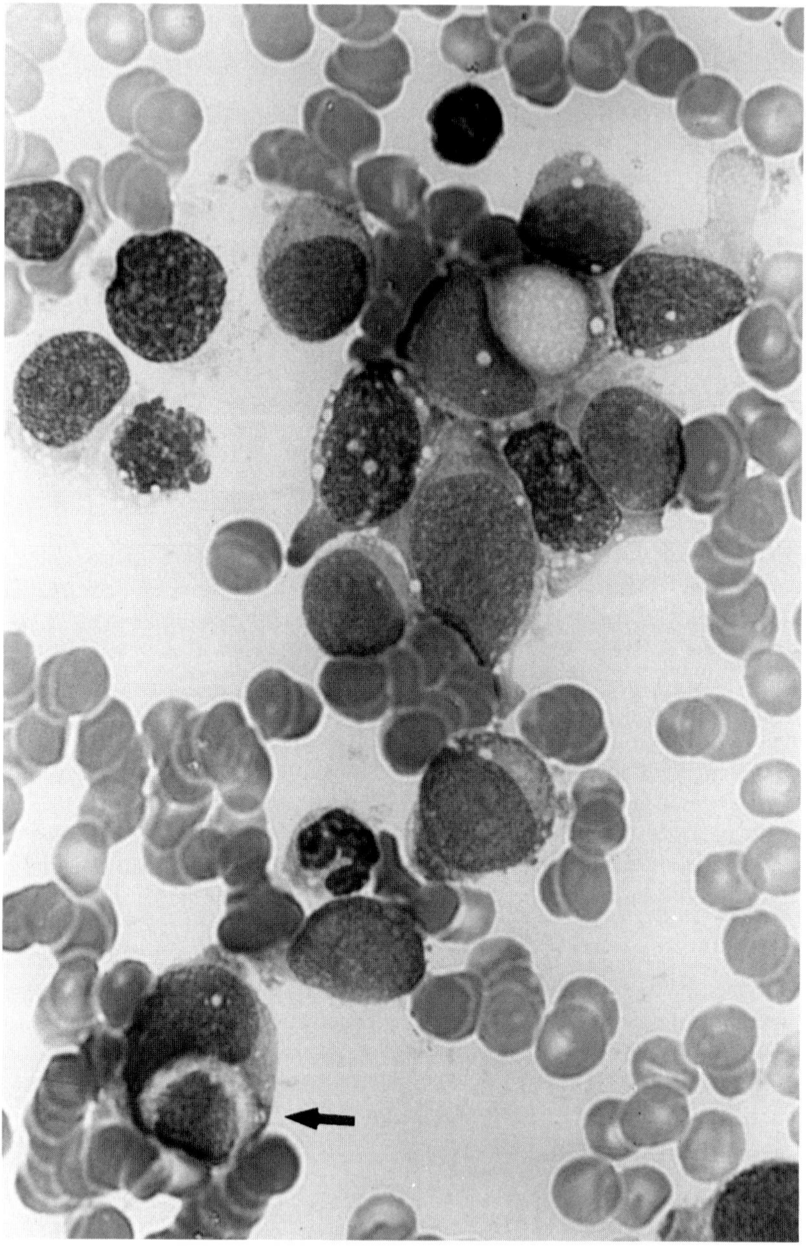

Figure 5 Metastatic tumor (rhabdomyosarcoma). There is phagocytosis of one tumor cell by another (arrow). (W-G, ×800).

Table 1 Cytochemistries of Acute Leukemias

FAB type	Myeloperoxidase >3%	Sudan black B >3%	Platelet peroxidase by EM	TdT >40%	a=NBE (strong, diffuse >20%)	NASD-CAE (>3%)	PAS	MGP	Oil Red 0
FAB-L1	–	– (occ+)	–	+	– (may be weak, focal +)	–	+ (block pos., most cases)	+	– (occ+)
FAB-L2	–	– (occ+)	–	+	– (may be weak, focal +)	–	+ (block pos., most cases)	+	– (occ+)
FAB-L3	–	–	–	– (rare+)	– (may be weak, focal +)	–	– (rare+)	+	+
FAB-M1	+	+	–	– (occ +)	–	+/–	+/–	+/–	–
FAB-M2	+	+	–	– (occ +)	–	+/–	+/–	+/–	–
FAB-M3	+	+	–	– (occ +)	–	+/–	+/–	+/–	–
FAB-M4	+	+	–	– (occ +)	+	+/–	+/–	+/–	–
FAB-M5	+/–	+/–	–	– (occ +)	+	+/–	+/–	+/–	–
FAB-M7	–	–	+		–	–	+ (coarse granules)		
AUL	–		–		–	–	–	+/–	

Key
occ +: occasional positive cases
rare +: rare positive cases
TdT: Terminal deoxynucleotidyl transferase
a-NBE: alpha-naphthyl butyrate
NASD-CAE: naphthyl AS-D chloroacetate esterase
PAS: periodic acid-Schiff
MGP: methyl green-pyronine

arbitrary determination, however. The figure of 3% was chosen empirically so that the few normal residual myeloblasts in an ALL bone marrow would not result in the leukemia being classified as myeloid. We feel more comfortable when there are at least 5% myeloperoxidase-positive cells since we have seen cases of relapsing ALL and of mixed leukemia with 3% myeloperoxidase-positive blasts that had lymphoid surface markers and behaved clinically as ALL. The Sudan black B stain gives results very similar to the myeloperoxidase stain. We strongly prefer the myeloperoxidase stain, however, since we have found that the Sudan black B stain is positive in 1.6% of cases of pediatric ALL (Stass, Pui, Melvin, et al., 1984); others have also described occasional patients with Sudan black B positive lymphoid malignancies (Ho, Chan, and Todd, 1983), including some adult patients (Savage and Hoffman, 1983; Tricot et al., 1982).

Acute monocytic leukemia has a variable but generally low amount of myeloperoxidase activity. When the myeloperoxidase activity is low the cytochemical diagnosis of acute monocytic leukemia depends on a nonspecific esterase stain, such as α-naphthyl butyrate esterase (Li, Lam, and Yam, 1973) or α-naphthyl acetate esterase (with and without fluoride), which shows strong, diffuse positivity. This is very helpful for separating this type of leukemia from ALL, especially the FAB-L2 type. We have seen α-naphthyl butyrate activity in 25% of pediatric ALL patients (Stass, unpublished observation), but this should not cause diagnostic confusion, since in ALL the staining is focal and weak (Figure 6) in contrast to the diffuse, usually strong positivity in acute monoblastic leukemia. We would consider myeloperoxidase staining as the best available evidence for a myeloid lineage, and strong α-naphthyl butyrate staining as the best available evidence for a monocytic lineage, since monoclonal antibodies which were previously thought to be specific for myeloid or monocytic lineage have been identified in otherwise typical ALL (see Chapter 12).

In the same manner, the demonstration of platelet peroxidase in leukemic cells by electron microscopy (see Chapter 3) is the best available evidence for a megakaryocytic lineage. In both myeloblastic and monoblastic leukemias, there are instances in which the blasts are negative for cytochemistries at the light level but are myeloperoxidase positive at the ultrastructure level. In these cases, the primary granules containing myeloperoxidase are generally smaller than 250 nm. Granules less than this size cannot be visualized by light microscopy. Naphthyl AS-D chloroacetate esterase (NASD-CAE) (Yam, Li, and Crosby, 1971) is an enzyme expressed selectively in cells of the neutrophilic series. It is less sensitive than the myeloperoxidase stain in demonstrating that leukemic blasts are of myeloid origin. Spurious NASD-CAE positivity has been described in a single case of ALL (Keifer, Abromowich, and Stass, 1985) and can rarely be seen in acute monoblastic leukemia and acute erythroleukemia (Hayhoe and Quaglino, 1980).

The diagnosis of acute lymphocytic leukemia can often be made based on morphologic features. However, it should always be confirmed by cytochemical staining. ALL lacks cytochemical and morphologic features of myeloid leukemia (ALL

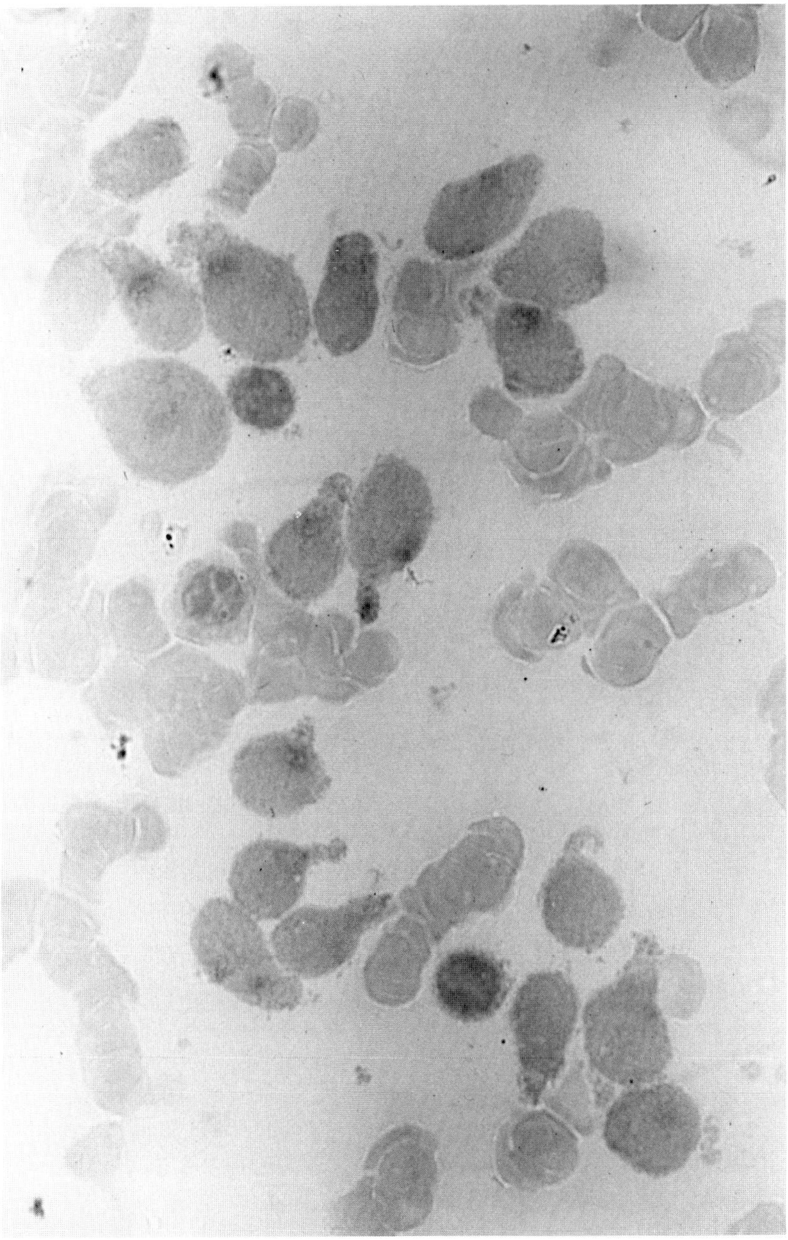

Figure 6 Acute lymphocytic leukemia, hand-mirror cell type. α-naphthyl butyrate stain from a case of hand-mirror ALL, showing weak, focal positivity in most of the blasts. (X800)

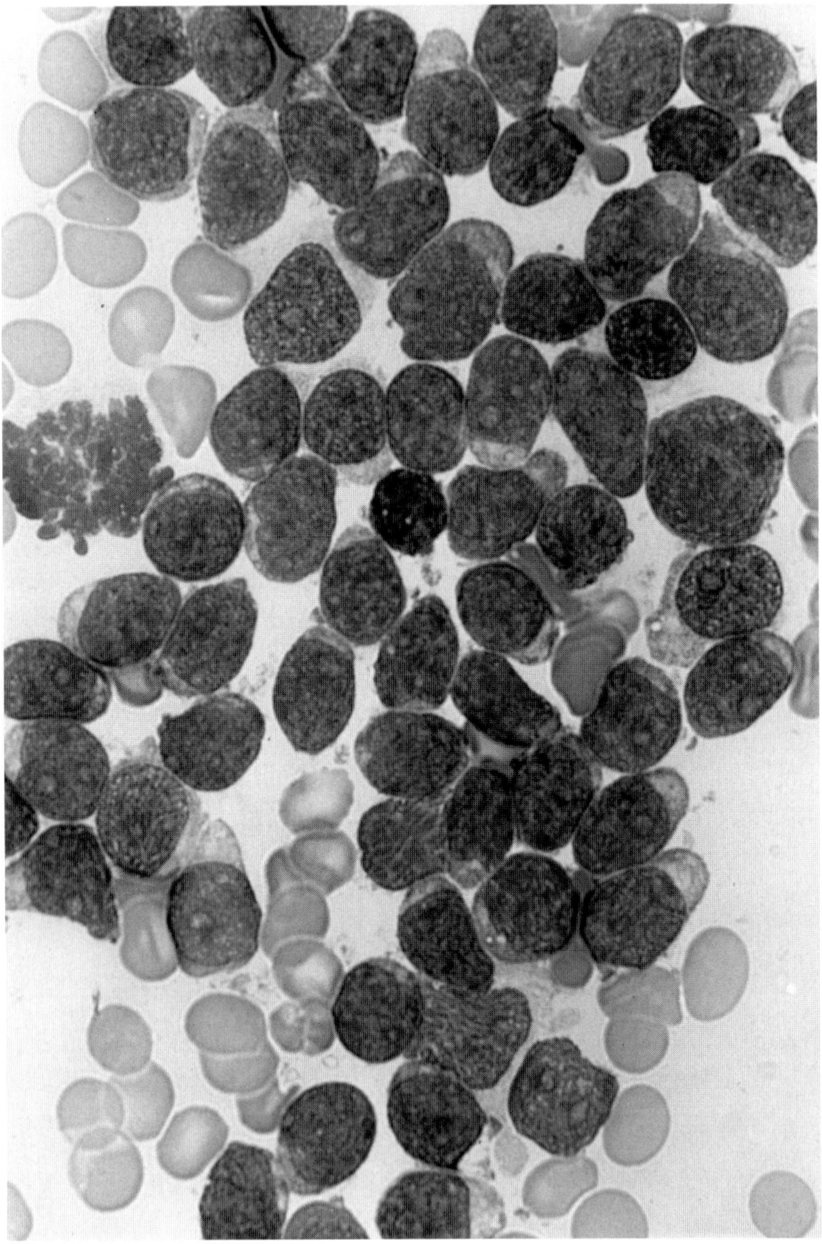

Figure 7a Acute lymphocytic leukemia, T-cell type. The case is FAB-L2. (W-G, ×800)

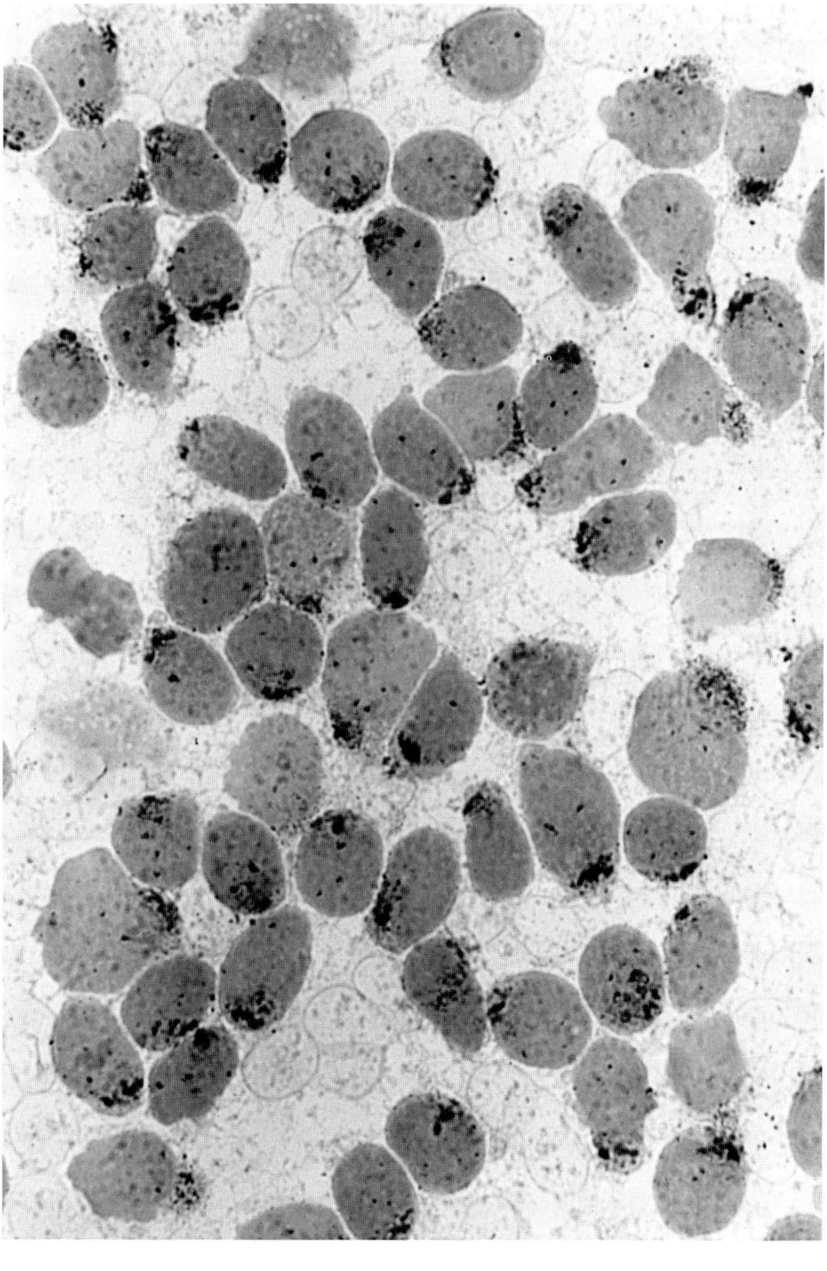

Figure 7b Acute lymphocytic leukemia, T-cell type. Acid phosphatase stain. There is intense focal positivity in nearly all the blasts. (×800)

is myeloperoxidase negative) and cytochemically is a diagnosis of exclusion. Stains for terminal deoxyribonucleotidyl transferase (TdT) are positive in 90-97% of cases of ALL, but we have noted many cases of AML that are TdT positive. The TdT in AML is usually in less than 40% of the blasts, but we have encountered cases of AML with more than 40% TdT-positive blasts. The PAS (Periodic acid-Shiff) stain shows a distinctive block positivity in most cases of ALL, but we have also seen rare cases of AML with PAS block positivity, so the finding of PAS block-positive blasts does not definitively establish the diagnosis of ALL. The degree of PAS positivity in ALL has been reported to be of prognostic significance by a number of authors, but this finding has also been challenged by multiple authors (see Lanham et al., 1985, for review). We feel that the degree of PAS positivity has no prognostic value independent of other known prognostic features (Lanham et al., 1985). Within the category of ALL, the acid phosphatase stain (Janckila et al., 1978) provides some information. Focal positivity in more than 50% of the leukemic cells is found in 90% of cases of T-ALL (Figure 7) and 10% or less of cases of non-B, non-T ALL (Catovsky et al., 1978); this stain may be of value when complete immunologic evaluation is not possible (Savage, Valenzuela, and Hoffman, 1981).

III. ACUTE NONLYMPHOCYTIC LEUKEMIAS

The following descriptions pertain to cases in which the diagnosis of ANLL has already been established, i.e. 30% or more of all bone marrow or peripheral blood cells are blasts and 3% or more of the blasts are myeloperoxidase positive or 20% or more show strong, diffuse α-naphthylbutyrate positivity. Further classification is then based on the proportions of granulocytic, monocytic, and erythroid elements in the bone marrow and peripheral blood. Cases with 50% or more erythroid cells (or 30% or more if the erythroid cells are particularly dysplastic) are FAB-M6. Cases with less than 20% monocytic cells are FAB-M1, M2 or M3. Cases with 20% or more monocytic cells are FAB-M4 or M5.

According to the revised October 1985 FAB proposal, the denominators for these calculations are the *nonerythroid cells* (NEC) in the bone marrow. Lymphocytes, plasma cells, mast cells and macrophages are excluded from these counts. Auer rods are most common in FAB-M2 and especially FAB-M3, but may be found in any of the acute myeloid leukemias, and their presence does not directly affect the classification of acute myeloid leukemias.

FAB-M1: Acute Myeloblastic Leukemia without Maturation

In FAB-M1, most of the cells are myeloblasts, with little tendency toward granulocytic maturation (Figure 8a). Less than 10% of the cells are progranulocytes or more mature granulocytes, and less than 20% are monocytic.

The blasts usually have rounded to oval nuclei and few cytoplasmic granules. Some cases are impossible to distinguish from FAB-L2 unless a myeloperoxidase stain is performed (Figure 8b).

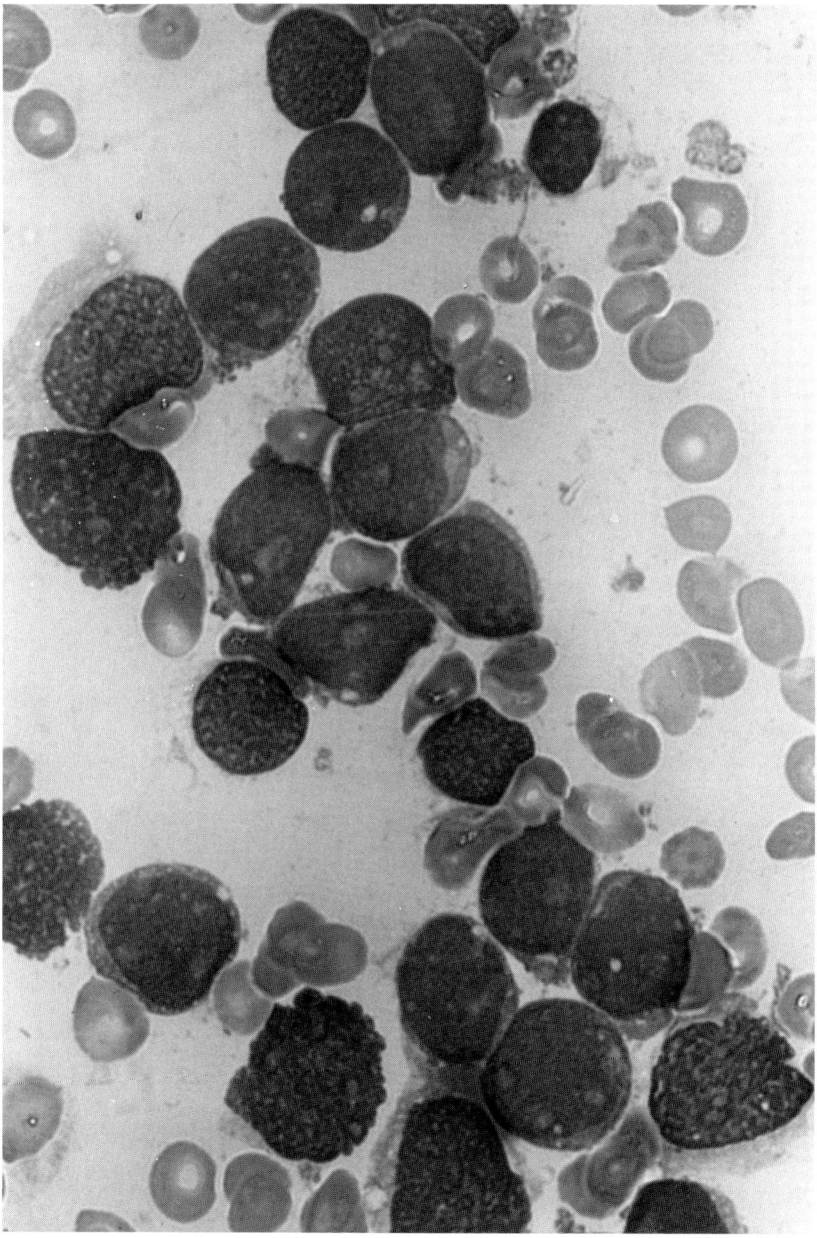

Figure 8a Acute myeloblastic leukemia (FAB-M1). Blasts are devoid of cytoplasmic granulation and are indistinguishable from those of FAB-L2. (W-G, X800)

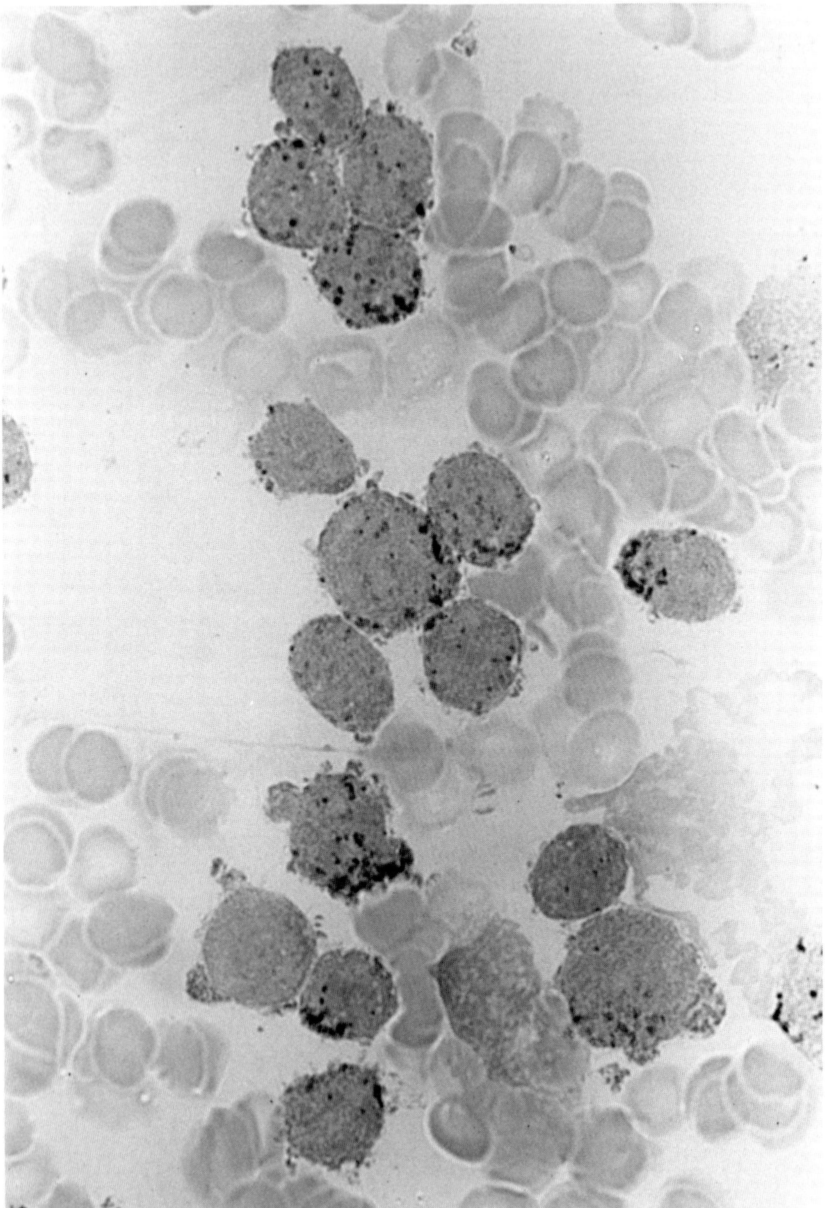

Figure 8b Acute myeloblastic leukemia (FAB-M1). Myeloperoxidase shows weak positivity in nearly all the blasts. (X800)

FAB-M2: Acute Myeloblastic Leukemia with Maturation

This category shows considerable morphologic heterogeneity; there is no single "typical" appearance for FAB-M2. The blasts are similar to those in FAB-M1, but may be larger and have a lower N/C ratio. The leukemic cells show evidence of granulocytic maturation with more than 10% progranulocytes or more mature granulocytes (Figure 9). Additionally, according to the October 1985 proposal, if greater than 10% of the NEC are "early maturing cells," the leukemia is classified FAB-M2. These early maturing cells show some cytoplasmic maturation without being recognizable as promyelocytes. This modification was devised to ensure that some cases of AML with t(8;21) previously classified as FAB-M1 could be classified with the majority of t(8;21) cases as FAB-M2. Less than 20% of the cells are monocytic cells (promonocytes plus monocytes). The promyelocytes may be abnormal but do not have the characteristic appearance of those in FAB-M3 (see below) and no faggot cells are present. Many cases of FAB-M2 show recognizable dysplasia of the maturing granulocytes, reflecting the fact that these cells are descendants of the leukemic blasts (Fearon et al., 1986). The nuclei may be hyposegmented, with a pseudo Pelger-Huet appearance, or may be ring-shaped, similar to rodent granulocytes (Staven et al., 1969). There may be abnormalities of granulation, including hypogranularity or enlarged pseudo Chediak-Higashi granules. Increased numbers of myeloperoxidase-deficient neutrophils have been described in AML, including 9/18 cases in one series (Bendix-Hansen, 1986). Auer rods may be found in mature granulocytes as well as in myeloblasts (Stass et al., 1984). Finally, there may be asynchrony between the development of the cytoplasm and the nucleus. Most commonly, this entails the findings of a blastic nucleus with prominent nucleoli in a cell with mature secondary granulation.

FAB-M3: Acute Promyelocytic Leukemia

FAB-M3 occurs most commonly in its hypergranular form, but also occurs in a variant or microgranular form (Bennett et al., 1980; Golomb et al., 1980; Edelman and Grossman, 1983). Both forms can be identified in Romanowsky-stained bone marrow smears. The diagnosis should be a morphologic one based on a pattern recognition; it is noteworthy that most cases of FAB-M3 have less than 30% blasts but that the number of progranulocytes is frequently greater than 75% (Stanley et al., 1985). The hypergranular form shows large numbers of abnormal progranulocytes, their enlarged granules frequently obscuring the nucleus (Figure 10). The variant or microgranular form shows a distinctive nuclear configuration in the majority of the leukemic cells: some nuclei are lobulated or reniform and others have an "apple core" shape (Figure 11). The cytoplasm shows a fine dusting of granules. The myeloperoxidase reactivity can be helpful in identifying this variant form of FAB-M3: the myeloperoxidase is intensely positive despite the lack of conspicuous cytoplasmic granulation. The α-naphthyl butyrate stain can be positive in some cases of FAB-M3 (Hayhoe and Flemans, 1982; Tomonaga et

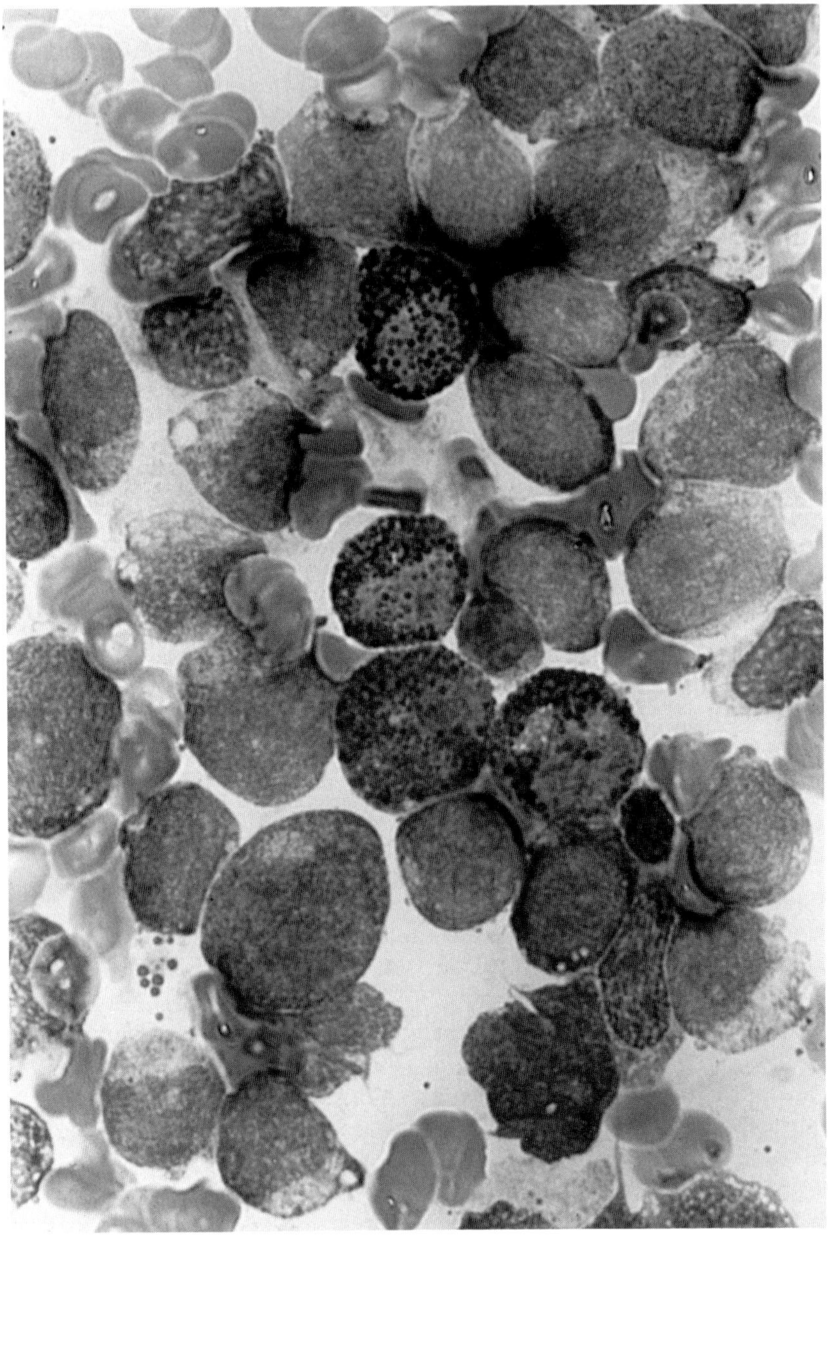

Figure 9a Acute myeloblastic leukemia (FAB-M2). Blasts, progranulocytes and an occasional eosinophilic myelocyte are present. (W-G, ×800)

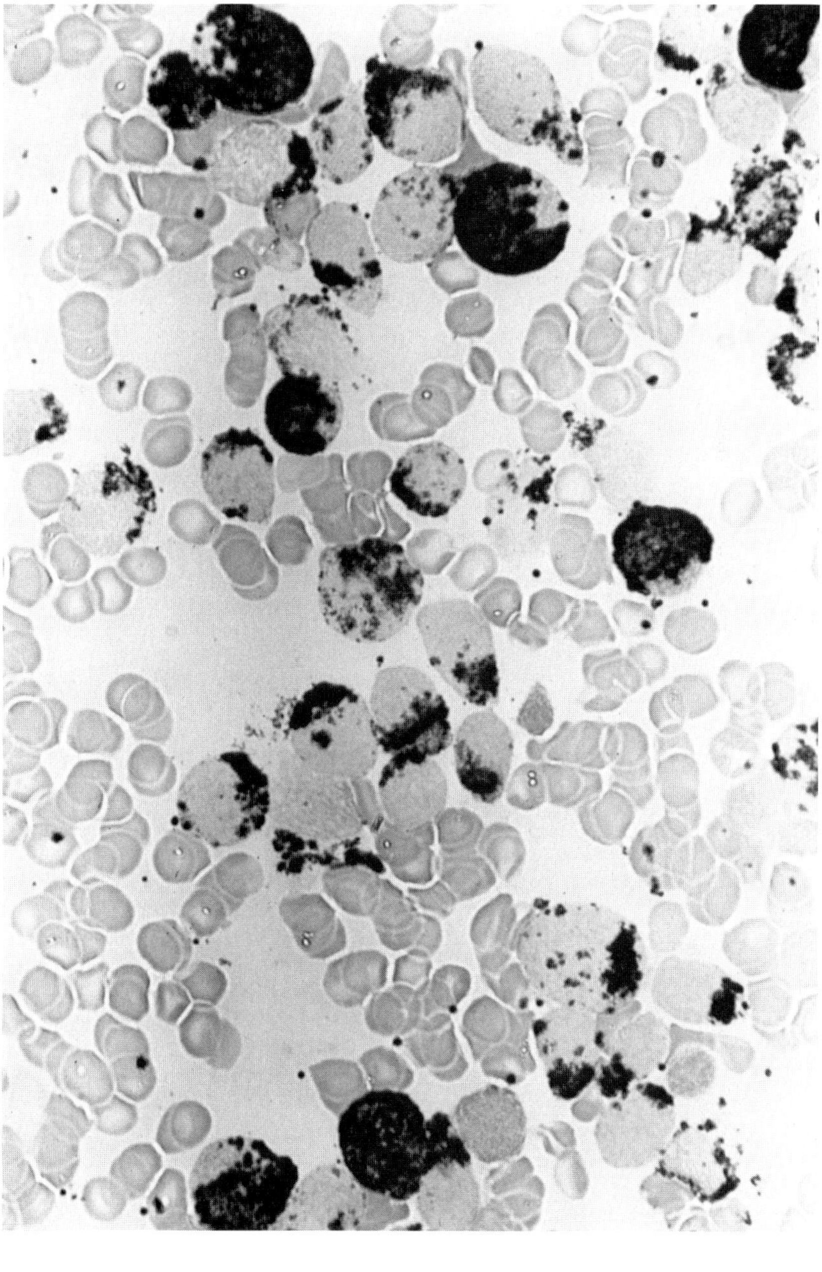

Figure 9b Acute myeloblastic leukemia (FAB-M2). Myeloperoxidase shows strong positivity in the progranulocytes and moderate positivity in the blasts. (X800)

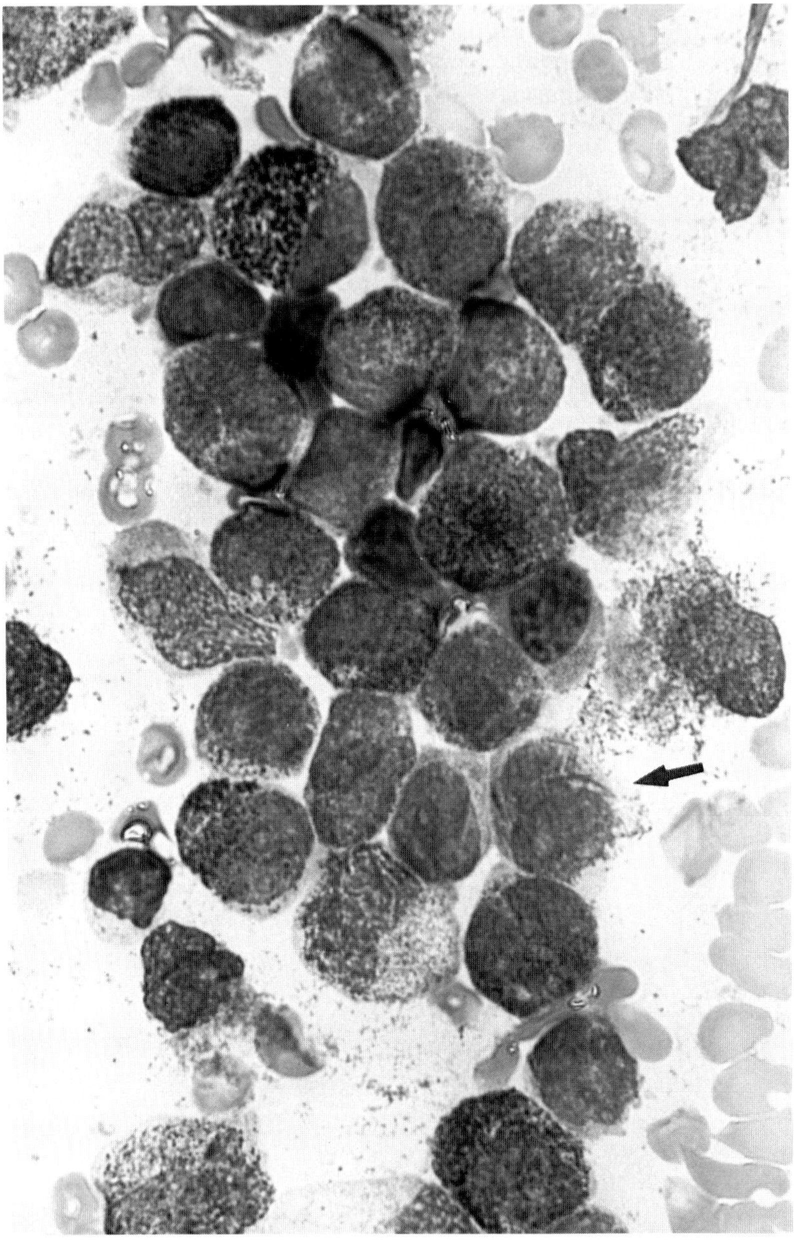

Figure 10 Acute progranulocytic leukemia (FAB-M3). Most of the cells are progranulocytes, some with enlarged granules obscuring the nucleus. A cell with multiple Auer rods is present (arrow). (W-G, X800)

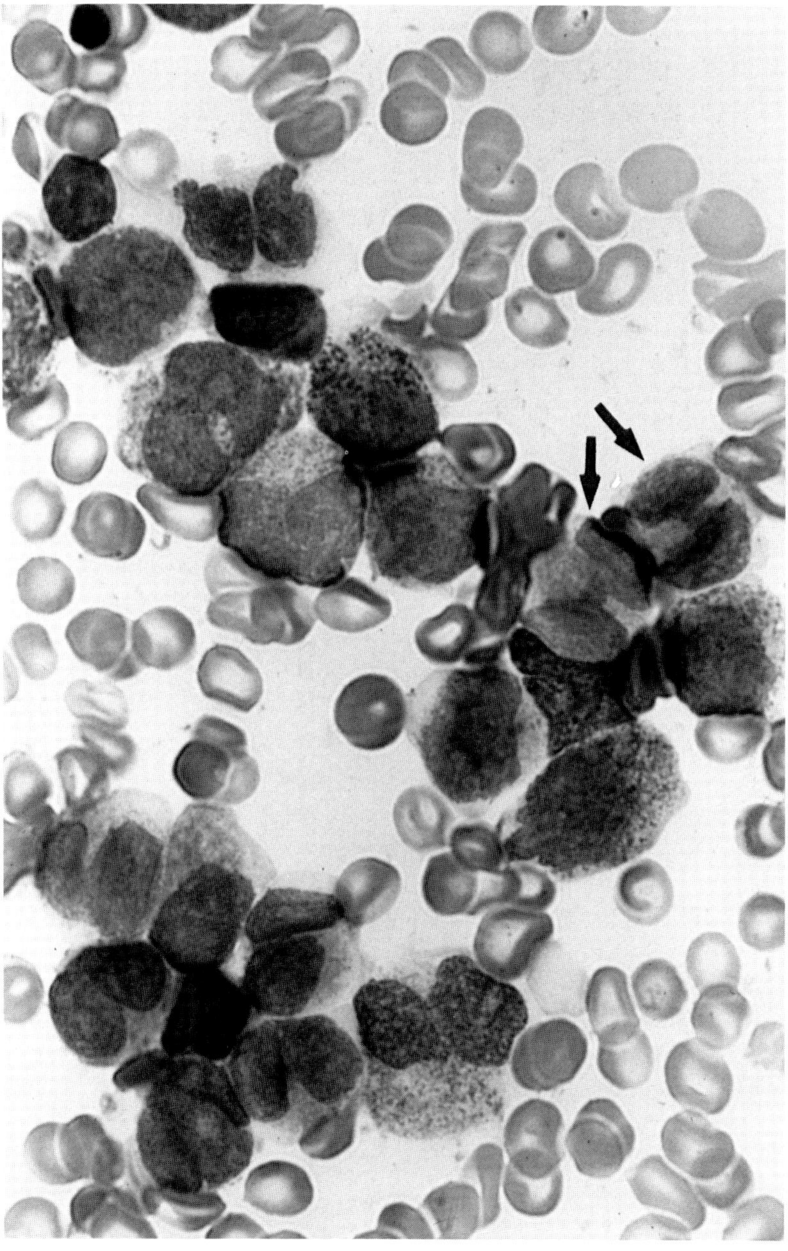

Figure 11a Acute progranulocytic leukemia (FAB-M3 variant). Nearly all the cells show nuclear lobulation. Occasional cells show an "apple core" nuclear configuration (arrows) (W-G, ×800).

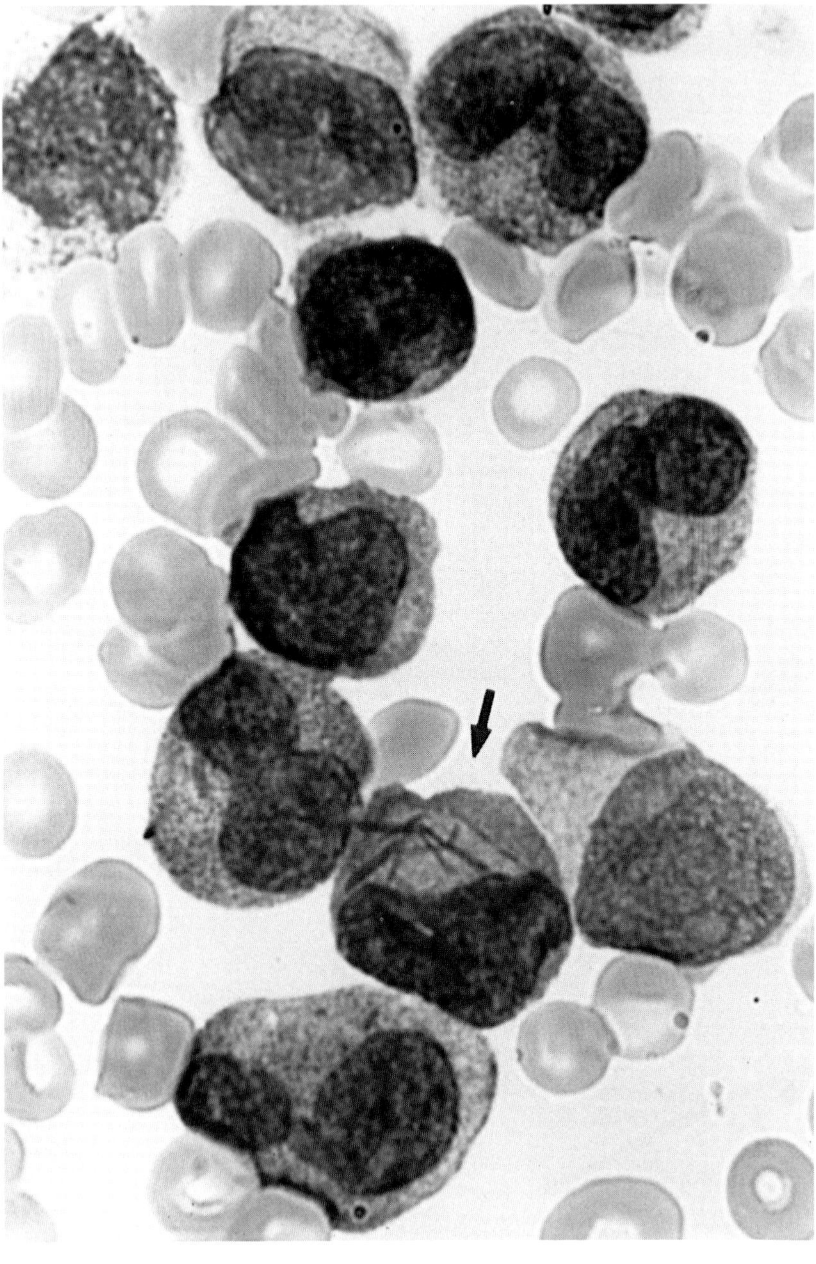

Figure 11b Acute progranulocytic leukemia (FAB-M3 variant). Multiple Auer rods are present in a leukemic blast (arrow). (W-G, ×1250)

al., 1985). This should not change the diagnosis, in our opinion. Cells containing multiple Auer rods (faggot cells) can usually be identified in both types of FAB-M3, although we have found occasional examples of hypergranular FAB-M3 where granulation was too heavy to allow identification of Auer rods. We have also found occasional cases of the microgranular variant in which we were unable to identify faggot cells. Small cells with "hyperbasophilic" cytoplasm can be found in many cases of FAB-M3 and can be the predominant cell type in some cases (McKenna et al., 1982). It is helpful to be aware that these cells can be found in FAB-M3, but they do not appear to be of any clinical significance.

Prompt recognition of FAB-M3 is critical so that the patients can be managed in ways directed toward minimizing risk of hemorrhage.

FAB-M4: Acute Myelomonocytic Leukemia

FAB-M4 shows differentiation along both granulocytic and monocytic pathways (Figure 12), with at least 20% myeloblasts and promyelocytes in the bone marrow and at least 20% monocytic cells in the bone marrow, peripheral blood, or both. The revised FAB proposals for the FAB-M4 require that both the bone marrow (BM) and peripheral blood (PB) show evidence of monocytic proliferation. If only one shows such evidence, bone marrow cytochemical tests or serum or urine lysozyme determinations are recommended to confirm the diagnosis. In most instances we use the α-naphthyl butyrate to document the presence of monocytes (Figure 12c). However, occasionally we have noted cases with a substantial monocytic component both by light and ultrastructure that are α-naphthyl butyrate negative. We do classify such cases as myelomonocytic. In some cases of FAB-M4, the populations of granulocytic and monocytic cells seem to be separate and distinct; in other cases, individual leukemic cells seem to be "hybrids" showing coexistent granulocytic and monocytic features morphologically or cytochemically. "Combined esterase" procedures have been done, in which individual leukemic cells have been shown to contain NASD-CAE, a neutrophil enzyme; and α-naphthyl butyrate, a monocyte enzyme (Kass, 1977; Lam, Li, and Yam, 1985; Li, Phyliky, and Yam, 1986; Yam, Li, and Crosby, 1971). It has been asserted that cases of FAB-M4 showing coexpression of neutrophilic and monocytic enzymes in individual cells frequently evolved through a preleukemic phase (Tavassoli, Shaklai, and Crosby, 1979). This is supported by the finding of similar coexpression of enzymes in myelodyplastic syndromes (Scott et al., 1983; Tavassoli, 1984).

A distinctive subtype of FAB-M4, which we will refer to as FAB-M4-E, is seen in association with abnormalities of chromosome 16, most commonly inv(16). The most striking feature of this subtype of leukemia is the presence of bone marrow eosinophils with interspersed large basophilic granules (Figure 13). By electron microscopy (EM), the eosinophils show abnormal granulation and, importantly, nuclear blebs (Dalton et al., 1985). A large monocytic component is morphologically apparent in all of these cases, but we have found α-naphthyl

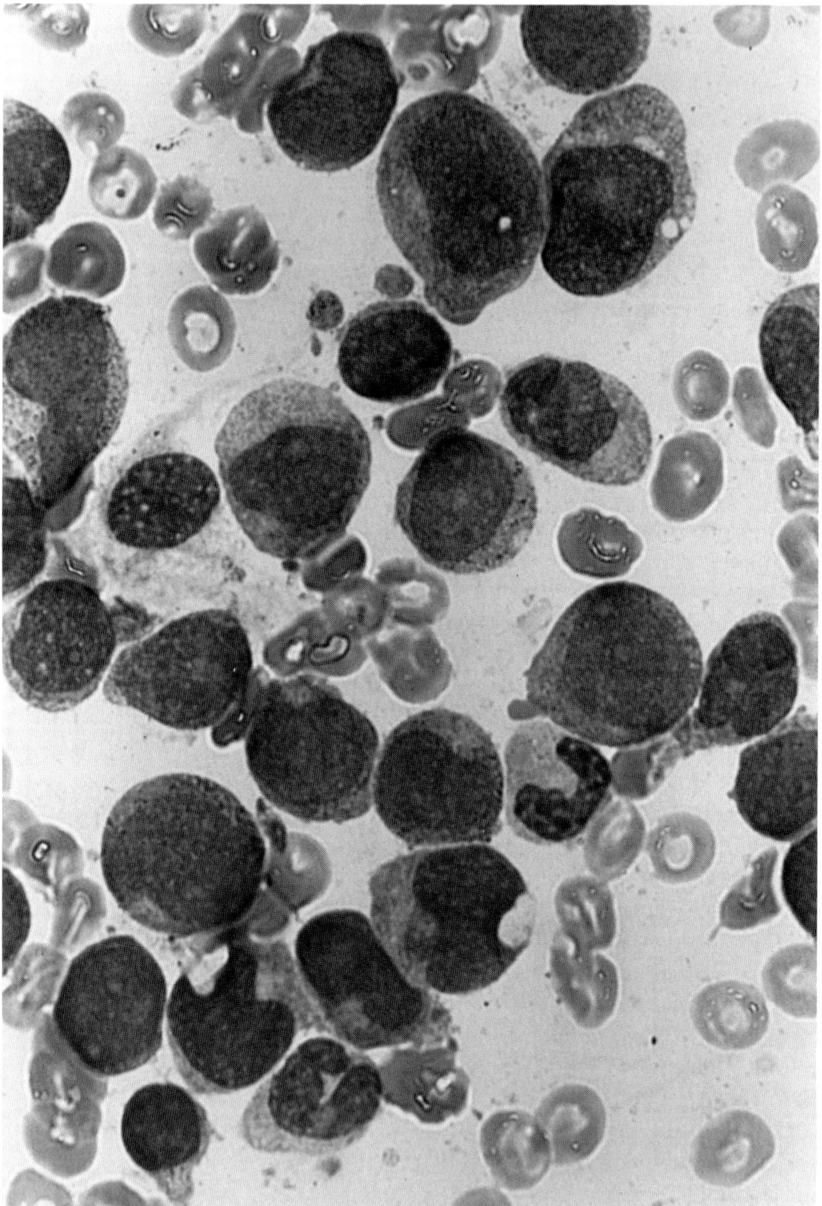

Figure 12a Acute myelomonocytic leukemia (FAB-M4). Both myeloid and monocytic blasts are present. (W-G, ×800)

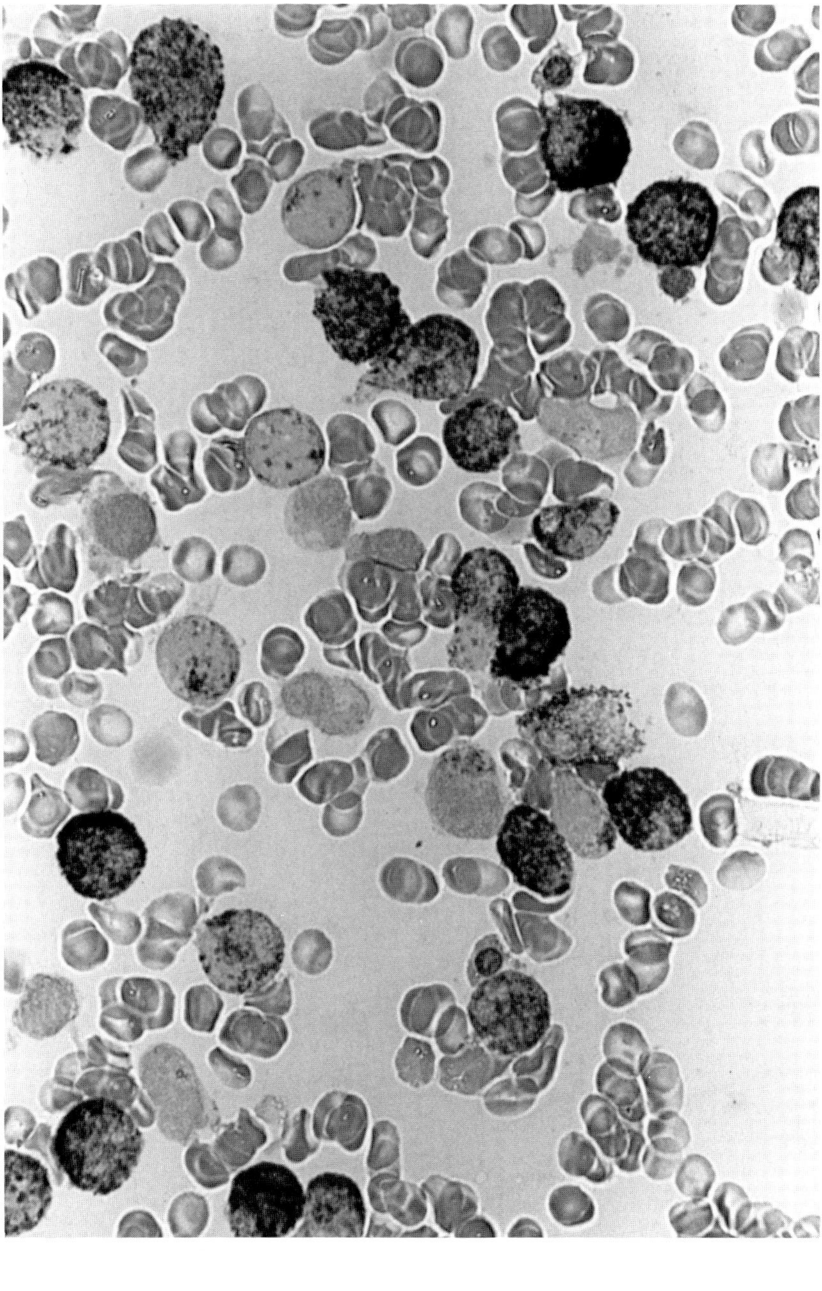

Figure 12b Acute myelomonocytic leukemia (FAB-M4). Myeloperoxidase stain is positive in nearly all the blasts. (X500)

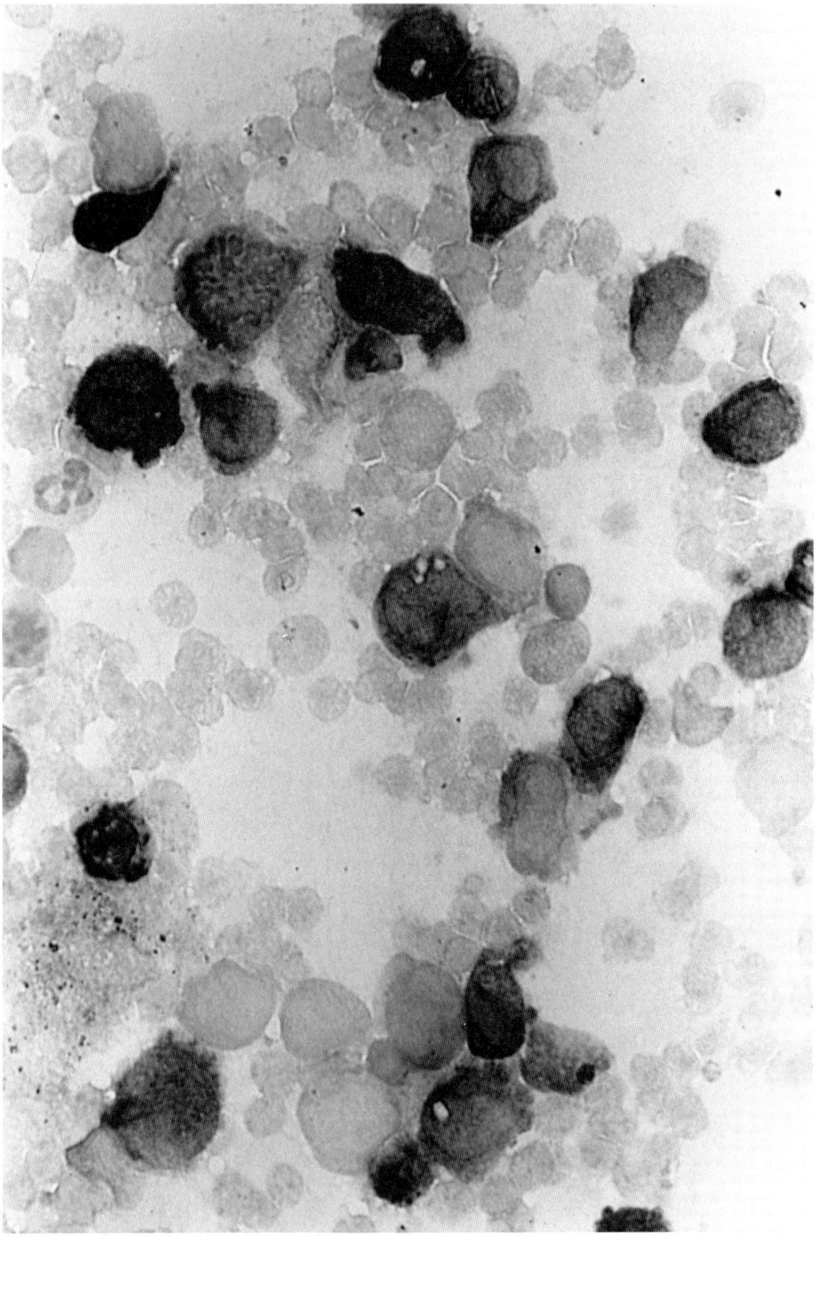

Figure 12c Acute myelomonocytic leukemia (FAB-M4). α-naphthyl butyrate confirms that there is a large monocytic component. (X500)

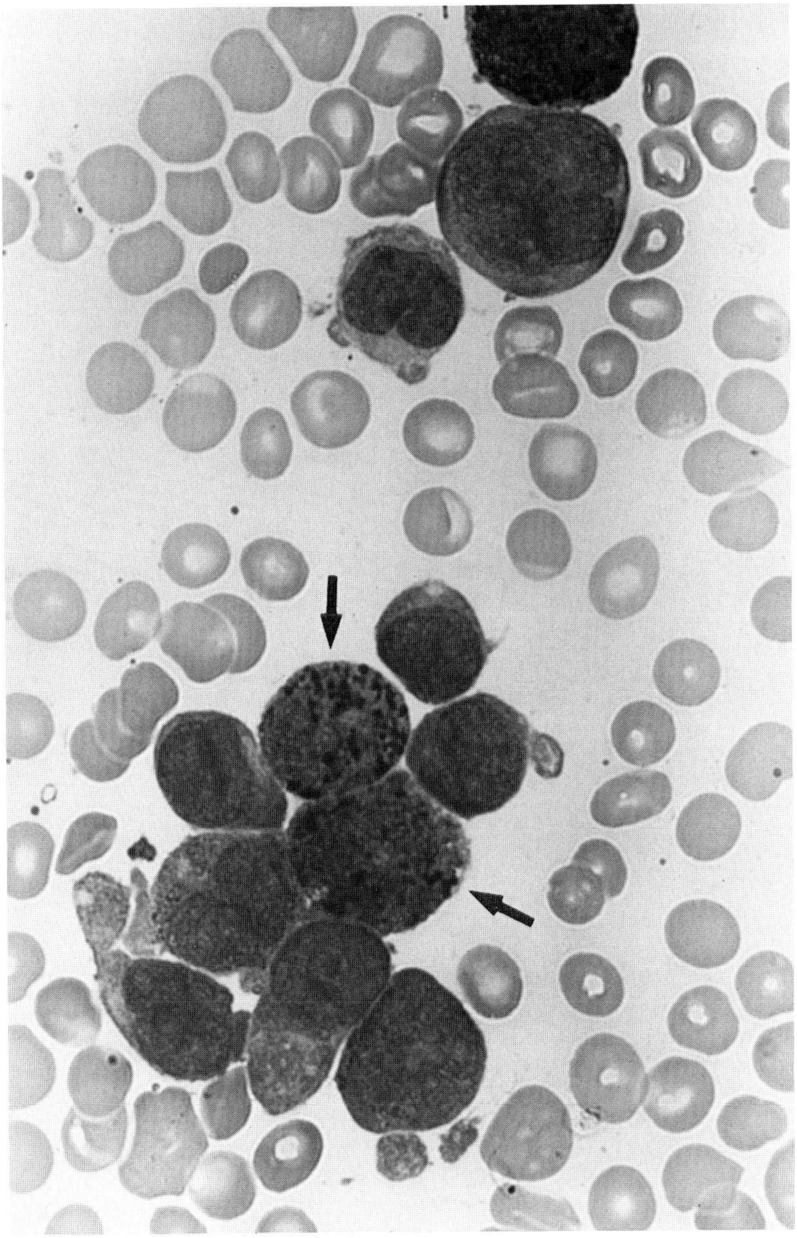

Figure 13a Acute myelomonocytic leukemia with eosinophilia (FAB-M4-E). Monocytoid blasts and two large eosinophils with basophilic granules are present (arrows). (W-G, ×800)

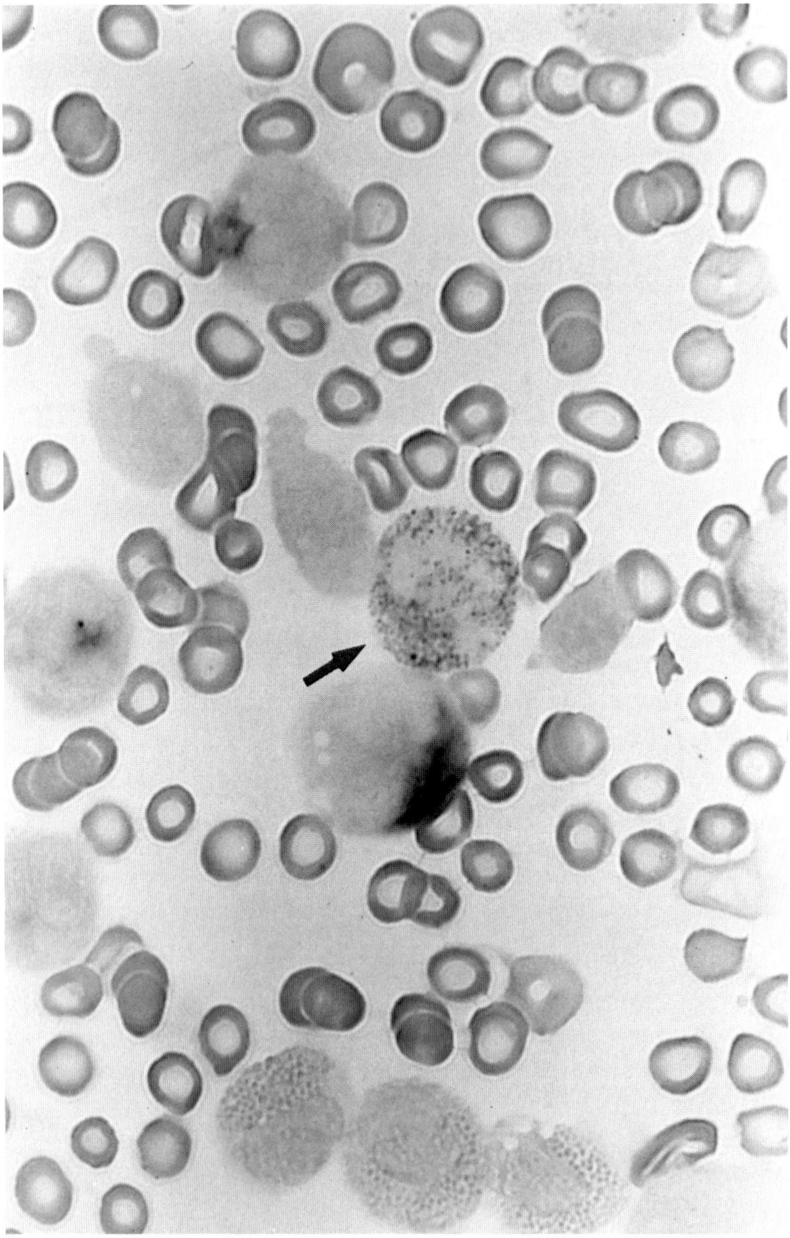

Figure 13b Acute myelomonocytic leukemia with eosinophilia (FAB-M4-E). NASD-chloroacetate esterase stain. An eosinophil shows positivity in its granules (arrow), an anomalous reaction. (X800)

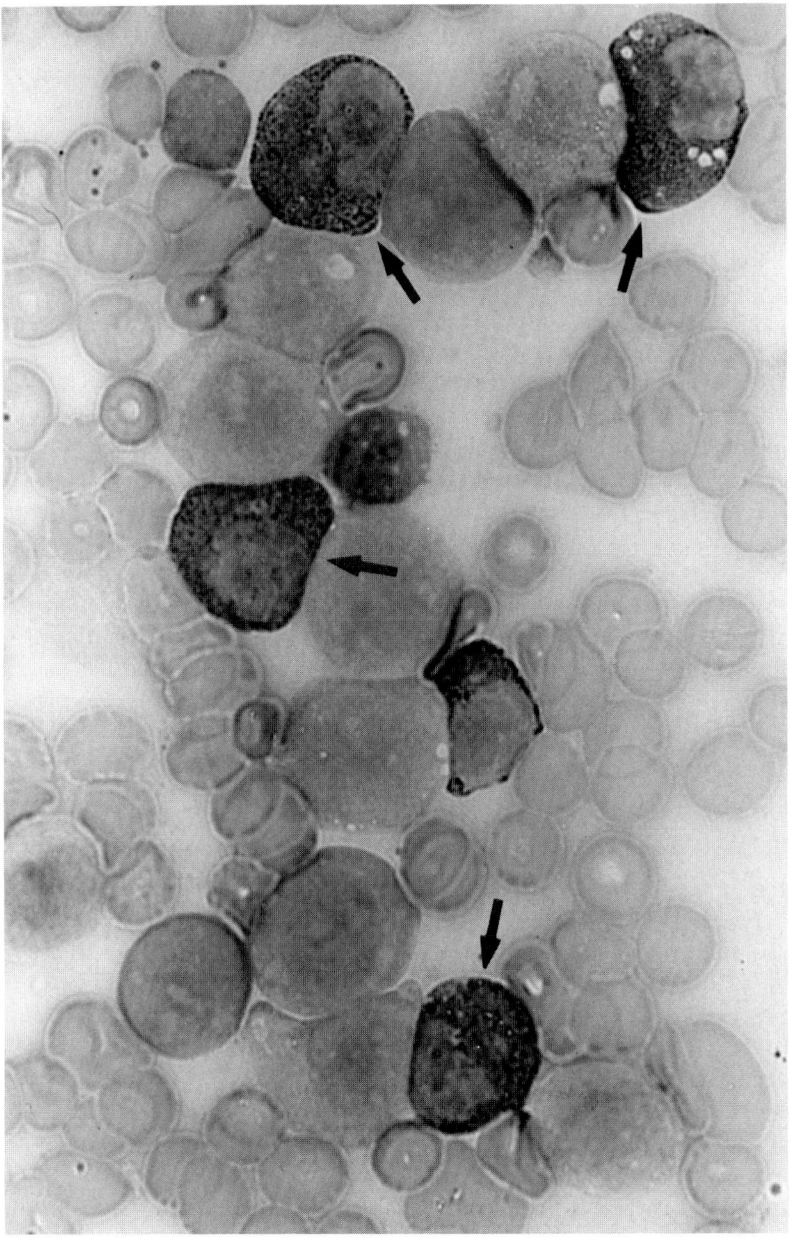

Figure 13c Acute myelomonocytic leukemia with eosinophilia (FAB-M4-E). PAS. Some eosinophils show positivity in their granules (arrows), an anomalous reaction. (X800)

butyrate positivity (defined as 20% of total bone marrow cells positive) in only about 25% of cases of FAB-M4-E (Dalton, submitted for publication). EM confirms that all the cases of FAB-M4-E have a substantial monocytic component. Others have also reported that the eosinophil granules in FAB-M4-E show anomalous positive staining with PAS and with NASD-CAE (Figure 13) (Bitter et al., 1984; Liso et al., 1977).

FAB-M5: Acute Monocytic Leukemia

In FAB-M5, the leukemic cells are large, have ample gray-blue cytoplasm (Figure 14), and may have cytoplasmic vacuoles or show phagocytosis of erythrocytes or platelets. Small salmon-colored granules are frequently present, and the granulation can be fairly intense in some cases. Many cases show a characteristic large owl's eye nucleolus and a folded nucleus. Auer rods may be present. Most cases show diffuse α-naphthyl butyrate esterase positivity (Figure 14c). Some cases show NASD-CAE positivity, an anomalous reaction for monocytic cells. Such NASD-CAE positivity does not cause us to change the diagnosis of FAB-M5 in an otherwise typical case. Both a poorly differentiated (M5a) and a differentiated (M5b) form of acute monocytic leukemia are recognized, although the two forms have not been shown to differ biologically. According to the October 1985 FAB revision, in M5a 80% or more of the monocytic cells are monoblasts, and in M5b, less than 80% are. We would like to point out that there are some cases of FAB-M5b where the bone marrow is virtually replaced by monocytic cells but where the proportion of blasts is less than 30%. In one series, only 5/14 cases classified as M5b had more than 30% bone marrow blasts (Stanley et al., 1985). The decision of whether to classify these leukemias as acute versus chronic can be a difficult one, and, as in FAB-M3, depends on the ability to recognize the distinctive overall morphologic picture.

FAB-M6: Erythroleukemia

FAB-M6 is an uncommon form of acute leukemia characterized by the proliferation of erythroid and myeloblastic elements. The original FAB proposal required that 50% or more of the BM cells be erythroid (or 30% if the erythroid cells are particularly dysplastic) and that 30% or more of the BM cells be blasts. The erythroid cells are dysplastic and can show multinuclearity (Figure 15a), nuclear irregularities (such as "clover leaf" forms), karyorrhexis, and Howell-Jolly bodies. They may be megaloblastic and may have cytoplasmic vacuoles. The PAS stain typically shows intense block positivity in the erythroid cells (Figure 15b). If vacuoles are present the PAS can be shown to be present within the vacuoles by ultrastructure (Schumacher and Stass, 1982). The maturing erythroid precursors may demonstrate a "blush" positivity in addition to the block positivity. The Prussian blue stain frequently shows ringed sideroblasts. Rare cases fail to show either abnormality, however. An EM feature that facilitates the identification of

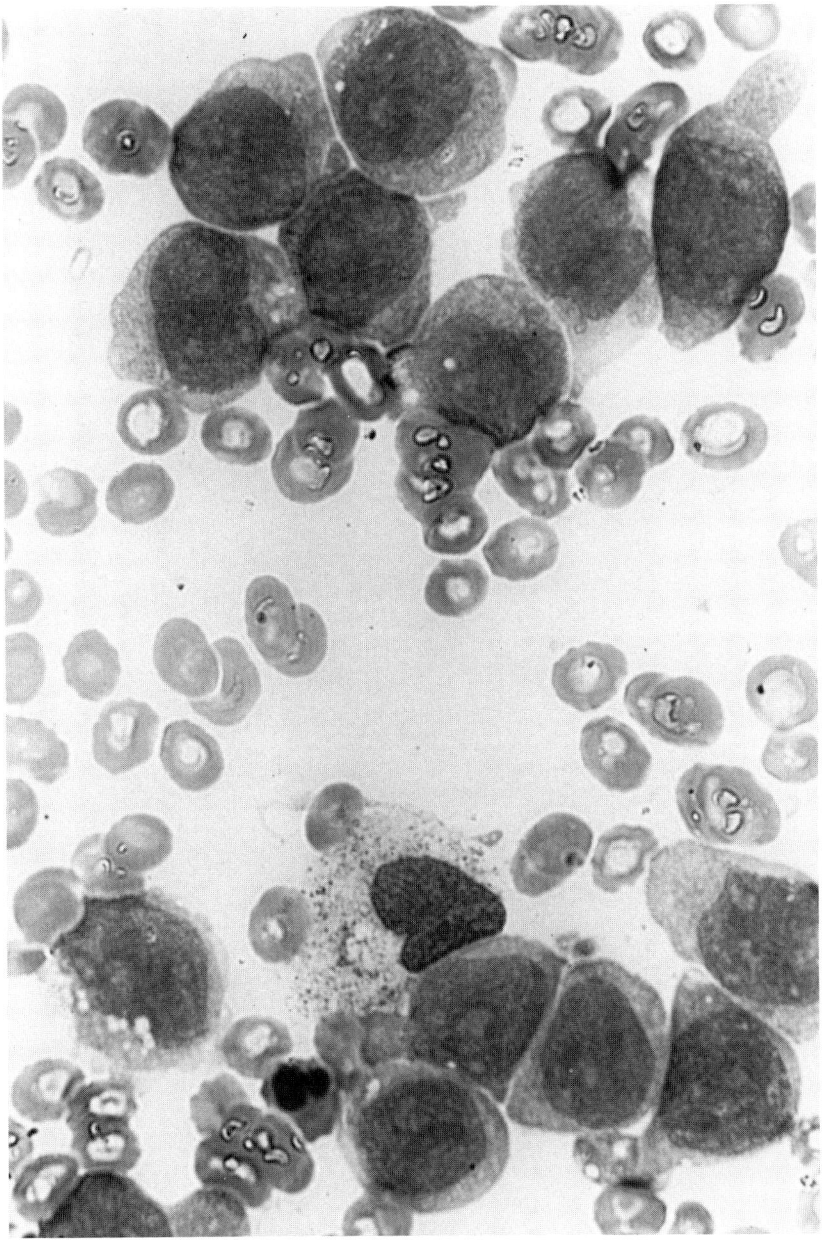

Figure 14a Acute monocytic leukemia (FAB-M5). Most of the cells are monoblasts, with a few cells showing folded nuclei. (W-G, ×800)

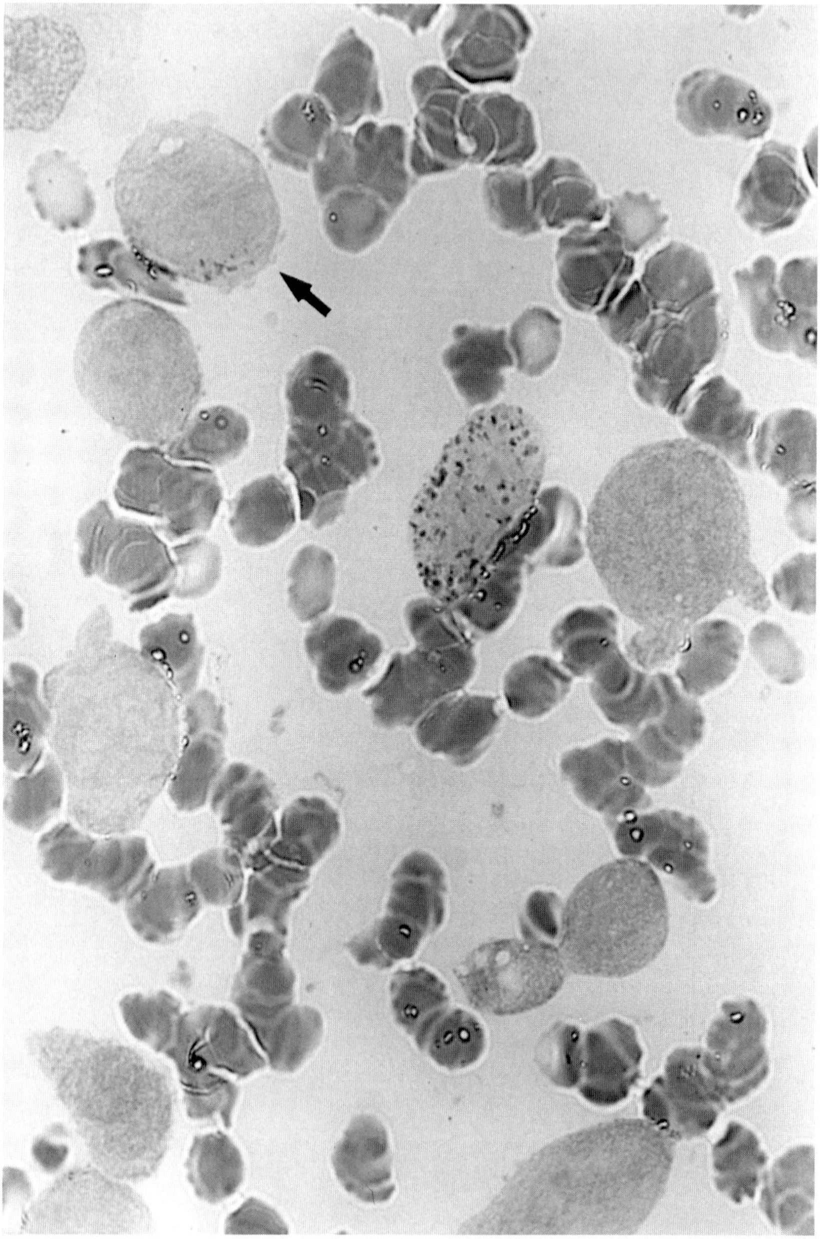

Figure 14b Acute monocytic leukemia (FAB-M5). Myeloperoxidase stain showing rare weakly positive blasts (arrows). (×800)

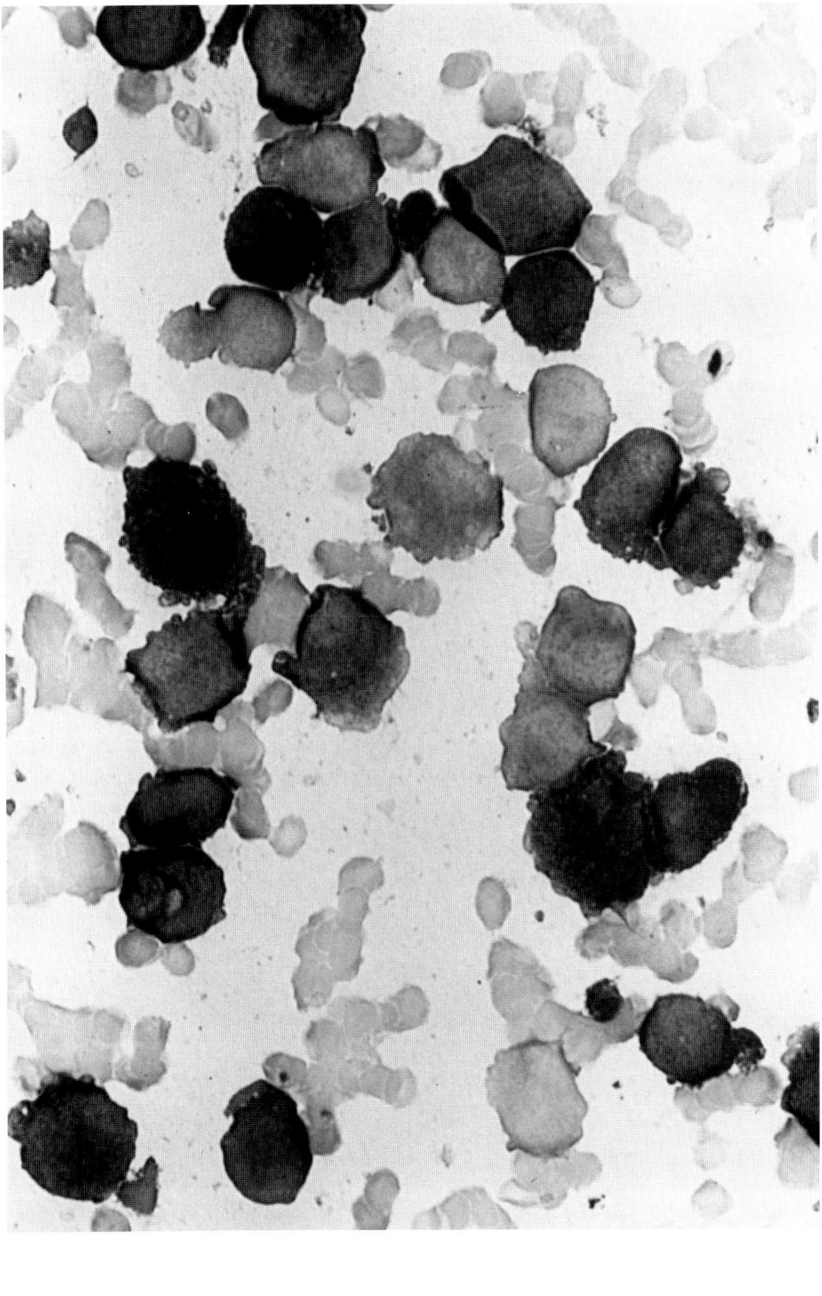

Figure 14c Acute monocytic leukemia (FAB-M5); alpha-naphthyl butyrate stain shows intense, diffuse positivity in the majority of the cells. (X500)

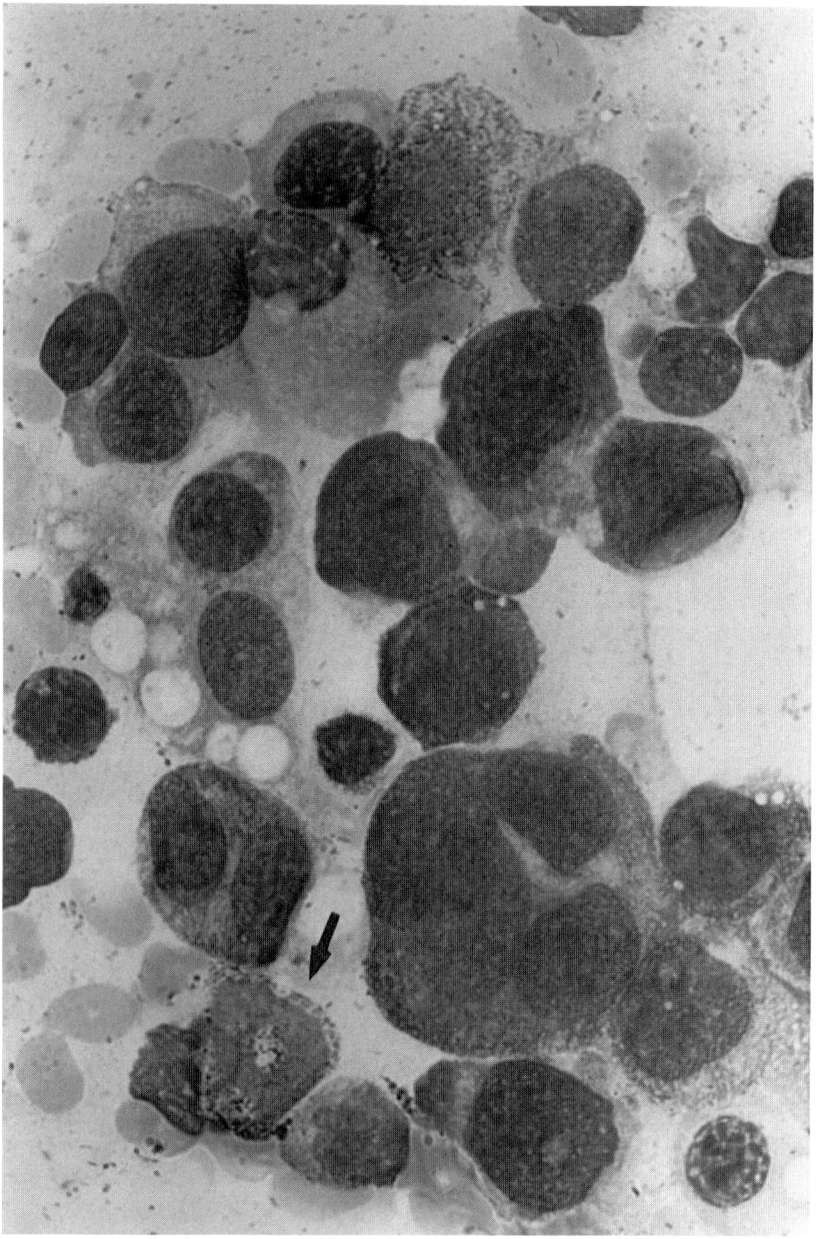

Figure 15a Erythroleukemia (FAB-M6). Multinucleated erythroid cells are present. Also note neutrophil with ring nucleus (arrow). (W-G, ×800)

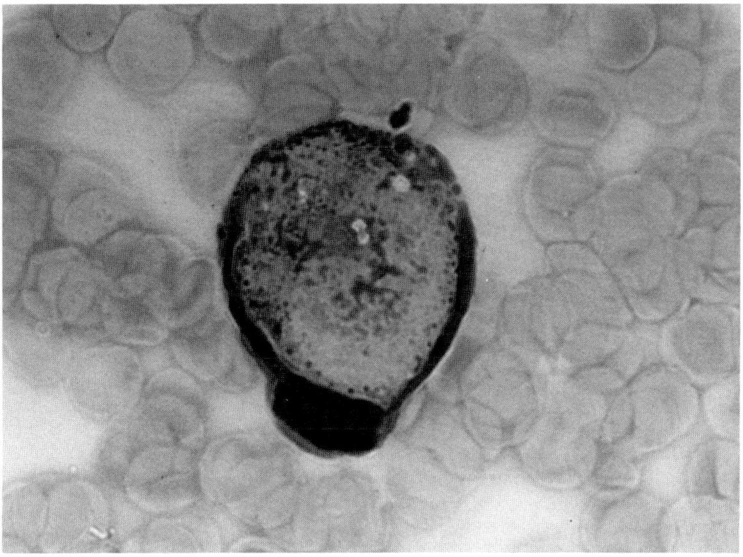

Figure 15b Erythroleukemia (FAB-M6). PAS stain showing ring of intense positivity. (X800)

leukemic cells as being of erythroid lineage is the presence of ferritin rhopheocytosis. The other component in FAB-M6 is myeloblastic. These blasts may be indistinguishable from those seen in FAB-M1 or M2, and Auer rods may be present. The myeloblastic element may eventually outstrip the erythroid element in some cases, producing a picture of FAB-M1, M2, or M4.

The revised FAB criteria of October 1985 would change the diagnosis of M6 substantially. First, the percentage of erythroid cells must be at least 50% of the bone marrow cells. Second, blasts must comprise 30% or more of the nonerythroid bone marrow cells to establish a diagnosis of FAB-M6. If the blasts are less than 30% of the NEC, the case probably represents one of the dysmyelopoietic syndromes.

FAB-M7: Acute Leukemia of Megakaryocytic Lineage

In our experience, this is a rare form of acute leukemia, although some authors have asserted that FAB-M7 accounts for up to 10% of ANLL. The diagnosis is usually complicated by the fact that marrow fibrosis prevents aspiration of sufficient cells for evaluation. The blasts may resemble lymphoblasts on W-G smears, but tend to be larger. The cytoplasm typically shows "budding" but this feature is not specific for FAB-M7 (Figure 16). The α-naphthyl acetate may show focal

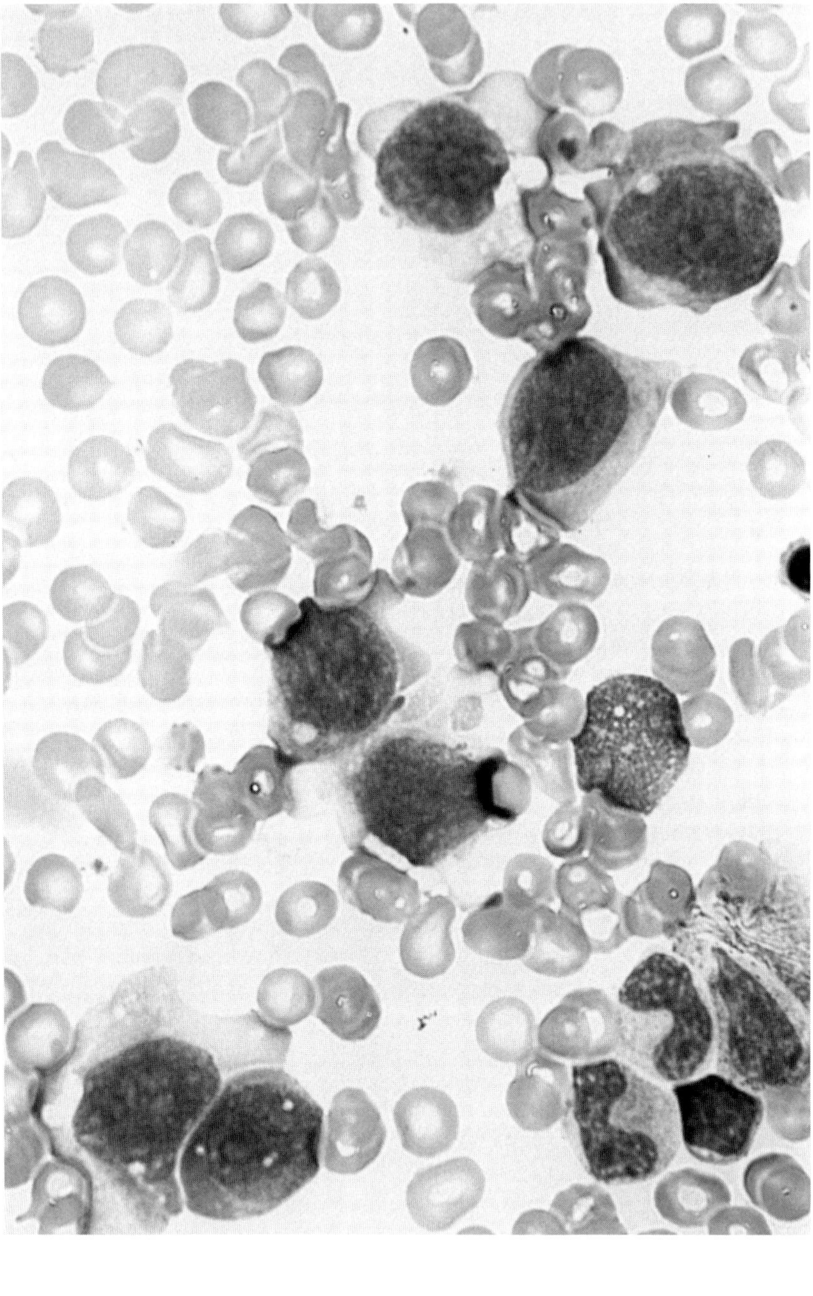

Figure 16 Acute leukemia of megabaryocytic lineage (FAB-M7). Several of the blasts show cytoplasmic "budding." (W-G, ×800)

positivity and the PAS stain may be positive, but again, these features are not definitive. The blasts may show a tendency to aggregate and should not be mistaken for metastatic tumor (Pui, Rivera, Mirro, et al., 1985). The FAB group has published criteria for the diagnosis of FAB-M7; in a departure from their previous approach, they recommend the diagnosis be confirmed either with EM demonstration of platelet peroxidase, or with immunologic studies to demonstrate factor VIII, or glycoprotein IB or IIB/IIIA on the surface of the blasts.

IV. ACUTE LYMPHOCYTIC LEUKEMIA

FAB-L1 and FAB-L2

The morphologic diagnosis of ALL is largely a diagnosis of exclusion: less than 3% of the blasts are myeloperoxidase positive and less than 20% show diffuse α-naphthyl butyrate positivity. The cytoplasm is light blue to blue, does not contain Auer rods, and generally lacks granulation, although "granular ALL" does occur (Stein et al., 1983). We feel it is important to use the myeloperoxidase stain rather than Sudan black because Sudan black can be positive in ALL. Even the myeloperoxidase stain can be positive in slightly more than 3% of the blasts in rare cases of ALL, cases that by immunologic and clinical parameters behave as otherwise typical ALL (Pui et al., 1984). Such cases highlight the arbitrary nature of the 3% myeloperoxidase-positive cutoff value. As mentioned earlier, α-naphthyl butyrate esterase is weakly and focally positive in 25% of pediatric ALLs (Figure 6) and should not cause diagnostic confusion. We have also seen punctate NASD-CAE positivity in a case of ALL (Keifer, Abromowitch, and Stass, 1985) and it has been reported in normal lymphocytes (Heumann, 1983).

The TdT stain is positive in 90-97% of cases of ALL; this is one of the few positive findings in ALL, but its importance is diminished by the fact that a substantial number of cases of AML can have TdT positivity. The PAS stain shows block positivity against a fairly clean cytoplasmic background in most cases of pediatric ALL, but can also be block positive in ANLL.

The FAB group defined three morphologic types of acute lymphocytic leukemia: FAB-L1, the common morphologic type of ALL in childhood; FAB-L2, the most common morphologic type of ALL in adults; and FAB-L3, the rare (approximately 3%) B-cell, Burkitt's type acute leukemia. The FAB group reported that the morphologic categories of FAB-L1 and L2 had prognostic significance independent of other parameters, although this has been questioned by others.

In 1981, the FAB group devised a scoring system for classifying ALL as FAB-L1 or L2, with the aim of improving the precision of the classification. The system is based on the N/C ratio of the cells, the nucleoli, the shape of the nuclear membrane, and the cell size. If more than 75% of the cells have a high N/C ratio (>4:1), this feature is scored +1; if 25% or more of the cells have a low N/C ratio, it is scored −1. If 75% or more of the cells have zero to 1 small nucleoli, this feature is scored +1; if 25% or more of the cells have 1 or more prominent nucleoli, it is scored −1. If 25% or more of the nuclear membranes are irregular, this feature is scored −1. If 50% or more of the cells are larger than twice the diameter of a small lymphocyte, this feature is scored −1. The scores are then tallied. A score of 0 to +2 is defined as FAB-L1 (Figure 17), and a score of −1 to −4 is defined as FAB-L2 (Figure 18). To achieve good precision, we feel that a formal 100-cell differential should be performed for each of the features. However, this entails a considerable amount of effort considering that the prognostic information gained is of marginal value.

FAB-L3

The leukemic cells in FAB-L3 are typically very uniform in size and shape, and have moderate amounts of deep blue cytoplasm and prominent vacuolization (Figure 19). The vacuoles contain lipid and are Oil Red-0 positive, although FAB-L1 or L2 can also occasionally have Oil Red-0 positive vacuoles. FAB-L3 is morphologically indistinguishable from Burkitt's lymphoma, and most cases have the phenotype of B cells, although exceptions have been reported (Ganick and Findlay, 1980; Mangon et al., 1985). FAB-L3 may have the same chromosomal translocations as are found in Burkitt's lymphoma. The TdT and the PAS stains are usually negative in B-cell FAB-L3, though there are rare reports of positivity for TdT (Drexler et al., 1986; Shaw et al., 1978) and PAS (Schumacher, 1978). We have also seen a rare case of FAB-L3 that showed TdT positivity and PAS block positivity, but the cells lacked surface immunoglobulin, and showed more size heterogeneity and nuclear irregularity than the usual case of FAB-L3.

V. MISCELLANEOUS ACUTE LEUKEMIA

AUL: Acute Undifferentiated Leukemia

A few percent of cases of acute leukemia defy classification with currently available methods and are called "undifferentiated." This area of study is rather confusing because various criteria have been used for the diagnosis of AUL, and the criteria have changed as additional methods of characterizing leukemic cells have become available. We currently consider a case to be AUL when the blasts are negative for TdT, α-naphthyl butyrate, NASD-CAE, and are myeloperoxidase negative at the level of both light and electron microscopy. The blasts usually have moderate amounts of agranular cytoplasm, and have a very fine chromatin pattern by light microscopy and are very euchromatic by electron microscopy. We have found that some of these cases express myeloid-associated or lymphoid-associated surface markers, but we do not yet have enough confidence in the lineage specificity of these markers to base the lineage solely on immunophenotype data. Thus, in the absence of clear morphologic or cytochemical evidence for myeloid or lymphoid features, we have not used immunophenotype to define the lineage. Cases of AUL that are TdT positive have also been described. In these

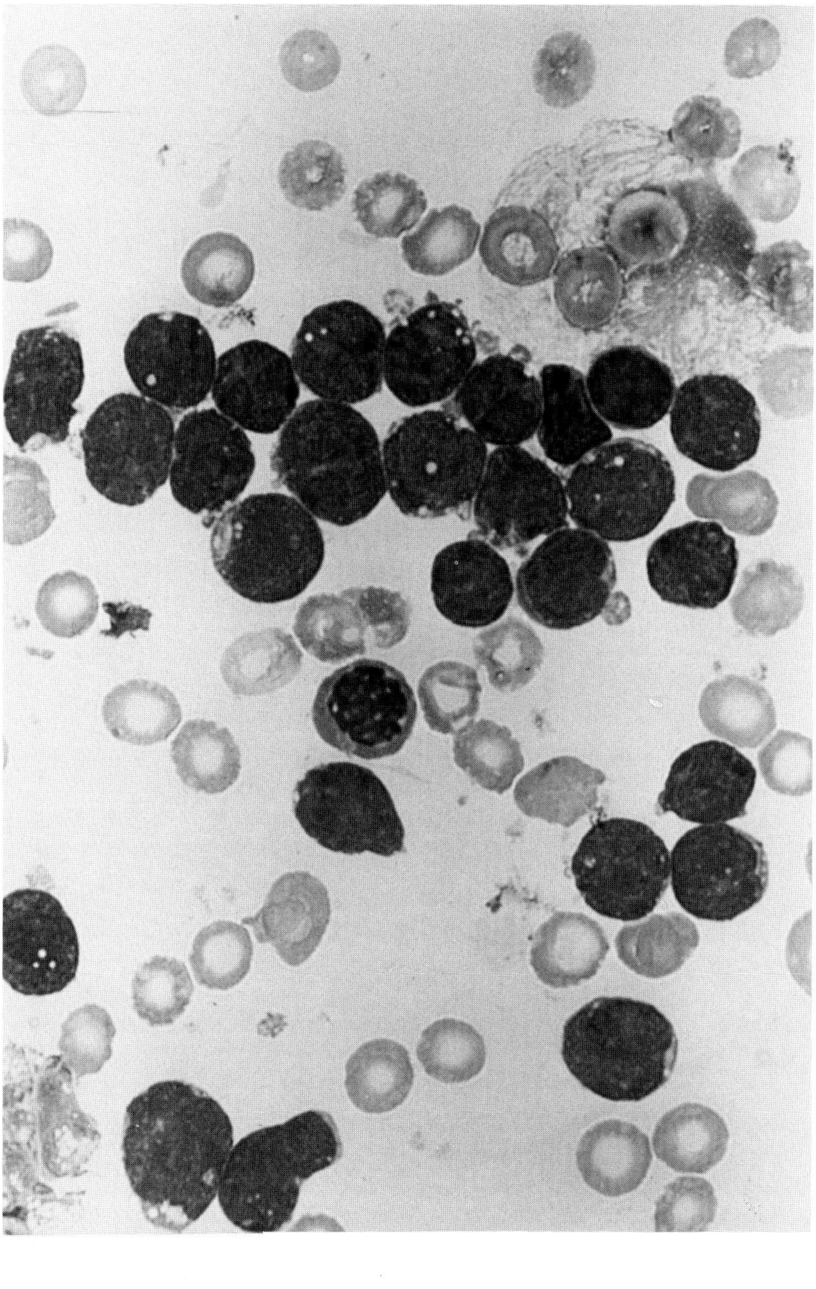

Figure 17a Acute lymphocytic leukemia (FAB-L1). Blasts have a high N/C ratio and inconspicuous nucleoli. (W-G, X800)

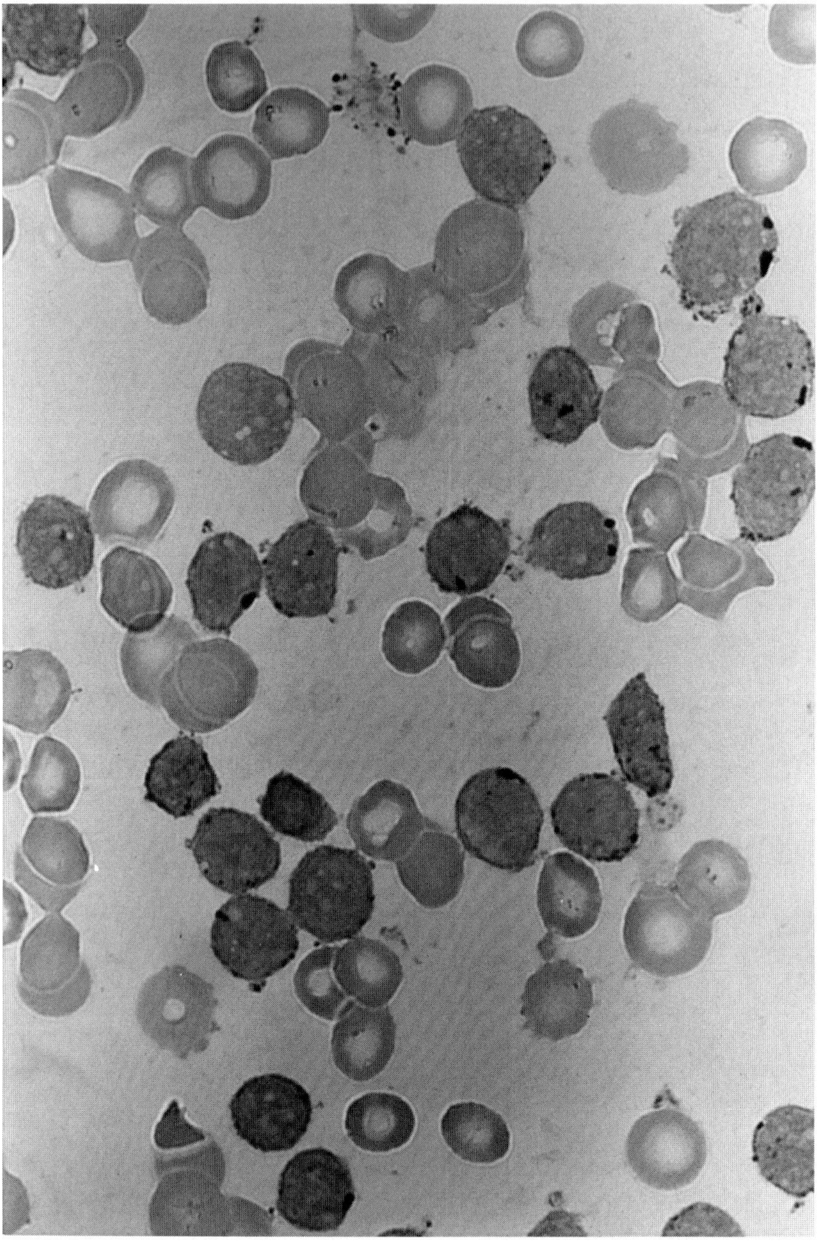

Figure 17b Acute lymphocytic leukemia (FAB-L1). PAS stain showing "block" positivity in many of the blasts. (×800)

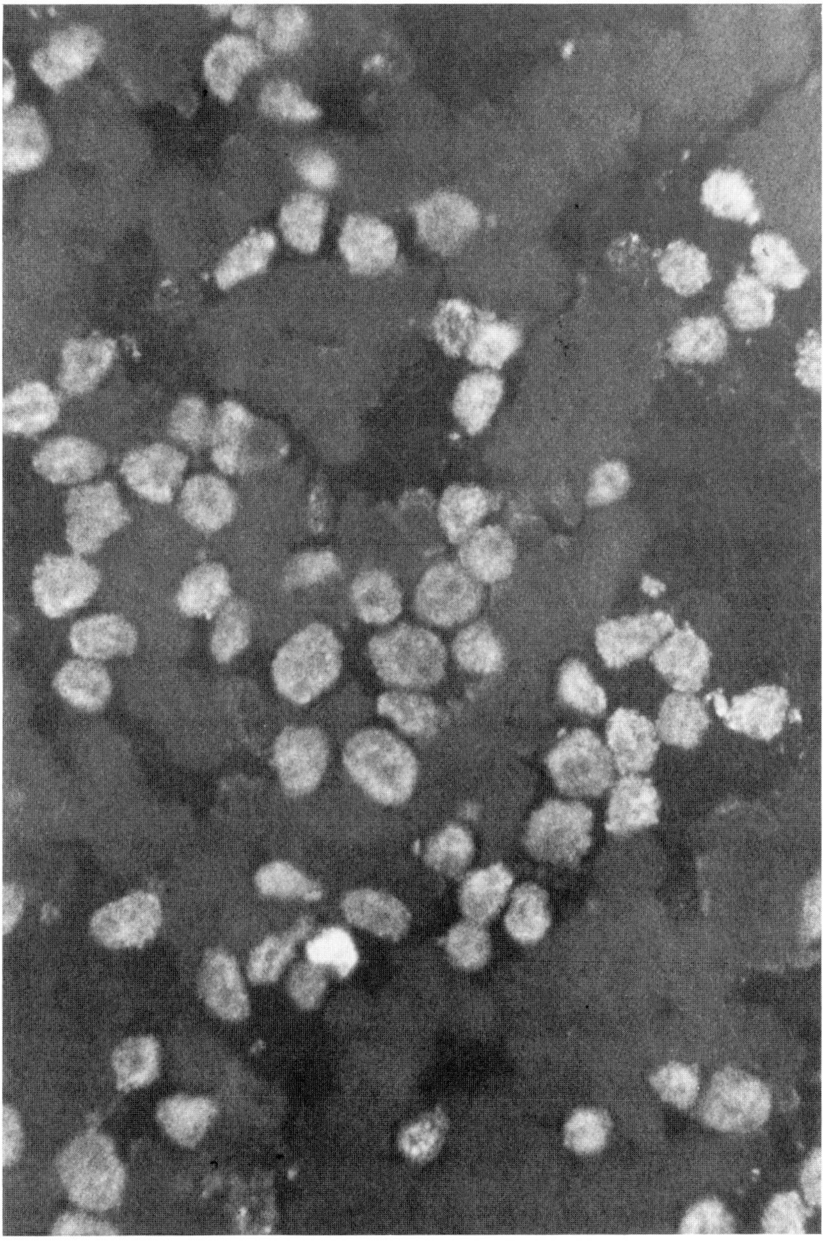

Figure 17c Acute lymphocytic leukemia (FAB-L1). TdT immunofluorescent stain showing nuclear positivity in more than 90% of the blasts. (×500)

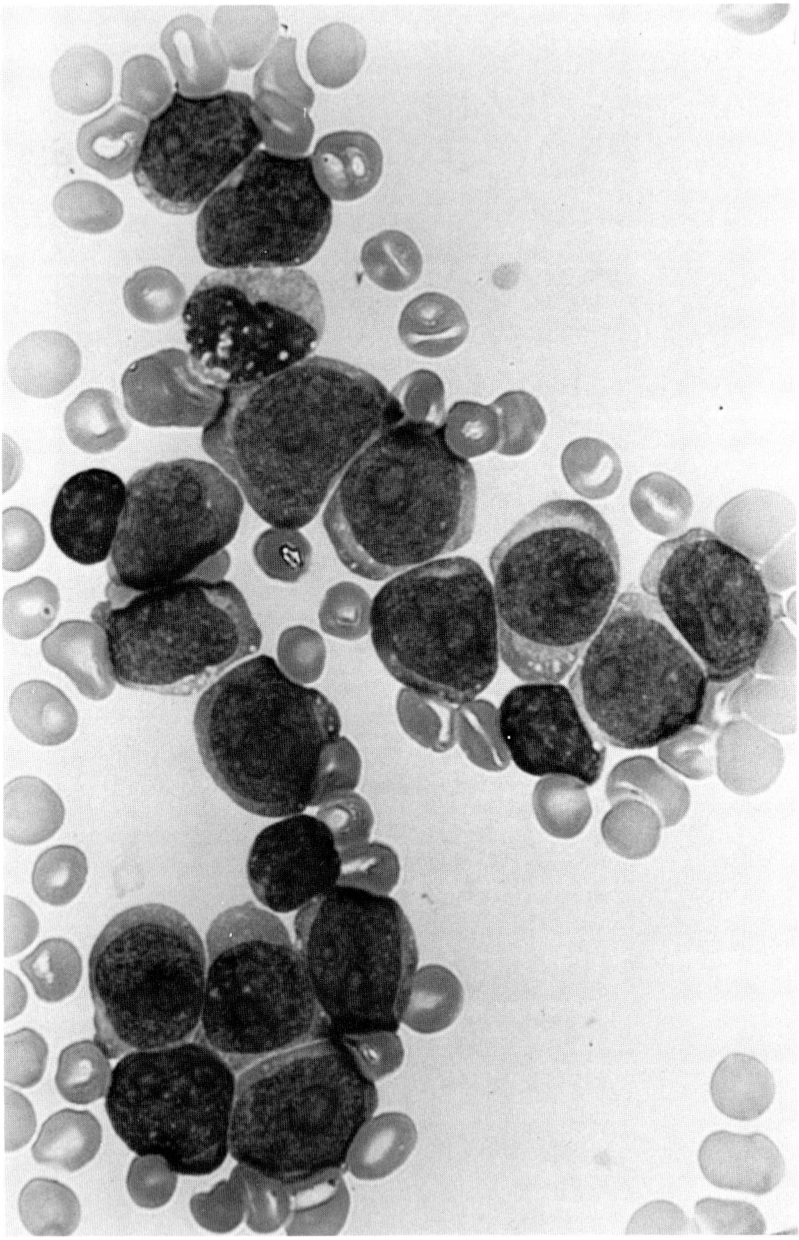

Figure 18 Acute lymphocytic leukemia (FAB-L2). Blasts have a low N/C ratio and prominent nucleoli. (W-G, X800)

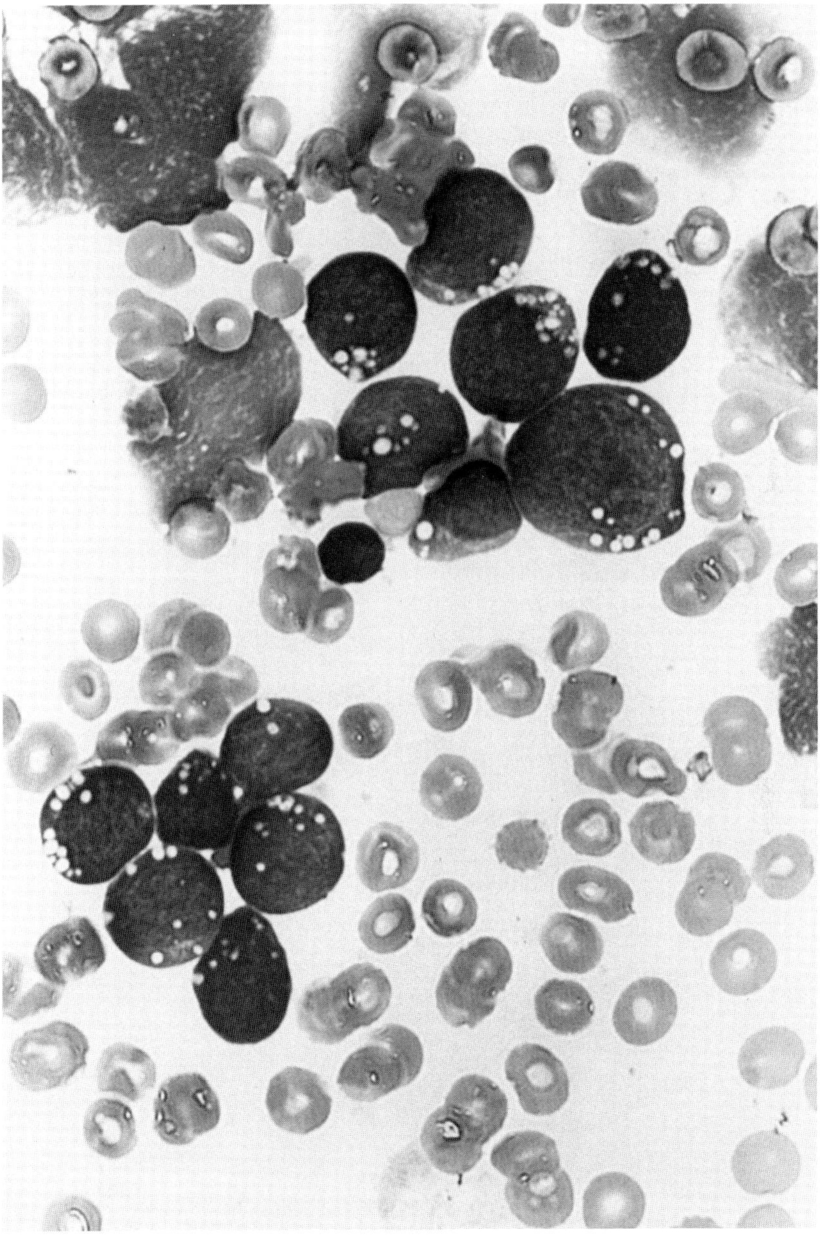

Figure 19 Acute lymphocytic leukemia (FAB-L3). Blasts are fairly uniform in size and have deep blue cytoplasm and vacuoles. (W-G, ×800)

cases, however, the observer is forced to differentiate between ALL and AUL on purely morphologic grounds, something that we find difficult to do reliably.

ALL: Hand-Mirror Variant

In this morphologic variant, the leukemic cells show a cytoplasmic tail or uropod, giving the cell a "hand-mirror" appearance (Figure 20) (Glassy, Sun and Okun, 1980; Gramatski et al., 1985; Schumacher, 1984; Schumacher et al., 1977, 1979; Sharp et al., 1979; Stass et al., 1978). Most cases are classified as FAB-L2, but we have also seen cases of FAB-L1, and L3 (Schumacher et al., 1978). An association between hand-mirror cell ALL and immune complexes related to baboon endogenous virus has been reported, but its significance is unclear (Stass, Phillips, Weislow, et al., 1980). It has been suggested that hand-mirror cell ALL in adults is a clinicopathologic syndrome characterized by a female predominance and an indolent clinical course for a year or more after diagnosis (Mazur et al., 1986).

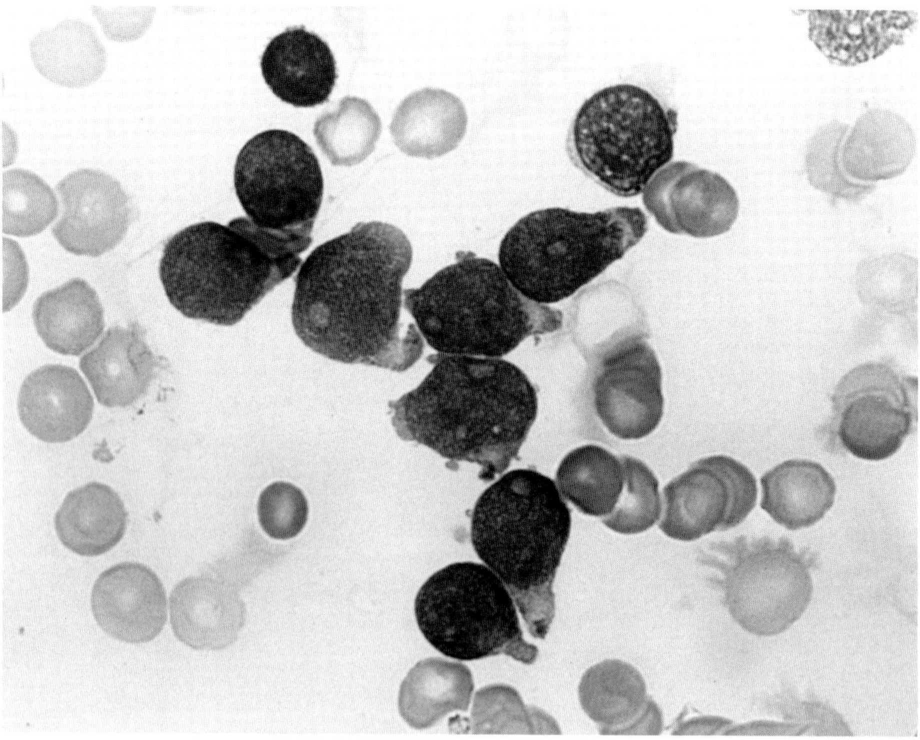

Figure 20 Acute lymphocytic leukemia, hand-mirror cell type. Nearly all the blasts have a projecting uropod. Classified as FAB-L2. (W-G, X800)

Hand-mirror cells have also been described in AML (Cerezo et al., 1984; Haider, Phillips, and Schumacher, 1982).

Prolymphocytic Leukemia

The distinguishing morphologic feature of this uncommon type of lymphocytic leukemia is the finding that most of the leukemic cells have a single large nucleolus surrounded by a rim of condensed chromatin (Figure 21). The chromatin pattern is described as intermediate between that of a mature lymphocyte and a lymphoblast (Kjeldsberg, Bearman, and Rappaport, 1980). The peripheral leukocyte count is usually greater than 100×10^9/L, splenomegaly is prominent, and lymphadenopathy is inconspicuous (Kraemer and Byrne, 1977). Galton, who first described the disorder (Galton et al., 1974), uses 55% circulating prolymphocytes as the defining criterion for prolymphocytic leukemia (Melo, Catovsky and Galton, 1986). B-cell phenotype is most common but T-cell phenotype is also reported (Bearman, Pangalis, and Rappaport, 1978; Chan et al., 1982; Polliack et al., 1984; Singh et al., 1978; Theil, Bavchinger, and Rodt, 1977; Woessner et al., 1978). Prolymphocytic leukemia is a unique disorder, and is felt to arise de novo; it seems to be distinct from the cases of CLL that show a "prolymphocytoid" transformation (Melo, Catovsky, and Galton, 1986). The onset of the disease may be sudden, similar to an acute leukemia, and the patients usually have a rapidly deteriorating course.

Acute Leukemia of Basophilic Lineage

In this rare type of acute leukemia, a fraction of the blasts contain variable numbers of myeloperoxidase-negative basophilic granules. The basophilic nature of the cells can be demonstrated by metachromatic staining with toluidine blue, or by electron microscopy. It may therefore be worthwhile to perform EM or a toluidine blue stain in any case where the leukemic blasts contain myeloperoxidase negative granules. Clinically, the patients may have associated urticarial or pigmented skin lesions (Wick, Li, and Pierre, 1982) and can also have a coagulopathy.

This leukemia is distinct from chronic myelogenous leukemia (CML) with expansion of the basophilic compartment, and the Philadelphia chromosome is not found in acute basophilic leukemia.

VI. BONE MARROW NECROSIS

Bone marrow necrosis (Figure 22) is occasionally seen in patients presenting with acute leukemia and usually manifests itself with bone pain, bone tenderness, and fever. Several studies in adults have shown that bone marrow necrosis is associated with a poor prognosis (Brown, 1972; Colvin et al., 1980; Kiraly and Wheby, 1976; Kundel et al., 1964; Nies et al., 1965). Bone marrow necrosis can also be seen in children with acute leukemia. In one series of five children with ALL and bone

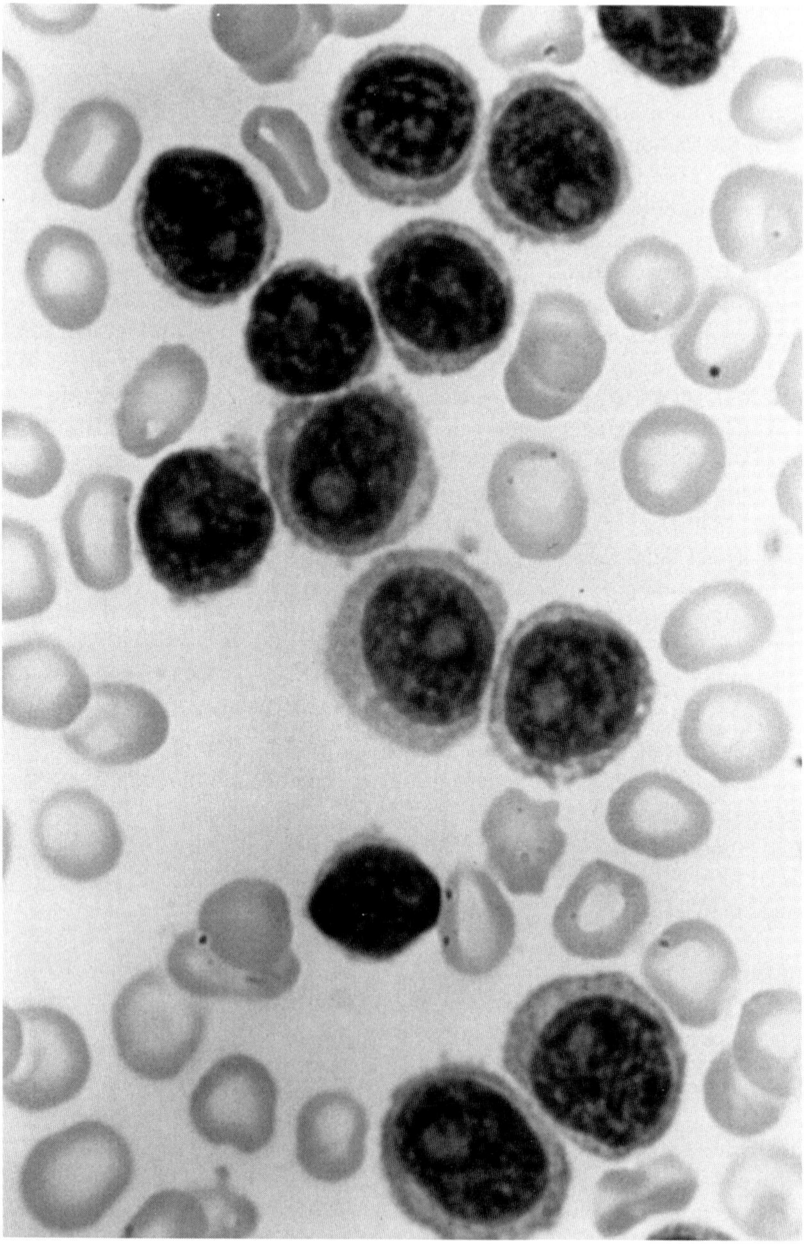

Figure 21 Prolymphocytic leukemia. All the cells show a prominent nucleolus surrounded by a rim of condensed chromatin. (W-G, ×1250)

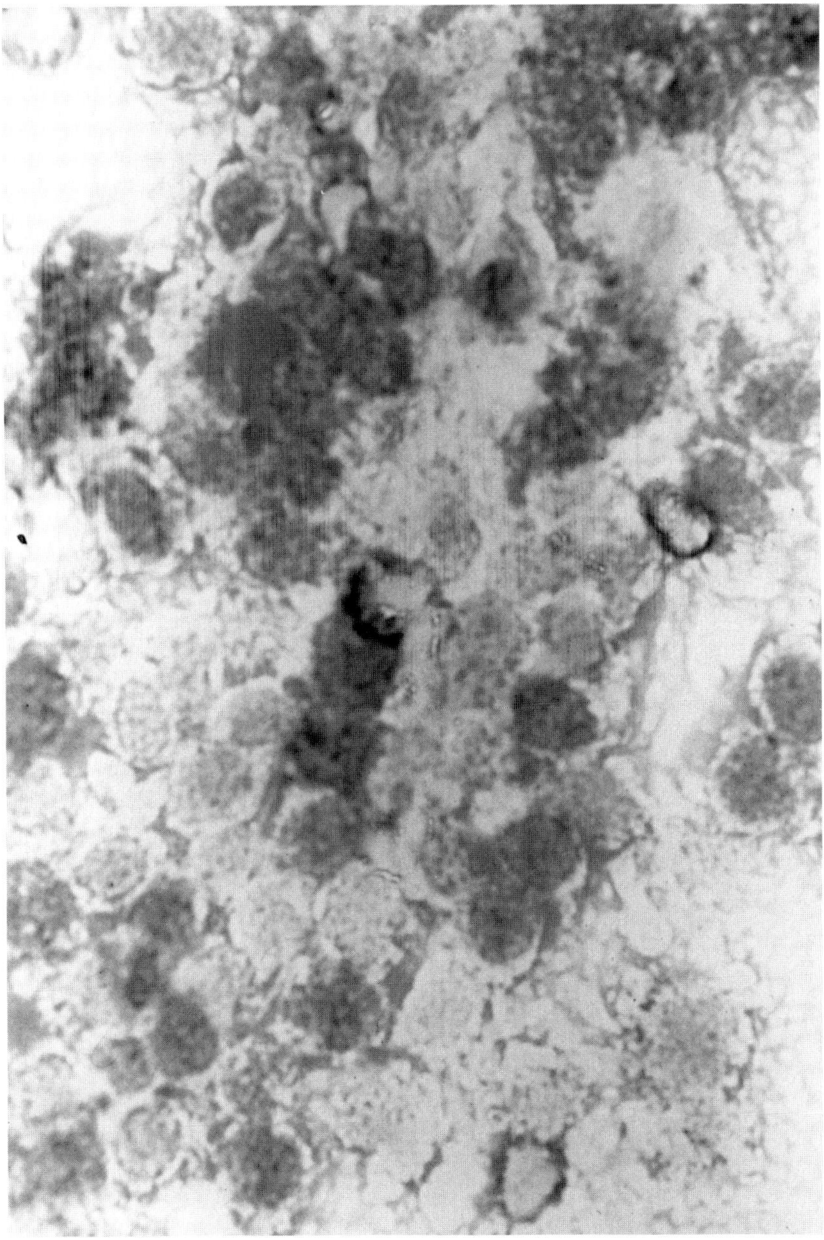

Figure 22 Bone marrow necrosis. No cellular detail can be discerned; only the outlines of the cells can be seen. (W-G, X500)

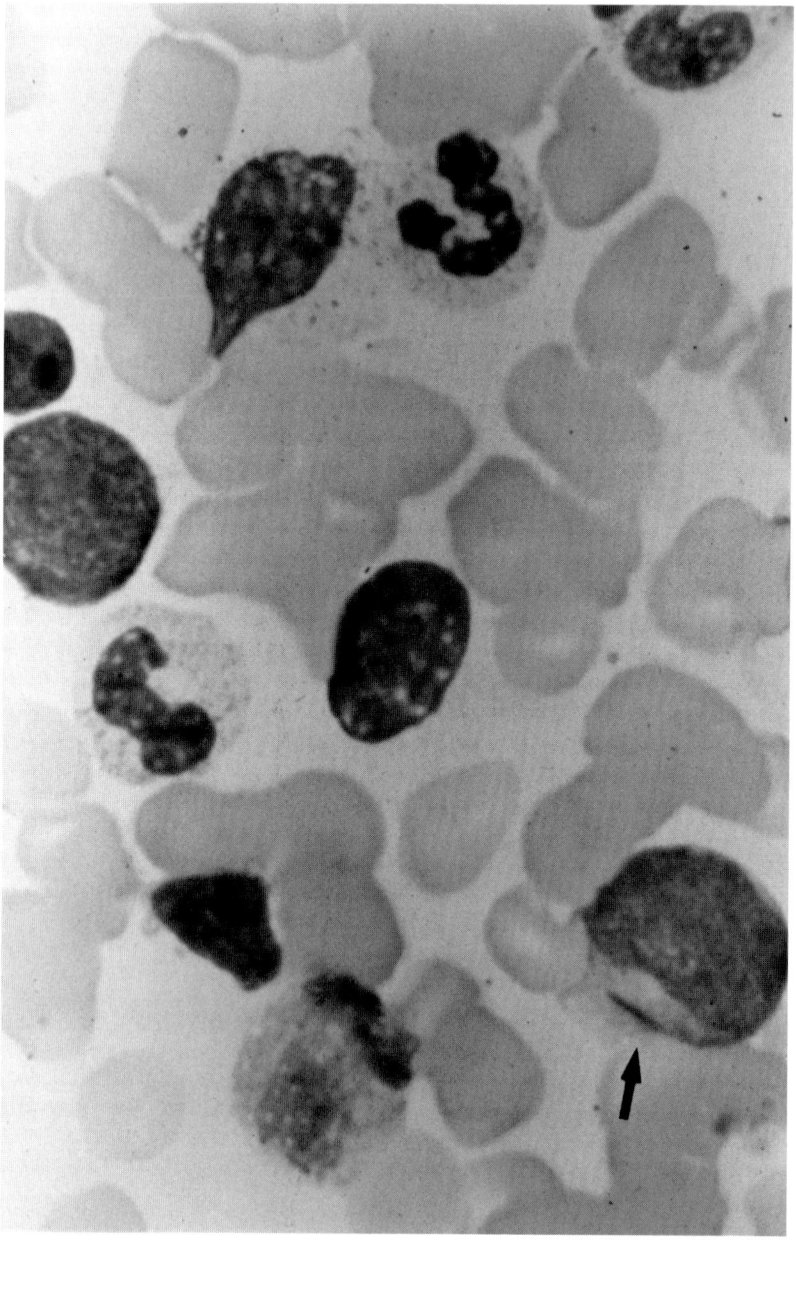

Figure 23 Blast with Auer rod. Post treatment bone marrow from an AML patient showing good maturation and only 1% blasts. Blast with an Auer rod (arrow) establishes that this patient has residual AML, however. (W-G, X1250)

marrow necrosis, all five achieved complete remission and did not seem to have a poorer prognosis than other children with ALL (Pui, Stass, and Green, 1985).

VII. REMISSION BONE MARROW

In a patient treated for acute leukemia, we consider complete remission to be present when peripheral blood counts approach the normal range; the bone marrow is normocellular and shows orderly maturation of granulocytic, erythroid and megakaryocytic elements; and no leukemic cells are identified irrespective of the blast count. In our institution, we require that the patient have a granulocyte count of 1.5×10^9/L, be able to sustain a hemoglobin of 11.0 g/dL, and have a platelet count of 100×10^9/L.

As mentioned, one of our criteria for remission is the absence of identifiable leukemic cells. The criteria for remission of less than 5% bone marrow blasts is arbitrary. This can be demonstrated by the leukemic cells in FAB-M3 and FAB-L3, which are quite distinctive and can be reliably identified even when present in small numbers. Similarly, when blasts containing Auer rods are identified, an unequivocal diagnosis of residual leukemia is usually possible even though the blast count may be 1% or less. This is demonstrated in a case of Auer rod positive FAB-M2 that had a remission marrow by all criteria including 1% blasts, but clearly demonstrated an Auer rods (Figure 23). The patient relapsed approximately 3 months after this bone marrow examination.

With other types of acute leukemia, it is frequently helpful to reexamine the original leukemic marrow concurrently with the possible remission marrow in order to key in on any additional morphologic clues the leukemic blasts may offer. Even though a definite diagnosis of residual leukemia may not be possible, this approach will maximize the diagnostic information obtained.

Pediatric patients, especially infants, who have never had leukemia, may have 5-10% lymphoblasts in their bone marrows; even some adults without leukemia have had up to 10% bone marrow blasts (Woessner et al., 1985). Increased TdT-positive lymphoblasts may be seen in idiopathic thrombocytopenic purpura (ITP) (Stass et al., 1980). In addition, a rebound lymphocytosis post therapy for ALL, usually beginning at 6 months and ending at 18 to 24 months, may be accompanied by a slight increase in the number of lymphoblasts. The key morphologic feature in all these instances is the predominance of mature lymphocytes in addition to the slight increase in blasts. Therefore, the finding of a few lymphoid blasts in pediatric patients with ALL should not be overinterpreted.

VIII. FUTURE DIRECTIONS

Morphologic and cytochemical evaluation of bone marrow smears remains the standard for the diagnosis and classification of acute leukemias. However, it is hoped that in the future, more biologically oriented classification systems will allow better understanding and improved management of these disorders. Careful application of current morphologic techniques will help make this transition a smooth and rational one.

REFERENCES

Abildgaard, C. F. (1980). Unique features of metastatic neuroblastoma in the bone marrow. *Am. J. Clin. Pathol.* 74:363-364.

Almanaseer, I. Y., Trujillo, Y. P., Taxy, J. B., and Okuno, T. (1984). Systemic rhabdomyosarcoma with diffuse bone marrow involvement. *Am. J. Clin. Pathol.* 82:349-353.

Bearman, R. M., Pangalis, G. A., and Rappaport, N. (1978). Prolymphocytic leukemia, clinical, histopathological and cytochemical observations. *Cancer* 42: 2360-2372.

Bendix-Hansen, K. (1986). Myeloperoxidase-deficient polymorphonuclear leukocytes. Longitudinal study during the preremission and the remission phase in acute myeloid leukaemia. Comparison to neutrophil alkaline phosphatase (NAP) activity. *Blut* 52:237-242.

Bennett, J. M., Catovsky, D., Daniel, M. T., Flandrin, G., Galton, D. A. G., Gralnick, H. R., and Sultan, C. (1976). Proposals for the classification of the acute leukemias (FAB co-operative group). *Brit. J. Haem.* 33:451-458.

Bennett, J. M., Catovsky, D., Daniel, M. T., Flandrin, G., Galton, D. A. G., Gralnick, H. R., and Sultan, C. (1980). A variant form of hypergranular promyelocytic leukaemia (M3). *Brit. J. Haem.* 44:169-170.

Bennett, J. M., Catovsky, D., Daniel, M. T., Flandrin, G., Galton, D. A. G., Gralnick, H. R., and Sultan, C. (FAB co-operative group) (1981b). The morphological classification of acute lymphoblastic leukemia: concordance among observors and clinical correlatives. *Brit. J. Haem.* 47:553-561.

Bennett, J. M., Catovsky, D., Daniel, M. T., Flandrin, G., Galton, D. A. G., Gralnick, H. R., and Sultan, C. (The FAB co-operative group). (1982). Proposals for the classification of the myelodysplastic syndromes. *Brit. J. Haem.* 51: 189-199.

Bennett, J. M., Catovsky, D., Daniel, M. T., Flandrin, G., Galton, D. A. G., Gralnick, H. R., and Sultan, C. (1985a). Criteria for the diagnosis of acute leukemia of megakaryocyte lineage (M7). *Ann. Int. Med.* 103:460-462.

Bennett, J. M., Catovsky, D., Daniel, M. T., Flandrin, G., Galton, D. A. G., Gralnick, H. R., and Sultan, C. (1985b). Proposed revised criteria for the classification of acute myeloid leukemia. *Ann. Int. Med.* 103:626-629.

Bitter, M. A., Le Beau, M. M., Larson, R. A., Rosner, M. C., Golomb, H. M., Rowley, J. D., and Vardiman, J. W. (1984). A morphologic and cytochemical study of acute myelomonocytic leukemia with abnormal marrow eosinophils associated with Inv(16) (p13q22). *Am. J. Clin. Path.* 81:733-741.

Bloomfield, C. D., and Brunning, R. D. (1985). The revised French-American-British classification of acute myeloid leukemia: Is new better? *Ann. Intern. Med.* 103:614.

Brown, C. H. III. (1972). Bone marrow necrosis: A study of seventy cases. *Johns Hopkins Med. J.* 131:189-203.

Catovsky, D., Greaves, M. F., Pain, C., Cherchi, M., Janossy, G., and Kay, H. E. M. (1978). Acid-phosphatase reaction in acute lymphoblastic leukaemia. *Lancet* I:749-751.

Cerezo, L., Head, D. R., Pullen, J., and Humphrey, B. (1984). The prevalence of hand-mirror cells in acute myeloblastic and lymphoblastic leukemia. *Am. J. Clin. Path.* 81:355-357.

Chan, W. E., Check, I. J., Haffner, L. T., Gordon, D., Whitsett, C., and Brynes, R. K. (1982). Prolymphocytic leukemia of helper cell phenotype: Report of a case and review of the literature. *Am. J. Clin. Path.* 77:643-647.

Colon-Otero, G., Li, C.-Y., Dewald, G. W., and White, W. L. (1984). Erythrophagocytic acute lymphocytic leukemia with B-cell markers and with a 20q− chromosome abnormality. *Mayo Clin. Proc.* 59:678-682.

Colvin, B. T., Revell, P. A., Ibbotson, R. M., and Turnbill, A. L. (1980). Necrosis of bone marrow and bone in malignant disease. *Clin. Oncol.* 6:265-272.

Dalton, W. T., Ahearn, M. J., Cork, A., Trujillo, J. M., Keating, M. J., McCredie, K. B., Freireich, E. J., and Stass, S. A. (1985). Nuclear blebs in eosinophils in the acute leukemia associated with inversion of chromosome 16[inv(16)(p13q22)]. *Blood* 66:234a.

Drexler, H. G., Messmore, H. L., Menon, M., and Minowoda, J. (1986). A case of TdT-positive B-cell acute lymphoblastic leukemia. *Am. J. Clin. Pathol.* 85:735-738.

Edelman, B. B., and Grossman, N. J. (1983). Microgranular acute promyelocytic leukemia—a case with multiple Auer rods demonstrable only after staining for chloroacetate esterase. *Am. J. Clin. Path.* 79:621-625.

Fearon, E. R., Burke, P. J., Schiffer, C. A., Zehnbauer, B. A., and Vogelstein, B. (1986). Differentiation of leukemia cells to polymorphonuclear leukocytes in patients with acute nonlymphocytic leukemia. *N. Engl. J. Med.* 315:15-24.

Galton, D. A. G., Goldman, I. M., Wiltshaw, E., Catovsky, D., Henry, K., and Goldenberg, G. J. (1974). Prolymphocytic leukemia. *Br. J. Haem.* 27:7-23.

Ganick, D. J., and Finlay, J. L. (1980). Acute lymphoblastic leukemia with Burkitt cell morphology and cytoplasmic immunoglobulin. *Blood* 56:311-314.

Glassy, E. F., Sun, N. C. J., and Okun, D. B. (1980). Hand-mirror cell leukemia. Report of nine cases and a review of the literature. *Am. J. Clin. Path.* 74:651-656.

Golomb, H. M., Rowley, J. D., Vardiman, J. W., Testa, J. R., and Butler, A. (1980). "Microgranular" acute promyelocytic leukemia: a distinct clinical, ultrastructural, and cytogenetic entity. *Blood* 55:253-259.

Gralnick, H. R., Galton, D. A. G., Catovsky, D., Sultan, C., and Bennett, J. M. (1977). N.I.H. conference: classification of acute leukemia. *Ann. Int. Med.* 87:740-753.

Gramatzki, M., Strong, D. M., Duval-Arnould, B., Morstyn, G., and Schumacher, H. R. (1985). Hand-mirror variant of acute lymphoblastic leukemia. Evidence for early T-cell lineage in two cases by evaluation with monoclonal antibodies. *Cancer* 55:77-83.

Grogan, T. M., Insalaco, S. J., Savage, R. A., and Vail, M. L. (1981). Acute lymphocytic leukemia with prominent azurophilic granulation and punctate acidic nonspecific esterase and phosphatase activity. *Am. J. Clin. Path.* 75:716-722.

Haider, Y. S., Phillips, T. M., and Schumacher, H. R. (1982). Acute myeloid leukemia with hand-mirror cells. *Arch. Pathol. Lab. Med.* 106:271-274.

Hayhoe, F. G. J., and Flemans, R. J. (1982). *Color Atlas of Hematologic Cytology*. John Wiley and Sons, New York, p. 69.

Hayhoe, F. G. J., and Quaglino, D. (1980). *Haematological Cytochemistry*. Churchill Livingston, New York, p. 167.

Head, D. R., Kennedy, P. S., and Goyette, R. E. (1979). Metastatic neuroblastoma in bone marrow aspirate smears. *Am. J. Clin. Pathol.* 72:1008-1011.

Heumann, D., Colombatti, M., and Mach, J.-P. (1983). Human large granular lymphocytes contain an esterase activity usually considered as specific for the myeloid series. *Eur. J. Immunol.* 13:254-258.

Ho, F. C. S., Chan, G. T. C., and Todd, D. (1983). Non-specificity of Sudan black B in the diagnosis of acute myeloid leukaemia. *Br. J. Haem.* 53:171-172.

Janckila, A. J., Li, C.-Y., Lam, K.-W., and Yam, L. T. (1978). The cytochemistry of tartrate-resistant acid phosphatase. Technical considerations. *Am. J. Clin. Path.* 70:45-55.

Kantarjian, H. M., Keating, M. J., Walters, R. S., Estey, E. H., McCredie, K. B., Smith, T. L., Dalton, W. T., Cork, A., Trujillo, J. M., and Freireich, E. J. (1986). Acute promyelocytic leukemia. M. D. Anderson Hospital experience. *Am. J. Med.* 80:789-797.

Kaplow, L. S. (1965). Simplified myeloperoxidase stain using benzidine dihydrochloride. *Blood* 26:215-219.

Kass, L. (1977). Esterase reactions in acute myelomonocytic leukemia. *Am. J. Clin. Path.* 67:485-488.

Keating, M. J., Smith, T. L., Gehan, E. A., McCredie, K. B., Bodey, G. P., Spitzer, G., Hersh, E., Gutterman, J., and Freireich, E. J. (1980). Factors related to length of complete remission in adult acute leukemia. *Cancer* 45:2017-2029.

Keating, M. J., Smith, T. L., Gehan, E. A., McCredie, K. B., Bodey, G. P., and Freireich, E. J. (1982). A prognostic factor analysis for use in development of predictive models for response in adult acute leukemia. *Cancer* 50:457-465.

Keifer, J., Abromowitch, M., and Stass, S. (1985). Chloroacetate esterase positivity in acute lymphoblastic leukemia. *Am. J. Clin. Path.* 83:647-650.

Kiraly, J. F. III, Wheby, M. S. (1976). Bone marrow necrosis. *Am. J. Med.* 60: 361-368.

Kjeldsberg, C. R., Bearman, R. M., Rappaport, H. (1980). Prolymphocytic leukemia: an ultrastructural study. *Am. J. Clin. Path.* 73:150-159.

Kraemer, H. J., and Byrne, G. E. (1977). *Prolymphocytic leukemia*. American Society of Clinical Pathologists Check Sample, Hematology No. H-89, pp. 1-5.

Kundel, D. W., Brecher, G., Bodey, G. P., and Brittin, G. M. (1964). Reticulin fibrosis necrosis in children: Three instances. *Blood* 23:526-544.

Lam, K.-W., Li, C. Y., and Yam, L. T. (1985). Simultaneous demonstration of nonspecific esterase and chloroacetate esterase in human blood cells. *Stain Technology* 60:169-172.

Lanham, G. R., Kalwinsky, D. K., Williams, D. L., Melvin, S. L., Harber, J. R., Motroni, T. A., and Stass, S. A. (1985). Periodic acid-Schiff stain in childhood acute lymphoblastic leukemia: Lack of independent prognostic value. *Am. J. Clin. Path.* 83:496-497.

Larson, R. A., Kondo, K., Vardiman, J. W., Butler, A. E., Golomb, H. M. Rowley, J. D. (1984). Evidence for a 15;17 translocation in every patient with acute promyelocytic leukemia. *Am. J. Med.* 76:827-841.

Larson, R. A., Williams, S. F., Le Beau, M. M., Bitter, M. A., Vardiman, J. W., and Rowley, J. D. (1986). Acute myelomonocytic leukemia with abnormal eosinophils and inv(16) or t(16;16) has a favorable prognosis. *Blood* 68:1242-1249.

Le Beau, M. M., Larson, R. A., Bitter, M. A., Vardiman, J. W., Golomb, H. M., and Rowley, J. D. (1983). Association of an inversion of chromosome 16 with abnormal marrow eosinophils in acute myelomonocytic leukemia. A unique cytogenetic-clinicopathological association. *N. Eng. J. Med.* 309:630-636.

Le Beau, M. M., Bitter, M. A., and Rowley, J. D. (1984). Letter to Editor. *N. Eng. J. Med.* 310:

Li, C. Y., Lam, K. W., and Yam, L. T. (1973). Esterases in human leukocytes. *J. Histochem. Cytochem.* 21:1-12.

Li, C.-Y., Phyliky, R. L., and Yam, L. T. (1986). Acute myelomonocytic leukemia: An unusual variant with both granulocytic and monocytic esterase in the leukemic cells. *Mayo Clin. Proc.* 61:104-109.

Liso, V., troccoli, G., Specchia, G., and Magno, M. (1977). Cytochemical "normal" and "abnormal" eosinophils in acute leukemias. *Am. J. Hematol.* 2: 122-131.

Mangon, K. F., Rauch, A. E., Bishop, M., Spiers, A. S. D., Larch, C., Scharfman, W. B. (1985). Acute lymphoblastic leukemia of Burkitt's type (L-3 ALL) lacking surface immunoglobulin and the 8;14 translocation. *Am. J. Clin. Pathol.* 93:121-126.

Mazur, E. M., Wittels, E. G., Schiffman, F. J., South, K., and Horner, R. J. (1986). Hand mirror cell lymphoid leukemia in adult. A distinct clinicopathologic syndrome. Case report and literature review. *Cancer* 57:92-99.

McKenna, R. W., Parkin, J., Bloomfield, C. D., Sundberg, R. D., and Brunning, R. D. (1982). Acute promyelocytic leukaemia: a study of 39 cases with identification of a hyperbasophilic microgranular variant. *Br. J. Haem.* 50:201-214.

Melo, J. V., Catovsky, D., and Galton, D. A. G. (1986). The relationship between chronic lymphocytic leukaemia and prolymphocytic leukaemia. *Br. J. Haem.* 63:377-387.

Nies, B. A., Kundel, D. W., Thomas, L. B., and Freireich, E. J. (1965). Leukopenia, bone pain, and bone marrow necrosis in patients with acute leukemia: A clinicopathologic complex. *Ann. Intern. Med.* 62:698-705.

Pollack, E. R., Miller, H. J., and Vye, M. V. (1981). Medulla blastoma presenting as leukemia. *Am. J. Clin. Pathol.* 76:98-103.

Polliack, A., Leizerowitz, R., Berrebi, A., Gamliel, H., Galili, N., Gurfel, D., and Catovsky, D. (1984). Prolymphocytic leukaemia: surface morphology in 21 cases as seen by scanning electron microscopy and comparison with B-cell CLL and CLL in "prolymphocytoid" transformation. *Br. J. Haem.* 57:577-584.

Potter, V. P., Sorell, M., Baglivo, J. A., Sather, H., and Miller, D. R. (1984). Prognostic significance of vacuoles in L1 lymphoblasts in childhood acute lymphoblastic leukaemia: a report from Children's Cancer Study Group. *Br. J. Haematol.* 56:215-222.

Pui, C., Dahl, G., Melvin, S., Williams, D., Peiper, S., Mirro, J., Murphy, S., and Stass, S. (1984). Acute leukemia with mixed lymphoid and myeloid phenotype. *Br. J. Haematol.* 56:121-

Pui, C.-H., Rivera, G., Mirro, J., Stass, S., Peiper, S., and Morphy, S. B. (1985). Acute megakaryoblastic leukemia: Blast cell aggregates simulating metastatic tumor. *Arch. Pathol. Lab. Med.* 109:1033.

Pui, C.-H., Stass, S., and Green, A. (1985). Bone marrow necrosis in children with malignant disease. *Cancer* 56:1522-1525.

Pui, C.-H., Mirro, J., Woodruff, L., Motroni, T., and Stass, S. (1986). Phagocytic activity and expression of myeloid-associated cell surface antigens by blast cells in acute lymphoblastic leukemia. *Med. Ped. Onc.* 14:12-16.

Raman, S. B. K., and VanSlyck, E. J. (1983). Nature of intracytoplasmic crystalline inclusions in myeloma cells (morphologic, cytochemical, ultrastructural, and immunofluorescent studies). *Am. J. Clin. Path.* 80:224-228.

Savage, R. A., Valenzuela, R., and Hoffman, G. C. (1981). Acid phosphatase staining pattern as an indicator of T-cell acute leukemia. *Am. J. Clin. Path.* 76:760-764.

Savage, R. A., and Hoffman, G. C. (1983). Sudan black positivity in non-myeloid leukaemia. *Br. J. Haem.* 54:494-495.

Schumacher, H. R. (1984). Hand-mirror cells: structure reflects function. *Am. J. Clin. Path.* 82:131-132.

Schumacher, H. R., Perlin, E., Miller, W. M., and Stass, S. A. (1977). Hand-mirror-cell leukaemia. *Lancet* I:655-656.

Schumacher, H. R., Rainey, T., Davidson, L., Simon, D., Strong, M., Creegan, W. J., Holloway, M. L., and Stass, S. A. (1978). American Burkitt lymphoma–hand-mirror variant. A detailed cytological, ultrastructural and immunologic markers investigation. *Am. J. Clin. Pathol.* 70:937-944.

Schumacher, H. R., Champion, J. E., Thomas, W. J., Pitts, L. L., and Stass, S. (1979). Acute lymphoblastic leukemia–hand mirror variant. An analysis of a large group of patients. *Am. J. Clin. Path.* 7:11-17.

Schumacher, H. R., and Stass, S. A. (1982). *Cytochemical, Biochemical and Immunological Markers in Acute Leukemias: Approach to Diagnosis.* Chicago: American Society of Clinical Pathologists.

Scott, C. S., Cahill, A., Bynoe, A. G., Ainley, M. J., Hough, D., and Roberts, B. E. (1983). Esterase cytochemistry in primary myelodysplastic syndromes and megaloblastic anaemias: demonstration of abnormal staining patterns associated with dysmelopoiesis. *Br. J. Haematol.* 55:411-418.

Sharp, J. W., Stass, S. A., Creegan, W. J., Pitts, L. L., and Schumacher, H. R. (1979). Acute lymphoblastic leukemia, hand-mirror variant. A detailed ultrastructural study. *Am. J. Clin. Path.* 72:551-558.

Shaw, M. T., Dwyer, J. M., Allaudeen, H. S., and Weitzman, H. A. (1978). Terminal deoxyribonucleotidyl transferase activity in B-cell acute lymphocytic leukemia. *Blood* 51:181-187.

Singh, A. K., Vaughan-Smith, S., Sawyer, B. et al. (1978). Cell studies in prolymphocytic leukaemia. *Br. J. Haem.* 40:587-596.

Skoog, D. P. (1976). Acute lymphocytic leukemia with prominent azurophilic granules. American Society of Clinical Pathologists Check Sample, Hematology No. H-82.

Stanley, M., McKenna, R. W., Ellinger, G., and Brunning, R. D. (1985). Classification of 358 cases of acute myeloid leukemia by FAB criteria: analysis of clinical and morphologic features. In *Chronic and Acute Leukemias in Adults*, C. D. Bloomfield (Ed.). Martinus Nijhoff, Publishers, Boston, 147-174.

Stass, S. A., Perlin, E., Jaffe, E. S., Simon, D. R., Creegan, W. J., Robinson, J. J., Holloway, M. L., and Schumacher, H. R. (1978). Acute lymphoblastic leukemia–hand mirror cell variant: A detailed cytological and ultrastructural study with an analysis of the immunologic surface markers. *Am. J. Hematol.* 4:67-77.

Stass, S. A., Miller, W., Schumacher, H. R., Keneklis, T. P., and Bollum, F. J. (1980). Terminal-deoxynucleotidyl-transferase in idiopathic thrombocytopenic purpura. *Arch. Pathol. Lab. Med.* 104:493.

Stass, S. A., Phillips, T. M., Weislow, O. S., Perlin, E., and Schumacher, H. R. (1980). Antigen-antibody complexes related to the baboon endogenous virus in patients with acute lymphoblastic leukemia–hand mirror variant. *Blood* 56:661-

Stass, S. A., Lanham, G. R., Butler, D. Williams, D. L., Peiper, S. C., Kalwinsky, D. K., and Dahl, G. V. (1984). Auer rods in mature granulocytes: A unique morphologic feature of acute myelogenous leukemia with maturation. *Am. J. Clin. Pathol.* 81:662-665.

Stass, S. A., Pui, C.-H., Melvin, S., Rovigatti, U., Williams, D., Motroni, T., Kalwinsky, D., and Dahl, G. V. (1984). Sudan black B positive acute lymphoblastic leukaemia. *Br. J. Haem.* 57:413-421.

Staven, P., Hjort, P. F., Vogt, E., and vander Hagen, C. B. (1969). Ring-shaped nuclei of granulocytes in a patient with acute erythroleukemia. *Scand. J. Haem.* 6:31-32.

Stein, P., Peiper, S., Butler, D., Melvin, S., Williams, D., and Stass, S. A. (1983). Granular acute lymphoblastic leukemia. *Am. J. Clin. Path.* 79:426.

Tavassoli, M., Shaklai, M., and Crosby, W. H. (1979). Cytochemical diagnosis of acute myelomonocytic leukemia. *Am. J. Clin. Path.* 72:59-62.

Tavassoli, M. (1984). Combined esterases in acute myelomonocytic leukaemia. *Br. J. Haem.* 57:178.

Theil, E., Bauchinger, M., and Rodt, H. (1977). Evidence for monoclonal proliferation in prolymphocytic leukemia of T-cell origin. A cytogenetic and quantitative immunoautoradiographic analysis. *Blut* 35:427-436.

Tomonaga, M., Yoshida, Y., Tagawa, M., Jinnai, I., Kuriyama, K., Amenomori, T., Yoshioka, A., Matsuo, T., Nonaka, H., and Ichimaru, M. (1985). Cytochemistry of acute promyelocytic leukemia (M3): Leukemic promyelocytes exhibit heterogeneous patterns in cellular differentiation. *Blood* 66:350-357.

Tricot, G., Broeckaert-Van Orshoven, A., Van Hoof, A., and Vernilglen, R. R. (1982). Sudan black B positivity in acute lymphoblastic leukaemia. *Br. J. Haem.* 51:615-621.

Trujillo, J. M., Cork, A., Ahearn, M. J., Youness, E. L., and McCredie, K. B. (1979). Hematologic and cytologic characterization of 8/21 translocation acute granulocytic leukemia. *Blood* 53:695-706.

Wheeler, M. S., Wilson, E. C., and Stass, S. A. (1981). Erythroleukophagocytosis cells—a nonspecific finding. *Am. J. Clin. Pathol.* 75:266-267.

Wick, M. R., Li, L.-Y., and Pierre, R. V. (1982). Acute nonlymphocytic leukemia with basophilic differentiation. *Blood* 60:38-45.

Woessner, S., LaFuente, R., Sans-Sabrafen, I. (1978). Prolymphocytic leukaemia of T-cell type: immunological, enzymatic and ultrastructural morphometric characteristics. *Br. J. Haem.* 39:9-15.

Woessner, S., Sans-Sabrafen, J., Laufuente, R., Florensa, L. (1985). Asymptomatic bone marrow infiltration by blast cells. *N. Eng. J. Med.* 312:1129.

Yam, L. T., Li, C. Y., and Crosby, W. H. (1971). Cytochemical identification of monocytes and granulocytes. *Am. J. Clin. Path.* 55:283-290.

Yanagihara, E., Naeim, F., Gale, R. P., Austin, G., and Waisman, J. (1980). *Am. J. Clin. Path.* 74:345-349.

Youness, E., Barlogie, B., Ahearn, J., and Trujillo, J. M. (1980). Tumor cell phagocytosis: Its occurrence in a patient with medulloblastoma. *Arch. Path. Lab. Med.* 104:651-653.

3

Electron Microscopy as an Aid to the Diagnosis and Characterization of Acute Leukemia

MICHAEL J. AHEARN *The University of Texas System Cancer Center, M. D. Anderson Hospital and Tumor Institute, Houston, Texas*

I. INTRODUCTION

The application of electron microscopy to the diagnosis of hematopoietic disorders has proven to be a useful tool in the classification of those leukemias whose light microscopic morphology and cytochemistries are negative or equivocal (Breton-Gorius et al., 1973; Catovsky, 1977; Glick et al., 1980; Jansson et al., 1980; and Schmalzl et al., 1973). The modification of processing techniques has reduced the specimen preparation time for ultrastructural analysis from several days to a few hours and increased the feasibility of utilizing this technology in a routine diagnostic context (Bencosme and Tsutsumi, 1970; Carr and Toner, 1977; Estes and Apicella, 1969; Fujita et al., 1977; Hayat and Giaquinta, 1970; and Rowden and Lewis, 1974).

Several classical treatises have documented the major cellular ultrastructural alterations observed in hematopoietic malignancies (Bessis, 1973b; Cawley and Hayhoe, 1973). Beginning in 1951, Bessis and coworkers described a number of ultrastructural pathological features which appear to be peculiar to the leukemic cells (e.g., nuclear blebs, pseudoviral inclusion bodies, extensive microfibrils, and splinter-form granules) (Bessis, 1951; Bessis and Breton-Gorius, 1969). In many instances, these ultrastructural observations reaffirmed the disordered and asynchronous pattern of maturation called "cellular anarchy" that was observed at the light microscopic level.

Recently, the application of both cytochemical and immunological staining techniques to the ultrastructural study of hematopoietic tissue has expended significantly the capacity of the electron microscopist to identify poorly differentiated leukemic cells. Numerous studies have demonstrated that myeloperoxidase activity, not discernable by light microscopic resolution, may be visualized ultrastructurally (Marie et al., 1979; O'Brien, Catovsky, and Costello, 1980; Palakavongs et al., 1977; Youness et al., 1980). In addition, the platelet peroxidase (PPO) reaction has been used as a definitive marker for megakaryocytic lineage. Application of ultrastructural techniques for other enzyme delineation, such as tartrate-resistant acid phosphatase in hairy cell leukemia and nonspecific esterase in monocytic leukemia, are often helpful adjuvants in diagnostic hematology.

In a similar manner, the ability of immunoelectron microscopy to detect membrane and cytoplasmic antigens using monoclonal antibodies has provided a greater sensitivity than that possible by standard light microscopic immunofluorescence (Marie et al., 1982). This has been particularly true in evaluating the subtle details of reactivity in closely related stages of cell maturation (Polli, Zola, and Catovsky, 1984). Additionally, the combination of standard electron microscopic cytochemistry and immunoelectron microscopic techniques offer the advantage of simultaneously demonstrating the presence of peroxidase-labeled cytoplasmic enzymes in cells marked for specific membrane antigens by colloidal gold particles. The application of these new methodologies in diagnostic hematology has resulted in an even further reduction of those cases remaining in the undifferentiated category of leukemia following electron microscopic analysis.

In this chapter we present the salient ultrastructural features of the major subtypes of human acute leukemia, using the French, American and British (FAB) classification scheme; also we discuss the ultrastructural features of some less common acute leukemia subtypes (Bennett et al., 1976).

II. ACUTE NONLYMPHOCYTIC LEUKEMIA (ANLL)

A. Acute Myelogenous Leukemia-M1

Ultrastructurally, the leukemia myeloblasts in cases of AML-M1 are usually of medium size (12-15 μm) and, due to the absence of maturation, do not exhibit the pronounced nucleo-cytoplasmic asynchrony that is characteristic of other AML subtypes (Figure 1). The round to oval nucleus is usually large and centrally located with a diffuse reticular, fine-grained euchromatic pattern. The one to two nucleoli present are markedly hypertrophied and of variable size and morphology (Glick, 1976; Glick et al., 1980; Smetna, Gyorkey, and Busch, 1969). In most cases, nuclear bodies, believed to be rudimentary nucleoli, appear as small spheres of circular fibrils in close proximity to the nucleoli. Although not diagnostic for neoplastic cells, the latter structures do appear in higher frequency in leukemic myeloblasts (Krishan, Uzman, and Hedley-Whyte, 1967).

Occasionally, blebs or pockets occur on the nuclear surface (Figure 2). These cellular alterations, which in our experience are associated with cytogenetic abnormalities, are formed by projections of the nuclear membrane in a manner that is reminiscent of pinocytosis by the plasma membrane. Variable cytoplasmic material is included within these blebs, but it is isolated from the rest of the nucleus

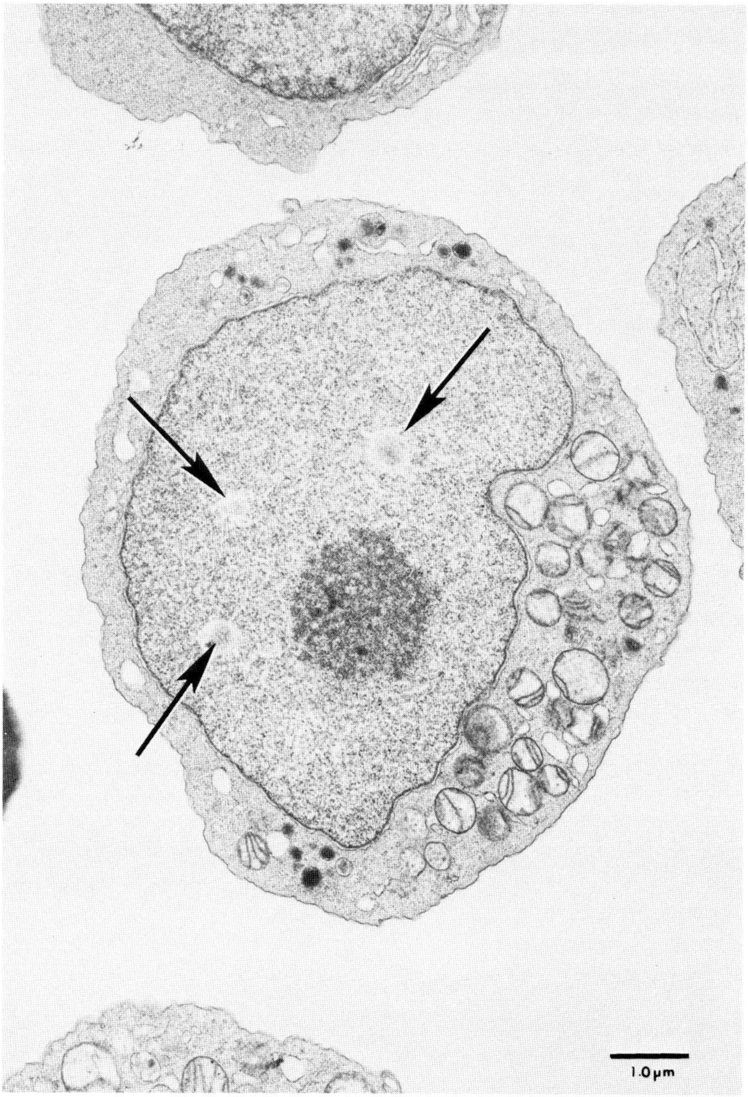

Figure 1 This myeloblast from the bone marrow of a patient with acute myelogenous leukemia (AML-M1) demonstrates a fine grained euchromatic nucleus with a distinct nucleolus. Nuclear bodies (arrows) composed of circular fibrils enclosing a number of central dense particles are noted. The cytoplasm exhibits peroxidase positive primary granules after incubation in Graham and Karnovsky's medium.

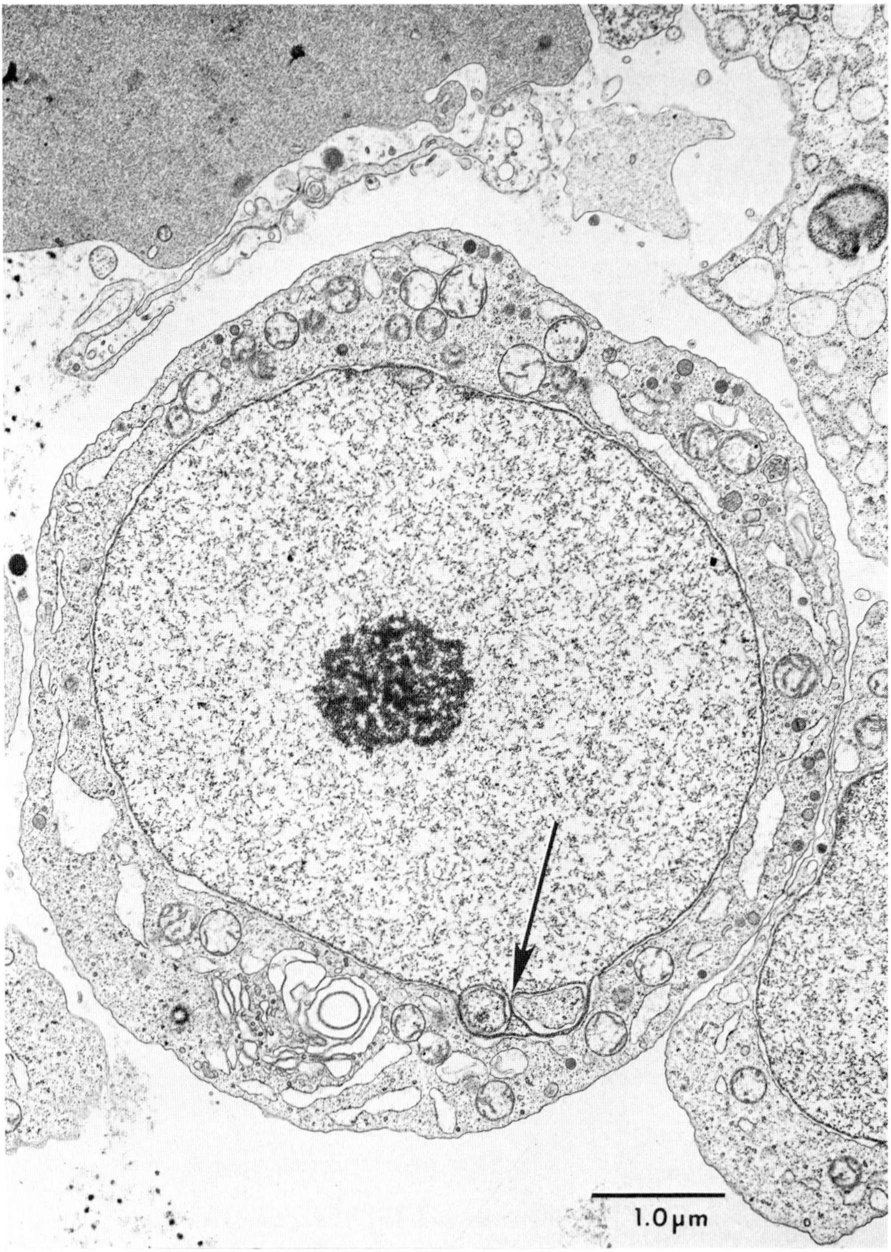

Figure 2 Two adjacent nuclear blebs are seen in this myeloblast from a patient with AML-M1. These structures may enclose a variety of cytoplasmic constituents.

by the presence of the double-layered nuclear membrane (McDuffie, 1967). As will be discussed later in the chapter, the association of nuclear blebs with cytogenetic abnormalities has also been observed in other subtypes including M2 (Ahearn et al., 1974) and M4b (Dalton et al., 1985). The cytoplasm of these leukemic blasts contain limited organelles. Polyribosomes are diffusely distributed in the cytoplasm. Profiles of endoplasmic reticulum are sparse and primitive in development. Mitochondria appear rounded and are uniformly dispersed. Occasionally, these structures may be damaged; however, with present tonicity-controlled fixation, this does not appear as a prominent feature (Hayat, 1986). The Golgi apparatus is usually poorly developed and does not exhibit dilated vesicles.

The primary granules are infrequent and therefore not observed in every cell section. Because of their small number and size they are often not identifiable by light microscopy and can only be observed at the ultrastructural level. Electron microscopic cytochemistry utilizing diaminobenzidine to stain myeloperoxidase is useful in delineating the primary granules in these cases (Schmalzl et al., 1973). Prior to its deposition in primary granules, myeloperoxidase formation can be visualized first in the perinuclear space, then later in the endoplasmic reticulum, and finally (Figure 3) on the concave surface of the Golgi, where it is collected in the azurophilic granules (Bainton, Ullyot, and Farquhar, 1971).

B. Acute Myelogenous Leukemia-M2

In the FAB AML-M2 subtype (Figure 4) the asynchrony in differentiation of nucleus and cytoplasm becomes more apparent as cellular maturation increases; although some M1 subtype blasts are observed. Cells classified as blasts on the basis of nuclear morphology will frequently demonstrate cytoplasmic structures more typically observed in progranulocytes. In striking contrast to their normal counterparts, both blasts and progranulocytes in this subtype demonstrate marked heterogeneity in the size and composition of these granules. The common expression of myeloperoxidase, nevertheless, indicates that they do correspond to primary granules (Bainton, Ullyot, and Farquhar, 1971), and their abnormal aggregation most likely contributes to the large pathological granules characteristically seen in these cases. The crystalloid cores in some of the granules are noted to break through the membrane, giving rise to even more bizarre shapes (Figure 5). Autophagic vacuoles, which are seldon found in nonmalignant myeloblasts, are reported to fuse with these azurophilic granules and contribute to the subsequent formation of Auer rods, parallel tubular structures which demonstrate a variable ultrastructural periodicity from 60-120 Å. The similarity of cytochemical staining support the concept that Auer rods are derived from primary granules (Figure 6) (Hayhoe and Cawley, 1972; White, 1967). Additionally, it has been noted that genesis of Auer rods is more frequent in those blast cells with the abundant cytoplasm and granules characteristically seen in AML-M2 (Freeman, 1966).

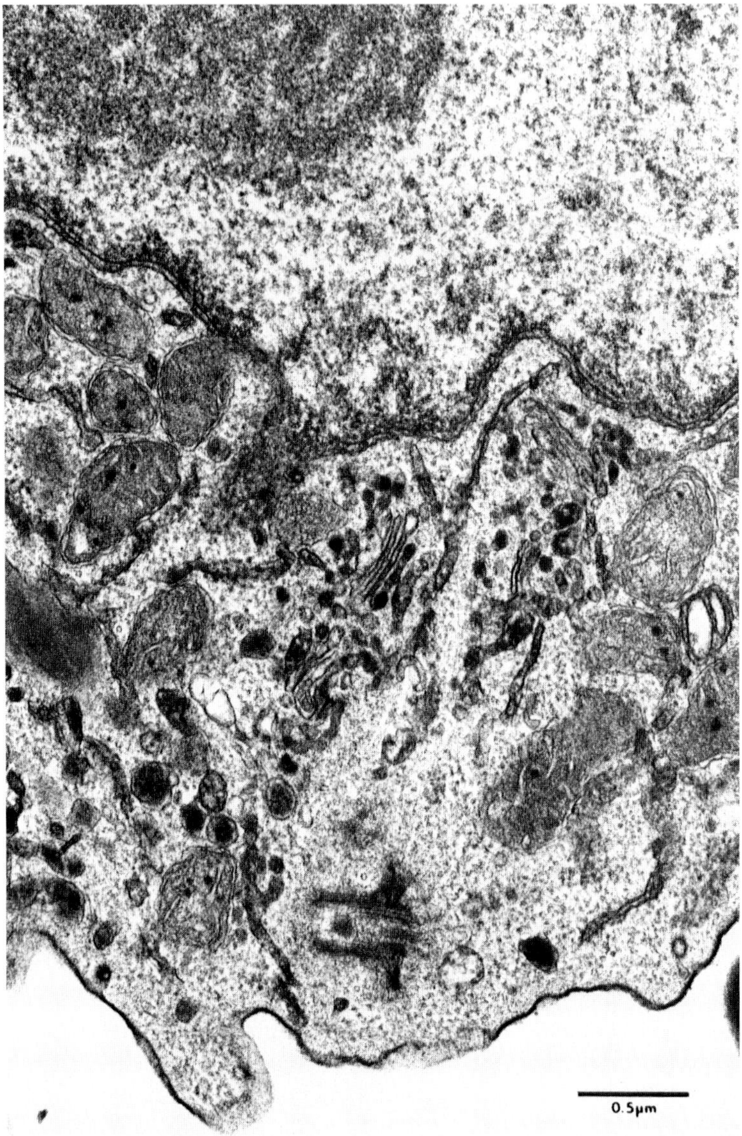

Figure 3 Myeloperoxidase localization is noted in this early myeloblast from the bone marrow of a patient with AML. The dense reaction product demonstrates peroxidase activity in the endoplasmic reticulum, the Golgi apparatus and in newly formed primary granules.

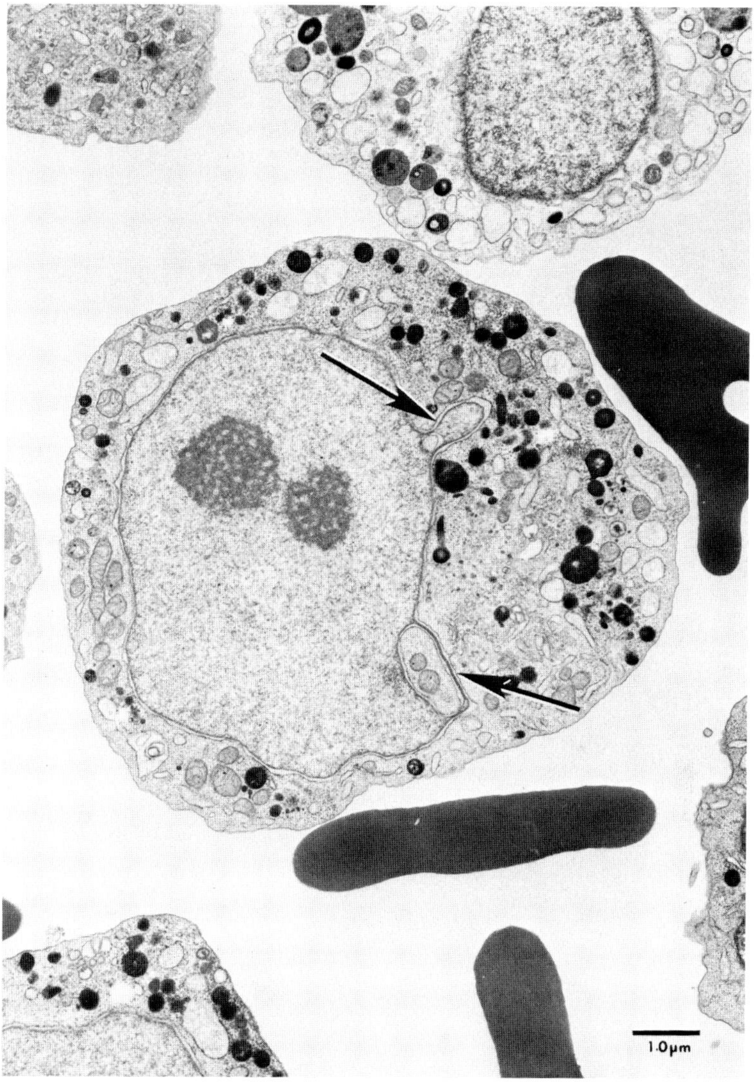

Figure 4 The primitive euchromatic nucleus of this myeloblast from the bone marrow of a patient with AML-M2 contrasts sharply with its more differentiated cytoplasm. Distinct nucleoli are noted. Nuclear blebs (arrows) are present. The dense-staining peroxidase-positive primary granules exhibit considerable morphological variation.

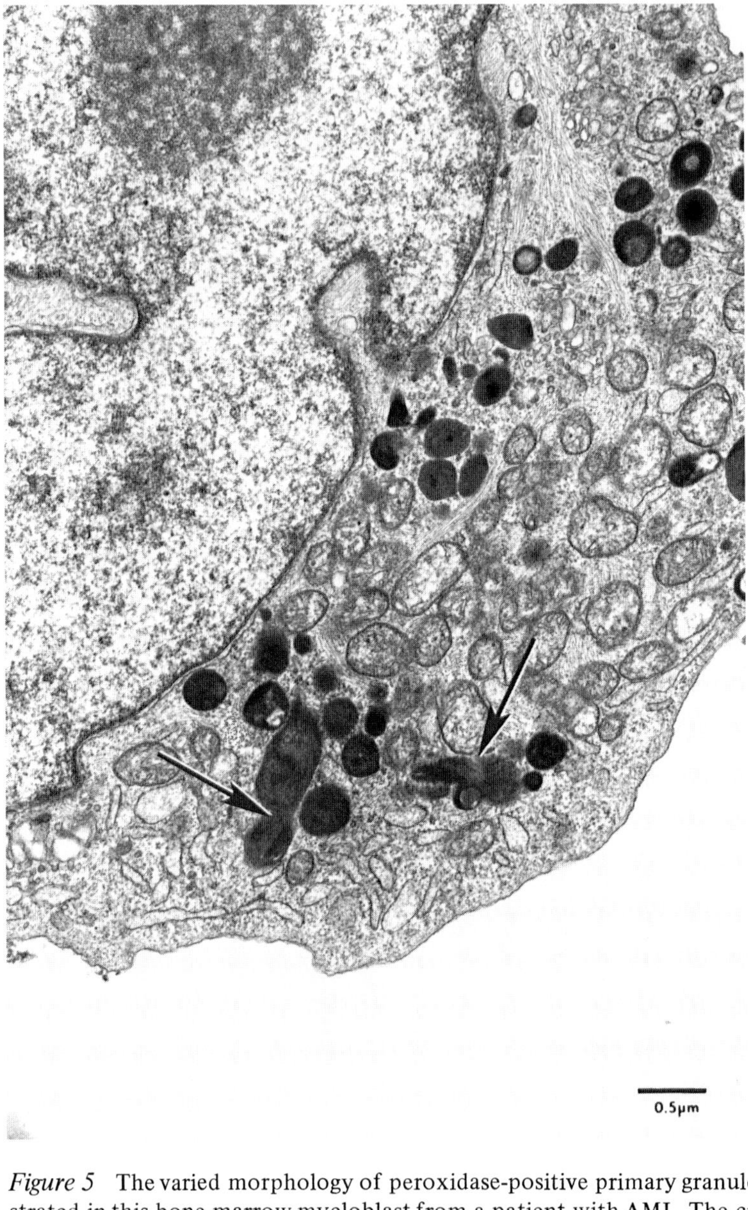

Figure 5 The varied morphology of peroxidase-positive primary granules are illustrated in this bone marrow myeloblast from a patient with AML. The crystalloid cores of some granules appear to break their limiting membrane and contribute to the bizarre shapes noted in these cells.

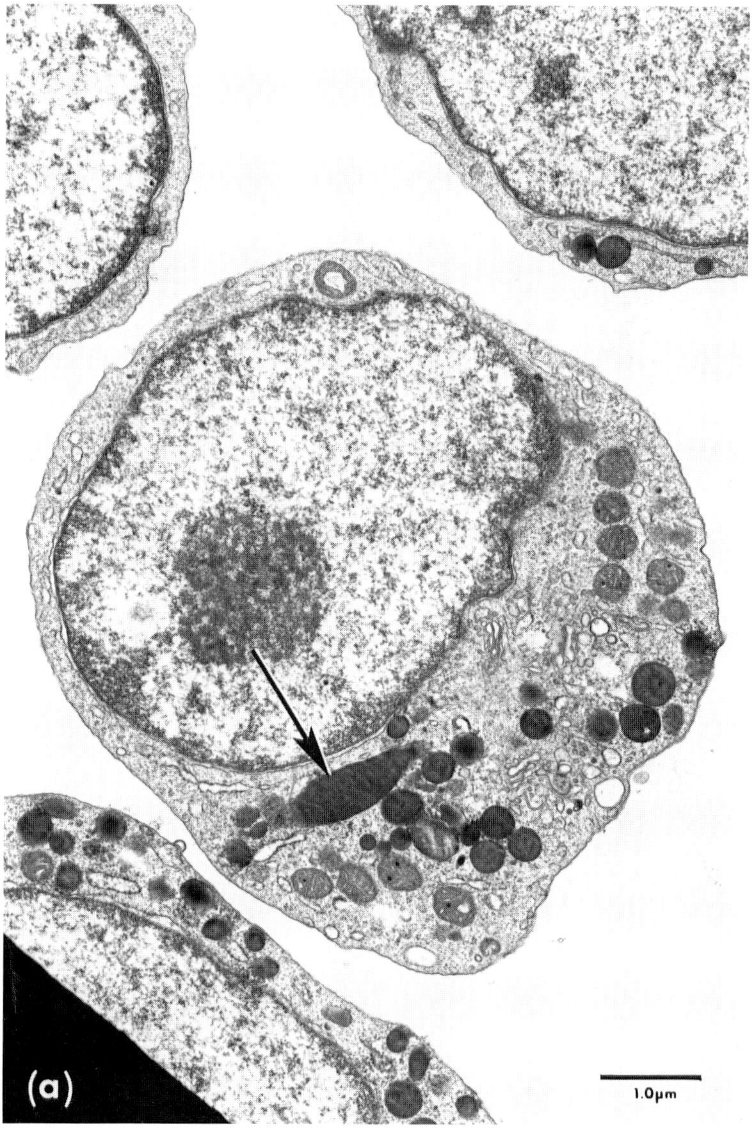

Figure 6 (a) This myeloblast exhibits a similar staining intensity in the Auer body (arrow) and primary granules following incubation in the Graham and Karnovsky medium. (b) The characteristic 60-120 Å periodicity of the Auer bodies as well as the presence of dense aggregates within their structure can be observed in this higher magnification micrograph.

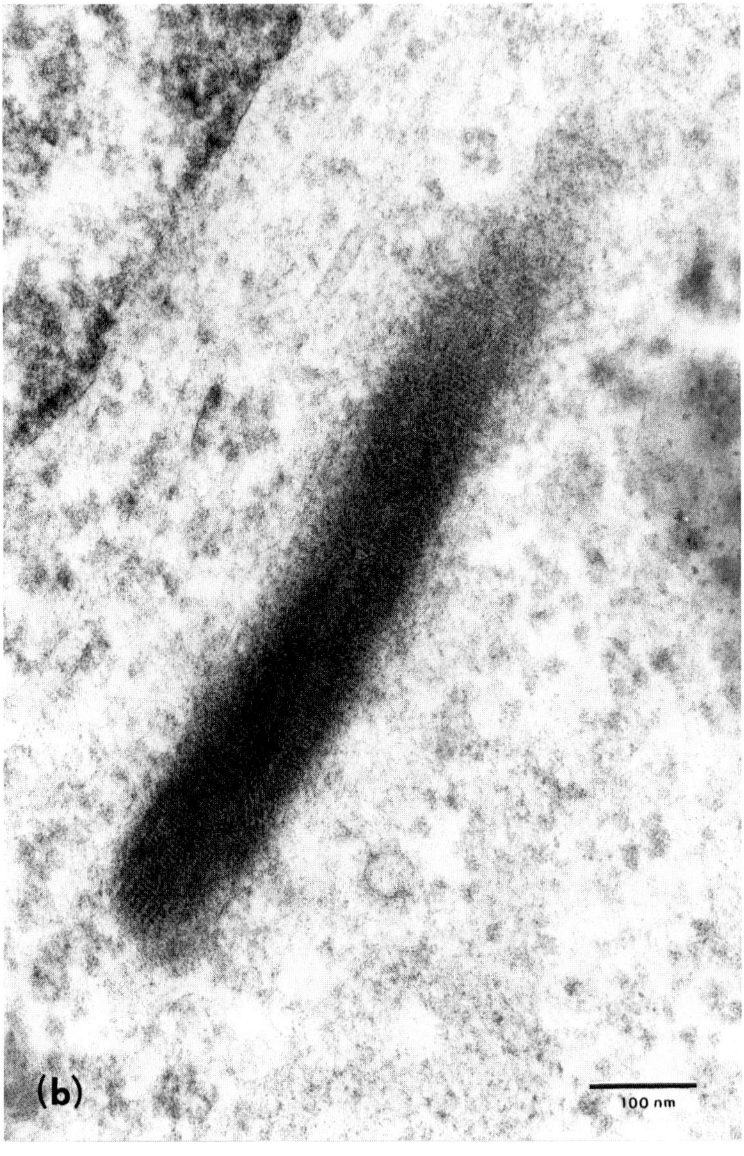

Figure 6 (*continued*)

C. Acute Promyelocytic Leukemia-M3 and M3 Variant

The striking hemorrhagic tendency (disseminated intravascular coagulation, or DIC), frequently observed in patients with AML-M3 disease, has contributed a great deal to the recognition of this form of leukemia as a distinct entity. This subtype of AML is characterized by a proliferation of abnormal promyelocytes rather than myeloblasts. The leukemic promyelocytes (Figure 7a) are characteristically 15-20 μm in diameter. The nucleus is lobulated, reniform and exhibits a clumped heterochromatin pattern associated with a more differentiated cell. One to two condensed nucleoli are evident. The cytoplasm demonstrates dilated multilaminar cisternae of endoplasmic reticulum and dense coarse granules varying in size from 140 to 1000 nm in diameter (Parkin and Brunning, 1978; Albarracin and Haust, 1971).

Abnormally large rod-shaped structures have been identified as splinter-form granules by electron microscopy. They are considered a characteristic cytological feature of acute promyelocytic leukemia. These splinter-form granules on longitudinal section appear as membrane-bound bundles of tubules (Figure 7b). The varying density with which these tubules are packed has given rise to the terminology "light" and "dark-form" splinters. In general, the density of these structures is not as great as that observed in Auer rods. On cross-section, the splinter-form granules show a crystalloid structure with a periodicity of 200-250 Å (Figure 7c). Cytochemically, at the ultrastructural level, a majority of these structures demonstrate positive acid phosphatase and peroxidase staining reactions; however, some splinters may be observed which are clearly peroxidase negative (Figure 8).

A variant (V) of the classical acute promyelocytic leukemia (APL) has been designated as AML-M3V by the FAB classification system. The cells (Figure 9) typically exhibit the features observed in cases of AML-M3 disease with the exception of granule size, which is characteristically less than 250 nm (Golomb et al., 1980). Although too small to lie within the limit of light microscopic resolution, these granules are easily observed by electron microscopy (Rajnoldi et al., 1981). Their morphology does not support reports suggesting a heterogenous myeloid and monocytic pattern of cellular differentiation for this subclassification of AML (Edelman and Grossman, 1983; Stavem, et al., 1981; Tomonaga et al., 1985). Rather, the peroxidase-positive microgranules many times appear asymmetrical and do not exhibit evidence of a lucent area inside their limiting membrane.

Ultrastructural analysis may be useful as a diagnostic adjuvant to identify the AML-M3V subtype, which carries the same risk of disseminated intravascular coagulation as AML-M3 disease.

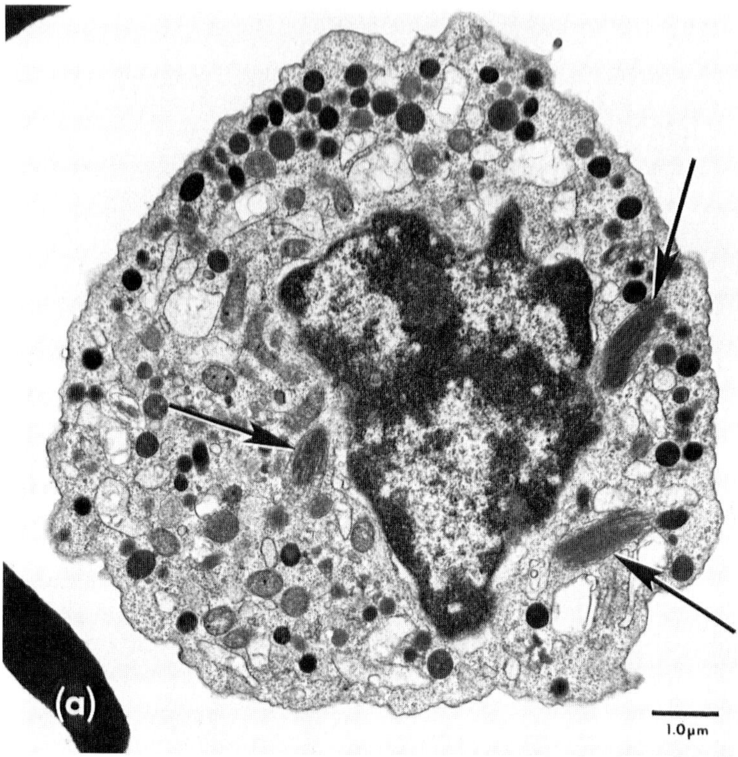

Figure 7 (a) This promyelocyte from the bone marrow of a patient with acute promyelocytic leukemia (AML-M3) exhibits characteristic dilated cisternae of endoplasmic reticulum as well as the presence of "splinter-form" granules (arrows). (b) The enlargement of a "splinter-form" granule reveals that the structures are membrane-bound and may stain positively with the Graham and Karnovsky medium. (c) On cross-section the "splinter-form granule is observed to have a crystalloid-type structure.

D. Acute Myelomonocytic Leukemia-M4

Electron microscopic studies have improved our ability to recognize both the myeloid and monocytic malignant elements in some cases of acute myelomonocytic leukemia (AMML). As a result, the frequency of this disease (FAB AMML-M4) is now found to be greater than initially suspected. The myeloblastic element in AMML-M4 is similar to that observed in AML-M1 and M2. In AMML-M4

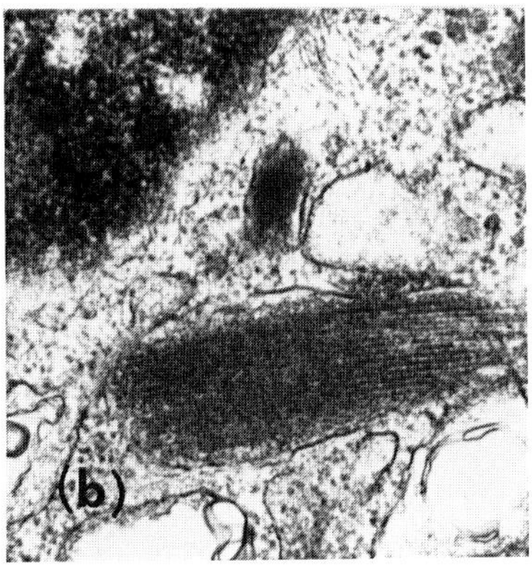

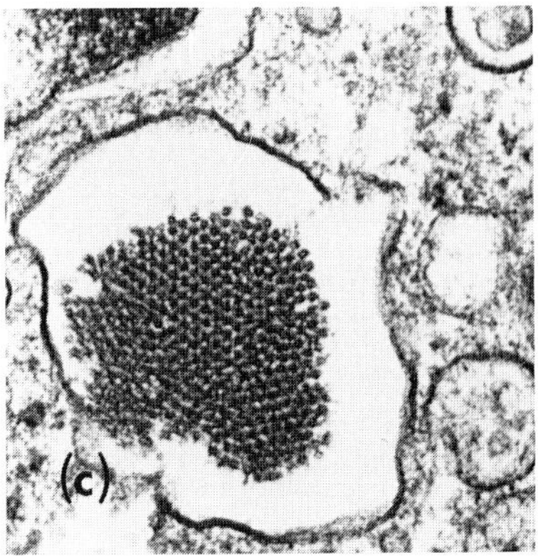

the marrow contains 12-14 μm promonocytes and a lesser population of monoblasts characterized by irregular nuclei exhibiting coarse-grained chromatin and a single large nucleolus (Figure 10). Cases in which α-naphthyl butyrate esterase staining is negative by light microscopy can be demonstrated to contain a monocytic component based on ultrastructural morphology. In addition, the absence or low levels of peroxidase staining reaction in the granules of some malignant monocytes, as well as a reduction in granule number associated with asynchronous differentiation, many times masks identification of these cells at the light microscopic level.

Ultrastructural cytochemistry, on the other hand, is capable of detecting peroxidase reactivity in monocytic granules of most AMML-M4 cases. The morphology of these granules by electron microscopy is smaller and more uniform in size than those observed in the varying number of myeloblastic elements present. Characteristically, the monocytic granules exhibit a clear or lucent area inside their limiting membrane. Although occasional monocytic elements are noted lacking peroxidase activity (Cawley and Hayhoe, 1973), these cells may reflect early stages of granule formation or defects in enzyme production associated with the malignant process.

Additionally, at the ultrastructural level acid phosphatase (AP) (Polliack and Leizerowitz, 1983) and nonspecific esterase (Payne et al., 1980) have been demonstrated in monocytic granules. In early monoblasts, AP activity is noted to precede myeloperoxidase (MPO) staining in the membrane-bound granules (O'Brien, Catovsky, and Costello, 1980), whereas the esterase reaction does not exhibit a clear relationship to any membrane-bound granules.

Distinctive bundles of 60-80 Å microfibrils are frequently noted to occur in the cytoplasm of monocytic elements in both AMML-M4 and AML-M5 disease

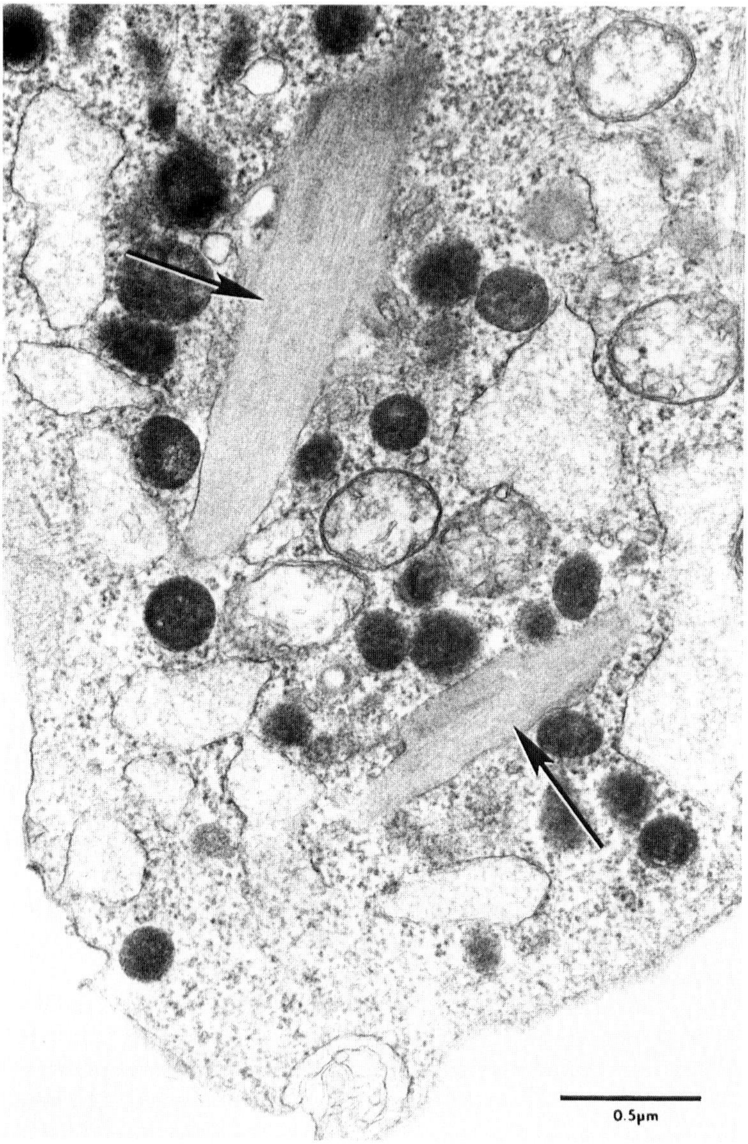

Figure 8 The "splinter-form" granules (arrows) observed in this promyelocyte from the bone marrow of a patient with AML-M3 are peroxidase negative following incubation in the Graham and Karnovsky medium although surrounded with positive-staining primary granules.

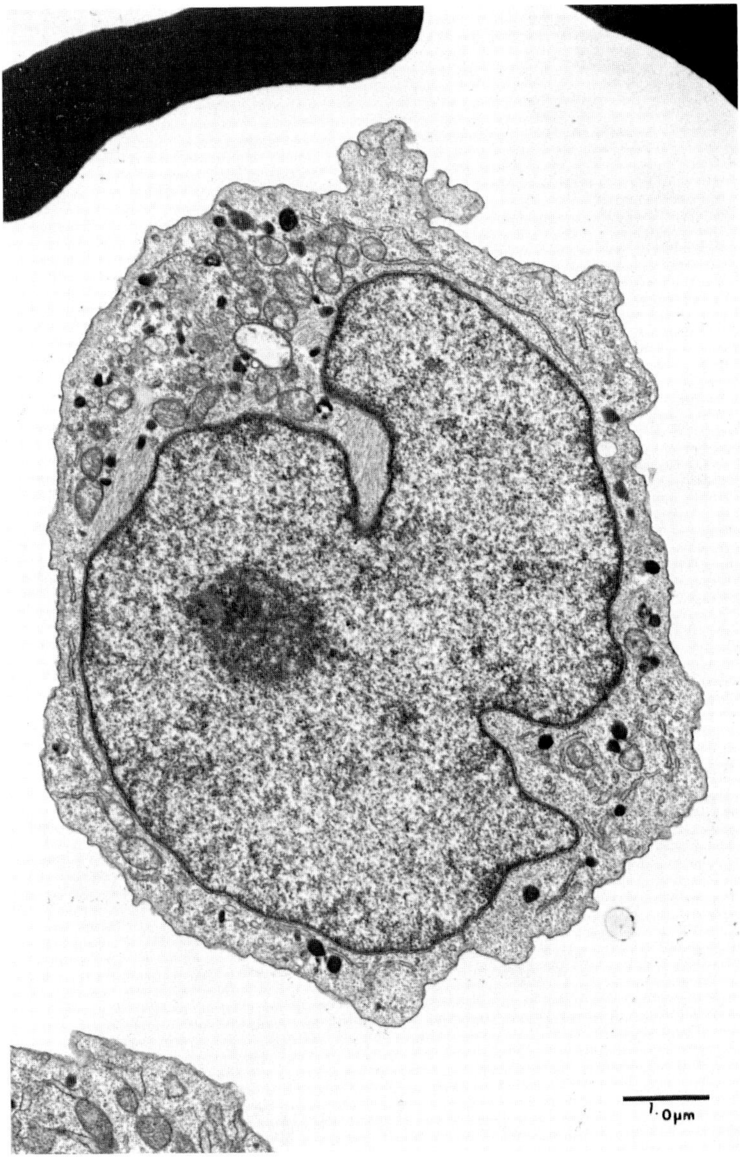

Figure 9 This promyelocyte from the bone marrow of a patient with AML-M3V exhibits microgranules which are typically less than 250 mm in diameter and, therefore, below the level of light microscopic resolution.

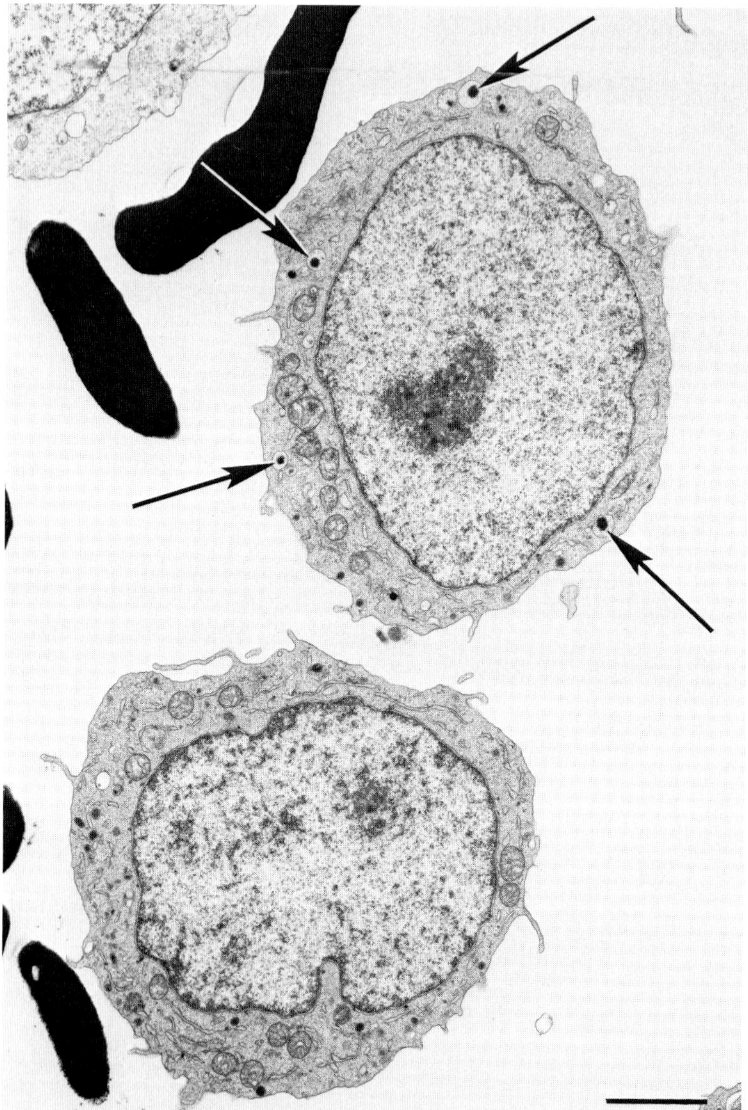

Figure 10 Bone marrow cells from a patient with acute myelomonocytic leukemia (AMML-M4) demonstrating both the presence of a monoblast with uniform circumscribed "bull's eye" granules (arrows) and an immature myeloid cell with developmental granule formation.

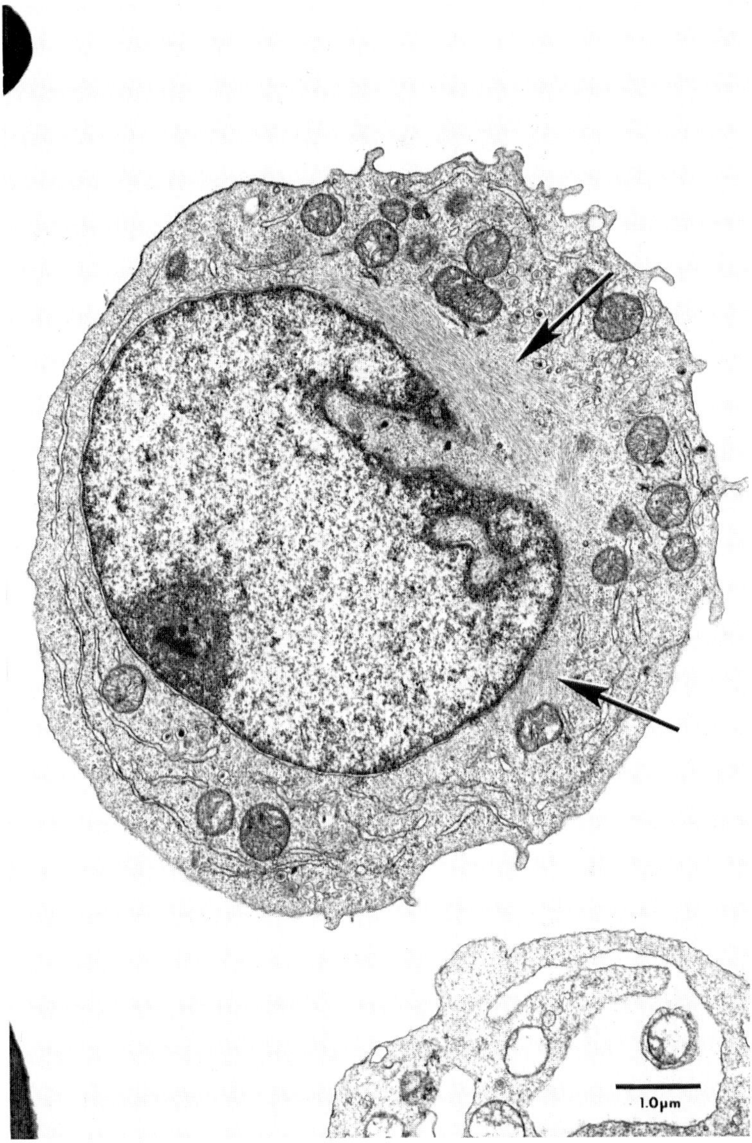

Figure 11 The microfibrils (arrows) noted in the cytoplasm of this immature leukemic monocyte frequently occur in bundles located in the juxtanuclear region.

(Figure 11). These structures may occupy extensive cytoplasmic area and are often observed in the juxtanuclear area.

A subset of AMML (FAB M4b) has been described which shows a consistent abnormality associated with bone marrow eosinophils and the presence of a unique chromosome abnormality, inv(16) (p13q22) (Bitter et al., 1984). Ultrastructurally, the immature eosinophils are distinguished by lack of a central crystalloid in their specific granules and the presence of intermixed basophil-type granules. A consistent ultrastructural feature in this AML-M4b subtype is the high frequency of nuclear blebs noted on the abnormal eosinophils (Figure 12) (Dalton et al., 1985).

E. Acute Monocytic Leukemia-M5

The round, oval, or kidney-shaped nuclei of monoblasts in AML-M5 are primarily euchromatic, and even in relatively undifferentiated cases, examples of irregularity in nuclear outline may be observed (Figure 13). The nucleoli are large and loosely structured. The cytoplasm of these cells contain minimal organelles (Shaw, 1980). Characteristic granules (.05-.10 μm) are frequently seen only in small clusters, which may not be present in all cell sections. These granules exhibit a clear halo between their electron-dense core and the limiting membrane. Cytoplasmic inclusions resembling ribosomal lamella complexes (RLC) are occasionally noted in the monoblasts of these AML-M5 patients (Figure 14). Unlike those inclusions which have also been observed in normal monocytes (Bessis, 1973a), the RLC complex has been reported only in neoplastic cells, most commonly hairy cell leukemia (Begin, Osborne, and Mackay, 1981; Brunning and Parkin, 1975).

F. Acute Erythroleukemia-M6

Electron microscopic analysis of erythroblasts in cases of AML-M6 reveal 12 to 16-μm diameter cells, which contain large nuclei with dispersed euchromatin (Figure 15). The nuclear outline is round to oval with slight irregularity. A large single nucleolus is present. The cytoplasm contains densely packed ribosomes, profiles of endoplasmic reticulum and more numerous mitochondria than noted in normal erythroblasts. Mitochondrial accumulation of ferruginous micelles resembling those noted in sideroblastic anemia may be observed (Glick, 1976). Frequently, by light microscopy, the erythroid alterations in this subtype may be completely overshadowed by more obvious abnormalities in the myeloid series. At the ultrastructural level, however, the presence of cytoplasmic glycogen deposits (Hayhoe and Cawley, 1972), increased numbers of mitochondria with ferruginous deposits (Kamiyama, 1971), asynchrony in nucleocytoplasmic differentiation, as well as rhopheocytosis are helpful in identifying undifferentiated erythroblasts. Electron microscopic study reveals that erythroblasts often contain

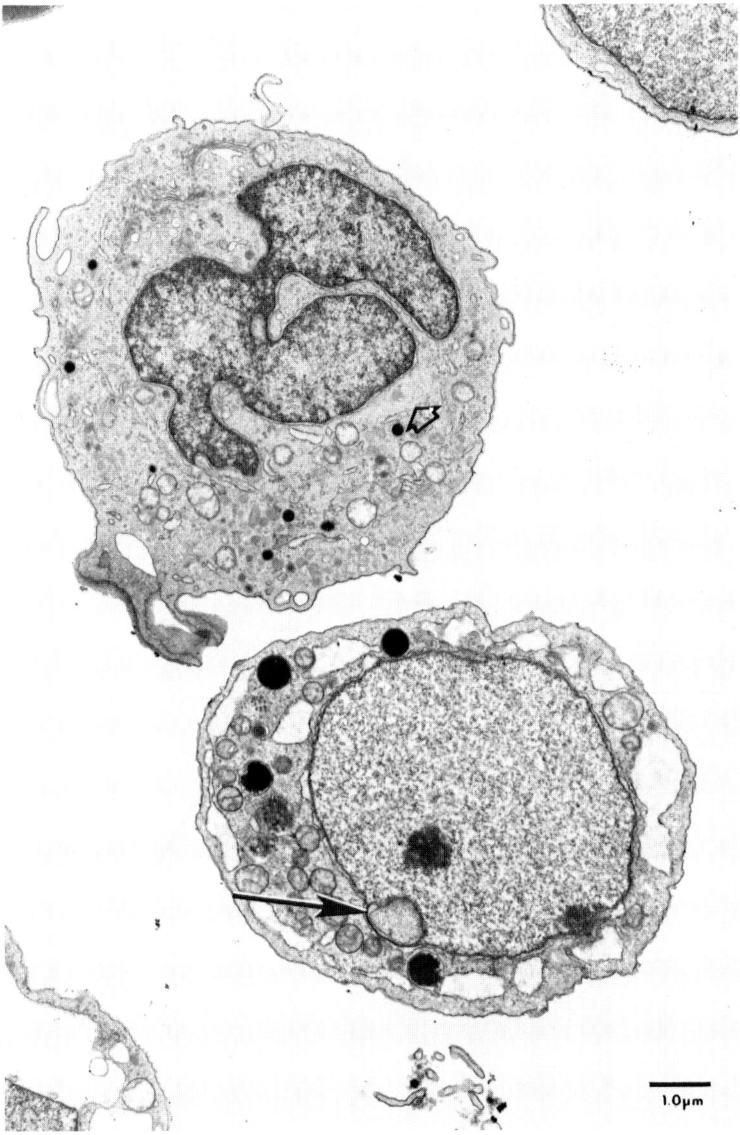

Figure 12a These bone marrow cells from a patient with AMML-M4b exhibit ultrastructural abnormalities in both the monocytic element and in the immature eosinophil. Bundles of microfibrils (open arrow) are noted in the promonocyte, and a bleb (solid arrow) is present on the blastlike nucleus of the asynchronously differentiating eosinophil.

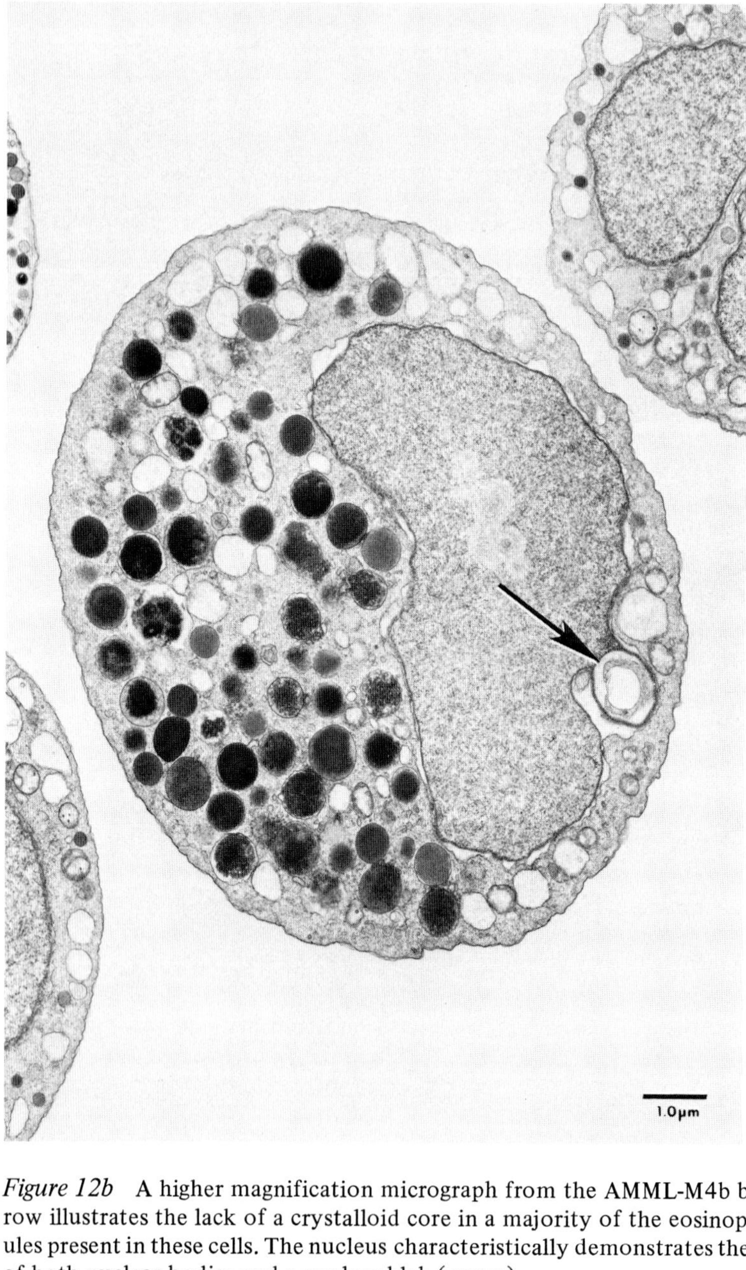

Figure 12b A higher magnification micrograph from the AMML-M4b bone marrow illustrates the lack of a crystalloid core in a majority of the eosinophil granules present in these cells. The nucleus characteristically demonstrates the presence of both nuclear bodies and a nuclear bleb (arrow).

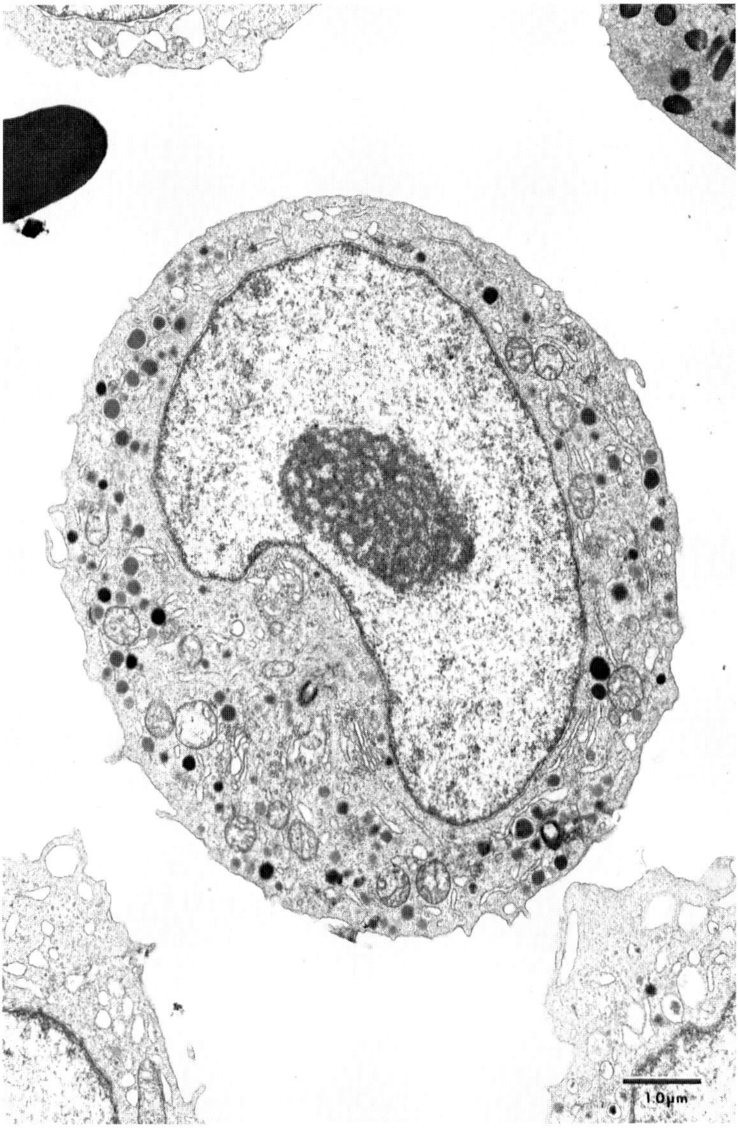

Figure 13 This monoblast from the bone marrow of a patient with acute monocytic leukemia (AML-M5) exhibits asynchrony of nuclear/cytoplasmic differentiation. The kidney-shaped euchromatic nucleus contains a large well-developed nucleolus. The cytoplasmic "bull's eye" granules display reactivity for myeloperoxidase after incubation in the Graham and Karnovsky medium.

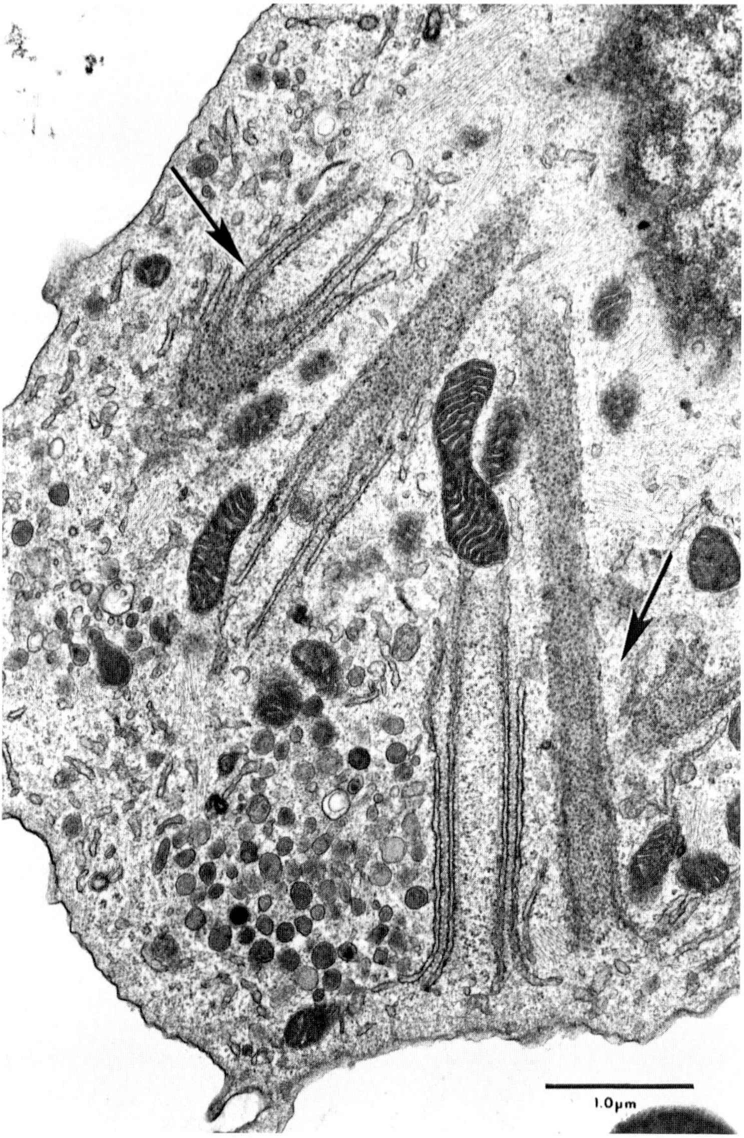

Figure 14 Variable profiles of ribosome-lamellar complex (arrows) are seen in the cytoplasm of the leukemic monoblast. These configurations appear to correspond to oblique and longitudinal sections of a hollow cylindrical structure.

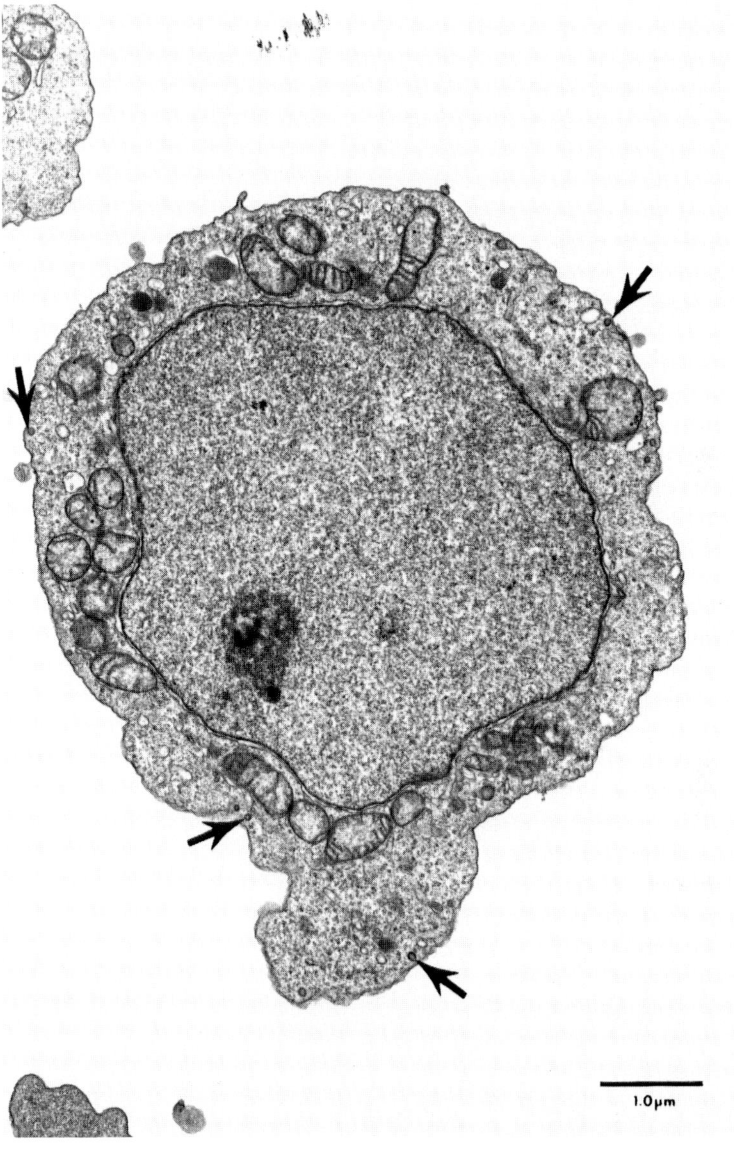

Figure 15 A proerythroblast from the bone marrow of a patient with acute erythroleukemia (AML-M6). The nucleus is devoid of heterochromatin condensation and contains a distinct nucleolus. The cytoplasm is marked by increased numbers of mitochondria, rhopheocytosis (arrows) and scattered glycogen particles.

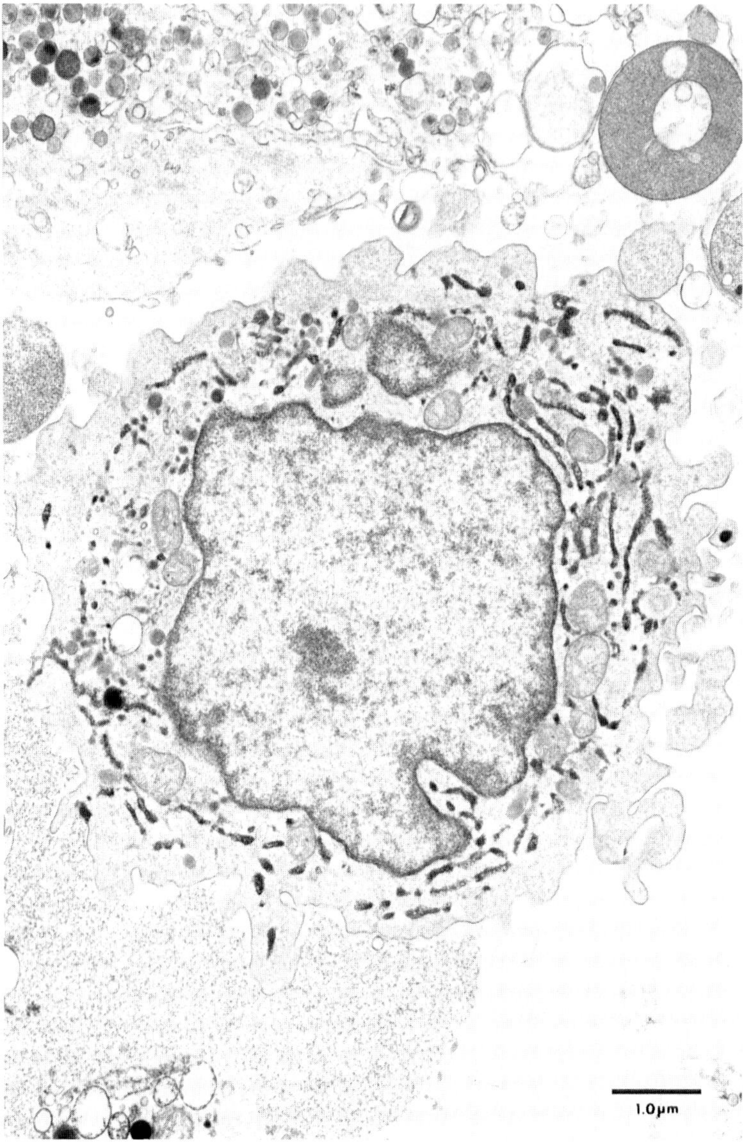

Figure 16 Incubation in diaminobenzyidine (DAB) prior to fixation reveals platelet-peroxidase (PPO) activity in the endoplasmic reticulum of this megakaryoblast from the bone marrow of a patient with myeloproliferative disease. The enzyme activity in these cells is not localized in either the Golgi or primary granules.

cytoplasmic vacuoles that are PAS positive in contrast to the lipid-containing vacuoles observed in cases of ALL-L3.

G. Acute Megakaryoblastic Leukemia-M7

Megakaryoblasts, as viewed by electron microscopy, usually display a high nucleocytoplasmic ratio. The large nucleus, with a delicate chromatin pattern, is round or oval and contains one or two nucleoli. Cytoplasmic organelles include a well-developed Golgi, short strands of rough endoplasmic reticulum, and limited mitochondria. Neoplastic megakaryocytes and their precursors may be identified by the asynchronous development of the cytoplasm, which frequently demonstrates scattered granules with "bull's eye" appearance and early evidence of a demarcation system (Koike, 1984) (Mirchondani and Palutke, 1982).

Application of the platelet peroxidase staining reaction (PPO) has assisted the recognition of these early precursors (Figure 16). Both the Roels technique (unfixed cells) and the Anderson technique (tannic acid/paraformaldehyde/glutaraldehyde) utilize diaminobenzidine as the electron-dense peroxidase stain which is localized in the endoplasmic reticulum and the perinuclear space of early megakaryoblasts and not in the Golgi region or granules (Bain et al., 1981; Breton-Gorius et al., 1978).

Combined studies utilizing both the PPO reaction and immunological staining for megakaryoblasts' surface glycoproteins indicate that the PPO appears positive prior to detection of the IIB/IIIA glycoprotein complex (Tabilio et al., 1984).

Micromegakaryocytes are occasionally observed in cases of chronic granulocytic leukemia exhibiting transformation (Bain et al., 1977; Efrati et al., 1979). These cells are 6-11 μm in diameter. They exhibit an elevated nuclear/cytoplasmic ratio. The euchromatic nuclei typically exhibit clefts or folds on their surface. There is minimal heterochromatin margination at the internal nuclear membrane. One to two small nucleoli are present. The cytoplasm contains scattered ribosomes, mitochondria, small segments of endoplasmic reticulum, and a few granules (Breton-Gorius et al., 1973). The ultrastructural PPO reaction is extremely useful in identifying the lineage of these microblasts that, by conventional morphology, may appear to be of lymphoid origin (Bain et al., 1981).

III. ACUTE LYMPHOCYTIC LEUKEMIA (ALL)

A. Acute Lymphocytic Leukemia-L1

Ultrastructurally, the typical leukemic lymphoblasts in ALL-L1 disease (Figure 17) are small (7-8 μm) and rather uniform in size. There is an increased nuclear-cytoplasmic ratio. A nuclear indentation may be evident in some cell sections. The nuclear chromatin is typically coarse in texture and demonstrates variable degrees of heterochromatin pattern and margination. There are typically one to two nucleoli that are reticulated in appearance. The cytoplasm in general is agranular

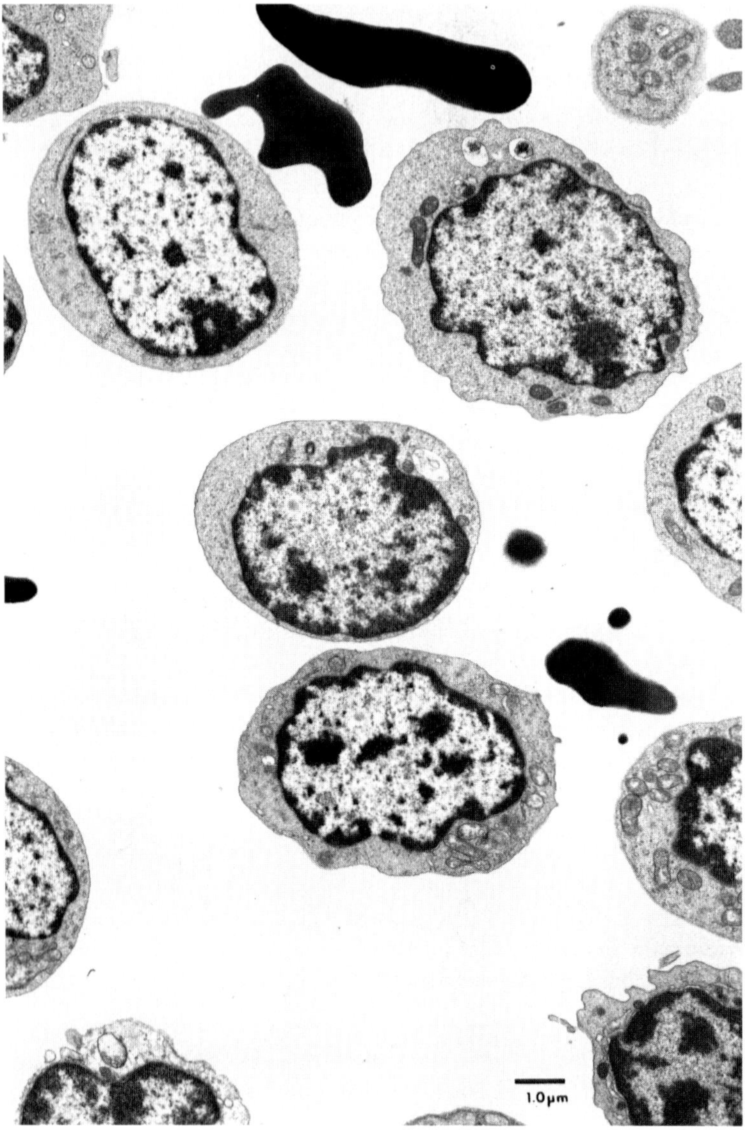

Figure 17 These uniform-sized lymphoblasts from the bone marrow of a patient with acute lymphocytic leukemia (ALL-L1) are characterized by a high nuclear/cytoplasmic ratio, peripheral heterochromatin condensation in the nuclei, and indistinct nucleoli. The cytoplasm is sparse and organelles are limited to small mitochondria, ribosomes and scattered profiles of rough endoplasmic reticulum.

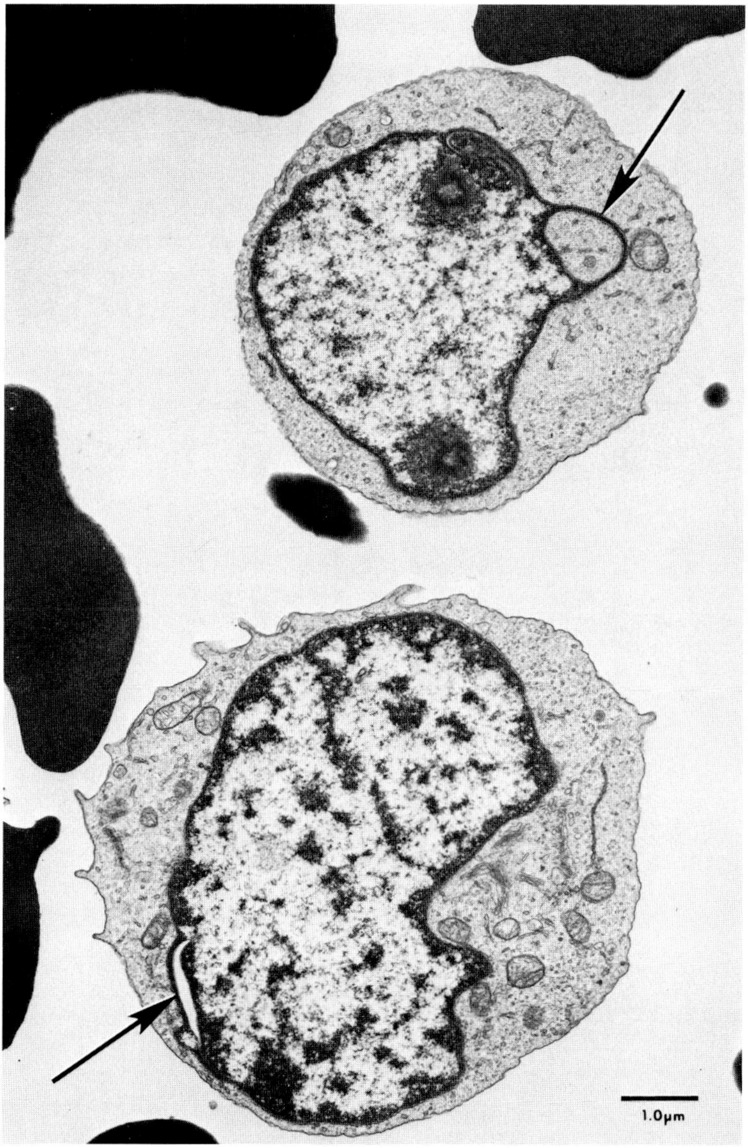

Figure 18 Arrows indicate the presence of a nuclear bleb (upper cell) and a nuclear cleft (lower cell) in the bone marrow lymphoblasts from a patient with ALL-L1. These structures are frequently noted in the leukemic cells of these individuals.

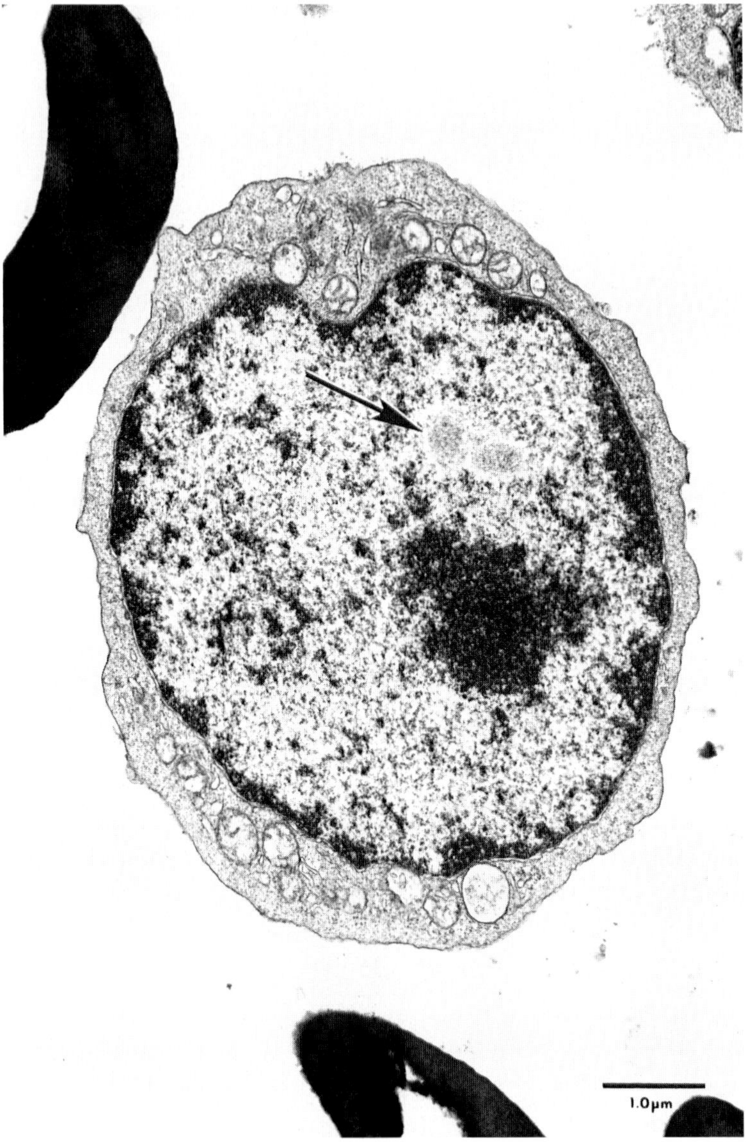

Figure 19 The nucleus of this lymphoblast from a case of ALL-L1 demonstrates dense heterochromatin pattern and the presence of two nuclear bodies. These spherical bodies are also noted in significant numbers in other types of acute leukemia.

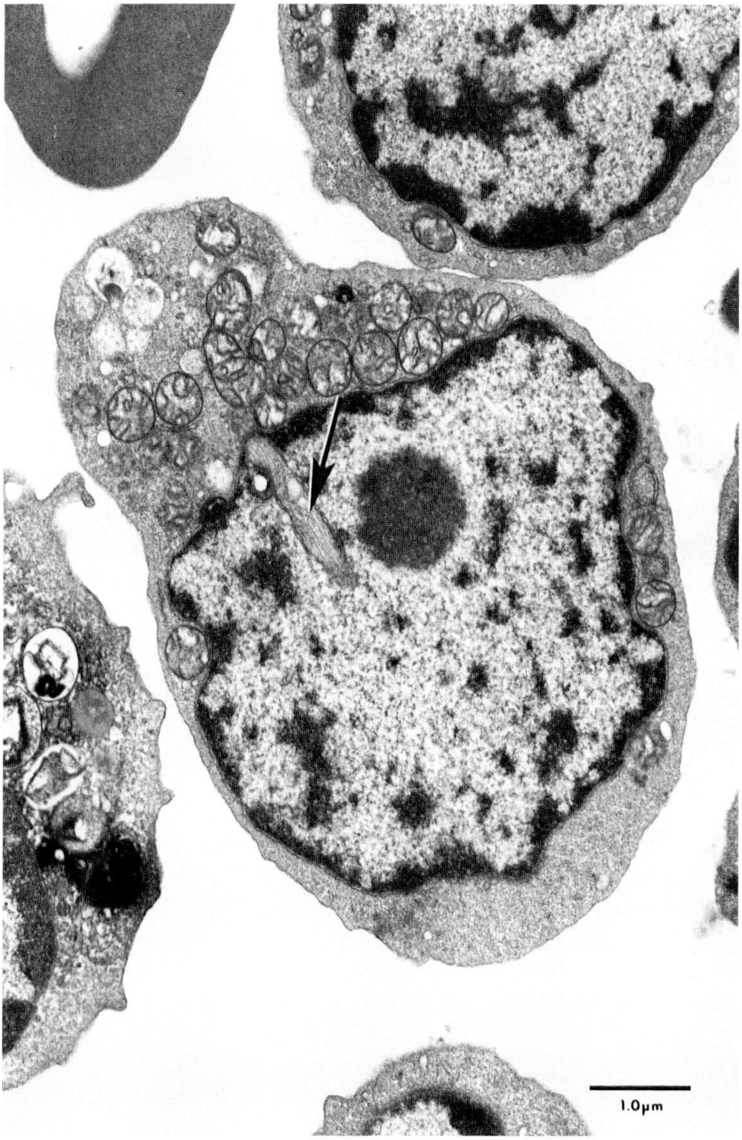

Figure 20 Although the nuclear outline is usually regular in ALL-L1, folding and indentation may be observed in thin sections of these blasts. Bundles of cytoplasmic fibrils (arrow) are frequently localized in this area.

and demonstrates the presence of large mitochondria and restricted amounts of endoplasmic reticulum.

Malignant associated features such as nuclear blebs or clefts (Figure 18), nuclear bodies (Figure 19), and bundles of microfilaments (Figure 20) are readily apparent in these cells by electron microscopy.

B. Acute Lymphocytic Leukemia-L2

Lymphoblasts from the bone marrow of patients classified as ALL-L2 are characterized by their heterogeneity in size (Figure 21). In addition to the small lymphoblasts observed in L1 cases, larger blasts up to 14 μm are noted. These larger blasts usually exhibit an increased cytoplasmic area and increased number of organelles, with the exception of profiles of endoplasmic reticulum, which are relatively scarce. The nuclei of these larger blasts exhibit a more pronounced indentation and a more varied heterochromatin pattern than observed in ALL-L1. One to two large, prominent nucleoli are noticeable in these cells. ALL-L2 is not specific for T-cell disease, but many T-cell leukemias have an L2 morphology. Combined cytochemical and immunological studies reveal that T-cell malignancies demonstrate higher levels of acid phosphatase staining than observed in B-cell disease (Brouet et al., 1976). The localization of alpha-naphthyl acid esterase in these T cells is most likely related to the increased lysosomes (Zicca et al., 1981).

Using peroxidase-labeled antibodies directed against T-cell subpopulations simultaneously with ultrastructural cytochemistry, OKT8 positive suppressor cells are found to contain Golgi and related lysosomal granules. OKT4 positive helper cells, on the other hand, have a less prominent Golgi and relatively few granules (Polliack and Leizerowitz, 1983).

C. Acute Lymphocytic Leukemia-L3

The homogeneous medium-sized blasts cells that characterize ALL-L3 disease display a round or oval nucleus, with or without indentation. The nuclear chromatin demonstrates heterochromatin pattern and margination. One to two nucleoli are present. The most striking diagnostic feature of these blasts is the presence of prominent cytoplasmic lipid-containing vacuoles (Figure 22). Ultrastructurally, these cells are indistinguishable from the classic Burkitt's lymphoma cell and usually exhibit similar B-cell surface immunoglobulins and a high incidence of translocations between chromosomes 8 and 14 (t8;14). This is the only subtype of ALL that clearly is associated with a specific immunophenotype. Recently a case of ALL-L3, confirmed by electron microscopy, has been reported that does not express either the surface immunoglobulin or the cytogenetic abnormality (Mangan et al., 1985). We have also seen a similar case.

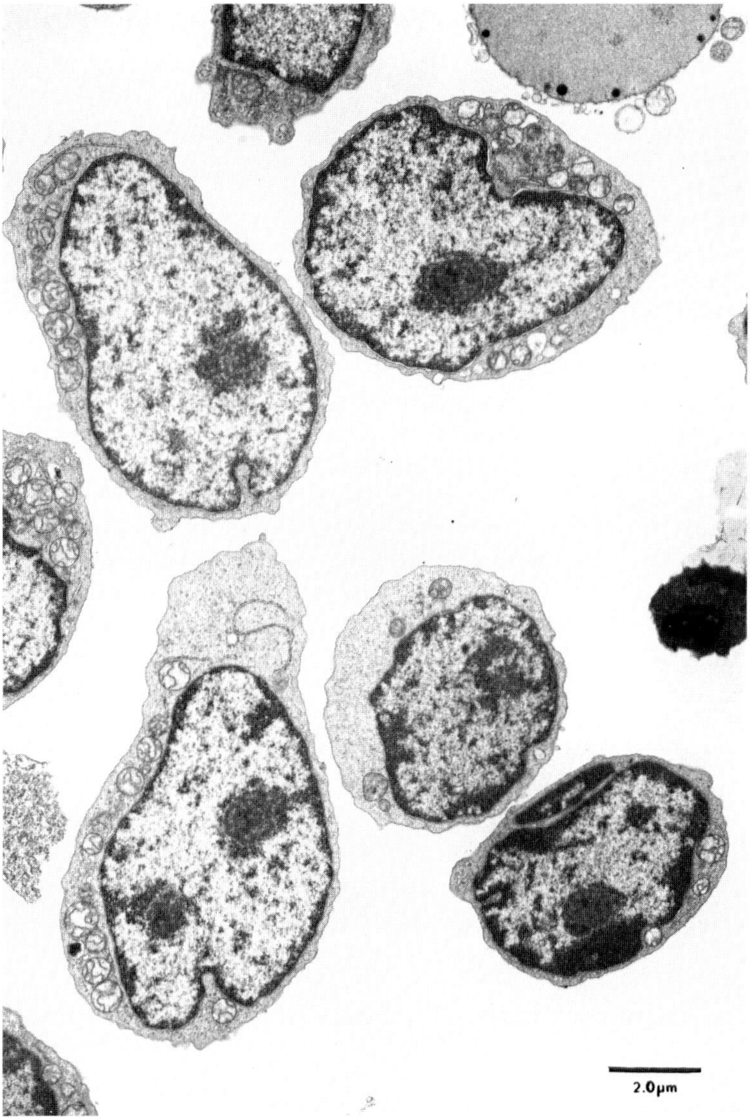

Figure 21 Bone marrow lymphoblasts from a patient with ALL-L2, exhibiting heterogeneity in cell size. The larger blasts display moderate amounts of cytoplasm, distinct heterochromatin pattern in the nuclei, and large, prominent nucleoli.

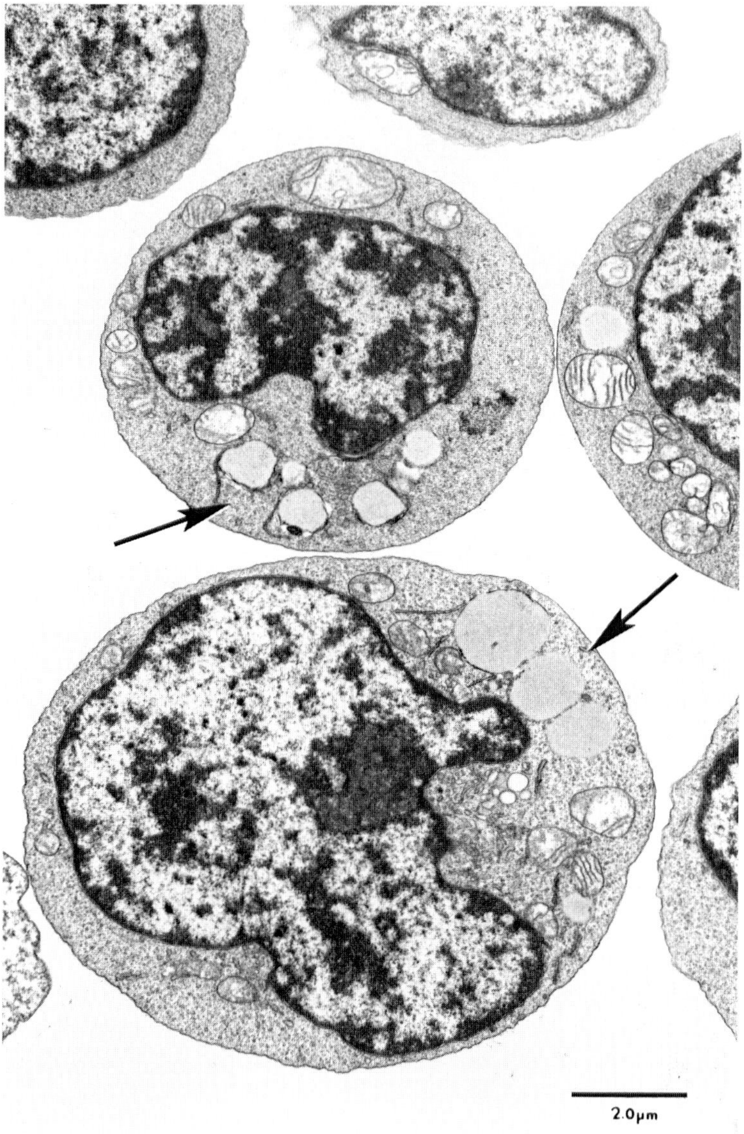

Figure 22 These medium-sized blast cells from the bone marrow of a patient with ALL-L3 demonstrate the presence of characteristic lipid-containing vacuoles in their abundant cytoplasm. Large mitochondria with irregular cristae, rare profiles of endoplasmic reticulum, and numerous ribosomes are noted.

IV. MISCELLANEOUS ACUTE LEUKEMIAS

A. Plasma Cell Leukemia

Plasma cell leukemia may occur de novo as acute leukemia or as the terminal phase of multiple myeloma. In the latter case, it is reported to be a more frequent occurrence in those patients who have the IgD type of multiple myeloma (Kass, 1982).

Plasmablasts or plasma cell leukemia may be so undifferentiated at the light microscopic level that ultrastructural examination is essential to the detect the plasma cell origin.

Electron microscopic examination of aspirated bone marrow from these patients reveal medium-sized (12-14 μm) blast cells (Figure 23). The nucleus may be indented and irregular in shape with a predominance of euchromatin. A prominent nucleolus is evident. The cytoplasm contains well-developed parallel profiles of rough endoplasmic reticulum identical to that observed in cells from patients with multiple myeloma. The polysomes associated with the endoplasmic reticulum have been demonstrated to vary in aggregate size related to their characteristic monoclonal Ig production (Kitani et al., 1982; Yonezawa et al., 1982). Mitochondria frequently exhibit bizarre shapes, as well as alterations in the architecture of their internal christae (Djaldetti, 1984). The well-differentiated cytoplasmic organelles in these cells contrast sharply with their immature nuclei (Bassan, Gutmann, and Djaldetti, 1981). Occasionally, precipitated immunoglobulin with the appearance of rods is noted in the cytoplasm. This material can be confused with Auer rods at both the light and electron microscopic level but is peroxidase negative and does not have the periodicity associated with Auer rods.

B. Prolymphocytic Leukemia

Prolymphocytic leukemia (PLL) was first described as a lymphoproliferative disorder in 1974 (Galton et al., 1974). The malignancy exhibits a pronounced leukocytosis with large numbers of circulating prolymphocytes. Ultrastructural examination of these prolymphocytes reveals a cell 9-12 μm in diameter. The round or oval nucleus usually contains small indentations on the surface and is characterized by heavy peripheral condensation of heterochromatin. One or two large, prominent immature nucleoli, often showing nucleolonema, are commonly observed. These structures appear asynchronous with the degree of chromatin condensation present in the nucleus. Indeed, the simultaneous appearance of the large nucleolus and the heavy patterned heterochromatin distinguish these malignant cells from those of chronic lymphocytic leukemia or acute lymphoblastic leukemia. The cytoplasm of the PLL cell contains few polyribosomes, short segments of rough endoplasmic reticulum, variable numbers of mitochondria and a poorly developed Golgi apparatus (Kjeldsberg, Bearman, Rappaport, 1980).

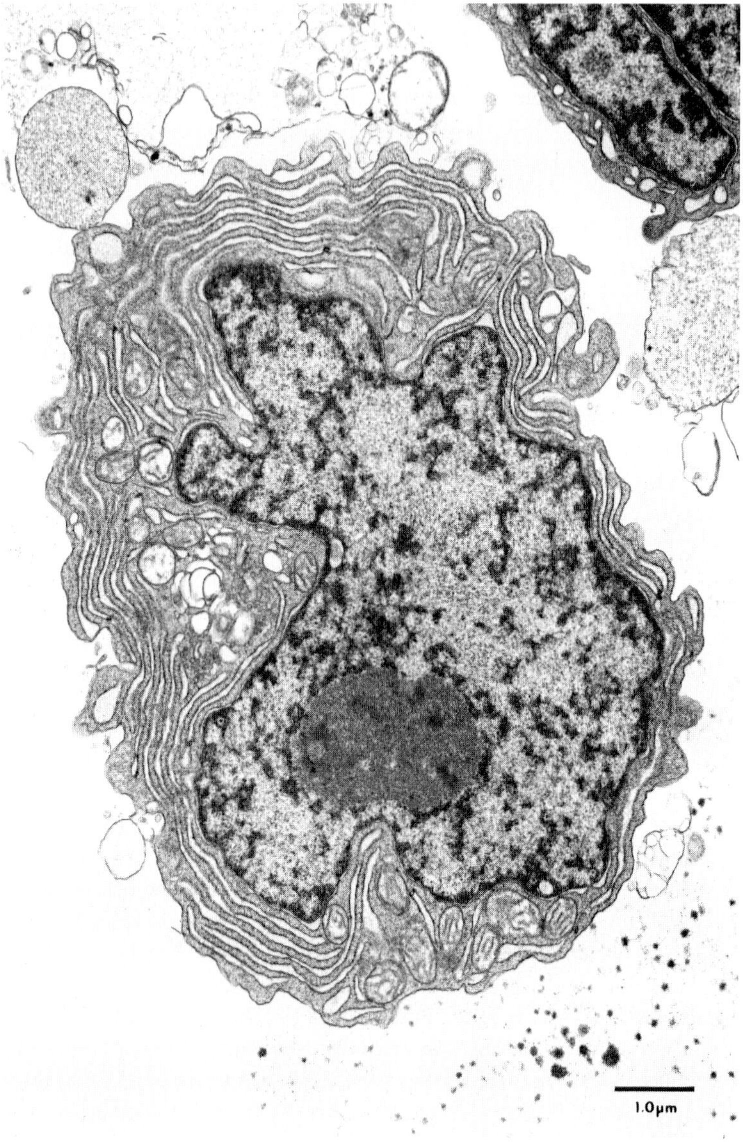

Figure 23 This bone marrow blast cell from a case of plasma cell leukemia exhibits a large, irregular-shaped nucleus with a prominent nucleolus. Several grossly distended mitochondria are present among the abundant cisternae of rough endoplasmic reticulum which characterizes the cytoplasm of this cell.

Granulelike structures of varying size and electron density have also been reported in the prolymphocyte cytoplasm (Costello et al., 1980). Some of these structures may represent residual phagocytized material. Prolymphocyte phagocytosis of erythrocytes and other cellular elements has been described (Martelli et al., 1980).

C. Acute Undifferentiated Leukemia

This subclass includes those blasts cells which, ultrastructurally, are myeloperoxidase- and platelet-peroxidase-negative and without any clear nuclear or cytoplasmic morphology that would permit classification according to the FAB cooperative group (Polli et al., 1985). The cells are typically 8-12 μm in diameter. The nuclear-cytoplasmic ratio is variable. The round nuclei exhibit uniform euchromatin and a distinct nucleolus. The cytoplasmic organelles are limited to ribosomes, scant profiles of endoplasmic reticulum, and a few mitochondria (Figure 24). Cases of acute leukemia that are undifferentiated by light microscopy with negative cytochemistry and the absence of lineage associated antigens can be documented to be myeloid based on the presence of ultrastructural peroxidase (Youness et al., 1980).

D. Acute Mixed Lineage Leukemia (AMLL)

Acute mixed lineage leukemia is often associated with the t(4;11) chromosome rearrangement or the presence of the Philadelphia chromosome. The morphological features of the leukemic blasts in cases with the t(4;11) abnormality have been reported to vary from lymphoid to myeloid (Parkin et al., 1982). Ultrastructural myeloperoxidase staining reveals that some lymphoid or undifferentiated-appearing blasts exhibit the presence of myeloid or monocytic granules (Childs et al., 1986). The Philadelphia-chromosome-positive acute leukemias have been shown to have mixed lineage; although myeloperoxidase is positive at the EM level, the cells exhibit the presence of lymphoid-associated surface antigens by light microscopy (Hirsch et al., 1986). These findings support the concept that a pluripotential stem cell is involved in this subset of acute leukemia.

E. Acute Lymphoblastic Leukemic Hand-Mirror Variant

The association of hand-mirror morphology with cells of lymphocytic origin is well established (McFarland, 1969; Norberg, Rydgren, and Stenstam, 1974; Rich, Wintrobe, and Lewis, 1929; Schumacher et al., 1977). Hand-mirror cells are most commonly associated with ALL (all FAB subtypes L1, L2, and L3) but have been noted also in AML. Stass (1978) has provided a detailed case study of this ALL variant in which morphological, cytochemical, and immunological surface markers confirmed the lymphoid features of the hand-mirror cell. Ultrastructurally the cells are 9-10 μm in size (Figure 25). The nuclear chromatin is coarse in texture

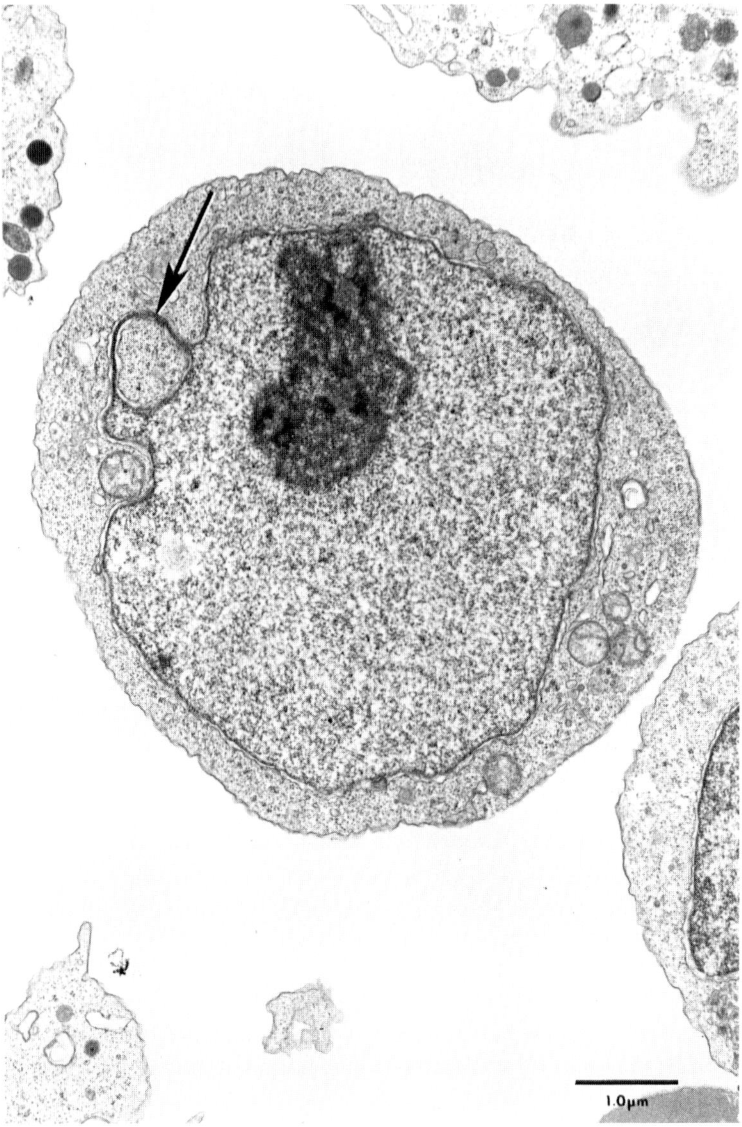

Figure 24 This primitive bone marrow cell from a patient with acute leukemia displays a completely undifferentiated appearance. The nuclear chromatin is uniformly euchromatic and a distinct nucleolus is present. Ultrastructural cytochemistry with both myeloperoxidase and platelet peroxidase are negative. Apart from the presence of abundant ribosomes, there is a paucity of organelles.

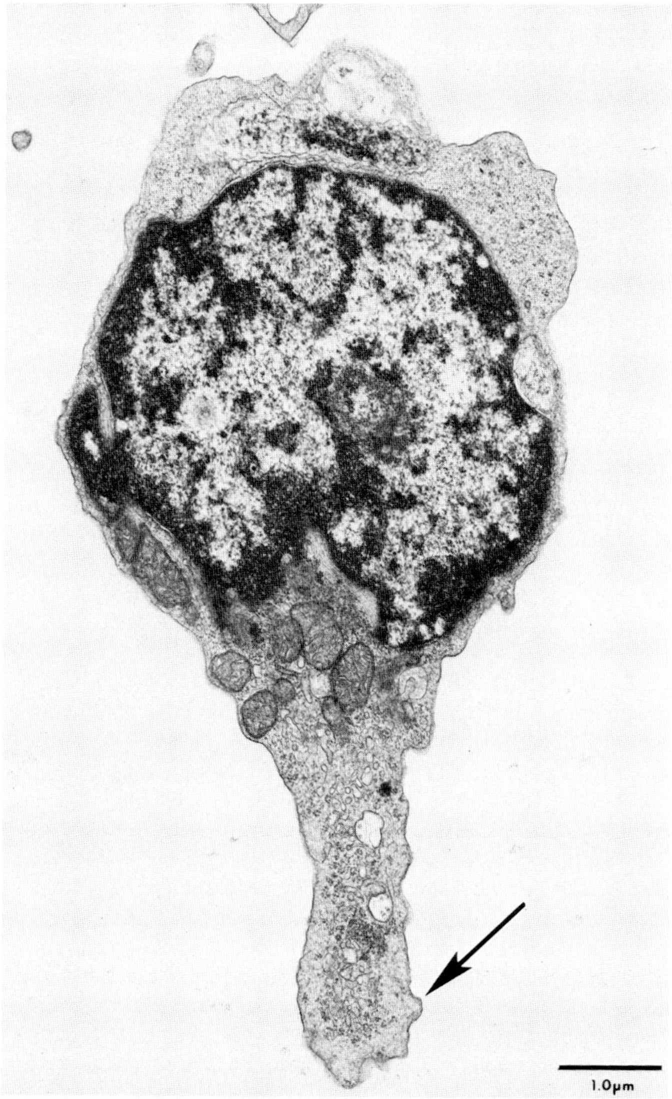

Figure 25 This hand-mirror cell from the bone marrow of a patient with ALL-L1 exhibits the typical ratio of long cell axis/short cell axis greater than 2. The abundant mitochondria are localized between the nucleus and the base of the uropod. Microtubules in cross-section are noted throughout the length of this cytoplasmic extension, which often exhibits microspikes (arrow) on its terminal end.

and demonstrates distinct heterochromatin margination. The cytoplasm contains a striking uropod extension with mitochondria clustered at its base. Microspikes can often be noted on the terminal end of the uropod. Glycogen is noted throughout the cytoplasmic area.

V. CONCLUSION

As illustrated in this chapter, ultrastructural morphology can be utilized as a useful adjuvant in diagnostic hematology. The application of EM cytochemistry, particularly the myeloperoxidase and the platelet peroxidase reaction, has proven to be a highly sensitive technique that has expanded significantly the capacity of the hematologist to identify the lineage of those cells that appear undifferentiated by light microscopy.

REFERENCES

Ahearn, M., Trujillo, J., Cork, A., Fowler, A., and Hart, J. (1974). The association of nuclear blebs with aneuploidy in human acute leukemia. *Cancer Res.* 34:2887-2896.

Albarracin, N., and Haust, M. (1971). Intravascular coagulation in prolyelocytic leukemia: A case study including ultrastructure. *Am. J. Clin. Pathol.* 55:677-685.

Bain, B., Catovsky, D., O'Brien, M., Spiers, A., and Richards, H. (1977). Megakaryoblastic transformation of chronic granulocytic leukemia: An electron microscopy and cytochemical study. *J. Clin. Path.* 30:677-685.

Bain, B., Catovsky, D., O'Brien, M., Grant-Prentice, H., Lawlor, E., Kumaran, T., McCann, S., Matutes, E., and Galton, D. (1981). Megakaryoblastic leukemia presenting as acute myelofibrosis—a study of four cases with the platelet-peroxidase reaction. *Blood* 58:206-213.

Bainton, D., Ullyot, J., and Farquhar, M. (1971). The development of neutrophilic polymorphonuclear leukocytes in human bone marrow: Origin and content of azurophil and specific granules. *J. Exp. Med.* 134:907-921.

Bassan, H., Gutmann, H., Djaldetti, M. (1980). Ultrastructural characteristics of the plasma cells of a patient with nonsecretory meyloma and plasma cell leukemia. *Acta. Haemat.* 66:129-133.

Begin, L., Osborne, B., and Mackay, B. (1981). Monocytic leukemia with cutaneous involvement: Ultrastructural observations on unusual cytoplasmic complexes. *Ultrastr. Pathol.* 2:11-18.

Bencosme, S., and Tsutsumi, V. (1970). A fast method for processing biologic material for electron microscopy. *Lab. Invest.* 23:447-450.

Bennett, J., Catovsky, D., Daniel, M., Flandring, G., Galton, D., Gralnick, H., and Sultan, C. (1976). Proposals for the classification of the acute leukemias. *Br. J. Haematol.* 33:451-464.

Bessis, M. (1951). Etude au microscope electronique des leucocytes normaux et leucemiques. *Acta First International Cancer Congress* 7:646-649.

Bessis, M. (1973a). The reticulo-histocytic system and the monocyte. In *Living Blood Cells and Their Ultrastructure*. (Translated by R. I. Weed.) Springer-Verlag, New York, pp. 447-517.

Bessis, M. (1973b). Malignancies of cells of the granulocytic series. In *Living Blood Cells and Their Ultrastructure*. (Translated by R. I. Weed.) Springer-Verlag, New York, pp. 568-598.

Bessis, M., and Breton-Gorius, J. (1969). Pathologie et asynchronisme de developpement des organelles cellulaires au cours des leucemies aigues granulocytaires. *Nouvelle Revue Francaise d'Hematologie* 9:245-256.

Bitter, M., Le Beau, M., Larson, R., Rosner, M., Golomb, H., Rowley, J., and Vardiman, J. (1984). A morphologic and cytochemical study of acute myelomonocytic leukemia with abnormal marrow eosinophils associated with inv (16) (p13q22). *Am. J. Clin. Pathol.* 81:733-741.

Breton-Gorius, J. (1974). Apport de la microscopie electronique dans la classification cytologique des leucemies aigues. *Bull. Cancer* 61:367-376.

Breton-Gorius, J., Daniel, M., Fandrin, G., and Kinet-Denoel, G. (1973). Fine structure and peroxidase activity of circulating micromegakaryoblasts and platelets in a case of acute myelofibrosis. *Br. J. Haematol.* 25:331-339.

Breton-Gorius, J., Reyes, F., Duhamel, G., Najman, A., and Gorin, N. (1978). Megakaryoblastic acute leukemia: Identification by the ultrastructural demonstration of platelet peroxidase. *Blood* 51:45-59.

Brouet, J., Valensi, F., Daniel, M., Flandrin, G., Preud'homme, J., and Seligman, M. (1976). Immunologic classification of acute lymphoblastic leukaemias: Evaluation of its clinical significance in a hundred patients. *Br. J. Haematol.* 33:319-328.

Brunning, R., and Parkin, J. (1975). Ribosome lamella complexes in neoplastic hematopoietic cells. *Am. J. Pathol.* 79:565-578.

Carr, I., and Toner, P. (1977). Rapid electron microscopy in oncology. *J. Clin. Pathol.* 30:13-15.

Catovsky, D. (1977). Immunologic cell markers in acute leukemia: classification of acute leukemia. *Ann. Intern. Med.* 87:740-753.

Cawley, J., and Hayhoe, F. (1973). Acute myeloblastic (granulocytic) leukemia (AGL) and acute myelomonocytic leukemia. In *Ultrastructure of Haemic Cells: A Cytological Atlas of Normal and Leukemic Blood and Bone Marrow*, W.B. Saunders Co. Ltd., London, pp. 156-214.

Childs, C., Ahearn, M., Trujillo, J., Ruben, J., Cork, A., Walters, R., and Stass, S. (1986). Lineage heterogeneity in acute leukemia with the t(4;11) abnormality: Implications for acute mixed lineage leukemia. *Am. J. Clin. Path.* 86:403.

Costello, C., Catovsky, D., O'Brien, M., and Galton, D. (1980). Prolymphocytic leukemia: An ultrastructural study of 22 cases. *Br. J. of Haematol.* 44:389-394.

Dalton, W., Ahearn, M., Cork, A., Trujillo, J., Keating, M., McCredie, K., Freireich, E., and Stass, S. (1985). Nuclear blebs in eosinophils in acute leukemia associated with inversion of chromosome 16 [Inv(16) (p13q22)]. *Blood* 66:234a.

Djaldetti, M. (1982). Mitochondrial abnormalities in the cells of myeloma patients. *Act Haemat.* 68:241-249.
Djaldetti, M. (1984). Plasma cell leukemia: Ultrastructural aspects in diagnosis. In *Human Leukemias*, A. Polliack (ed.). Martinus Nijhoff Publishing Co., Boston, pp. 309-326.
Edelman, B., and Grossman, N. (1983). Microgranular acute promyelocytic leukemia: A case with multiple Auer rods demonstrable only after staining for chloroacetate esterase. *Am. J. Clin. Pathol.* 79:621-625.
Efrati, P., Nir, E., Yaari, A., Berrebi, A., Kaplan, H., and Dvilanski, A. (1979). Myeloproliferative disorders terminating in acute micromegakaryblastic leukemia. *Br. J. Haematol.* 43:79-86.
Estes, L., and Apicella, J. (1969). A rapid embedding technique for electron microscopy. *Lab. Invest.* 20:159-163.
Freeman, J. (1966). Origin of Auer bodies. *Blood* 27:449-510.
Fujita, K., Yamada, K., Sato, T., Takagi, I., and Sakashita, T. (1977). A rapid method for embedding biological tissues in a low viscosity epoxy resin "Quetol 651" for electron microscopy. *J. Electron Microsc.* 26:165-166.
Galton, D., Goldman, J., Wiltshaw, E., Catovsky, D., Henry, H., and Goldenberg, G. (1974). Prolymphocytic leukaemia. *Br. J. Haematol.* 27:7-23.
Glick, A. (1976). Acute leukemia: Electron microscopic diagnosis. *Seminars Oncol.* 3:229-241.
Glick, A., Paniker, K., Flexner, J., and Collins, R. (1980). Acute leukemia in adults. *Am. J. Clin. Pathol.* 73:459-470.
Golomb, H., Rowley, J., Vardiman, J., Testa, J., and Butler, A. (1980). Microgranular acute promyelocytic leukemia: A distinct clinical, ultrastructural and cytogenetic entity. *Blood* 55:253-259.
Hayat, M., and Giaquinta, R. (1970). Rapid fixation and embedding for electron microscopy. *Tissue Cell* 2:191-195.
Hayat, M. (1986). Fixation. In *Basic Techniques for Transmission Electron Microscopy*, Academic Press, New York, pp. 31-55.
Hayhoe, F., and Cawley, J. (1972). Acute leukemia: Cellular morphology, cytochemistry and fine structure. *Clinics in Haematol.* 1:49-62.
Hirsch, C., Trujillo, J., Cork, A., Ahearn, M., Ruben, J., Keating, M., McCredie, K., Freireich, E., Walters, R., Dalton, W., and Stass, S. (1986). Philadelphia chromosome positive acute leukemia: Evidence for mixed lineage. *Am. J. Clin. Path.* 86:402-403.
Jansson, S., Gripenberg, J., Vuopio, P., Teerenhovi, L., and Anderson, L. (1980). Classification of acute leukemia by light and electron microscope cytochemistry. *Scand. J. Haematol.* 25:412-416.
Kamiyama, R. (1971). An electron microscopic study of erythroleukaemia with special reference to the structure of erythroblasts. *Acta Pathol. Japan* 21:231-243.
Kass, L. (1982). Plasma cell leukemia. In *Leukemia Cytology and Cytochemistry*, J.B. Lippincott, Philadelphia, pp. 232-239.
Kitani, T., Yonezawa, T., Imanaka, T., Hiraoka, A., and Nasu, T. (1982). Ultrastructural analysis of membrane-bound polysomes in human myeloma cells. *Blut* 44:51-63.

Kjeldsberg, C., Gearman, R., and Rappaport, H. (1980). Prolymphocytic leukemia: An ultrastructural study. *Am. J. Clin. Pathol.* 73:150-159.

Koike, T. (1984). Megakaryoblastic leukemia: The characterization and identification of megakaryoblasts. *Blood* 64:683-692.

Krishan, A., Uzman, B., and Hadley-Whyte, E. (1967). Nuclear bodies: A component of cell nuclei in hamster tissues and human tumors. *J. Ultrastruc. Res.* 19:563-572.

McDuffie, G. (1967). Nuclear blebs in human leukemia cells. *Nature* 214:1341-1344.

Mangan, K., Rouch, A., Bishop, M., Spiers, A., Lorch, C., and Scharfman, W. (1985). Acute lymphoblastic leukemia of Burkitt's-type (L-3 ALL) lacking surface immunologlobulin and the 8:14-translocation. *Am. J. Clin. Pathol.* 83:121-126.

Marie, J., Vernant, J., Dreyfus, B., and Breton-Gorius, J. (1979). Ultrastructural localization of peroxidase in undifferentiated blasts during the blast crisis of chronic granulocytic leukemia. *Br. J. Haematol.* 43:549-558.

Marie, J., Perrot, J., Boucheux, C., Zittoun, J., Martyre, M., Kaybanda, M., Rosenfeld, C., Mishal, Z., and Zittoun, R. (1982). Determination of ultrastructural peroxidase and immunologic membrane markers in the diagnosis of acute leukemias. *Blood* 59:270-276.

Martelli, M., Falini, B., Tabilio, A., and Velardi, A. (1980). Prolymphocytic leukaemia with erythrophagocytic activity. *Br. J. of Haematol.* 46:141-142.

Mirchondani, I., and Palutke, A. (1982). Acute megakaryoblastic leukemia. *Cancer* 50:2866-2872.

Norberg, B., Rydgren, L., and Stenstam, M. (1974). Amoeboid movement configuration. A cell configuration observed in tumour cells from 3 cases of bone marrow neoplasia. *Scand. J. Haematol.* 13:294-304.

O'Brien, M., Catovsky, D., and Costello, C. (1980). Ultrastructural cytochemistry of leukaemic cells: Characterization of the early small granules of monoblasts. *Br. J. Haematol.* 45:201-298.

Palakavongs, P., Teichberg, S., Vinciguerra, V., Degnan, T., and Sinlaratana, P. (1977). Ultrastructural cytochemical analysis of blastic transformation of chronic myelocytic leukemia. *Blood* 49:535-547.

Parkin, J., and Brunning, R. (1978). Unusual configurations of endoplasmic reticulum in cells of acute promyelocytic leukemia. *J. Natl. Cancer Inst.* 61:341-348.

Parkin, J., Arthur, D., Abramson, C., McKennia, R., Kersey, J., Heideman, R., and Brunning, R. (1982). Acute leukemia associated with the t(4;11) chromosome rearrangement: Ultrastructural and immunologic characteristics. *Blood* 60:1321-1331.

Payne, B., Kim, H., Pangalis, G., Rothman, A., and Rappaport, H. (1980). A method for the ultrastructural demonstration of nonspecific esterase in human blood and lymphoid tissue. *Histochem. J.* 12:84-94.

Polli, N., Zola, H., and Catovsky, D. (1984). Characterization by ultrastructural cytochemistry of normal and leukemic myeloid cells reacting with monoclonal antibodies. *Am. J. Clin. Pathol.* 82:389-395.

Polli, N., O'Brien, M., Tavares de Castro, J., Matutes, E., San Miguel, J., and Catovsky, D. (1985). Characterization of blast cells in chronic granulocytic leukemia in transformation, acute myelofibrosis and undifferentiated leukemia, I: Ultrastructural morphology and cytochemistry. Br. J. Haematol. 59:277-296.

Polliack, A., and Leizerowitz, R. (1983). Cytochemistry and ultrastructure in lymphoma and leukemia: Utility in the diagnosis of leukemias and the recognition of subtypes of lymphoproliferative disorders. *Hematol. Oncology.* 1: 110-126.

Rajnoldi, A., Ferrari, M., Secchi, G., Uderzo, C., and Masera, G. (1981). Atypical acute promyelocytic leukemia (M3 variant): description of two cases. *Acta Haematol.* 65:44-49.

Rowden, G., and Lewis, M. (1974). Experience with a three hour electron microscopy biopsy service. *J. Clin. Pathol.* 27:505-510.

Schmalzl, F., Huhn, D., Asamer, H., Rindler, R., and Braunsteiner, H. (1973). Cytochemistry and ultrastructure of pathologic granulations in myelogenous leukemia. *Blut* 27:243-260.

Schumacher, H., Robinson, J., Creegan, W., Perlin, E., and Miller, W. (1977). Hand-mirror-cell leukemia. *Lancet* 8012:655-656.

Shaw, M. (1980). Monocytic leukemia. *Human Pathol.* 11:215-227.

Smetna, K., Gyorkey, F., and Bush, H. (1969). On the ultrastructure of nucleoli in human leukemic myeloblasts. *Exp. Cell Res.* 58:303-311.

Stass, S., Perlin, E., Jaffe, E., Simon, D., Creegan, W., Robinson, J., Holloway, M., and Schumacher, H. (1978). Acute lymphoblastic leukemia—hand-mirror cell variant: a detailed cytological and ultrastructural study with an analysis of the immunological surface markers. *Am. J. Hematol.* 4:66-67.

Staven, P., Rorvik, T., Blichfeldt, P., and Hagen, C. (1981). Differing form of variant of hypergranular promyelocytic leukaemia (M3) or transition between M3 and monocytic leukemia? *Scand. J. Haematol.* 26:149-152.

Tabilio, A., Vainchenker, W., Van Haecke, D., Vinci, G., Guichard, J., Henri, R., Reyes, F., and Breton-Gorius, J. (1984). Immunological characterization of the leukemic megakaryocytic line at light and electron microscopic levels. *Leukemia Research* 8:769-781.

Tomonaga, M., Yoshida, Y., Tagawa, M., Jinnai, I., Kuriyama, K., Amenomori, T., Yoshioka, A., Matsuo, T., Nonaka, H., and Ichimaru, M. (1985). Cytochemistry of acute promyelocytic leukemia (M3): Leukemic promyelocytes exhibit heterogeneous patterns in cellular differentiation. *Blood* 66:350-357.

White, J. (1967). Fine structure demonstration of acid phosphatase activity in Auer bodies. *Blood* 29:667-682.

Yonezawa, T., Kitani, T., Tamaki, ?., Kanayama, Y., Hiraoka, A., and Tarui, S. (1982). Immunoglobulin production and secretion in Bence Jones protein myeloma and "nonsecretory" myeloma. *Blut* 45:121-129.

Youness, E., Trujillo, J., Ahearn, M., McCredie, K., and Cork, A. (1980). Acute unclassified leukemia: A clinicopathologic study with diagnostic implications of electron microscopy. *Am. J. Hematol.* 9:79-88.

Zicca, A., Leprini, A., Cadoni, A., Franzi, A., Ferrarini, M., and Grossi, C. (1981). Ultrastructural localization of alpha napthyl acid esterase in human T lymphocytes. *Am. J. Pathol.* 105:40-46.

4

Flow Cytochemistry in the Diagnosis of Acute Leukemia

BENJAMIN DREWINKO *The University of Texas System Cancer Center, M. D. Anderson Hospital and Tumor Institute, Houston, Texas*

I. INTRODUCTION

The H-6000 hematology analyzer* is an automated instrument that provides, in addition to rapid, accurate, and precise measurements of traditional hematology parameters (WBC and RBC counts, hematocrit), a differential count on 10^4 WBC separated into categories that are equivalent to those recognized on the basis of morphological criteria (1-5). This machine-made WBC differential count is effected by a combination of technological innovations in flow cytometry mechanics, and cytochemical (peroxidase content) and physical (light scattering) quantitative measurements. Because of these unique characteristics, the H-6000 instrument can theoretically provide diagnostic, prognostic and monitoring functions for patients with hematopoietic malignancies. As the normal WBC in the peripheral blood are replaced by an ever-increasing number of abnormal elements, the instrument analyzes, registers and computes these cells under criteria established for the normal WBC. This process results in an altered distribution of "normal" cell categories as well as in the appearance and preponderance of new cell classes—large unstained cells (LUC) and cells with high peroxidase content (HPX)—as well as new parameters (for example, mean peroxidase or MPA) that may serve as indicators of the nature and extent of the abnormal state.

This chapter describes the flow cytochemical patterns and changing parameters associated with the major entities of acute leukemia, and demonstrates the usefulness of automated WBC differentials in the diagnosis and prognostic evaluation of the peripheral blood of patients with such diseases.

Studies were effected on the peripheral blood of 118 patients admitted to M. D. Anderson Hospital with the diagnosis of acute leukemia; 68 patients had not

---

*Manufactured by Technicon Instruments Corp., Tarrytown, N.Y., 10591.

been treated and 50 patients had received some form of chemotherapy within the days preceding our evaluation. Of the untreated patients, 36 had acute granulocytic leukemia; 25 had acute lymphocytic leukemia, and 7 patients were diagnosed as having hairy cell leukemia (HC). Of the 50 treated patients, 27 had acute granulocytic leukemia and 23 had acute lymphocytic leukemia. Serial follow-up determinations were obtained on 32 previously treated and on 22 untreated patients during the first course of chemotherapy. Of the patients with available sequential follow-up determinations, 19 (14 with granulocytic and 5 with lymphocytic leukemia) had evaluations performed on days 11, 12, or 13 post-induction chemotherapy and were utilized to examine the general validity of using the ratios of LUC to lymphocytes obtained on such days as predictors of remission induction (6,7). In addition, blood was collected from 50 healthy volunteers (31 males) ranging in age from 18 to 71 years.

Laboratory hematology workup at M. D. Anderson Hospital for patients with presumed leukemia includes a complete automated hematology survey and a peripheral blood WBC differential count (8). All cases are segregated according to the French-American-British (FAB) classification (9). For our study, an aliquot of the peripheral blood obtained for routine laboratory hematology evaluation was also processed through the H-6000 automated hematology analyzer within 4 hours of the venipuncture.

The study included extensive statistical analysis of data. Analysis of variance of mean values and ranks (Kruskal-Wallis tests) were used for discriminatory analysis of WBC, MPA, HPX and LUC among the leukemia categories (10). Student-Newman-Keuls mean rank tests were used to compare means of leukemia categories. Logarithmic transformations (base 10) were made to stabilize variances over leukemia categories as is common with this type of data so that the analysis of variance was also performed comparing log harmonic means. Student's t test and Mann-Whitney rank test were utilized for evaluation of LUC to lymphocyte ratios on days 11 through 13 as predictors of remission.

II. FLOW CYTOCHEMICAL CYTOMETRY

The H-6000 is the only available fully automated hematology analyzer that utilizes the principles of flow cytometry to provide, in addition to the eight traditional CBC parameters, a five-part WBC differential count based on cell size and cytochemical characteristics. The instrument requires 400 μL of blood, which are processed in a series of manifolds. Within the "alkaline peroxidase" manifold, RBC are lysed and WBC enzymes are fixed and stained cytochemically for peroxidase. The flow stream of fixed and stained cells is analyzed by an electro-optical system axially positioned around a common tungsten-halogen light source. Signals are analyzed by the Signal Processing and Decision Logic circuit, which classifies cells into categories equivalent to those identified morphologically in the peripheral blood. Cells are segregated on the basis of light scatter characteristics, which reflect cell size, and light absorption, which measures peroxidase content; basophils are identified on the basis of 2-color analysis following Alcian blue staining in a separate manifold. This procedure produces a 2-dimensional diagram (abscissa = light absorption; ordinate = light scatter), which identifies each cell category by the position of the dots in the diagram (Figure 1). The display has a superimposed grid with fixed and moving thresholds. The two fixed vertical thresholds designate the lower (A_L) and the arbitrarily set upper (A_H) limits of light absorption, while the two-fixed horizontal thresholds specify the lower (S_L) and upper (S_H) limits of light scatter. Because there are considerable interindividual variations in the distribution of peroxidase content in WBC, an analog signal output analyzer applied to the peroxidase absorbance channel determines the peak of this frequency distribution; the analysis automatically sets two additional mobile tracking thresholds, low ($A'_L = 0.75 \times$ peak) and high ($A'_H = 1.3 \times$ peak), which traverse the S_H abscissa.

RBC stroma and platelets are represented by a cluster of dots that appears in the lower left corner of the display in the area bound by the S_L and A_L limits. Lymphocytes are encompassed in the area delineated by S_L, A_L, and S_H. Monocytes (and basophils), identified by their low peroxidase content, will appear in the region delineated by A_L and the low tracking threshold A'_L, while the majority of neutrophils are encompassed between A'_L and A'_H. Eosinophils appear in the region below the S_H threshold because their high peroxidase content attenuates this light scatter and makes them appear smaller than their true size. Dots located in the upper left corner (above S_H and to the left of A_L) represent the so-called large unstained cells, LUC, which usually comprise variant monocytes or lymphocytes, and blasts.

The presence of the tracking thresholds and the analysis on which they are based provide additional parameters. Determination of the peak value of the peroxidase content distribution originates the "mean peroxidase activity" (MPA) function, which can be calculated manually (in volt units) as v/0.75, where v is the distance of A_L to A'_L along the S_H abscissa. Cells represented to the right of the A'_H have a comparatively (sometimes inordinately) higher amount of peroxidase and are classified as WBC with high peroxidase content (HPX). When the peroxidase content of the entire WBC population is low, the width of the distribution may be retained, but the lower tracking threshold, A'_L, may approach (within 1.2 volt units), or merge with, A_L. In this case, the instrument will print a signal (flag) LPX (low peroxidase) in the printout display. When the total number of cells with peroxidase activity is low (i.e., neutropenia or cells with a flat, markedly abnormal distribution of peroxidase content), the interval bound by a 50% limit about the peak value will not register at least 100 cells/second. In this case, the

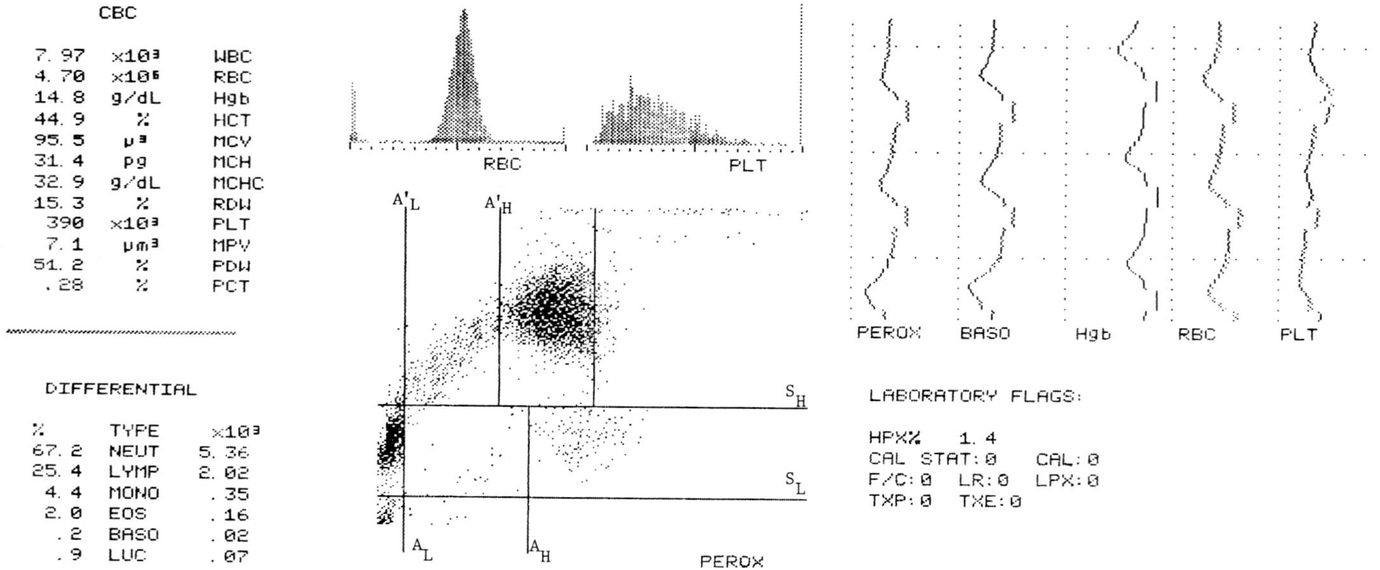

Figure 1 Schematics of an H-6000 dot display indicating fixed and moving thresholds as well as clusters of specific blood-formed elements.

instrument will print another flag, LR (low rate), to alert the operator about this abnormality.

III. FLOW CYTOCHEMICAL PATTERNS IN ACUTE LEUKEMIA

The H-6000 analysis of the peripheral blood of 50 healthy donors displayed the anticipated conventional normal values for all formed elements (WBC, RBC, and platelet counts; hemoglobin; hematocrit; and RBC indices). The median MPA value was 4.0 with a range of 2.8 to 4.6; HPX values ranged from 0.8% to 5.0%; and the proportion of LUC ranged from 0.5% to 3.3% (Table 1). Lymphocytes represented 31.3% ± 6.5% of the differential WBC count.

The peripheral blood of patients with untreated acute leukemia displayed the typical abnormalities of this disease (leukocytosis, and erythro- and thrombocytopenia) as well as characteristic changes in the light scatter and peroxidase absorption properties of the WBC, which permitted a qualified segregation of these specimens according to the FAB classification. With few exceptions, granulocytic leukemias had higher WBC counts, lower MPA values, and higher HPX results than lymphoid leukemias (Table 1) ($p < 0.00001$ for all parameters). In fact, both MPA and HPX values were sufficient to discriminate between these two types of leukemias, especially when the median results (instead of mean values) were considered. With the exception of M3 leukemias, with an inherent high value of peroxidase content conferred by the large number of primary granules present in these malignant blasts, all other granulocytic leukemias had significantly lower ($p < 0.001$) MPA than the blood of normal individuals. In contrast, lymphocytic leukemias had equal or larger MPA values than normal ($p < 0.001$). Ranking of the MPA value for each entity at a significance level of 0.05 is represented in Figure 2. Thus, M1, M4, M5, and M2 leukemias are clearly different from the other entities and from normal individuals. M1 and M5 leukemias presented HPX values slightly but significantly higher than normal; M2, M3 and M4 leukemias showed HPX values severalfold higher than normal. In contrast, lymphoid leukemias showed low HPX values, closer to the lower limit of the normal range. The median values of LUC were very high only for M4 and M5 leukemias and tended to the lower limit of normal in M2 and M3 leukemias. All other leukemias showed median LUC values that were only slightly to moderately (but always significant statistically) above normal. M-type leukemias had normal or below normal proportions of lymphocytes while, with extremely rare exceptions (L1 = 0/12; L2 = 2/12), both L1 and L2 leukemias had "lymphocyte" differential counts at least twice than normal (mean values of 83.6% and 76.5%, respectively) ($p < 0.0001$). Ratios of LUC to lymphocytes for all acute leukemias, and even for lymphocytic leukemia subtypes, were noncontributory. LR and LPX alerts were erratic and unreliable in flagging abnormal peroxidase distributions. Only 53% of all leukemias were flagged by the LR alarm (M2 and M3 subtypes were rarely recognized by this method) and only 9% of all cases were flagged with the LPX alarm; no case of lymphoid leukemia was tagged by this analysis.

Table 1 H-6000 Analysis of the Peripheral Blood of Untreated Acute Leukemia Patients

Leukemia type	N	WBC ($\times 10^3$) Mean	Median	SD	Range	Mean Peroxidase Activity (MPA) Mean	Median	SD	Range
M1	6	22.6	13.3	20.2	1.3-52	2.5	2.0	1.2	1.1-4.3
M2	9	50.8	44.4	39.4	11.7-114	2.8	2.6	1.2	1.5-4.4
M3	6	39.0	17.9	47.7	0.9-124	4.0	3.4	0.9	3.2-5.6
M4	9	29.4	27.4	22.6	3.6-65.7	2.4	2.1	1.0	1.1-3.9
M5	6	32.3	17.8	34.2	2.9-92.5	2.7	2.3	1.0	1.7-4.3
L1	12	84.7	13.4	129.2	1.1-365.6	4.3	4.2	0.5	3.5-5.6
L2	12	30.0	9.8	31.6	3.5-92.1	4.6	4.6	0.8	3.8-6.5
Hairy cell	7	14.8	17.1	9.2	5.6-31.2	3.7	3.8	0.6	2.8-4.6
Normal	50	6.6	6.5	1.7	3.7-10.7	4.0	4.0	0.4	2.8-4.6

LR = low rate; LPX = low peroxidase.

Our single case of untreated L3 leukemia (not shown on Table 1) showed no distinguishing characteristics: WBC, 7.4K/μL; MPA, 4.6; HPX, 6.9; LUC, 2.9; and lymphocytes, 32.6%.

The dot display of cell size vs. peroxidase content for each case showed fairly consistent patterns that may be used to segregate the peripheral blood of patients with acute leukemias along morphologically equivalent guidelines (9). Figure 3 shows a representative scattergram of a case with M1 leukemia, characterized by a high proportion of LUC and an HPX population within normal limits. Some M1 cases may display a high proportion of "monocytes"; in many instances, such cells, clustered between A_L and A'_L, are not true monocytes, but blasts with very low levels of lysosomal myeloperoxidase. Figure 4 shows the diagram of an M2 leukemia; these leukemias are characterized by high to very high HPX values, and low numbers of LUC because the instrument recognizes the blasts as cells with increased peroxidase content and classifies than as "neutrophils." For the same reason, many such blasts will also be located within the "monocyte" compartment, since they contain a lesser amount of peroxidase than those classified as "neutrophils."

A representative case of an M3 leukemia is shown in Figure 5: low LUC and invariably high HPX. The high peroxidase content of the progranulocytes decreases the light scatter to such a degree that it makes some of the blasts appear smaller, cross the upper scatter threshold (S_H), and become classified as "eosinophils." In cases of "microgranular" M3 leukemias (11,12), the dots do not cross

High Peroxidase Content (HPX)(%)				Large Unstained Cells (LUC)(%)				LR	LPX
Mean	Median	SD	Range	Mean	Median	SD	Range	N(%)	N(%)
6.8	5.8	4.6	1.4-13.3	6.8	8.4	4.5	0.6-11.8	4(67)	1(17)
30.7	37.2	16.1	6.7-58.5	7.4	1.7	12.1	0.1-32.9	1(11)	2(22)
34.8	24.0	24.9	4.7-77.1	0.9	0.9	0.6	0.3-2.0	1(17)	0
21.7	18.8	16.8	4.4-52.6	17.0	14.4	14.5	0.8-34.2	6(67)	2(22)
8.3	3.9	8.1	0.9-22.2	31.2	25.1	13.9	13.2-48.4	5(83)	1(17)
1.4	1.5	0.6	0.3-2.5	4.6	3.7	3.9	0.3-14.0	8(66)	0
1.9	1.8	1.0	0.5-3.6	8.0	5.2	5.5	1.6-18.3	7(58)	0
1.1	0.7	0.9	0.2-2.6	14.3	6.0	16.7	1.9-39.3	4(57)	0
2.1	1.9	0.9	0.8-5.0	1.5	1.4	0.6	0.5-3.3	–	–

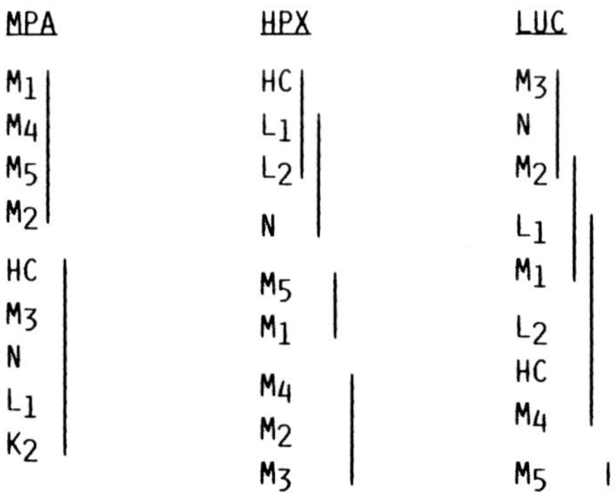

Figure 2 ANOVA analysis of parameters detailed in Table 1. N, normal; HC, hairy cell leukemia; (L and M)$_{i...n}$, lymphocytic or myelocytic FAB classification. Side bars include groups for which there is no statistically significant difference at the 0.05 level. The order of disease entity listed under each parameter reflects the degree of dissimilarity within a group and the rank of distinction with respect to the other groups.

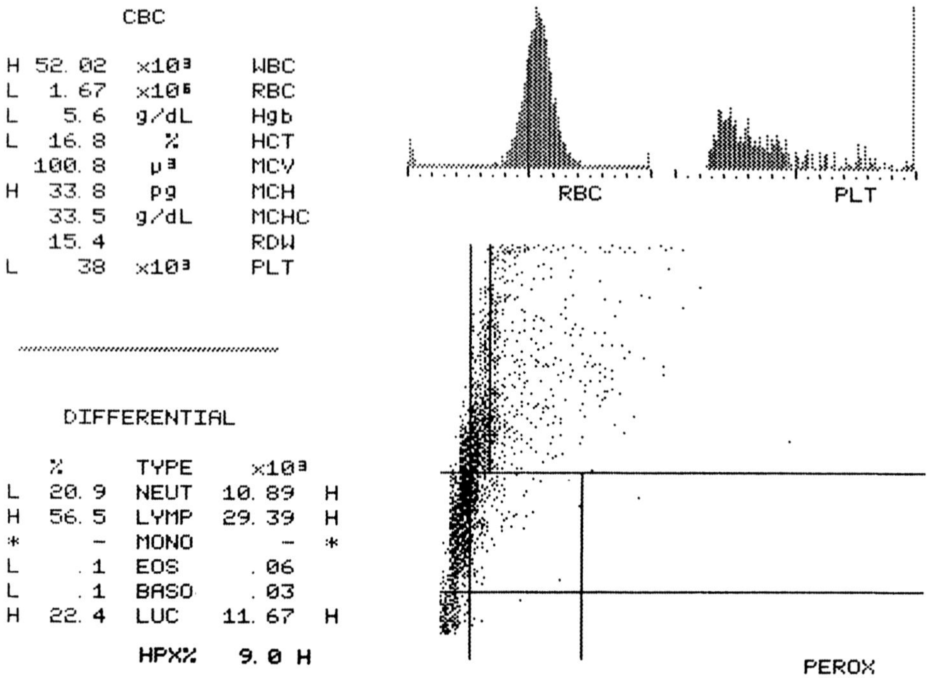

Figure 3 Representative scattergram (peroxidase vs. light scatter) of a patient with M1 leukemia.

S_H and are confined to the upper half of the area bound by S_H and A'_H, in the midst of the HPX region. True nonmalignant eosinophilia is reflected by a cluster of dots neatly encased between the upper and lower scatter thresholds without extending into the HPX area.

M4 leukemias (Figure 6) are characterized by a large LUC population, a considerable monocytic component, and a more modest HPX proportion. This pattern is frequently similar to that of an M1 leukemia except that cases with M4 leukemia often present cells in the area bound by A_L and A'_L, a display seen rather rarely in M1 leukemia. M5 leukemias are characterized by a tilted, elongated cluster of dots that starts in the lymphocyte box and crosses the A_L boundary, reaching the upper limit of the plot (Figure 7). This characteristic generates a large number of LUC and a large proportion of "monocytes," because these blasts have only slight peroxidase activity. In other cases, monoblasts will be identified as "neutrophils" because the tracking thresholds shift to the left and delete the monocyte box. Many small monoblasts devoid of significant peroxidase activity are classified by the instrument as "lymphocytes" on the basis of

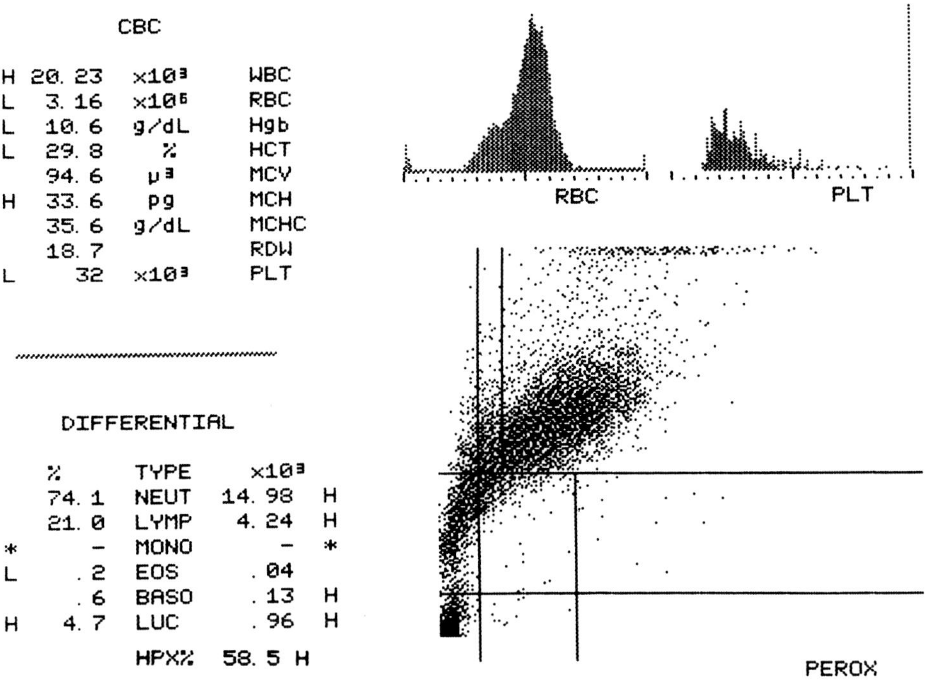

Figure 4 Representative dot display of a patient with M2 leukemia.

size (scatter) alone. The HPX component is only slightly elevated or even within normal limits.

L1 and L2 leukemias present similar patterns: a large cluster of points located primarily in the "lymphocyte" region and extending to the lower third of the LUC compartment. Infrequently, these dots may cross the A_L boundary but, in contrast to M5 leukemias, almost never reach the upper limit of the plot (Figures 8 and 9). Ratios of LUC to lymphocytes are similar for both types of leukemias, and HPX values are essentially within normal limits. The single case of untreated L3 leukemia that we analyzed showed dot display characteristics similar to those of the preceding lymphocytic leukemias. Most hairy cell leukemias (Figure 10) show a typical, almost pathognomonic pattern: a vertical cluster of points extending from the lymphocytic to the LUC box due to the almost equal increment of "lymphocytes" and LUC with only a rare point crossing the A_L boundary.

Following induction treatment, flow cytochemical patterns change enormously and become more difficult to interpret, particularly because chemotherapy

CBC

H	51. 15	x10³	WBC
L	2. 98	x10⁶	RBC
L	8. 6	g/dL	Hgb
L	27. 3	%	HCT
	91. 4	µ³	MCV
	28. 9	pg	MCH
L	31. 7	g/dL	MCHC
	18. 0	%	RDW
L	61	x10³	PLT
	7. 5	µm³	MPV
	62. 9	%	PDW
	. 05	%	PCT

DIFFERENTIAL

	%	TYPE	x10³	
	77. 3	NEUT	39. 55	H
L	4. 2	LYMP	2. 16	
	6. 2	MONO	3. 16	H
H	10. 8	EOS	5. 53	H
	. 5	BASO	. 25	H
	1. 0	LUC	. 50	H

HPX% 40 9 H

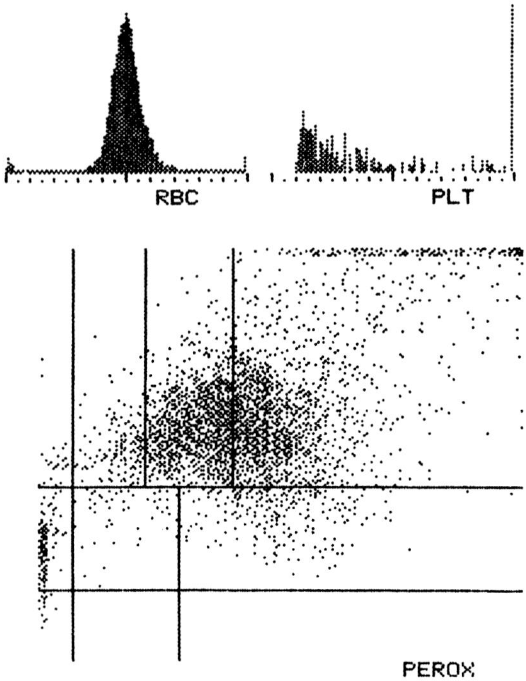

Figure 5 Representative scattergram of a patient with typical M3 leukemia.

may affect the size and peroxidase content of both malignant and normal cells. An increase of LUC is almost always seen following treatment for acute leukemia but these cells are not necessarily blasts, and frequently consist of larger, atypical lymphocytes, monocytes, or both. Such LUC can also be seen in patients with solid tumors following severe myelosuppressive chemotherapy. Generally, an LUC fraction of less than 7% and a low HPX fraction represent the effects of chemotherapy on normal cells, while larger proportions of LUC, and, in the case of M2 through M5 leukemias, larger fractions of HPX, are highly suggestive of true blasts.

Successful chemotherapy in M1 leukemias originates a rather typical sequence of cytochemical patterns: LUC decrease in parallel with the WBC count; LUC continue to stay low even when the WBC as well as the RBC and platelet count commence to rise. HPX cells, usually low in M1 leukemias, drop to almost zero and stay low throughout the course of treatment. In some patients, the proportion of HPX may increase slightly at the time of, and after, the nadir of the WBC

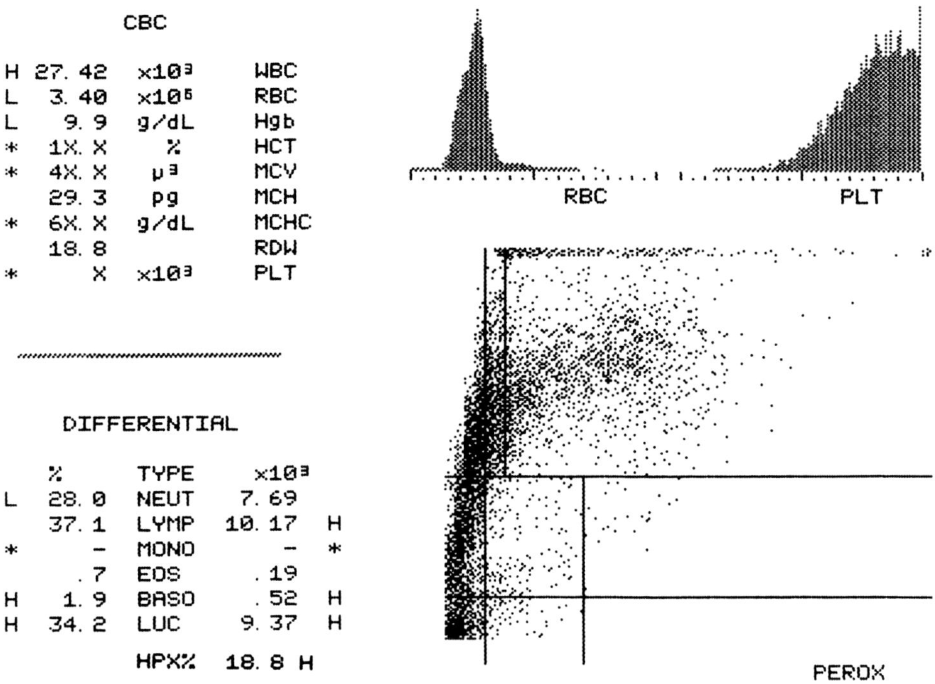

Figure 6 Representative scattergram of a patient with M4 leukemia.

count. M2 leukemias also show typical cytochemical patterns following chemotherapy. These leukemias are characterized by high WBC counts, low LUC fractions, and very high HPX fractions. Successful induction is characterized by a consistent decrease in all three parameters. In particular, a declining WBC count is accompanied by a sharply diminishing HPX fraction, which prognosticates remission. In some instances, the recovering blood contains a larger proportion of LUC than the untreated counterpart, possibly as a reflection of chemotherapy-induced disturbance in myeloperoxidase production. The pattern of M3 leukemias follows an almost identical sequence as that of M2 leukemias. Successful induction results in a sharp decline of HPX and "eosinophils"; failing patients continue to display high proportions of these two elements.

All six patients with M4 leukemia that we followed with consecutive measurements of flow cytochemical patterns failed to enter remission during the follow-up period (first induction course). The sequence of changes was uniform for all: untreated M4 leukemias were characterized by high WBC counts, and elevated LUC and HPX values; after initiating chemotherapy, values for all three parameters

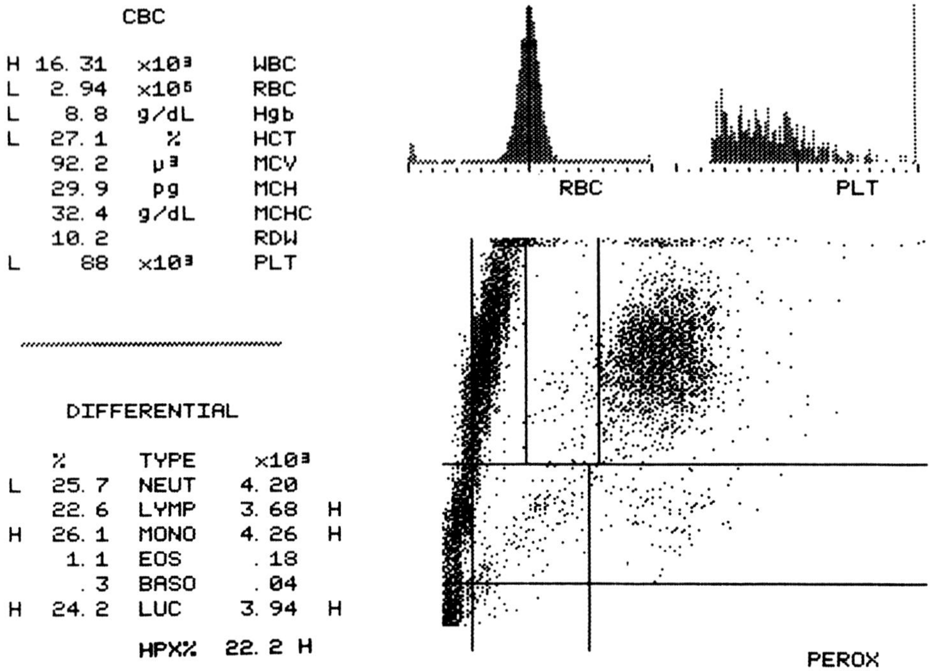

Figure 7 Representative dot display of a patient with M5 leukemia.

initially declined in parallel. However, while the WBC count continued to decrease, HPX or LUC or both stabilized at a high borderline normal or supranormal value. Recurrence (following the WBC count nadir) was heralded by a concomitant elevation of WBC counts and LUC or, more commonly, HPX.

M5 leukemias, characterized by large increments of WBC counts, LUC, and "lymphocytes" and decreased or occasionally slightly above normal HPX values also followed a rather uniform pattern. Induction therapy rapidly lowered the WBC count but the proportion of LUC and "lymphocytes" stayed elevated. Values of LUC above 8% and greater than 30% "lymphocytes" (independent of the WBC count, even with values below 1000 WBC/μl) were always associated with a relapsed marrow following marrow recovery. Sometimes, these patients presented transient elevations of HPX (possibly indicating the rebound of a clone of normal granulocytes) but these values rapidly decreased when the marrow rebounded with a high proportion of LUC (which were recognized as blasts by microscopy). The only M5 case that we followed into remission had a rapid decrement of LUC (to less than 8%) and a more gradual decrease for "lympho-

CBC

H	57.93	$\times 10^3$	WBC
L	4.19	$\times 10^6$	RBC
L	10.3	g/dL	Hgb
L	32.1	%	HCT
L	76.6	μ^3	MCV
L	24.6	pg	MCH
	32.2	g/dL	MCHC
	18.5	%	RDW
	195	$\times 10^3$	PLT
	7.0	μm^3	MPV
	57.7	%	PDW
	.14	%	PCT

DIFFERENTIAL

	%	TYPE	$\times 10^3$	
L	10.3	NEUT	5.95	
H	75.5	LYMP	43.72	H
L	.7	MONO	.43	
	1.3	EOS	.76	H
H	1.6	BASO	.95	H
H	10.6	LUC	6.11	H
		HPX%	1.9	

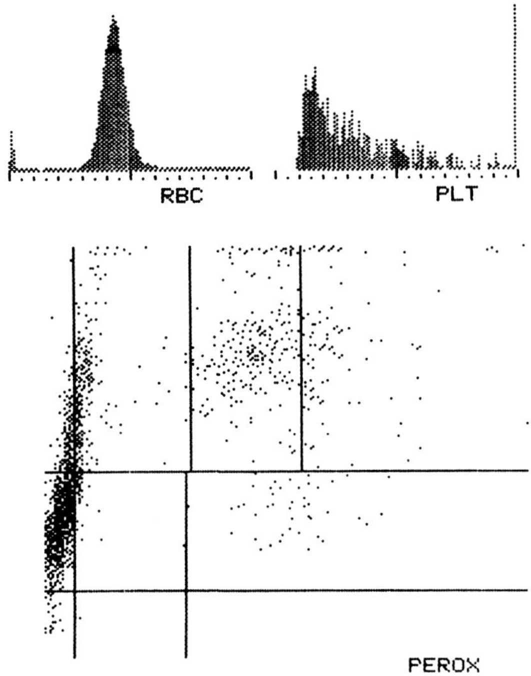

Figure 8 Representative scattergram of a patient with L1 leukemia.

cytes," a transient moderate increase in HPX and, finally, a trend for all values to return to normal limits when the WBC and platelet count recovered.

The post-induction treatment sequence of changes for both L1 and L2 leukemias were identical: an immediate drop in WBC and LUC, the latter frequently reaching normal limits. However, unless the "lymphocyte" count approached or fell below 50%, the patient would not enter remission and, upon recovery of the WBC count, the blood would, again, contain large numbers of "lymphocytes" and LUC (identified as blasts microscopically). For patients entering remission, the drop in WBC counts and LUC values was accompanied by a slower but steady decrease in "lymphocytes" and an almost invariable moderate increase in HPX. The latter decreased to normal values upon bone marrow recovery and clinical remission. It must be indicated that occasional patients showed spikes in LUC values upon attaining or passing the WBC count nadir; however, these were transient and always below 7%, and probably reflected chemotherapy-induced changes. The only case of L3 leukemia we could follow had changes similar to

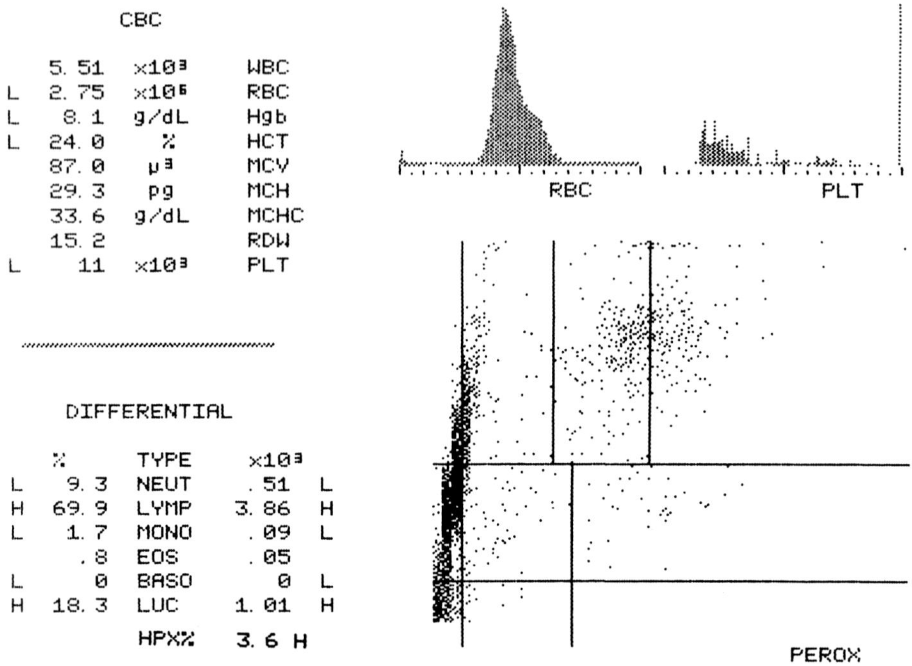

Figure 9 Representative dot display of a patient with L2 leukemia.

those described for the preceding lymphocytic leukemias entering remission, but changes in "lymphocyte" and LUC proportions were not as dramatic (probably because the original values were not as high as those of the L1 and L2 leukemias), and the HPX spike was higher. The sequence of changes of hairy cell leukemias when cytotoxic therapy was instituted followed the pattern of lymphoid leukemia: a rapid drop of WBC and LUC, and a slower decrease of "lymphocytes." If the latter stayed above 70%, the patient did not enter remission.

Arnstrom and associates have suggested that the ratios of LUC to lymphocytes analyzed on day 12 after chemotherapy could be used as prognostic markers of remission (6,7). We evaluated 19 patients for whom we had sequential patterns. However, because of a variety of academic, procedural and administrative reasons, we were unable to collect a population with homogeneous treatments that could always be measured on day 12. Virtually all of the M patients had chemotherapy protocols based on AMSA, vincristine and prednisone with the addition of either the traditional low- or the new high-dose cytosine arabinoside (ara-C). One patient received VP-16 and cytoxan, and 2 received interferon. Similarly,

CBC

H	31. 23	x10³	WBC
L	2. 98	x10⁶	RBC
L	9. 2	g/dL	Hgb
L	27. 2	%	HCT
	91. 1	µ³	MCV
	30. 9	pg	MCH
	33. 9	g/dL	MCHC
	22. 9	%	RDW
L	58	x10³	PLT
	9. 5	µm³	MPV
	67. 2	%	PDW
	. 06	%	PCT

DIFFERENTIAL

	%	TYPE	x10³	
L	1. 0	NEUT	. 31	L
H	59. 4	LYMP	18. 55	H
L	. 2	MONO	. 07	L
L	. 1	EOS	. 02	L
L	. 1	BASO	. 02	
H	39. 3	LUC	12. 27	H
		HPX%	. 2	

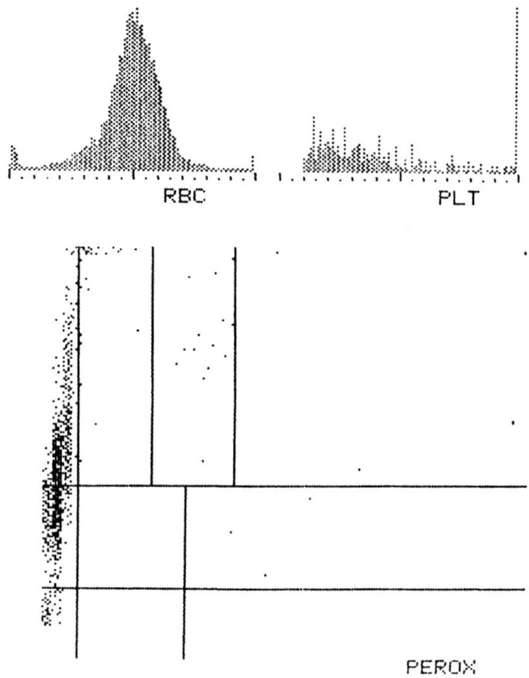

Figure 10 Representative dot display of a patient with hairy cell leukemia.

our L patients had either high or low dose ara-C, plus methotrexate, vincristine, daunomycin, prednisone, dexamethasone and/or cytoxan. Similarly, we elected to evaluate results on days 11 or 13 when a flow cytochemical pattern was unavailable on day 12. Eight patients (6M; 2L) eventually entered remission, and 11 (8M; 3L) failed to enter remission (although some eventually did with additional courses of chemotherapy). The ratios of LUC to lymphocytes for those entering remission ranged from 0.000 to 0.260 (mean 0.049), while those of nonremitting patients ranged from 0.006 to 2.013 (mean 0.102). These results were not statistically significant either by the Student's or the Mann-Whitney tests ($p > 0.2$ and $p > 0.05$ respectively). Since M2 and M3 leukemias do not usually contain large numbers of LUC, we deleted the 6 patients with these diseases leaving 6 responding patients (4 with granulocytic, 2 with lymphocytic) and 7 nonresponding individuals (4 with granulocytic; 3 lymphocytic), which again showed no statistically significant difference ($p > 0.2$ and $p > 0.1$, respectively).

IV. CONCLUSION

Several reports have presented the performance characteristics of the H-6000 as an automated hematology quantifier of traditional CBC parameters (1,3,5,13-15). However, few reports have described the additional capabilities of this instrument as an automated differentiator of cell classes equivalent to those recognized on classical morphological attributes and the relevance of utilizing this analytical proficiency for enhanced diagnostic and monitoring functions in hematopoietic disease (1,2,4,5,16). Other investigators have previously discussed the value of the preceding model, the Hemalog D, in the diagnosis and followup of patients with leukemia (1,4,6,7,13,15,17-24,36), but this concept has not yet become widely utilized. Our report demonstrates that the H-6000 automated analyzer can, indeed, serve as a rapid and flexible tool for provisional diagnosis in hematopoietic malignancies including preliminary classification according to FAB criteria, while awaiting the traditionally definitive (morphological) conclusions. In addition, its intrinsic capabilities provide new valuable parametric quantifications that can be utilized with other sophisticated measurements to predict and to follow the outcome of therapeutic intervention. The typical patterns serve to differentiate these leukemic entities and the sequential changes in the new parameters, MPA, HPX and LUC, are useful to follow the course of disease, independent of the classic microscopic examination. It can be anticipated that additional, formal, and larger studies may yet uncover new ways of utilizing this information and will provide corroborative support to our present contentions. For instance, Swan already proposed the usefulness of the MPA in the evaluation of disease (20), but it is only after our study that its discriminatory value has been demonstrated. Our data, however, are somewhat at variance with the reports of other investigators who also studied acute leukemias with the Hemalog D (4,13-15,19,22,24,36). In our experience, the two alarms, LR and LPX, were useless in flagging disease as their rate of appearance was no greater than chance (i.e., 50%). Similarly, LUC were inadequate by themselves to demonstrate blasts as several granulocytic blasts were registered as HPX due to the characteristics of the peroxidase content distribution. This discrepancy could be ascribed to the different instruments used in the analysis (H-6000 vs. Hemalog D) but also to the bias in leukemic cases selected by these investigators who had a heavy preponderance of leukemic types that contain large numbers of LUC (e.g., M1, L1). Our analysis of the LUC to lymphocytic ratios following induction chemotherapy showed numerical results similar to those reported by the Danish investigators (6,7); but, in contrast, our data was not statistically significant. This discrepancy could be attributed to the fact that their studies included a more homogeneous population than ours and was always evaluated on day 12. Additional evaluations in larger numbers of patients are required to definitely establish the value of this parameter.

Our primitive attempts to introduce automated, machine-assisted criteria in the diagnosis and follow up of patients with acute leukemia must by necessity be met with utmost opposition* by traditional hematologic morphologists (1, 19,25,26). However, the arguments for this resistance must be placed in the historical perspective that even Ehrlich's demonstration that "white cells" could indeed be differentiated into colorful elements was met with skepticism and discredit (27), that diagnostic concordance of acute leukemia among traditional morphological evaluators varies from 56% (almost pure chance) to 70% (28-30), and that even when the FAB cooperative group reported their experience with lymphocytic leukemia (31), concordance increased only to a dubious 84% (by accepting 6 agreements and one disagreement among 7 observers). These are not unexpected failures of the human observer "instrument" and are accepted as unavoidable errors in medical practice. In contrast, machines provide significantly enhanced precision in the parameters they measure compared to the human observer. Thus, we can conceive that judicious selection of these now-reliable parameters will result in an improvement of the quality of patient care that will not be hindered by the limitations of the human sensory capabilities.

V. ADDENDUM

At the time of preparing this manuscript, we are also evaluating the latest version of automated flow cytochemical instrumentation, the H*1 flow cytometer, also manufactured by Technicon Instruments Corp. of Tarrytown, N.Y. (32-35). This system is a fully automated analyzer that uses 100 μL of blood to provide high speed measurements of traditional hematology parameters (e.g., WBC counts, hemoglobin [HGB] concentration levels), computations of newly accepted parameters (such as platelet volume distributions), and a complete WBC differential count equivalent to the traditional morphological classification. Revolutionary innovations in fluidics, reagents, and analytical mathematics provide a variety of useful indicators of hematological abnormalities (for example, flagging of red blood cell [RBC] morphological changes), and map displays of RBC volume vs. HGB content, and WBC size vs. peroxidase content. Further classification of leukocytes is performed in a basophil/lobularity (BASO) channel by stripping the cytoplasm from all WBC except basophils; a laser light scattering system quantifies basophils by their large, low-angle scatter and classifies the remaining cell nuclei as mononuclear or polymorphonuclear cells based on wide-angle light scatter of nuclear lobularity. WBC flags are generated based on cellular distributions in

*"There is nothing more difficult to take in hand, more perilous to conduct, or more uncertain in its success, than to take the lead in the introduction of a new order to things. Because the innovator has for enemies all those who have done well under the old conditions and lukewarm defenders in those who may do well under the new."–*Machiavelli*

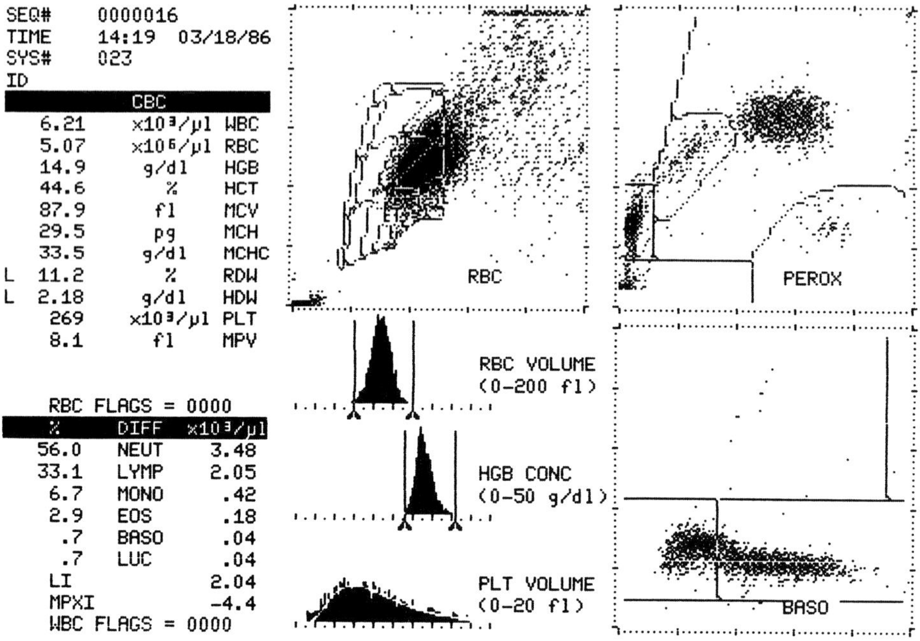

Figure 11 Facsimile of a printout of a normal blood specimen analyzed by the H*1. (See text for description.)

both the peroxidase (perox) and the BASO channels (suspected WBC left shifts, presence of blasts, variant lymphocytes, and/or nucleated RBC).

Figure 11 gives the typical arrangement of a routine screen display from the H*1 of a normal blood specimen. To the left of the display are the parametric CBC and WBC differential counts presented in tabular form. Included are values for 2 new parameters: lobularity index (LI) and mean peroxidase index (MPXI). The upper central portion exhibits a contour map of RBC size vs. HGB content, while the lower portion reveals distribution histograms for RBC volume, HGB concentration, and platelet volume. If desired, the H*1 can present a screen, similar in all aspects to this one, but with the upper middle portion displaying the table of morphology flags (highlighted with a + mark when abnormal) instead of the contour map. Finally, the right portion of the display presents the scattergrams for cell size vs. peroxidase content (perox plot), and size vs. structure of cytoplasm-stripped WBC (BASO plot). The particular locations of each WBC entity in each such plot have been described elsewhere (34). The peculiar shape in the BASO plot of the cluster with a bulky head agglomerating mononuclear

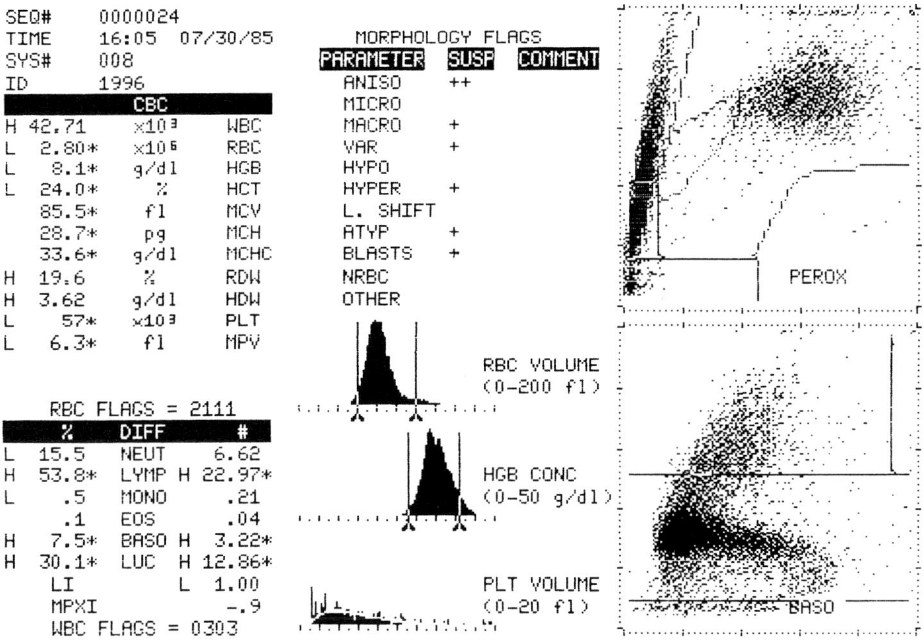

Figure 12 Printout of an H*1 analysis of a patient with L1 leukemia.

(MN) cells, a narrow neck, and an elongated body that comprises the polymorphonuclear (PMN) cells has been colloquially described as that of a "caterpillar."

Figure 12 presents a rather typical display of a case with L2 leukemia. The perox plot reveals a large cluster extending from the lymphocyte to the LUC region with only a small remnant of normal neutrophils. The BASO plot reveals the most interesting feature: an inclined trailing of dots issuing directly from the head of the cytogram into the basophil region (thus yielding equivocally high basophil counts). This pattern has been noted in 3 of 6 untreated L1 leukemias and in 6 of 9 untreated L2 leukemias. Interestingly, every one of these cases of ALL had WBC counts greater than 20 K/μL and frequently surpassing 100 K/μL. All of the cases with no trailing had WBC counts lower than 20 K/μL and frequently lower than 5 K/μL. Yet, because many of the cases with high WBC counts were analyzed in the H*1 after a 1:5 or 1:10 dilution with autologous plasma, the actual number of WBC presented to the machine was similar to that of the cases with lower WBC counts and no trailing. Thus, we conclude that the trailing is not the result of a high WBC count's being a limiting factor for the surfacting agents, but reveals a true association between resistance to cytoplasmic stripping and high WBC counts. If this resistance of the cell membrane and cytoplasm of blasts to be lysed in vitro reflects a similar resistance to be destroyed in vivo by normal cell aging or immunosurveillance processes, it would provide an explanation for the high WBC counts observed for these patients; thus, the finding would offer an additional prognostic marker for this disease, since high WBC counts are a poor prognostic sign for patients with ALL.

Thus, the enhanced performance of the H*1 instruments and the new vistas opened by the novel technology make this flow cytometric-based instrument a futuristic technological advance in the field of automated laboratory hematology and make the trend for "hematology beyond the microscope" (1,21) an impending reality.

REFERENCES

1. Simson, E. (ed.) (1984). *Hematology Beyond the Microscope*. Technicon Instruments Corporation. Health/Communication/Projects, Inc., Tarrytown, N.Y.
2. Panke, T. (1984). Workshop on interpretation of Technicon H6000 system reports in diagnosis of disease. In *Hematology Beyond the Microscope*, E. Simson (ed.). Technicon Instruments Corporation, Health/Communication/Projects, Tarrytown, N.Y., pp. 123-130.
3. Hosty, T. A., Harris, L. G., Stonacek, S. M., and Frazier, B. (1982). Evaluation of an automated continuous-flow hematology instrument: The Technicon H6000. *J. Clin. Lab. Automat.* 6:408-415.
4. Reicher, V., and Barclay, J. E. (1983). *Innovative Technology in Automated Haematology for Improved Patient Care*. Gorges-les-Gonesse, France, 1983.
5. Corash, L. (1983). Automated leukocyte differential analysis by flow cytochemistry. *Laboratory Medicine* 14:503-508.
6. Arnstrom, S., Ralgkian, E., Winkel, P., and Nissen, N. I. (1985). The relative merit of various cytochemical quantities and manual differential count in predicting remission following chemotherapy of patients with de novo acute myeloblastic leukemia. *Am. J. Clin. Path.* 83:73-76.
7. Winkel, P., Olesen, T., and Nissen, N. I. (1982). Automated cytochemistry in the prediction of remission following chemotherapy of patients with de novo acute myeloblastic leukemia. *Am. J. Clin. Path.* 77:50-53.
8. Drewinko, B., and Bollinger, P. B. (1984). The modern, high volume, computer-assisted clinical hematology laboratory. In *Clinical Laboratory Annual*. H. A. Homburger and J. G. Batsakis (ed.). Appleton-Century-Crofts, Norwalk, CN, pp. 133-175.
9. Bennett, J. M., Catovsky, D., Daniel, M. T., Flandrin, G., Galton, D. A. G., Gralnik, H. R., and Sultan, C. (1976). Proposals for the classification of the acute leukemias. *Br. J. Haemat.* 33:451-458.
10. Zar, T. H. (1984). *Biostatistical Analysis*. 2nd edition. Prentice-Hall, Englewood Cliffs, N.J.

11. Colomb, H. M., Rowley, J. D., Vardiman, J. W., Testa, J. R., and Butler, A. (1980). "Microgranular" acute promyelocytic leukemia: a distinct clinical, ultrastructural, and cytogenetic entity. *Blood* 55:253-259.
12. Savage, R. A., Hoffman, G. C., and Lucas, F. V. (1981). Morphology and cytochemistry of "microgranular" acute promyelocytic leukemia (FAB M3m). *Am. J. Clin. Path.* 75:548-552.
13. Ross, D. W., and Bardwell, A. (1981). Automated cytochemistry and the white cell differential in leukemia. In *Automation in Hematology: What to Measure and Why*. D. W. Ross, G. Brecher, and M. Bessis (eds.). Springer Verlag, Berlin, pp. 287-302.
14. Cairns, J. W., Healy, M. J. R., Stafford, D. M., Vitak, P., and Waters, D. A. W. (1977). Evaluation of the Hemalog D differential leukocyte counter. *J. Clin. Path.* 30:997-1004.
15. Peacock, J. E., Ross, D. W., and Cohen, M. S. (1982). Automated cytochemical staining and inflammation. *Am. J. Clin. Path.* 78:445-449.
16. Drewinko, B. (1984). Flow cytochemical patterns in human hematopoietic malignancies. In *Hematology Beyond the Microscope*, E. Simson (ed.). Technicon Instruments Corporation. Health/Communication/Projects, Inc., Tarrytown, N.Y., pp. 36-48.
17. Takubo, T., Kubota, Y., Oguma, S., Veda, T., Shibata, H., Nakamura, H., Masaoka, T., Yoshitake, J., and Ishigami, S. (1983). Classification of acute non-lymphocytic leukemia according to the distribution picture of peroxidase activity and cell size: correlation between the classification and therapeutic response. *Blood Cells* 9:501-512.
18. Kitahara, M., Eyre, H. J., and Simonian, Y. (1977). Simultaneous serial observations using the Hemalog D and manual leukocyte counts in leukemia. In *Advances in Automated Analysis*, E. C. Bartos (ed.). Mediad, Inc., Tarrytown, N.Y., pp. 335-339.
19. Fernbach, B. R., Ohnuma, T., Holland, J. F., and Gilbert, H. S. (1977). Automated cytochemical analysis of circulating cells in acute myelocytic leukemia. *Blood* 50:suppl 1, 190.
20. Swan, H. T. (1983). Four years experience of the contribution of automated cytochemistry to improved patient care. In *Innovative Technology in Automated Haematology for Improved Patient Care*. V. Reicher and J. E. Barclay (eds.). Gorges-les-Gonesse, France, pp. 51-58.
21. Bessis, M. (1984). Automation: Hematology beyond the microscope. In *Hematology Beyond the Microscope*. E. Simson (ed.). Technicon Instruments Corporation, Health/Communication/Projects, Inc., Tarrytown, N.Y., pp. 20-23.
22. Patterson, K. G., Cawley, J. C., Goldstone, A. H., Richards, J. D. M., and Janossy, G. (1980). A comparison of automated cytochemical analysis and conventional methods in the classification of acute leukemia. *Clin. Lab. Haematol.* 2:281-291.
23. der Ottolander, G. J., van der Burgh, F. J., Lopes Cardozo, P., Hermans, J., and Jansen, J. (1983). The Hemalog D automated differential counter in the diagnosis of hairy cell leukemia. *Leukemia Res.* 7:309-320.

24. Hinchliffe, R. F., Lilleyman, J. S., Burrows, N. F., and Swan, H. T. (1981). Use of the Hemalog D automated leukocyte differential counter in the diagnosis and therapy of leukaemia. *Acta Haematol.* (Basel); 65:79-84.
25. Wintrobe, M. M. (1984). Chairman's Remarks. In *Hematology Beyond the Microscope*. E. Simson (ed.). Technicon Instruments Corporation, Health/Communication/Projects, Inc., Tarrytown, N.Y., pp. 75-76.
26. Cranendonk, E., Abeling, N. G. G. M., Bakker, A., de Jong, M. E., van Gennip, A. H., and Behrendt, H. (1984). Evaluation of the use of the Hemalog D in acute lymphoblastic leukaemia and disseminated non-Hodgkin's lymphoma in children. *Acta Haemat.* 71:18-24.
27. Diggs, L. W. (1977). Highlights in the history of neutrophil counts. In *Differential Leukocyte Counting*. J. A. Koepke (ed.). College of American Pathologists, Chicago, pp. 1-9.
28. Head, D. R., Savage, R. A., Cerezo, L., Craven, C. M., Bickers, J. N., Hartrock, R., Hosty, T. A., Saiki, J. H., Wilson, H. E., Morrison, F. S., Coltman, C. A., and Hutton, J. J. (1985). Reproducibility of the French-American-British classification of acute leukemia: the Southwest Oncology Group experience. *Am. J. Hematol.* 18:47-57.
29. Dick, F. R., Armitage, J. D., and Burns, C. P. (1982). Diagnostic concurrence in the subclassification of adult acute leukemia using French-American-British criteria. *Cancer* 49:916-920.
30. Whittaker, J. A., Withey, J., Powell, D. E. B., Parry, T. E., and Khurshid, M. (1979). Leukaemia classification: a study of the accuracy of diagnosis in 456 patients. *Br. J. Haematol.* 41:177-184.
31. Bennett, J. M., Catovsky, D., Daniel, M. T., Flandrin, G., Galton, D. A. G., Gralnik, H., and Sultan, C. (1981). The French-American-British Co-operative Group. The morphological classification of acute lymphoblastic leukemia: Concordance among observers and clinical correlations. *Brit. J. Haematol.* 47:553-561.
32. Bollinger, P., Drewinko, B., Brailas, C., Smeeton, N., Groner, W., Simson, E., and Trujillo, J. M. (1986). The Technicon H*1 Hematology Analyzer: New Horizons in the Identification of Abnormal WBC Populations. *Proc. XXI Congress of Intl. Soc. Hemat.*, p. 636.
33. Bollinger, P. B., Drewinko, B., Brailas, C. D., Smeeton, N. A., Trujillo, J. M. (1987). The Technicon H*1–An Automated Hematology Analyzer for Today and Tomorrow: I. CBC Parameters. *Am. J. Clin. Path.* 87:71-78.
34. De Cresce, R. (1986). The Technicon H*1: A Discrete, Fully Automated Complete Blood Count and Differential Analyzer. *Lab. Med.* 17:17-21.
35. Drewinko, B., Bollinger, P., Brailas, C., Smeeton, N., Groner, W., Simson, E., and Trujillo, J. M. (1986). The H*1 Automated Blood Cytometer: The Hematology Analyzer for Today and Tomorrow. *Proc. XXI Congress Intl. Soc. Hematol.*, p. 282.
36. d'Omofrio, G., and Mango, G. (1984). Automated cytochemistry in acute leukemias. *Acta Haemat.* 72:221-230.

5

The Role of Cytogenetics in the Characterization of Acute Leukemia

Acute Lymphoblastic Leukemia and Acute Myeloblastic Leukemia

JACQUELINE WHANG-PENG and TURID KNUTSEN *National Cancer Institute, National Institutes of Health, Bethesda, Maryland*

I. INTRODUCTION

Do all leukemic cells have an abnormal karyotype? Does the cytogenetic study play an important role in the characterization of acute leukemia? These questions are frequently asked by oncologists; cytogeneticists are striving to provide the answers.

In 1902, Boveri proposed that malignant tumors could be due to an abnormal chromosome constitution; 58 years were to pass before there was any concrete evidence to support this theory and it came with the discovery of the Philadelphia chromosome (Ph^1) in chronic myelogenous leukemia (CML) in 1960 (Nowell and Hungerford, 1960).

Despite numerous studies, it was to be 10 more years before the introduction of banding techniques (Caspersson et al., 1968; Seabright, 1971) made possible the demonstration of nonrandom chromosomal abnormalities in a variety of malignancies. More recently, the high-resolution chromosome technique (Yunis, 1976) has allowed the precise identification of these abnormalities, including specific breakpoints involved in structurally altered chromosomes. These technical advances have increased the observed incidence of chromosomal abnormalities from 50% to nearly 100% in acute nonlymphocytic leukemia (ANLL) (Yunis, Bloomfield, and Ensrud, 1981) and revealed that many abnormalities are specific for a particular subgroup of leukemia. A review of hundreds of cases at the Third International Workshop on Chromosomes in Leukemia in 1980 (Third IWCL, 1981) emphatically demonstrated, for the first time, that the karyotype is an important independent prognostic factor in acute lymphocytic leukemia (ALL), one that correlates with survival even when other known risk factors, such as age, white blood cell count, and histologic type by French-American-British, or FAB, classification

(Gralnick et al., 1977) are considered. It was also found that children and adults with the same chromosomal abnormalities have the same response to treatment.

In view of the importance of identifying the specific cytogenetic abnormalities in regard to the various subclassifications of acute leukemia, we present in this paper, an up-to-date review of the reported findings, in the hope that we can facilitate the diagnosis, treatment, and prognosis of this type of malignancy.

II. MATERIALS AND METHODS

A. Materials

Cytogenetic studies of acute leukemia are usually confined to the bone marrow because it is the original site of involvement, and usually has a high mitotic activity. The aspirate can be processed directly or after one day of culture. In active cases, the peripheral blood can also serve as a source of mitotic leukemia cells, and if leukemic involvement is documented, several other tissues (e.g., lymph node, tumor mass, and spinal fluid) may also yield actively dividing neoplastic cells.

B. Methods

Culture

Bone marrow. A bone marrow aspirate of 0.25-0.50 mL is collected, without anticoagulants, from the iliac crest or sternum. In the direct procedure, the cells are immediately transferred to a 0.1-0.2 μg/mL Colcemid solution (made up in phosphate-buffered saline), where they remain for 30-60 minutes. They are then harvested as described below. The remaining cells are cultured for one day in RPMI 1640 medium supplemented with 15% fetal calf serum, penicillin-streptomycin (50 U or 50 mg/mL each), and glutamine (4 mM/mL).

Peripheral blood. The blood is collected with 20 units of preservative-free heparin and leukocyte-rich plasma is collected after gravity sedimentation. The cells are added to supplemented culture media (as described above) at a final concentration of $1\text{-}2 \times 10^6$ cells/mL and cultured for 1-3 days with or without mitogenic stimulation. The most common mitogen is phytohemagglutinin (PHA), which stimulates T cells, but other mitogens are now increasing in popularity: pokeweed (PWM), which stimulates both T and B cells; and lipopolysaccharides (LPS) and Epstein-Barr virus (EBV), which stimulate B cells.

Tumor nodules and lymph nodes. These tissues are minced with sterile scissors and the pieces forced through a 190 μm pore size mesh to obtain single-cell suspensions. The cell count is adjusted to 1×10^6/mL, and the cells are cultured for 1-3 days with or without stimulation.

Cerebrospinal fluid. Leukemic cells can be found in the spinal fluid in meningeal leukemia and will occasionally yield mitoses. The spinal fluid is collected and placed in a Colcemid solution, and is processed in the same manner as a direct bone marrow specimen.

Harvest

All cultured specimens are harvested following the same procedure. Mitotic arrest is achieved by adding Colcemid, at a final concentration of 0.1-0.2 μg/mL, for 30-90 minutes. The cells are then exposed to a hypotonic solution consisting of a 1:1 mixture of 1% sodium citrate and 0.075M KCl for 20 minutes, and subsequently are fixed with a 3:1 mixture of absolute alcohol and glacial acetic acid for 10 minutes, followed by one to several more changes of fixative. Slides are made using the air-dry technique.

Staining

The standard Giemsa stain is applied to one slide from each set and is used primarily to evaluate the incidence of aberrations such as breaks, fragments, rings, and minute chromosomes. Banding stains (Giemsa-trypsin, quinacrine, and C-banding) are used to determine the exact chromosomal abnormality involved in each particular neoplastic cell.

C. Nomenclature

The most recent publication specifying the proper cytogenetic nomenclature is *An International System for Human Cytogenetic Nomenclature (ISCN)* (1985). We will briefly mention here the most commonly used symbols. The upper (short) arm is designated the "p" arm and the lower (long) arm is the "q" arm. Each arm is divided into regions, bands, and subbands; e.g., the abbreviation 5q23.1 indicates the lower long arm of chromosome 5, region 2, band 3, and subband 1. Plus (+) or minus (−) symbols indicate gain or loss of the whole chromosome when placed in front of the chromosome number, and addition or deletion of the designated arm when placed after the chromosome. Other common symbols include der (derivative chromosome), dic (dicentric), dup (duplication), iso or i (isochromosome), ins (insertion), inv (inversion), mar (marker), r (ring chromosome), and t (translocation).

III. ACUTE LYMPHOCYTIC LEUKEMIA

According to the FAB classification, acute lymphocytic leukemia (ALL) can be divided into three morphological categories, L1, L2, and L3. ALL can be further categorized according to the immunologic surface markers as T−, B−, and non-T non-B ALL. In L1 ALL, the predominant cell is small with small or not visible nucleoli, and scanty cytoplasm; L2 ALL cells have large nuclei and the amount of cytoplasm is often abundant. Detailed chromosomal analysis has always been difficult in this disease, due in general to the stickyness of the chromosomes, which results in an ill-defined and blurred appearance (Whang-Peng et al., 1976). Most data have indicated that L1 and L2 ALL show similar chromosomal abnormalities. However, concentrated efforts by several laboratories produced enough data so that the participants at the International Workshop in Lund, Sweden in 1980, were able to subdivide L1 and L2 on the basis of cytogenetic abnormalities and were also able to correlate specific abnormalities with morphological and immunological markers, and clinical behavior.

A. Specific Abnormalities

Ph¹

Most cases of Ph¹ positive ALL have the immunologic phenotype of common or null-cell ALL and monoclonal antibody study has further identified the proliferative cells as being of pre-B origin. Only four cases of Ph¹ positive T-ALL have been reported: Louwagie et al., 1985 reviewed three published cases and presented a fourth case where the Ph¹ chromosome completely disappeared during remission; the patient was a 50-year-old male with an E+, TdT+, OKT 10+, OKT 8+, and Leu 9+ immunologic phenotype. The authors observed that the occurrence of T- and B-cell blast crisis in CML and the Ph¹ chromosome in T- and B-ALL support the theory of a common stem cell for the hematopoietic and immunopoietic systems. Ph¹ positive ALL occurs three times more frequently in adults than it does in children, and the reported percentages have ranged from 5.7% to 10% in children and from 17.0% to 33% in adults (Third IWCL, 1983; Priest et al., 1980; Bloomfield et al., 1980). In childhood ALL, Ph¹ positive patients are older and have a higher initial platelet and white blood cell count than patients without the Ph¹ chromosome. They usually respond to regular ALL treatment but the Ph¹ chromosome is a poor prognostic sign, and both the initial remission and length of survival are short; the latter is especially true in adult Ph¹ positive ALL (Priest et al., 1980; Sandberg et al., 1980). This particular chromosomal abnormality continues to be an unfavorable sign in ALL despite the great improvement in survival in this disease in recent years.

The cytogenetic findings in Ph¹ positive ALL are similar to those of Ph¹ positive CML (Third IWCL, 1981): 10% of the cases show a variant Ph¹ translocation and trisomy of chromosome 8 is one of the most common additional abnormalities. There are several important differences, however, including more frequent occurrence of less than 100% positiveness in the ALL bone marrow, and the disappearance during remission and reappearance upon relapse of the Ph¹ chromosome in ALL; in CML, the Ph¹ rarely disappears from the bone marrow at any time during the disease. However, recently it has been shown that the Ph¹ can be reduced and disappear with interferon therapy (Talpaz et al., 1986).

t(4;11)(q21;q23)

The translocation t(4;11)(q21;q23) is usually seen in L1 and L2 ALL and is seen in about 5% of all cases of ALL in adults and children. Kocova, Kowalczyk, and Sandberg (1985) reported 3 cases of their own and reviewed an additional 33 published cases; they noted that these patients constitute a subgroup of ALL with several specific characteristics. Almost all patients have a high white blood cell count, organomegaly, and a relatively short survival. Patients fall into two age groups, one 16 months or younger (55% of cases), and the other, 11 years or older, most being adults; only 2 cases have been between the ages of 3 and 8 years. Most cases have a pseudodiploid karyotype at the beginning of the disease with no other karyotypic abnormalities other than the t(4;11); some cases develop hyperdiploidy during relapse but a modal chromosome number exceeding 50 has not been described (one case did have a clone with 89 chromosomes). The cell type is preponderantly non-B, and some cases can be of monocytoid and/or myeloid origin and some mixed lineage. The involvement of chromosome 11 at band q23 is common in monocytic leukemia of the M4 and M5 acute nonlymphocytic leukemia (ANLL) classification, so it is not unexpected that this chromosome band is involved in monocytoid ALL. Parkin et al. (1982) studied the morphological, ultrastructural, and immunologic characteristics of the leukemic cells from 10 patients with t(4;11) ALL and concluded that the blasts represent a proliferation of an early myeloid progenitor cell, which can appear as either lymph or myeloid blasts. In another study of 7 children with t(4;11) ALL (Mirro et al., 1986), immunologic phenotyping suggested the leukemias were of B-cell origin; flow cytometric analysis, however, from 3 patients demonstrated the simultaneous expression of the lymphoid-associated antigen B4 (CD-19) and the myeloid-associated antigen My-1 (X-Hapten), and electron microscopy of the blasts from one of these patients showed ultrastructural characteristics of both lineages. These latter findings suggest that the cases with t(4;11) are not truly non-T, non-B ALL and are also not entirely of monocytoid/myeloid origin but rather that they arise as a result of leukemogenesis in a multipotent progenitor cell, which produces cells with characteristics of mixed lineage. In general, the prognosis in this group of patients is poor and complete remission, though often achieved, is of short duration (about 3 months); the median survival is approximately 8 months.

Other cases involving chromosomes 4 or 11 have been reported in ALL. A congenital chromosome anomaly, inv(11)(p15q13) was observed in a child with non-T, non-B, ALL antigen (CALLA) positive, Ia-positive, and Daudi-negative ALL (Cabrol et al., 1983). However, a review of another family, in which the father and 4 children had the same inversion, showed no history of neoplasia (Russell, Miller, and Killam, 1982). Another case reviewed by Cabrol, a case of ALL with t(1;4), which resulted in trisomy of the 4q12-q32 segment, was observed in a 7-year-old female who died 5 months after diagnosis without ever achieving a remission (Kowalczyk, Grossi, and Sandberg, 1984) and another case of ALL involving chromosome 4, t(4;12)(q22;p12) was reported at the Third IWCL (1981). It has been postulated that chromosome 4 may contain genetic material that is capable of initiating leukemogenesis after it has been rearranged via translocation to a new genomic environment (Esseltine et al., 1982).

Deletion 5q

Abnormalities of chromosome 5 have been described in a variety of malignant hematologic disorders, primarily preleukemia syndromes and ANLL, and they are usually the results of a deletion rather than the product of a translocation; the deleted portion involves the band segment q22q23. Deletion of 5q has only occasionally been reported in ALL and then usually in association with other abnormalities. Three patients with an unusual type of leukemia had a 5q− chromosome plus other individual chromosomal changes (Haas et al., 1985). The blast cells had a lymphoid morphology with correlating cytochemical staining, but immunological studies showed a pure myeloid pattern in 1 patient and a mixed lymphatic/myeloid marker profile in the other 2 patients. ALL therapy was unsuccessful in 2 patients (both died within 5 weeks without remission); the third patient survived for more than 8 years despite several relapses. The authors suggested that the 5q− is found only in a specific biphenotypic subset of leukemia. By combining immunologic and cytogenetic studies, it may be possible to identify otherwise indistinguishable forms of acute leukemia, which can lead to the early initiation of appropriate therapy.

Deletion 9p

A 4-year-old boy with T-ALL had both an interstitial deletion of 5q and a deletion of 9p with a karyotype of 46,XY,del(5)(q12q13),del(9)(p21) (Abe et al., 1979). He survived for 15 months following diagnosis and the authors observed that the clinical manifestations of his disease were similar to those seen in 7 T-ALL patients with monosomy 9 or deletion of 9p reported by Kowalczyk and Sandberg (1983). The common deleted segment in these patients was 9p21→pter. Deletion of 9p occurs in about 10% of patients with T-ALL and the clinical features common to this subgroup include a high leukocyte count with a high percentage of blasts, lymphadenopathy and splenomegaly, older age at diagnosis, and a survival about one year shorter than other types of childhood ALL.

t(8;14) and 14q+

Virtually all cases of t(8;14) ALL are of the L3 (Burkitt's) variety and B-cell phenotype. It has a high male-to-female ratio, is seen more frequently in adults than in children (Third IWCL, 1983), and the mean survival is short (about 5 months). A majority of cases have pseudodiploid karyotypes with few additional abnormalities. A 14q+ without the 8q− has also been observed in ALL. Nine cases with 14q+ were studied at the Third IWCL: 56% had null-cell ALL and 44% had B-ALL; the karyotypic pattern in these patients was more complex than in patients with t(8;14) and in many cases the donor chromosome involved in the translocation to chromosome 14 could not be identified. The other translocations seen in Burkitt's lymphoma, t(2;8)(p13;q24) and t(8;22)(q24;q11), have also been reported in L3 ALL (Hecht et al., 1983; Chaganti et al., 1983). Immunoglobulin expression was correlated with the different translocations. The kappa chain genes are located on chromosome 2 and the translocations involving breakpoints at 2p13 and 8q24 expressed these genes, as predicted; the predicted expression of the lambda chain genes on chromosome 22 also held in the case involving t(8;22). One case of common ALL with a pre-B-cell phenotype had both t(8;14)(q24;q32) and t(14;18)(q23;q21) (Mufti et al., 1983). The latter abnormality is usually confined to follicular lymphoma.

Monosomy 7

Hypodiploidy with monosomy 7 is unusual in ALL, and monosomy 7 was only reported in 4% of the aneuploid cases at the Third IWCL in 1980 (Third IWCL, 1981). Two cases of ALL with deletion of chromosome 7 had a history of radiation exposure: (a) a 53-year-old survivor of the Hiroshima bomb blast who survived for only 4 months after the initial diagnosis despite aggressive combination chemotherapy (Stricker and Linker, 1983), and (b) a patient with Ph^1 positive ALL who had received prior radiation therapy (Mandel et al., 1977).

Chromosome 19 Translocations

Pre-B ALL is sometimes distinguished by another specific chromosomal abnormality, t(1;19)(q23;p13). Although there was originally a debate as to whether it was the p or q arm of chromosome 19 that was involved, it has now been resolved, through the use of high resolution chromosome banding, that the specific translocation in all these cases is t(1;19)(q23;p13.3) (Michael, Garson, and Gallen, 1985). Some of the clinical features of this subgroup are very similar to those of null-cell ALL, but the lymphoblasts are characterized by the presence of cytoplasmic μ chain (CIg) expression and the patients have a low white blood cell count on presentation. Williams et al. (1984) first described the t(1;19)(q23;p13.3) in 7 of 23 cases with pre-B-cell phenotype and L1 ALL. These patients showed higher rates of cell proliferation than patients with other translocations or no translocation; each of the 7 patients was strongly positive for CIg and 6 of the 7 had the $CALLA^+$, $HLA\text{-}DR^+$ phenotype. Early aggressive relapse, meningeal involvement, and short survival was seen in 4 of 10 reported cases (Carroll et al., 1984); it has been suggested that this type of patient receive early aggressive chemotherapy and CNS prophylaxis. In a study of 124 consecutive patients with ALL, 5 patients with pre-B ALL and t(1;19) were observed to have achieved complete remission and had survivals ranging from 4 to 21+ months (Michael, Levin, and Garson, 1984). In 4 of these patients the t(1;19) was present at diagnosis and in the fifth patient, who had Ph^1 positive ALL, it appeared at first relapse. The most recent study was that of Pui et al. (1986), who found t(1;19) in 16 (23%) of 70 patients with pre-B ALL, and different translocations in 11 of the remaining patients. They noted that a translocation was one of four presenting features which conferred an increased risk of treatment failure in pre-B ALL; the other three features were pseudodiploidy, black race, and higher lactic dehydrogenase.

Of the four, pseudodiploidy was the strongest factor for predicting relapse. Other clinical features in these 70 patients were similar to those seen in common ALL.

Chromosome 19 has also been involved in translocations with other chromosomes in ALL. A case of childhood T-ALL with t(11;19)(q23;p11) was reported by Knuutila et al. (1985); the patient responded well to conventional treatment and had not relapsed at the 6 month followup. In a report of t(10;19)(q26;q13) in non-T, non-B ALL in an adult female, De Braekeleer et al. (1985) reviewed the literature on other translocations involving chromosome 19 in ALL and found: (a) one case of t(11;19)(q23;p13) in a series of 114 leukemic children; (b) one case of non-T, non-B ALL L1 with t(1;19)(q21;q13) in a series of 50 ALLs; and (c) t(7;19)(q11;q13) in an 11-year-old boy with ALL that showed some features of pre-B ALL. Of the 234 ALL cases studied at the Third IWCL in 1980 (Third IWCL, 1981), only 4 involved chromosome 19, either at band p13 or q13.

Sex Chromosomes

Abnormalities of the X chromosome have been reported in about two dozen cases of ALL, all but a few involving numerical changes, such as loss of an X chromosome in hypodiploid clones and extra X chromosomes in hyperdiploid clones (Mitelman, 1985). Translocations between the X and autosomes has been seen in 2 cases and deletion of the X in a pseudodiploid clone, del(X)(q25) (Mitelman, 1985). Figure 1 shows another deletion of the X, 47,XY,del(X)(q23) in a case of ALL.

Mitelman (1985) lists 10 reported cases involving abnormalities of the Y chromosome, 6 cases of −Y, one case of +Y, 2 cases with deletions of the Y, del(Y)(q11) and del(Y)(q12), and one case involving translocation, t(Y;1).

B. Ploidy in ALL

Near-haploidy represents a unique subgroup of ALL, one in which each leukemic cell contains only about 26-28 chromosomes. It is extremely rare and of the 234 cases with abnormal karyotypes at the Third IWCL in 1980 (Third IWCL, 1981), only 2 such cases (less than 1%) were found: one had a modal number of 27 chromosomes and the other had 28 chromosomes. None of the 331 cases in our ALL series had near-haploidy (Whang-Peng et al., 1976). A review of the literature from 1978 to the present reveals an additional 10 cases. These patients had several common findings. All were under the age of 18 years. Cases in which surface markers were studied had the common ALL surface marker. Disomy of chromosome 21 was seen in 8 of the 10 cases. Five patients had 26 chromosomes: 4 of them had disomy 21, 3 had disomy 14, one had disomy 18, and the patient with monosomy 21 had disomy of chromosomes 6 and 18. These findings strongly suggest that chromosome 21 is necessary for the survival and function of these malignant cells and that disomy of chromosome 14 or 18 is important in malignant transformation. In 1982, Sandberg, Wake, and Kohno reviewed the literature

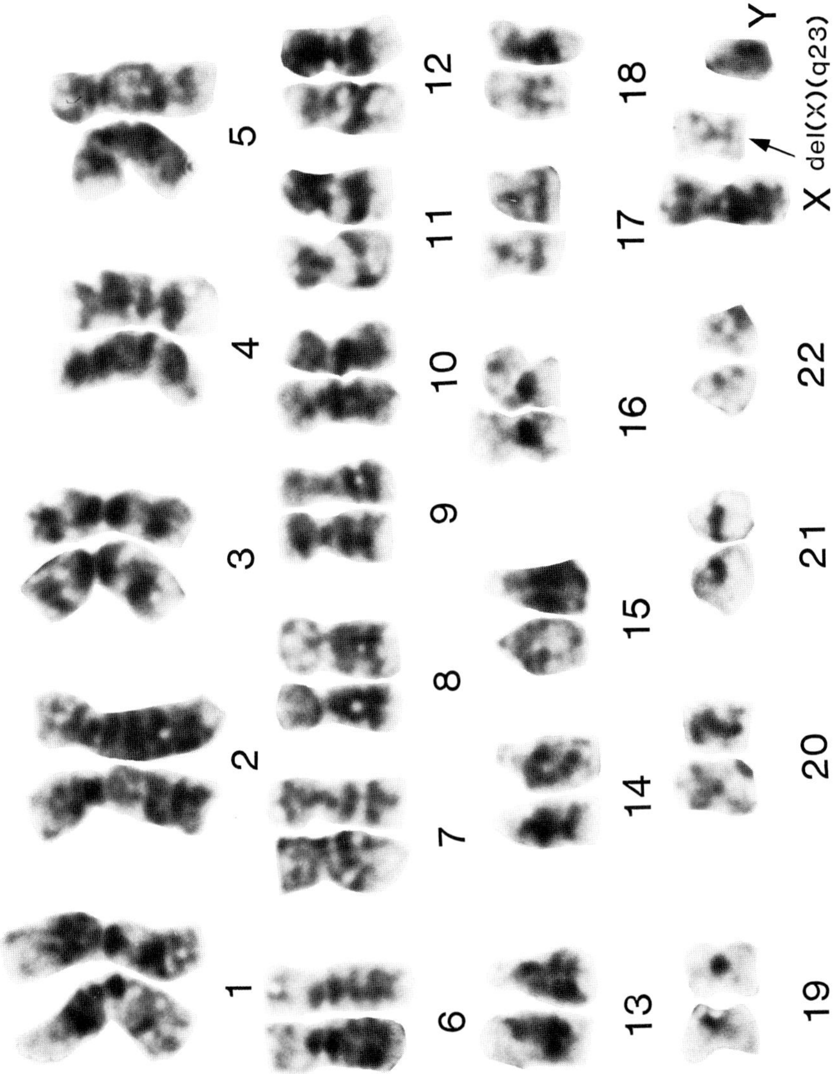

Figure 1 Karyotype from the bone marrow of a patient with ALL, 47,XY,+del(X)(q23).

reporting near-haploidy and severe hypodiploidy in ALL and CML in lymphoid blast crisis and found a total of 13 cases of ALL. Not a single case of ANLL has as yet been reported with near-haploidy, but the relationship between this phenomenon and lymphoid leukemia remains to be determined. Oshimura, Freeman, and Sandberg (1977) suggested that the most likely cause of near-haploidy is multipolar mitosis. Perhaps the formation of haploid genomes makes possible the expression of recessive genes, which results in the loss of regulatory control of growth and differentiation of lymphoid cells; it is not known, however, if near-haploidy results from or precedes malignant transformation. All cases had evidence of the coexistence of normal diploid cells or hyperdiploid cells in the bone marrow. These cells may be necessary to the survival of the near-haploid cells. All cases had low hemoglobin (median 7.8), 90-100% blasts in the bone marrow, and high white blood cell counts. A short remission (median, 6 months) and a short survival (median, 10 months) was characteristic of this group of patients. The severity of the disease indicates that intensive therapy, including bone marrow transplantation, should be emphasized in the treatment of these patients.

Severe hypodiploidy (30-36 chromosomes) is also a rare occurrence in ALL. Only 3 such cases (0.87%) were found in the 346 cases reported by the Third IWCL (1983); 1 case (0.74%) was observed in the 136 cases in another series (Williams et al., 1982). Detailed clinical and cytogenetic findings have been reported for only 4 cases. These patients were much older (52-67 years) than the patients with near-haploidy. Morphologically, their leukemic cells were characterized by sparse cytoplasm and a coarse chromatin pattern in the nucleus, and the blasts were usually periodic acid-Shiff (PAS) positive; all 4 patients had null-cell or common ALL. Survival in the 2 cases in which it was reported was 10 months and 19 months.

Untreated hyperdiploid patients were divided into two groups at the Third IWCL (1983), one with 47-50 chromosomes and the other with more than 50 chromosomes. These two groups showed a big difference in survival. Patients with more than 50 chromosomes had the best prognosis of all groups, with a median survival of 34 months; the median survival of the 47-50 chromosome group was 15 months; for patients with normal karyotypes it was 24 months. Of the 28 patients with 47-50 chromosomes, 87% had null cell-ALL, and the most common chromosomes abnormalities were +21, +13, +4, +8, and +18; there were relatively few structural changes, only one of which, i(1q), was seen in more than one patient. A total of 31 patients had more than 50 chromsomes. Two-thirds of the patients were children, and all were of the null-cell type (non-T, non-B); 96% were either FAB L1 or L2 (equal proportions of each). Trisomy 21 was again the most common abnormality, followed by (in decreasing frequency) +6, +18, +14, +4, +10, +13, +15, +17, and +X. Few structural changes were seen; they involved unidentified markers in 22 patients and other rearrangements in 8 patients. Constitutional chromosome abnormalities were seen in 7 patients, the most frequent being +21.

A total of 13 of our 331 ALL patients (3.9%) showed some tetraploidy or near-tetraploidy (Whang-Peng et al.,1976). In the 7 patients with tetraploidy (including one patient with endoreduplication), it was seen in 12-87% of the cells. In the 6 patients with near-tetraploidy, the number of involved cells ranged from 25% to 95%. The median initial remission duration for this group was 17 months and the median survival was 36 months. This compared favorably with the other ALL patients in the series. Another reported case (Trujillo et al.,1971), however, had a survival of only one month, despite intensive therapy.

Chromosome translocations have been shown to exert a strong independent influence on the effect of treatment in ALL (Williams et al., 1986). In a 6-year followup study of 125 patients with chromosome abnormalities, 30 of the 45 patients with a translocation failed therapy, while of the 116 without translocations, only 27 failed therapy; it was also estimated that only 14% of the patients with translocations remain in complete remission at 3 years. Patients with pseudodiploidy had the highest frequency (58%) and patients with 51 or more chromosomes had the lowest frequency (0) of translocations. When compared to other chromosome abnormalities (such as chromosome number) and other variables such as mediastinal mass, age, sex, race, cell markers, FAB type, etc., translocation was found to be the strongest single factor in predicting the outcome of treatment; it was also observed to increase the risk of treatment failure by six times.

C. Congenital ALL

Congenital leukemia is rare but cytogenetic studies have been performed in a number of cases. In our ALL series of 1976 (Whang-Peng et al., 1976), 5 of 331 patients were under the age of 1 year at the time of diagnosis, and 4 of these 5 patients showed aneuploidy; those patients had considerably shorter survivals (median, 14 months; range, 2-15 months) than did the rest of the group as a whole (median, 26 months; range, 2 weeks-204+ months). Studies of 15-month-old identical twins (Chaganti et al., 1979), one of whom was asymptomatic at the time of admission, showed identical abnormal clones, 47,XY,del(1)(q22), +mar2. This observation provided strong evidence that the leukemic cells populating their bone marrows originated in a single cell in one twin; this cell proliferated and subsequently migrated into the other twin via shared circulation.

Abe et al. (1983) reported a case of acute blastic leukemia in a 5-week-old infant with an interstitial deletion in 11q and insertion of this segment into the terminal region of 19p, ins(19;11)(p13;q13q23). They also reviewed 28 published cases of congenital leukemia, 7 of whom had ALL; 6 of the 7 had t(4;11)(q13 q23), and 1 had t(1;22;4) and other alterations, none involving chromosome 11.

Of the total of 29 cases, 14 had abnormalities of 11q, indicating that the long arm of chromosome 11 is very frequently involved in congenital leukemia and that the specific translocation t(4;11)(q13;q23) is characteristic of congenital ALL.

D. Prolymphocytic ALL

Prolymphocytic leukemia (PLL) is predominantly a B-cell type leukemic lymphoma. It is characterized by a high WBC, splenomegaly, and an aggressive course. Three cases have been reported with a deletion of chromosome 3, del(3)(p13) (Juliusson et al., 1985; Pittman and Catovsky, 1983). Sadamori et al. (1983), however, reported five cases of PLL with t(6;15), none of which had any chromosome 3 abnormalities. This has led to a suggestion that geographic distribution is a factor in the chromosomal abnormalities of PLL. Interestingly all cases had abnormalities of chromosomes 14, 18, and 22.

E. Discussion

Infrequently, cases of acute mixed leukemias are reported (several were reviewed by Neame et al., 1985). Some cases show distinct populations of lymphoid and myeloid cells, a few cases have shown biphenotypic expression of lymphoid and myeloid markers on the same cells, and others have shown sequential conversion of ALL to acute myeloid leukemia or vice versa (the second leukemia may be a consequence of therapy). The cases with two distinct populations may indicate malignant transformation of both lymphoid and myeloid lineages, and cells with biphenotypic expression may represent the disordered differentiation of a multipotential stem cell. These distinctions are made possible by the refinement of techniques using immunologic markers and monoclonal antibodies.

One group (Cuttner et al., 1984) was able to demonstrate that 13 patients with acute leukemias that were difficult to classify appeared to have a disease representing a leukemic transformation among early cells of the monocyte lineage, with cells less mature than seen in either acute myelomonocytic leukemia (FAB-M4) or acute monoblastic leukemia. All patients were TdT (terminal deoxyribonucleotidyl transferase) positive, had mature or early monocyte lineage antigens, and intense Ia antigen expression detected by monoclonal antibodies. TdT is usually considered to be diagnostic of lymphoid differentiation, but in these cases it was interpreted as indicative of the primitive state of the cells in the differentiation sequence.

Allogeneic bone-marrow transplantation, preceded by ablative chemotherapy, is now an accepted form of treatment in ALL. In several cases, leukemia has been noted in the donor cells (reviewed by Newburger et al., 1981). The most likely explanation for this phenomenon is the infection of these cells by some agent, possibly a virus, that was not eliminated by chemotherapy and irradiation. In some of these cases, the same abnormal karyotype was seen in the recipient's original leukemic cells and the transformed donor's cells.

IV. ACUTE NONLYMPHOCYTIC LEUKEMIA

In contrast to ALL, numerous large studies have been reported on the cytogenetics of acute nonlymphocytic leukemia, or ANLL (Testa and Rowley, 1980; Bernstein et al., 1982; Shiraishi et al., 1982; Second International Workshop on Chromosomes in Leukemia, 1979 [1980]; Conjalka et al., 1983; Larson et al., 1983; Yunis, 1984). This is due to the fact that it is much easier to obtain analyzable metaphases from ANLL bone marrow, either from direct preparations or short-term cultures of aspirates, or from peripheral blood containing leukemic cells.

Using the results obtained with the standard Giemsa-trypsin banding techniques, patients with ANLL have been divided into three categories, based on the karyotypic findings: normal (NN), a mixture of normal and abnormal (AN), and totally abnormal (AA). The NN category includes patients with only normal cells or cells with nonclonal abnormalities; the AN category consists of patients with both karyotypically normal cells and cells with clonal abnormalities; and AA category patients have only cells with clonal abnormalities. Both AN and AA patients are considered to be cytogenetically abnormal, and the two categories combined account for about 50% of all ANLL patients. A study employing methotrexate synchronization, however, reported chromosomal abnormalities in 93% of ANLL patients (Yunis et al., 1984). Another technique for producing long chromosomes is that employing flurodeoxyuridine (FdU) synchronization of bone marrow cultures; it was introduced by Webber and Garson (1983) and, since the DNA synthesis block produced by FdU can be completely reversed by the addition of bromodeoxyuridine (BrdU) or thymidine, it has the advantage of not requiring the time-consuming cell washing necessary for MTX synchronization. It also generally produces a much higher mitotic yield than does the MTX procedure and results in the loss of fewer cells. Both procedures increase the length of the chromosome and improve the quality of the metaphase spread. They are, however, time-consuming techniques and are not yet widely used in oncologic cytogenetics.

At the Fourth International Workshop on Chromosomes in Leukemia, 1982 (Fourth IWCL, 1984), ANLL was divided into 8 categories, based on their FAB classifications:

- M0: ANLL but diagnosis of ALL cannot be excluded
- M1: Acute myeloblastic leukemia without maturation
- M2: Acute myeloblastic leukemia with maturation
- M3 (M3V): Acute promyelocytic leukemia and hypogranular variant (M3V)
- M4: Acute myelomonocytic leukemia
- M5: Acute monocytic leukemia
- M6: Acute erythrocytic leukemia
- M7: Acute megakaryocytic leukemia
- M8: definitely ANLL but not otherwise classifiable.

The Fourth International Workshop presented a tremendous amount of valuable data. Not only did the participants subclassify their 956 patients according to the FAB system, they were also able, via computer analysis, to determine the clinical significance of the cytogenetic abnormalities and their relationship to risk factors, response to treatment, and survival. Below are listed the clinical findings of the abnormalities in specific chromosomes, as reported at the workshop.

A. Specific Abnormalities

Chromosome 1

A total of 26 de novo cases had abnormalities of chromosome 1. The sex ratio in these patients showed a predominance of males (5:1) and the age peak was between 60 and 70 years. The most frequent type of ANLL was M5 (25%), followed by M2 (16%) and M1 (14%). There was no correlation between the type of chromosome abnormality and breakpoints and the FAB type, but breakpoints were predominantly located on the short arm, near the centromere at p11 for cases of trisomy 1q, and in the terminal area at p36 (33→36) for cases with reciprocal translocations. Survival in patients with chromosome abnormalities is short; death occurred during induction and early relapse in 80% of the cases.

Chromosome 3

Abnormalities of chromosome 3 were reported in 24 patients at the workshop. No consistent FAB classifications or specific breakpoints were noted in these patients and they were distributed as follows: M2 (8 patients), M4 (6 patients), M1 (4 patients), M6 (2 patients), M8 (2 patients), M3 (1 patient), and M5 (1 patient). The most consistent anomaly was t(3;5), with breakpoints at 3q21-25 and 5q31-34; this translocation was seen in 3 patients with M2 ANLL. Werner-Favre, Engel, and Beris (1985) reported a fourth case of M2 ANLL with t(3;5). A total of 17 translocations between Chromosome 3 and other chromosomes (including chromosomes 1, 2, 3, 6, 7, 11, 12, 13, and 21) were observed in the 24 patients at the workshop. Figure 2 shows a translocation between chromosomes 3 and 17, t(3;17)(p21;q13), from a patient with AMMoL.

There have been several reports linking abnormalities of chromosome 3 with platelet abnormalities. An insertional translocation between homologous number 3 chromosomes was reported in a patient with M4 and thrombocythemia (Rowley and Potter, 1976) and in 1979, the same group (Sweet, Golomb, Rowley, and Vardiman) reported a second case with thrombocythemia in ANLL; the authors postulated that a region on the long arm of chromosome 3 is concerned with regulation of thrombopoiesis. Bitter et al. (1985), in a report of 14 ANLL patients and a review of 14 cases from the literature with abnormalities of the long arm of chromosome 3 reinforced the original proposal that structural rearrangements involving chromosome bands 3q21 and 3q26 are associated with

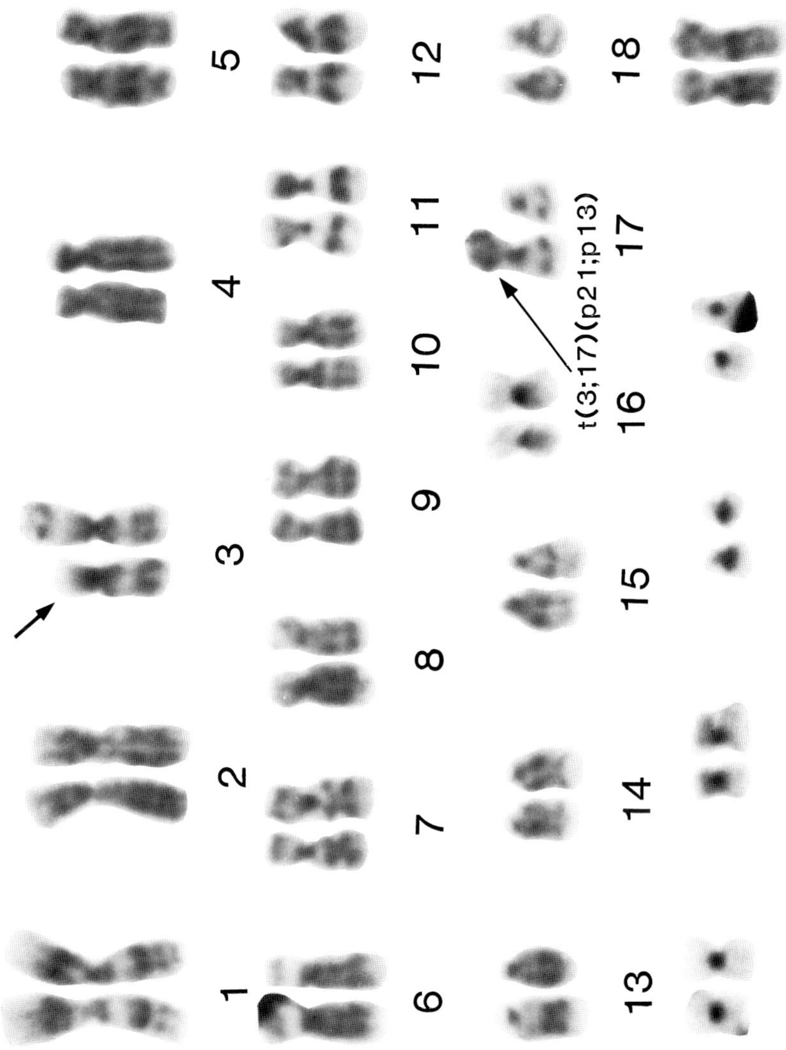

Figure 2 A bone marrow karyotype showing 46,XX,t(3;17)(p21;p13) in acute myelomonocytic leukemia.

unusually high platelet counts accompanied by morphological abnormalities of thrombopoiesis in ANLL, a disease which is generally associated with pancytopenia. The most common 3q abnormalities noted in these patients were inv(3q), t(3q-;3q+), ins(3;3), and ins(3;5).

Deletion of Chromosome 5q22-33 or q33

A deletion of Chromosome 5 was first described in 1974 (Van Den Berghe et al.) as a consistent finding in some cases of refractory anemia. Subsequently, Van Den Berghe (1977) noted that when additional chromosomal changes appear, patients with 5q- are in the process of developing subacute or acute myelogenous leukemia. Wisniewski and Hirschhorn (1983) recently reviewed the data on 105 patients with 5q-, the majority of whom had refractory anemia, polycythemia vera, acute myelogenous leukemia, or leukemia secondary to lymphoma; less common disorders with 5q- included multiple myeloma, myelofibrosis, and myeloid metaplasia. The type of the deletion varied (interstitial deletion resulting in the loss of band q13-15 to q31-32, or terminal deletion of material distal to q14-15 or q22-31), but study of the overlapping areas revealed that in all cases the deletion is defined by band q22 proximally and band q31 distally. The presence of the 5q- appears to be a poor prognostic sign. Of the 105 patients surveyed in the review, 38 presented with overt leukemia and an additional 21 patients were known to have developed leukemia subsequent to a different disorder. In patients with a history of polycythemia vera, lymphoma, or other less common conditions, the 5q- abnormality was almost always associated with hematological changes of a transitional or terminal nature. Survival was generally poor in overt leukemia patients treated with chemotherapy.

A total of 4% of the ANLL patients studied at the Fourth IWCL in 1982 (Fourth IWCL, 1984) had 5q- abnormalities. Four different breakpoints were noted and the participants proposed that all deletions were interstitial in nature. The incidence of the various breakpoints were as follows: q14 or q15q33 (56%), q11 or q12q33 (33%), q22q33 (11%). The critical region was q22 to q33 or q34. Additional abnormalities were observed in 85% of the cases, the most common being loss of a number 7 chromosome, which was seen in 28% of the cases.

t(6;9)(p23;q34) and del(6)(q23)

In 1976, two cases of ANLL were reported to have the translocation t(6;9)(p23; q34) (Golomb, Vardiman, and Rowley, 1976) and, to date, a total of 10 such patients have been published in the literature (Fleischman et al., 1983; Sandberg et al., 1983; Schwartz et al., 1983; Vermaelen et al., 1983; Kao, Reine, and Miletello, 1984) (Figure 3). In all 10 cases, the t(6;9) was the sole abnormality. The FAB classification of these 10 cases were M2 (5 patients), M3 (1 patient), M4 (1 patient, and unclassified (3 patients). In two additional ANLL patients reported in the paper by Fleischman and colleagues (1983), abnormalities involving a break-

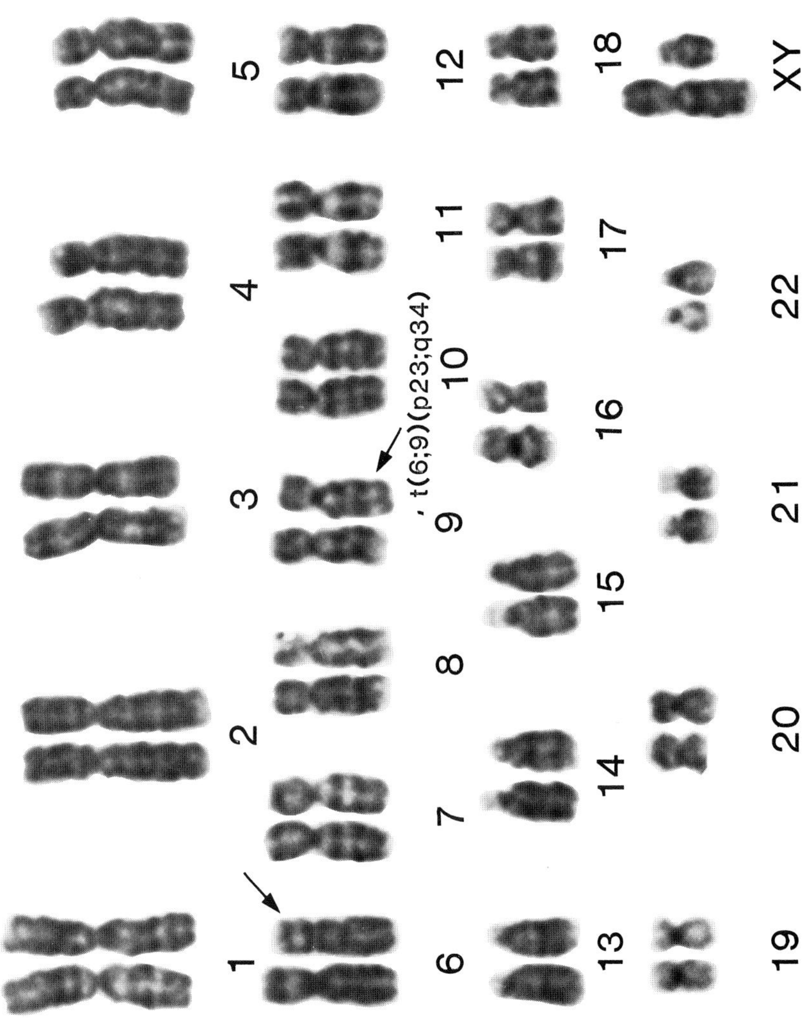

Figure 3 A karyotype demonstrating 46,XY,t(6;9)(p23;q34) in a case of M2 ANLL with eosinophils. (Courtesy of Y. S. Kao.)

point at 6p23 were noted; the karyotypes were 46,XXp–,t(X;6)(p11;p23) and 46,XY,t(2;11)(p21;q25),2der(6),t(6;17)(p23;q11),del(17)(q11); the former patient had M4 and the latter had M3 ANLL.

Of these 12 cases, only 2 were able to achieve complete remission; the others obtained either a partial remission or none at all. The age ranged from 5 to 51 years (average 40 years) and the average survival was 5 months. The median age for adult ANLL patients as a whole is about 49 years and the mean survival time from diagnosis is 7.7 months (9.2 months for those with normal karyotypes and 6.4 months for those with chromosomal abnormalities) (Schwartz et al., 1983); the patients with t(6;9), therefore, appear to be younger but have a similar survival to other ANLL patients.

Monosomy 7

Freireich et al. (1964) first described 3 cases of a syndrome characterized by refractory anemia, thrombocytopenia, granulocytic hyperplasia of the bone marrow, low or absent leukocyte alkaline phosphatase, and a missing C group chromosome; all 3 patients eventually developed myelomonocytic leukemia after preleukemic phases of 1-6 years' duration. Macdougall et al. (1974) later identified the missing chromosome as a number 7. Gyger, Bonny, and Forest (1982) reported that the most consistent feature of monosomy 7 is ". . . an increased susceptibility to bacterial infections related to a preleukemic dyshemopoiesis. . ." and that development of ANLL after this preleukemic syndrome of childhood suggests the involvement of a stem cell already committed to myeloid differentiation. Early detection of this chromosomal abnormality in children with repeated episodes of infection should lead to earlier, and hopefully, successful treatment of this syndrome.

Several families with genetic diseases have been shown to have a high incidence of monosomy 7 and ANLL. Two sisters with Fanconi's anemia, whose initial cytogenetic studies showed normal karyotypes with increased chromosomal breakage, subsequently developed ANLL after, or coincident with, the emergence of monosomy 7; a third sibling died of apparent sepsis (Stivrins et al., 1984).

Several cases of cerebellar ataxia were seen in another family with monosomy 7: the proband had monosomy 7 and died of ANLL after a 4-year course of pancytopenia, and the proband's father and all 4 siblings had cerebellar ataxia. One brother with C-group monosomy died with hypoplastic anemia and another brother died of ANLL; a sister had unexplained anemia (Li et al., 1981). In another kindred in which hematologic diseases appeared to be a maternally transmitted trait, 8 of 14 members in one generation had ANLL or aplastic anemia alone or terminating in ANLL; monosomy 7 or group C monosomy was seen in 3 of the patients, all of whom presented with aplastic anemia (Chitambar, Robinson, and Glode, 1983).

At the Fourth IWCL in 1982 (Fourth IWCL, 1984), monosomy 7 was the most common aberration in ANLL and was seen in 43 patients. The most common abnormalities associated with monosomy 7 were monosomy 5 (8 cases), 5q− (10 cases), and monosomy 17 (13 cases); all except 2 cases had either −5 or 5q−. Other aberrations were also seen in some of these patients.

Of 14 patients with "pure" monosomy 7 reported by Pasquali et al. in 1982, 5 had M2, M4, or M6 ANLL, and the remaining had dysmyelopoietic syndrome (acquired idiopathic sideroblastic anemia, refractory anemia with excess blasts, or chronic myelogenous leukemia). The authors reviewed 64 cases from the literature and found the following diagnoses: preleukemic dysmyelopoietic syndromes, 32 cases (10 evolved to acute leukemia); AML, 21 cases; AMMoL, 6 cases; APL, 2 cases; erythroleukemia, 2 cases; and myelofibrosis with extramedullary hematopoiesis, 1 case. When this data was combined with all known cases in the literature, the authors determined that a total of 88 cases of monosomy 7 as the sole anomaly have been reported, 49 of which had a preleukemic syndrome. The authors were able to identify three characteristics common to patients with monosomy 7: (1) a preleukemic phase in most cases, which eventually terminates in ANLL; (2) morphological abnormalities of red cells and granulocytes including deficient granulation, decreased or absent myeloperoxidase activity, and Pelger-Huet-like abnormal monocytoid appearing myelocytes and band forms in the peripheral blood; and (3) fairly consistent quantitative and qualitative abnormalities involving all cell lines in the bone marrow. Recurrent infections are frequent, response to chemotherapy in the ANLL phase is poor, and survival is short.

Chromosome 8

At the Fourth IWCL in 1982 (Fourth IWCL, 1984), chromosome gain most frequently involved chromosomes 8 and 21. Of the 354 patients with de novo ANLL and abnormal karyotypes, 36 (10.2%) had an extra chromosome 8. Trisomy 8 (+8) was observed in all FAB subgroups of ANLL in the following (decreasing) order of frequency: M4, M2, M5, M1, M3, and M6; 92% of the cases were 20 to >60 years old (median 58 years). A complete remission was seen in 43% of the patients and the median survival with +8 was 6 months (patients with a normal karyotype had a median survival of 10 months).

Nearly all patients with the translocation t(8;21)(q22;q22) have ANLL of the M2 variety, which is characterized by myeloid maturation and a low neutrophil alkaline phosphatase level (Kamada et al., 1981). At the Fourth IWCL in 1982 (Fourth IWCL, 1984), 7% (44 cases) of the cases with de novo ANLL had t(8;21), representing 18% of the M2 cases. This group had a large excess of male patients (33/44) and a high incidence of loss of a sex chromosome: −Y in 28 of the 33 males and −X in 7 of the 11 females. A study of one female patient by Levan and Mitelman (1979) showed that the missing chromosome was the inactive X.

The incidence of t(8;21) may show geographic variation: it was seen in 7% of the 660 consecutive ANLL patients studied at the Fourth IWCL in 1982 (Fourth IWCl, 1984) (these cases came from all over the world) but several centers showed a much higher incidence, e.g., 37.5% in Japan, 50% in London, and 62.5% in Johannesburg, South Africa.

Clinical data at the Workshop revealed that t(8;21) ANLL patients have a higher rate of remission (75%) than M2 patients as a whole (49.3%) but not a greatly increased median survival (9.5 versus 8.5 months, respectively). Also, patients with loss of a sex chromosome or total aneuploidy did not appear to have a poorer prognosis. Sakurai, Kaneko, and Abe (1982) have observed that acquisition of additional autosomal abnormalities at relapse signals a poor prognosis in these patients.

Variant forms of the 8;21 translocation have occasionally been reported. For example, Pasquali and Casalone (1981) reported one such case and reviewed three other cases from the literature; the translocations and FAB classification were as follows: t[inv(2);8;21] (2p11;2q13;8q22;21q22) (M2); and t(8;17;21)(q22;q23;q22) (AMMoL-M4); t(8;11;21)(q22;p15;q22) (M2); and t(1;8;21)(q32;q22;q22) (M2). Pasquali and Casalone noted that the breakpoints on chromosomes 8 and 21 were the same as in the standard translocation (at 8q22 and 21q22) and that involvement of a third chromosome did not appear to affect the prognosis.

In-situ hybridization studies of proto-oncogenes c-mos and c-myc in t(8;21) ANLL have recently been reported (Diaz et al., 1985). The results showed that c-mos, located at 8q22, remains on chromosome 8 and that c-myc, located at 8q24, is translocated to the 21q+ chromosome. Southern blot analysis of the DNA demonstrated no rearrangement of c-mos, even though it lies close to the breakpoint at 8q22.

Chromosome 9

Abnormalities of chromosome 9 were seen in 30 patients at the Fourth IWCL in 1982 (Fourth IWCL, 1984) and included translocation, deletions, one inversion, monosomy, and trisomy. Translocation was the most frequent abnormality (14 of 30 patients) and three different ones were noted: t(9;11)(p21 or p22;q23) in M5, t(6;9)(p21 or p23;q34) in M2, and t(9;22)(q34;q11) in M1.

Mecucci et al. (1984) studied 16 patients and reviewed another 10 patients with interstitial deletions of 9q. This deletion is found almost exclusively in myeloproliferative disorders and is rarely the sole abnormality. In more than one-third of cases it has been associated with t(8;21) and occurred as a secondary event. Although the breakpoints are variable, the deletion appears to be an interstitital one and does not involve the region containing the c-abl oncogene.

Ph^1

A Ph^1 chromosome, indistinguishable from the one observed in CML, also occurs in patients with ANLL. The incidence of the Ph^1, however, is lower in ANLL than in ALL: a rate of <1% (3 of 660 de novo cases) was observed at the Fourth IWCL in 1982 (Fourth IWCL, 1984) and 9.9% (12/121) by Sasaki, Kondo, and Tomiyasu (1983). Of the 12 patients reported by the latter group, 8 had M1 ANLL, which accounted for 24.2% of M1 cases (8/34), and 4 had M2 ANLL, 6.7% of M2 cases (4/60); a Ph^1 chromosome was seen in none of the 26 cases with M3, M4, or M5 ANLL. A median survival of 40 weeks was seen for these 12 patients as a group (31 weeks for Ph^1 positive M1 and 59 weeks for M2 patients). Detailed analyses were reported for 10 patients in this study. A rate of 6-65% karyotypically normal cells was seen at the initial examination in 7 patients and the remaining 3 patients were 100% Ph^1 positive; followup studies in 5 cases demonstrated an increase of normal cells to 80-100% during remission. In 5 cases, the Ph^1 translocation was the sole abnormality. Sasaki, Kondo and Tomiyasu (1983) also discussed the findings in other reports and observed that among 33 banded cases from the literature, the Ph^1 translocation was the standard type, t(9;22), in 27 cases and involved unusual or complex translocation in 6 cases. In combining results from their 12 patients and the 33 cases from the literature, Sasaki, Kondo, and Tomiyasu (1983) found that additional karyotypic changes were observed in about half of the cases, the most common being −7 (18.6%), $+Ph^1$ (9.4%), and +8 (6.9%). These additional changes differ in type and in frequency from those seen in Ph^1 CML and Ph^1 ALL.

t(4;11)

As discussed in the ALL section above, acute leukemia with t(4;11) represents a distinct subgroup characterized by hyperleukocytosis, poor response to therapy, poor prognosis, and blast morphology varying from lymphoid to myeloid, with some cells showing characteristics of both cell types. Although reported in adults, t(4;11) occurs more frequently in infants and children. Daeschner et al. (1985) reported one such case which showed a unique chromosomal rearrangement with insertion of the 11q23 band into the 4q21 region, ins(4;11)(q21;q23); the usual rearrangement is a reciprocal translocation involving the same breakpoint. The patient was an 8-week-old Latin American male whose initial bone marrow diagnosis was L1 ALL, PAS and TdT positive, and negative for nonspecific esterase and myeloperoxidase activity. After one course of treatment, the bone marrow contained 60% blasts, which were strongly positive for myeloperoxidase, and negative for PAS and TdT activity; the cells had remained negative for E rosettes and surface immunoglobulin and the bone marrow was diagnosed as M1 ANLL. The ins(4;11) was seen both during the lymphoid and the myeloid phases. The authors suggested that patients with a seemingly normal karyotype but with a clinical picture similar to t(4;11) may represent subtle versions of this translocation such as the one reported in their study.

Chromsome Segment 11q

Abnormalities involving 11q have been reported in a variety of malignancies, including lymphoma, acute leukemia, and in some small-round-cell tumors of childhood, notably Ewing's sarcoma and peripheral neuroepithelioma (Vermaelen et al., 1983a; Whang-Peng et al., 1986). Vermaelen's group observed 11q abnormalities in 13 of 365 consecutive ANLL cases (7.9% of cases with abnormal karyotypes); deletions of 11q involved bands q14-q22 and translocation sites were noted at bands q14, q22, and q24; the majority of cases involved a breakpoint at band q23. Combining their 13 patients with 41 ANLL cases from the literature, they found that 15 had deletions only, 2 had both deletion and translocation, 36 (67%) had translocations only; and 1 had i(11q). The partner chromosome involved with 11q varied considerably and included chromosomes (in order of descending frequency) 10, 13, 19, 1, 6, 9, 17, and 8, 11, 12, 22, and the X; there was one isochromosome of 11q and one t(11;11)(q22;qter). Abnormalities of 11q were present in 33 de novo ANLL patients studied at the Fourth IWCL, 1982 (Fourth IWCL, 1984): 21 had translocations, 11 had deletions, and one had an isochromosome of 11q. In both studies, acute monocytic (M5) and acute myelomonocytic (M4) leukemia predominated: of the 33 patients at the Workshop, 20 had M5 and 5 had M4 ANLL. In the Vermaelen study, the median age was 49 years (range, 4 months to 83 years) and common clinical findings included hepatosplenomegaly, lymph node enlargement, and bleeding; most patients were refractory to treatment.

Abnormalities of 12p

A total of 15 ANLL patients reported at the Fourth IWCL in 1982 (Fourth IWCL, 1984) had abnormalities involving chromosome segment 12p: 3 patients had deletions and 12 had translocations. The breakpoints varied along the arm but most were in the terminal portion; translocations involved several different chromosomes and only two were identical, t(1;12)(p36;p12) in 2 cases of M5. All FAB classifications were involved except M3 and no correlation was noted between FAB type and specific breakpoints or chromosome translocation partner. The median survival for these 15 patients was 2 months (range, 0.1-18.7 months).

Trisomy 13

Trisomy 13 as the sole chromosomal abnormality has been reported in 4 patients with leukemia (2 had ANLL), all reported or reviewed by Hsu et al. (1979); all 4 had a short survival. The authors suggested that trisomy 13 may be a nonrandom chromosome abnormality associated with malignancies of hematopoietic pluripotent stem cells.

t(15;17) Acute Promyelocytic Leukemia

In 1977, Rowley, Golomb, and Dougherty noted a consistent translocation, t(15; 17), in acute promyelocytic leukemia (APL; FAB-M3). An example of t(15;17) is shown in Figure 4. This abnormality has an unusual feature in that it shows an

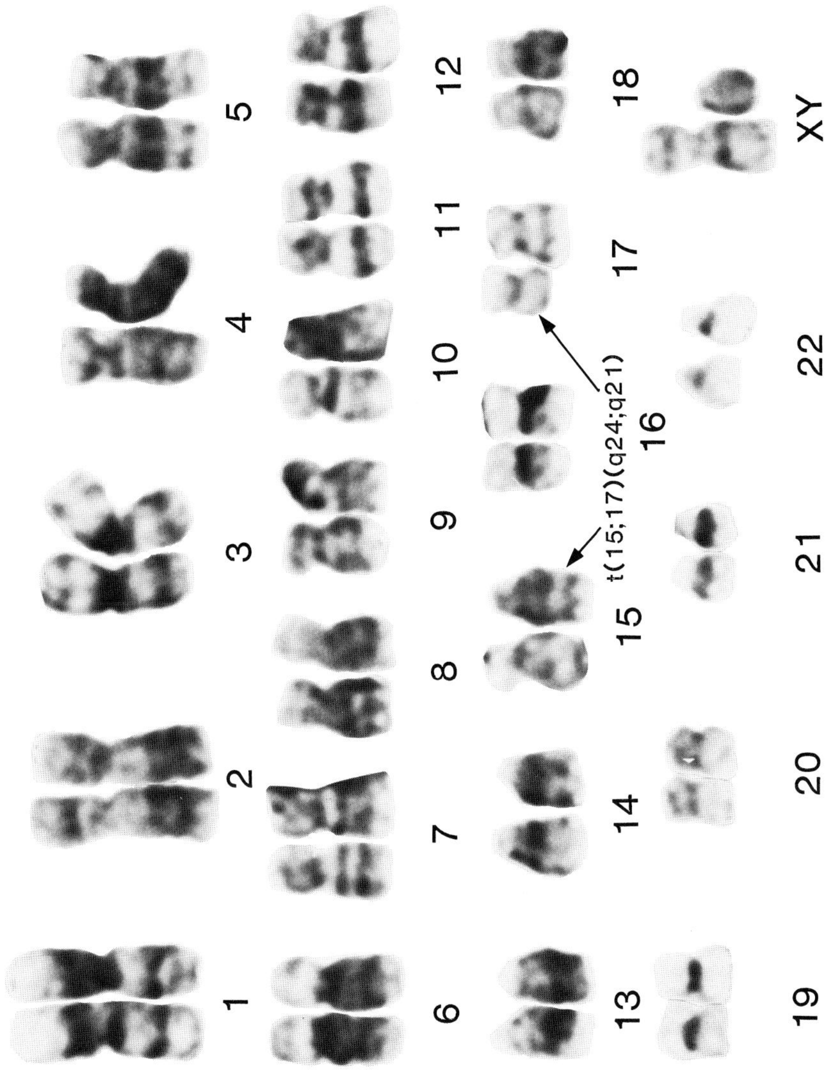

Figure 4 A karyotype from a one-day bone marrow culture demonstrating 46,XY,t(15;17)(q24;q21) in a patient with acute progranulocytic leukemia.

uneven geographical distribution. At the Fourth IWCL in 1982 (Fourth IWCL, 1984) t(15;17) was seen in: 100% of the cases from Chicago, Minneapolis, Belgium, France, Finland, Sweden, and the Netherlands; in a high proportion of the cases from Japan, South Africa, and Australia; a low proportion of the cases from Italy; and in none of those from England, Germany, or Rochester, New York. This variation could be truly due to geographic differences or exposure to different causative agents, or it could be due to the quality of the chromosome preparation (this small translocation is difficult to detect in the poor preparations which are common in APL) or the timing of the harvest (direct possessing or after 1-2 days in culture).

A total of 61 de novo patients were studied at the Workshop: 29 were males and 32 were females, 54 were diagnosed as M3 and 7 as M3 variant (microgranular), and the median age was 31 years (range, 1-69 years). Of the 61 patients, 43 (70%) had t(15;17), 3 had other chromosomal abnormalities without t(15;17), and 15 (25%) had normal karyotypes; 10 of the 43 (22%) with t(15;17) had additional abnormalities. All 3 patients without t(15;17) showed hyperdiploidy and 2 of the 3 had trisomy 8. Detailed evaluation of breakpoints was possible in only 45 of the cases available for review: they were determined to be at 15q22 and 17q12 or 21, but the participants agreed that they could be even more proximal on each chromosome.

Translocations involving chromosome 17 and chromosomes other than 15 have been reported in APL. Two such cases were reported by Yamada et al. (1983): one had 46,XX,t(7;17)(q36;q22) and another had 46,XY,t(1;17)(p36;q21). Complex translocations involving chromosomes 15 and 17 have also been described: Ohyashiki et al. (1985) reported one case with 47,XX,+X,t(1p+;5q−;15q+;17q−). The authors also noted that i(17q−) is also seen in APL without t(15;17), and they postulated that it is the breakpoint at band 17q12 which plays an important role in the development of APL. Oncogene determinations in this region should therefore be done.

Inversion 16 and del(16)(q22)

Inversion 16 is a recently reported cytogenetic subtype (Figure 5). It was first described as del(16)(q22) by Arthur and Bloomfield in 1983 as the sole karyotypic abnormality in the pretreatment bone marrow of 5 patients with ANLL and marrow eosinophilia ranging from 8% to 54% (none of the other 55 patients in the series had more than 4% marrow eosinophils). Of 61 ANLL patients studied by Hogge et al. (1984), all 6 patients with AMMoL and abnormal bone marrow eosinophils (1-24%) had a pericentric inversion of chromosome 16, inv(16)(p13q22) (5 patients), or a t(16;16)(p13.1;q22) (1 patient). One case with M1 ANLL had a rearrangement of chromosome 16 at band p13 but no abnormal eosinophils were observed. In a third report (Le Beau et al., 1983), 18 patients with inv(16)(p13q22) were identified from a group of 308 patients with de novo

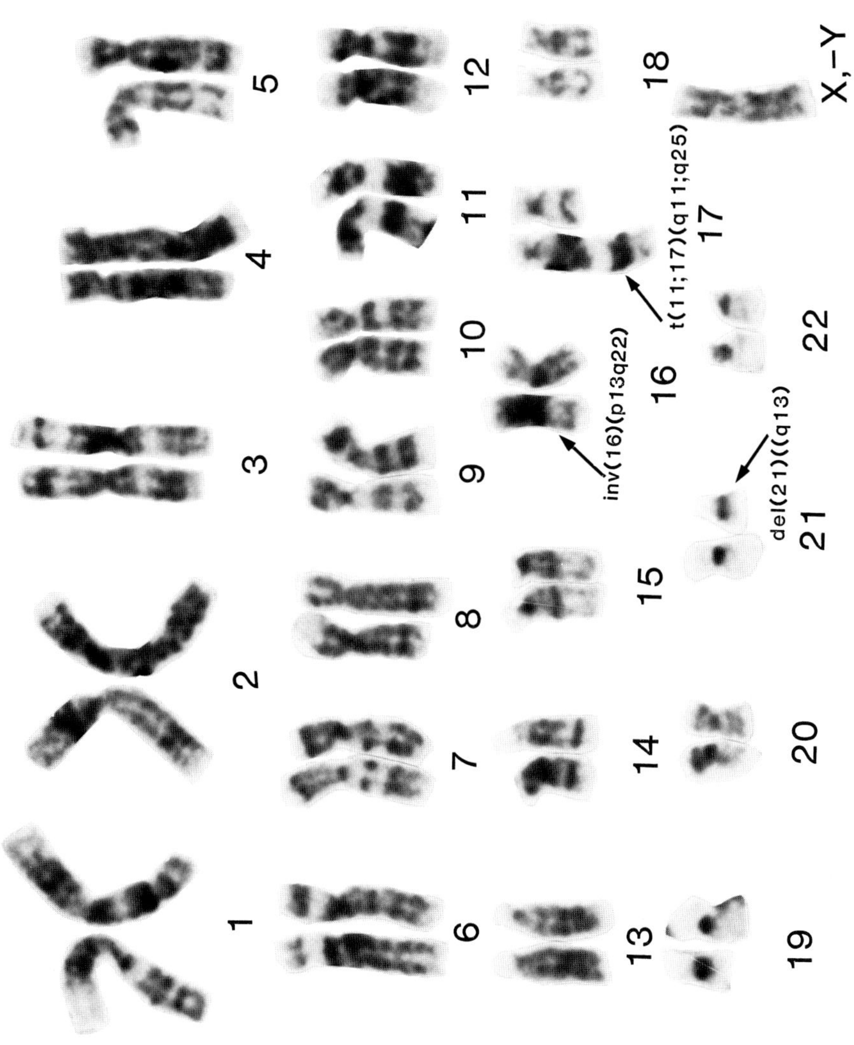

Figure 5 A karyotype from the bone marrow of a patient with acute myelomonocytic leukemia following a myelodysplastic syndrome with marrow eosinophilia, 45,X,−Y,t(11;17)(q11;q25), inv(16)(p13q22),del(21)(q13).

ANLL. All 18 had acute myelomonocytic leukemia (M4) and eosinophils with abnormal morphology, cytochemical staining, and ultrastructure. Of the 17 treated patients, 13 achieved complete remission and 10 were still in first remission at the time of the report.

Other types of ANLL show eosinophilia and in order to more clearly define the syndrome, hematologists at the Fourth IWCL in 1982 (Fourth IWCL, 1984) investigated the 42 such cases (5% of the total cases) at the Workshop: 16 were M2 (M2Eo), 25 were M4 (M4Eo), and one was M5b. None of the M2Eo patients with abnormal karyotypes had chromosome 16 abnormalities and, significantly, there was almost no overlap in the other chromosomal abnormalities between these two FAB types. Twelve of the 24 M4Eo patients had abnormalities of chromosome 16, 5 with del(16)(q22) and 7 with the inv(16); no significant morphologic differences were noted between the two. These four reports describe a unique cytogenetic clinicopathological subtype of ANLL, M4Eo, one with a favorable prognosis with standard antileukemic therapy.

Deletion 20q

In 1984, Davis et al. reviewed the findings in 20 patients with del(20q): there were 8 preleukemia patients, 6 ANLL, 3 polycythemia vera, 1 agnogenic myeloid metaplsia, 1 CML, and 1 case of pancytopenia. In 16 patients the break was near the centromere (20q1101), and in 4 patients it was at the distal part of this band (20q1109). Of the 6 patients (5 males and 1 female) with ANLL, 2 had M1, 1 had M2, and 3 had M6. Each had had cytopenia for 2-3 years before referral but none had received chemotherapy or radiation therapy; their ages ranged from 66 to 80 years, and the median survival for the group was 2 months (range, 1-18 months). Cytogenetic studies revealed a picture of total aneuploidy (AA) in 3 patients and mixed aneuploidy/normal diploidy in the other 3 patients; only one patient had chromosomal changes in addition to the 20q−. None of the ANLL patients had a breakpoint at 20q1109. Of the 43 patients from the literature reviewed by the authors, 11.6% had ANLL and in the 148 patients with ANLL studied at the Mayo Clinic, only 2.7% had 20q−. No clinical differences were noted among the patients with 20q− when they were compared to other patients having similar disorders but without a 20q−.

Sex Chromosome Anomalies

Structural abnormalities involving the X chromosome have been reported only sporadically in ANLL. Debiec-Rychter et al. (1985) described a case of ANLL in a 10-year-old girl with a 46,X,i(Xq) clone; the DNA replication pattern showed highly asynchromous inactivation of the isochromosome arms. In a review of the literature, the authors found only 2 other cases of ANLL and X chromosome abnormalities, one with tdic(X;X)(q13;q13), and another with i(Xq).

Y chromosome loss in the bone marrow has been associated with the normal aging process in the human male (Pierre and Hoagland, 1972). However, loss of the Y also occurs in the cells of younger males whose marrow cells are involved in leukemogenesis. In 6 cases of ANLL studied by Abe et al. (1980), the missing Y was the only chromosomal abnormality at diagnosis and it persisted throughout the course of the disease; 2 patients had 100% 45,X cells, the rest had a mixture of normal 46,XY and 45,X cells. The 45,X cells were not involved in karyotypic evolution; rather, the leukemic process seemed to involve the 46,XY cells instead of the 45,X cells. The authors felt that the existence of a missing Y picture conferred a benign clinical course on patients with ANLL.

At the Fourth IWCL in 1982 (Fourth IWCL, 1984), loss of a sex chromosome was frequently seen in association with t(8;21): −Y in 28 of 33 (70%) males and −X in 8 of 12 (60%) female patients. The survival in these patients was not poor in either the AA or the AN category.

Double Minutes

Double minute chromosomes (DMs) are paired chromatin structures without centromeres. They are very rare in leukemia. Hartley and Toolis (1980) reported one such case and reviewed the literature; DMs have been observed in one case of preleukemia, two cases of acute leukemia, one of which showed mixed myeloid-lymphoid characteristics, and in the authors' case of ANLL. The latter case was that of a 78-year-old female who had DMs in 50% of her bone marrow and blood cells; the DMs disappeared from both tissues following chemotherapy and did not reappear during relapse.

B. Ploidy in ANLL

Approximately 25% of aneuploid cases in ANLL display hypodiploidy, but marked hypodiploidy (<43 chromosomes) is unusual. A few cases have been reported and were reviewed by Como, Sarna, and Sparkes (1979) in their report of a case of acute undifferentiated leukemia with 42 chromosomes and several rearrangements. No uniform pattern was noted among the various patients and the clinical significance of hypodiploidy in ANLL is still unknown.

Tetraploid and near-tetraploid clones are also rare and, again, only a few cases have been reported. In a series of 841 patients with hematologic disease, Borgstrom, Vuopio, and de la Chapelle (1976) reported only 11 patients with greater than 10% polyploid mitoses. They found polyploid clones in 7 of their ANLL cases. Testa et al. (1983) described two cases, both with mixtures of normal diploid and abnormal tetraploid clones: one had 46,XY (7.5%)/ 90,XX,−Y,−Y,−11, t(8;21),t(8;21),+mar (92.5%) and M2 ANLL; and the other had 46,XY (20%)/ 93,XXYY,+mar(extra small) (80%) and AML with immature blasts. Survival in patients with tetraploidy have been poor: Borgstrom's 7 patients had a median survival of 2 months (range, 1-41 months); only Testa's patient, with t(8;21), which usually confers a good prognosis, had an extended survival (almost 2 years).

C. Erythroleukemia

No specific abnormalities have been observed in erythroleukemia (EL), but, except for t(15;17) and t(8;21), nearly all the nonspecific abnormalities seen in

ANLL occur in this type (classified as FAB-M6). The most common are increased polyploidy, chromosome breakage, ring chromosomes, dicentric chromosomes, and random structural abnormalities involving various chromosomes. EL accounts for less than 10% of ANLL cases and generally is seen in patients more than 50 years of age.

Several interesting cases have been reported. Gibas, Becher, and Sandberg (1983) described a case with a high degree of polyploidy, a dominating hypotetraploid clone (81-82 chromosomes), and extensive structural rearrangements, including del(3)(p11), t(16;16)(q13;q13), 8q+, del(1)(q21), +t(12;16)(p13;q13), and a ring and quadriradial chromosome, each observed in one cell; chromosomes 21 and 22 were mono- or disomic in most metaphases, whereas other chromosomes were predominantly tri- or tetrasomic. A case of EL in a 9-year-old male showed hypotetraploidy (mode, 72 chromosomes) with tetraploidy of several chromosomes, and the following structural rearrangements: t(2;15), t(8;?;13), t(11;14); i(16p), t(15;18), 6p−q−, 5 unidentified markers, and −Y. A short remission was achieved but the patient quickly relapsed, and died within 5 months of diagnosis (Douglass and Freeman, 1983). Two other cases of EL in elderly males showed hypodiploid karyotypes (Werner-Favre et al., 1983; Li et al., 1983): one had a 45,XY,−5,−7,−18,−19,−21,+17, +i(21q),+mar1,+mar2 and the other a 43,XY,−2,−4,−9,−15,−19,−20,+3mar karyotype (two of the marker chromosomes had homogeneously staining regions); both patients died within 4 months of diagnosis.

In his book, Sandberg (1980) lists 125 cases of EL, 18 of whom had polyploidy ranging from 10% to 50% of the metaphases. Of the 32 patients with M6 leukemia listed in the Fourth IWCL in 1982 (Fourth IWCL, 1984), 10 had normal karyotypes; no specific abnormalities were noted in these patients except that the frequency of 5q− was higher (15%) than in other FAB classifications (2%-8%); pseudodiploidy was seen in 5 patients and a total of 12 patients showed abnormalities of chromosomes 5 and/or 7 (−5, 5q−, −7, and 7q−). Trent et al. (1983) reported the karyotypic analysis and clinical features of 6 patients with EL, 5 of whom had substantial numerical and structural abnormalities. The modal chromosome numbers ranged from 45 to 61 with 32-100% abnormal cells; 12-17% polyploidy was seen in 2 patients and 3 patients had ring chromosomes. The most common abnormalities were monosomy 7 (4 patients) and monosomy 16 (3 patients). Remission durations in these patients were short, and the median survival was slightly more than one year.

D. Megakaryoblastic Leukemia

Megakaryoblastic leukemia is classified as FAB-M7 ANLL, and is sometimes preceded by other hematologic disorders such as myelofibrosis and CML. Of the 8 reported cases with cytogenetic studies, several have involved chromosome 21, and 2 have had a Ph^1 chromosome.

Pui et al. (1982) reported acute megakaryoblastic leukemia with intrinsic platelet dysfunction in a 3-year-old boy with a constitutional ring 21 chromosome; the leukemic cells showed a karyotype of 46,XY,+C,−D,−E,+large ring, all of which were absent in remission at which time the constitutional ring 21 was observed. Published reports reviewed by the authors revealed thrombocythemia in 3 of 4 patients with the congenital r(21) syndrome, suggesting that the r(21) was related to the persistence of platelet dysfunction seen in their patient after induction of complete remission. Three other cases of acute megakaryoblastic leukemia in early childhood have been reported, 2 of whom showed chromosome 21 abnormalities. Sariban et al. (1984) observed a 13-month female with an abnormal clone of 51-52 chromosomes, 51,XX,+9,+15,+20,+21,+t(10;11)(p11;q12); the cells with 52 chromosomes had an additional +21. Chan et al. (1983) reported 2 cases, both females less than 2 years of age: one patient had an abnormality of chromosome 21 [52,XX,+6,+7,+12,+19,+21,+t(11q+;22q−)] and the other also had a hyperdiploid clone, 50,XX,−1,+2,+8,+1q−,1p−. Two cases of Down's syndrome with features suggestive of megakaryoblastic leukemia, both with trisomy 21, were reviewed, making a total of 5 cases of acute megakaryoblastic leukemia with acquired or constitutional abnormalities of chromosome 21.

E. Eosinophilic Leukemia

The classification of eosinophilic leukemia remains unclear but it is frequently considered a type of ANLL, although in some patients the initial diagnosis is that of a myeloproliferative syndrome.

A 69-year-old male had hypereosinophilic syndrome for 9 years that underwent malignant transformation to acute leukemia with eosinophilic features, at which time he developed a pseudodiploid clone, 46,XY,t(5;11)(p15;q13); nonbanding studies 6 months before had shown a normal karyotype (Yoo et al., 1984). Another case in which the leukemia was preceded by a myeloproliferative disorder (for two years), showed an i(17q) in all marrow cells (Lonnqvist et al., 1979). The authors noted that i(17q) had been found in 2 of 6 patients with eosinophilic leukemia reported in the literature; other abnormalities noted in these 6 patients included +8 (2 patients), +10, and a short Y. Trisomy 8 is one of the most common abnormalities in ANLL. A typical abnormality seen in M2 ANLL, t(8;21)(q22;q22), was observed in a 9-year-old female; 15 of 20 cells with t(8;21) were overlaid with eosinophilic granules, while no granules were seen in the karyotypically normal cells (Kaneko et al., 1983).

V. HAIRY CELL LEUKEMIA

Cytogenetic studies have only been reported in a few cases of hairy cell leukemia (HCL), due to the low mitotic rate of the neoplastic cells and their poor response to mitogens.

Using a lipopolysaccharide (LPS), a B-cell mitogen, Sadamori et al. (1983a) were able to demonstrate multiple chromosomal abnormalities in the peripheral blood cells from an 80-year-old female whose disease evolved from CLL to HCL: 40% of the cells had 44,X,−X,−7,−8,−10,+M1,+r(S),del(3)(p25), and 8% had del(6)(q23), 14q+, del(11)(:p15-q21:). A 6q− in HCL was previously described by Golomb, Lindgren, and Rowley (1978). Abnormalities of chromosome 14 have been reported in several other cases of HCL. Khalid et al. (1981) found no metaphases in LPS cultures but numerous abnormal metaphases in PHA-stimulated cultures from a 76-year-old male with HCL: 14% had 46,XY,3q+,14q− and 14% had 47,XY,+2. A 14q− was also reported in 2 cases studied by Berger et al. (1985): both cases showed pseudodiploid karyotypes with an interstitial deletion of 14q, del(14)(q22q32), in cultures stimulated by *Nocardia opaca*, a polyclonal B-cell activator. At least 4 cases have thus been published reporting involvement of the 14q arm; since HCL is a B-cell leukemia, it is possible that the heavy chain immunoglobulin located on 14q may therefore play an important role in this disease.

VI. ADULT T-CELL LEUKEMIA

Abnormalities of two chromosomes, 6 and 14, have been reported in several studies of adult T-cell leukemia/lymphoma. In a large Japanese study, Miyamoto et al. (1984) observed that 17 of 30 patients had trisomy 6 or 6q−. Deletions of 6q were also found in 6 of 11 patients studied by Whang-Peng et al. (1985a). All 6 patients with 6q− exhibited hypercalcemia, poor response to chemotherapy, and short survival, while patients without a 6q deletion had normal calcium levels and a more indolent course.

Although abnormalities involving 14q+ are frequently seen in B-cell malignancies, several reports have implicated the involvement of the 14q11 band in T-cell malignancies. Clare et al. (1986) studied 5 cases of lymphocyte malignancy, 3 of whom had ATL and one of whom had peripheral T-cell lymphoma; all showed structural rearrangements involving 14q11, each specific abnormality being seen in one patient: t(9;14)(q34;q11), t(11;14)(p11 or 13;q11), del(14)(q11), and inv(14)(q11;q32). The authors reviewed the literature and noted that 5 cases of ataxia telangiectasia had shown 14q− or Dq−, with breakpoints very similar in appearance to that at 14q11, and that analysis of T-cell disorders (primarily T-CLL or cutaneous T-cell lymphoma) with 14q11 abnormalities revealed that 8/17 were inv(14)(q11q32), and 8/17 involved translocations with other chromosomes: chromosome 9 (3 cases), 14 (2 cases), 4, 11, and 17 (one case each); one case may have had t(7;14). Since 10 of the 17 cases also involved band 14q32, this area could be important in T-cell malignancies as well. The gene for the α chain of the T-cell receptor has been mapped to the 14q11-12 region, further implicating this region in the development of T-cell neoplastic malignancies (Croce et al., 1985).

VII. CONSTITUTIONAL CHROMOSOME ABNORMALITIES

Constitutional chromosome abnormalities are occasionally seen in patients with acute leukemia. They accounted for 1.2% (8 cases) of the 660 de novo cases of ANLL reported at the Fourth IWCL in 1982 (Fourth IWCL, 1984) and were not associated with any specific FAB classification (M1/1 patient, M2/3, M3/1, M4/2, and M5/1). Trisomy 21 was seen in 2 patients: the patient with M1 had a leukemic karyotype of 47,XY,−7,+21,+r(7) and the patient with M2 had 50, XX,+6,+19,+21,+22. None of the four patients with translocations [2 with t(14;21) and one each with t(1;12) and t(3;6)] showed any acquired chromosomal abnormalities in their leukemic cells. Two patients had sex chromosome abnormalities: the patient with XXX acquired a t(1;11)(q21;q24) in leukemia and the patient with XYY acquired −7. Twenty-five percent of ALL patients with constitutional abnormalities have Down's syndrome, whereas 57% of ANLL patients with constitutional abnormalities have Down's syndrome.

VIII. SECONDARY LEUKEMIA

An increased incidence of secondary leukemia has paralleled the increase in long-term survival brought about by the development of successful but aggressive chemotherapy and radiotherapy regimens for various cancers. Unfortunately, secondary leukemia is characteristically preceded by extended periods of myeloproliferative or myelodysplastic states, hindering the establishment of a definite diagnosis and delaying appropriate treatment. Because it now seems that chromosome abnormalities appear early in the disease, the cytogenetic study can play an important role in diagnosis in these patients. In this section we confine our discussion to three studies.

In 1979, we (Whang-Peng, Knutsen, O'Donnell, and Brereton) published the findings in 7 cases of ANLL and one of MPD who were identified from a pool of 189 cases of non-Hodgkin's lymphoma and CLL treated primarily with extensive radiotherapy (4 also received some chemotherapy). All were cytogenetically abnormal and hypodiploidy was the most common abnormality; chromosome 7 abnormalities were seen in all 5 patients with banding studies (4 had −7) and abnormalities of chromosome 5 were seen in 3 patients. Figure 6 demonstrates deletion of chromosome 7, del(7)(q22), in a case of ANLL secondary to lymphoma. Cytogenetic abnormalities were noted long before a morphologic diagnosis of leukemia; e.g., in one patient, the diagnosis was not established until autopsy yet 98% aneuploidy had been observed in the marrow cells 4 months prior to death. In 4 patients, 25-100% aneuploidy was noted 7-41 months prior to a diagnosis of ANLL. These data suggest that the presence of aneuploidy in the bone marrow and in unstimulated peripheral blood cells may be a better indicator of malignant transformation than morphologic examination.

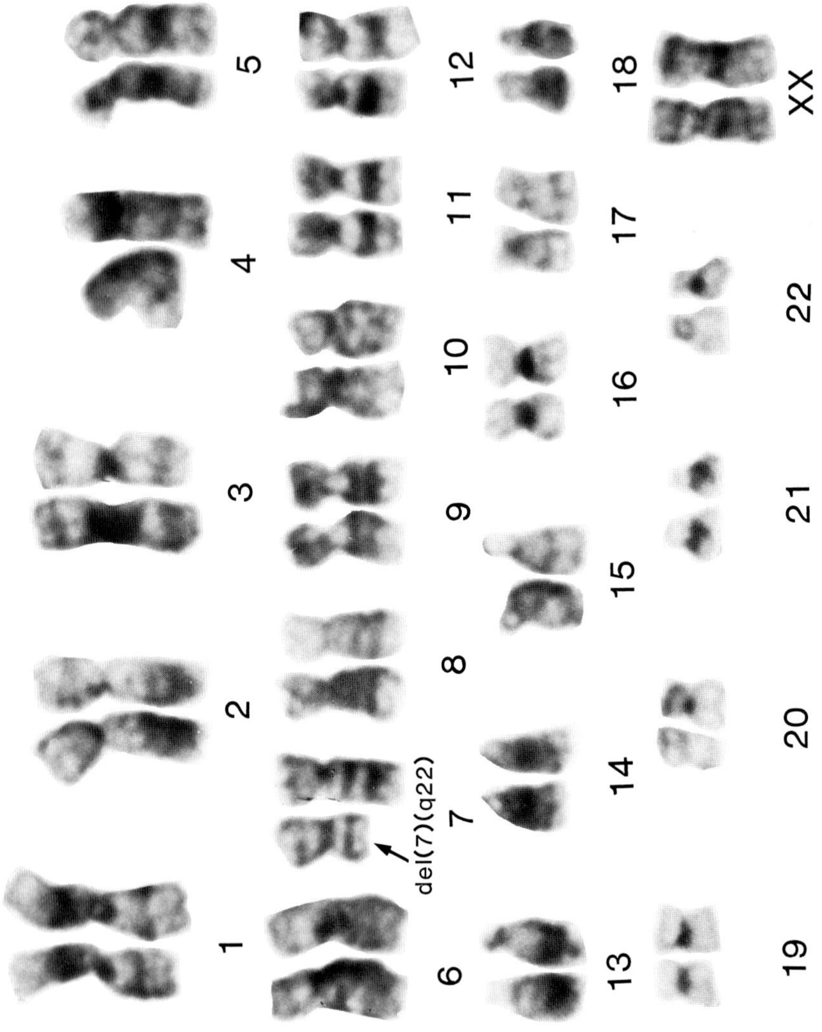

Figure 6 A karyotype from the bone marrow of a patient with AML secondary to poorly differentiated lymphoma showing deletion of chromosome 7, del(7)(q22).

At the Fourth IWCL in 1982 (Fourth IWCL, 1984), 56 patients were accepted in the secondary leukemia group and 14 patients were in the control group (patients who had a previous malignant disease not treated with cytotoxic therapy). The median age for the former was 58 years, and for the latter, 69 years. Of the 56 treated patients, 25% were NN (no abnormalities), 45% were AN, and 30% were AA, while the untreated group showed 29% NN, 64% AN, and 7% AA. The modal chromosome number in the treated group was hypodiploid in 35%, pseudodiploid in 40%, and hyperdiploid in 25% of patients, versus 50%, 30%, and 20%, respectively, in the control group. When categorized according to the FAB classification, both groups followed the same general pattern as ANLL patients as a whole, i.e., M2 was most common (37.5% in treated and 57.1% in untreated groups as compared to 31.5% in 883 submitted ANLL patients), followed by M4 (16%, 21.4%, and 20.9%, respectively). Chromosomes most frequently involved in abnormalities in the treated group were number 7 (15 cases), number 5 (15 cases), number 17 (10 cases), and number 1 (5 cases). The most common structural changes included 5q− (9 cases); 7q− (4 cases); and deletions of chromosome 17, due primarily to translocations with chromosomes 11 (4 cases), 1 (6 cases), 3 (3 cases), and 15 (3 cases). The most common numerical changes were −7 (11 cases), −5 (6 cases), and −17 (5 cases). Other abnormalities included ring chromosomes in 5 cases, DMs in 2 cases, and a possible HSR (homogeneously staining region) in 1 case.

Although the size of the control group was small, it still is fairly obvious that the type of abnormalities differed from those seen in the treated group and involved different chromosomes: chromosome 6 (4 cases), chromosome 22 (3 cases), and 2 cases each of chromosomes 3, 5, 8, and 16. Markers of unknown origin were observed in 3 cases and one case displayed a ring chromosome. Interestingly, no translocations were seen in any of the 14 control patients. Involvement of chromosomes 5 and 17, but not chromosome 7, was correlated with a shorter survival.

The Workshop study reported that in the 56 patients in the secondary leukemia group there was "no significant relationship between the diagnosis of the primary disease, the type of therapy given, and the nature of the karyotypic changes of the secondary leukemia. However, normal karyotypes were seen more often in patients who had received radiation only . . . rather than chemotherapy . . ., or both radiation and chemotherapy."

Sandberg et al. (1982) reported the results of their study on 20 patients with secondary leukemia and reviewed the cytogenetic findings from an additional 206 patients from the literature. Abnormalities most commonly involved chromosome 7 (29%), chromosome 5 (19%), chromosome 17 (17%), chromosome 3 (12%), chromosome 21 (10%), and chromosome 8 (9%). Another characteristic of secondary leukemia which set it apart from de novo ANLL was the ploidy level: hypodiploidy was twice as frequent as pseudodiploidy and hyperdiploidy combined in secondary leukemia, whereas in de novo ANLL the frequency of hypodiploidy and hyperdiploidy is about the same. Sandberg et al. (1982) felt that the evidence strongly suggests that the development of secondary leukemia is due to therapeutic agents; this view is supported by the fact that the chromosomal abnormalities in secondary leukemia resemble one another, regardless of the nature of the original neoplasm. It is possible, however, that the therapy merely accelerates a process that would have occurred spontaneously, or that it has allowed patients to live long enough to develop leukemia as part of their disease complex.

IX. CONCLUSION

A. Significance of Chromosome Abnormalities in Acute Leukemia

The relationship between chromosomal abnormalities and survival differs considerably in ALL and ANLL.

In an early study of 331 patients with ALL (Whang-Peng et al., 1976), aneuploidy was noted at diagnosis in 43% of the patients and in 54% at some stage of the disease. Patients less than one year old or more than 20 years of age had a high incidence of aneuploidy. The existence of chromosome abnormalities at diagnosis or later in the disease was not prognostically significant, but their persistence and the development of total aneuploidy indicated a poor prognosis. We proposed, therefore, that eradication of aneuploidy is essential for achievement of a long remission and eventual cure. The results from the 234 cases studied at the Third IWCL in 1980 (Third IWCL, 1981) were similar. The incidence of abnormal cases increased with patient age, adults having more chromosomal abnormalities than children 15 years old or younger. The percentage of children classified in the three groups, NN (this group also included patients with Ncl, nonclonal abnormalities), AN, and AA were 38%, 50%, and 12%, respectively; adults showed 31% NN, 44% AN, and 25% AA. Median survival in children was estimated at 25 months for the NN group and 24 months for the AN group. (Survival for the NN + Ncl and AA could not be estimated because the survival curve had not fallen below 50%.) Median survival for adults was estimated at 31 months for NN, 16 months for NN + Ncl, 9 months for AN, and 9 months for AA. At the 1983 update of the Fourth Workshop, the longest survivals (in decreasing length) were seen in patients with more than 50 chromosomes, deletion of 6q−, normal karyotypes, and pseudodiploidy; while the shortest survivals were seen in patients with 47-50 chromosomes, 14q+, t(4;11) and t(8;14). A review of the structural and numerical chromosome changes in relation to specific subtype of ALL, clinical characteristics, and prognosis is presented in Table 1.

In his book on cytogenetics and neoplasia (1980), Sandberg suggests that analysis of the karyotype is of prognostic value in ANLL. He found that patients who had never demonstrated normal metaphases in the marrow during the course of the disease (AA) had a median survival of only 1.2 months, while for those with both normal and abnormal cells (AN) the median survival was 7.2 months, and for those with only normal metaphases (NN) it was 9.1 months. Patients over 70 years of age had a very poor survival (median 0.7 months) regardless of the karyotype. By the time of the Fourth IWCL in 1982 (Fourth IWCL, 1984), survival for all groups was lengthened but the general pattern was the same: the median survival was 10 months in NN patients and 4 months in AA patients. In those patients with a mixture of normal and abnormal metaphases (AN), the percentage of normal metaphases had no effect on survival. The median survival in the different ploidy groups was 5 months for pseudodiploidy, 4 months for hyperdiploidy, and 5 months for hypodiploidy. (In 305 intensively treated patients the corresponding figures were 11, 13, and 18 months, respectively).

In contrast to the findings in de novo ANLL, karyotypic abnormalities appear to have little effect on survival in secondary leukemia: median survival for NN, AN, and AA patients were 3, 5, and 3 months, respectively.

B. Mutagenic and Carcinogenic Agents and Acute Leukemia

Several investigators have examined the published data on ANLL in an attempt to determine the extent and significance of occupational and environmental exposure to mutagenic and carcinogenic agents.

Mitelman, Brandt, and Nilsson (1978) compared two groups of adult ANLL in Sweden, 23 patients occupationally exposed to chemical, insecticide, and petrol products, and 33 patients with no history of such exposure. They found that M1 and M2 ANLL were more common in the exposed group while monocytic varieties were more common in the nonexposed group. No significant differences were seen in complete remission rate or median survival between the two groups, and patients with chromosome abnormalities had poorer prognoses than patients with normal metaphases in both groups. There were striking differences in the two groups, however, regarding the incidence and type of specific chromosome abnormalities: aneuploidy was seen in 24.2% of the nonexposed group and in 82.6% of the exposed group; the abnormal exposed group had a least one of four particular changes, −5, −7, +8, or +21, whereas none of the nonexposed patients had −7 or +8, and −7 and +21 were seen in only one patient each. None of the other abnormalities observed in the nonexposed group were seen in the exposed patients.

In a review article, Rowley (1982) speculated that ". . . those patients with AML (M1 and M2) de novo who have abnormalities involving #5 and 7 may have developed leukemia as a result of exposure to mutagenic agents. On the other hand, an extra #8, which is the most frequent change in all of the myeloproliferative disorders, may provide a general proliferative advantage to myeloid cells and may be less directly related to mutagen exposure."

Table 1 Cytogenetic Abnormalities in Acute Lymphocytic Leukemia

Karyotypic abnormality	Med. age	Surv. (mo.)	FAB Classif.			Surface markers			Clinical Comments
			L1	L2	L3	non-T, B	T	B	
Normal	15y	18	42%	51%	7%	74%	18%	9%	
t(1;19)(q23;q13)						pre-B			Low WBC, early aggressive relapse, meningeal involvement, short survival
del(3)(p13)								majority (PLL)	High WBC, splenomegaly, aggressive course
t(4;11)(q13;q23)	congenital					majority			High WBC, high CNS involvement, poor prognosis
t(4;11)(q21;q23)	14y	7	43%	50%	7%	88%	12%		High WBC, organomegaly, myeloid/lymphoid morphology and immunologic markers
del(5)(q22q23)									Usually bi-phenotypic, usually combined with other abnormalities, unfavorable prognosis
t(6;12)								majority (PLL)	High WBC, splenomegaly, aggressive course
del(6q)	6y	29	50%	50%		75%	25%		
Monosomy 7									History of radiation, usually secondary leukemia

t(8;14)(q24;q32) t(2;8)(p12;q24) t(8;22)(q24;q11)	22y	5	6%		94%			100%	CNS involvement, high WBC at diagnosis
del(9)(p21)	older	12					100%		High WBC, high % of blasts, lymphadenopathy, splenomegaly
t(9;22)(q34;q11)	6y 35y	14 13				>99% pre B	rare T		Unfavorable prognosis
14q+	33y	9	23%	54%	23%	56%		44%	High WBC, CNS involvement
Near-haploidy (<30 chromosomes)	all younger					100%			Rare; all had disomy 21, low Hg, high WBC and blasts, Unfavorable prognosis
Severe hypodiploidy (30-36 chromosomes)	19	14	29%	71%		80%	20%		Patients older, rather poor prognosis
Pseudodiploidy	18	21	32%	68%		74%	26%		
Hyperdiploidy									
a. 47-50 chromosomes	16	5-6	45%	55%		87%	13%		Unfavorable prognosis
b. >50 chromosomes	5	34	48%	48%	4%	100%			Higher ratio of females, best prognosis

PLL = prolymphocytic leukemia
WBC = white blood count
CNS = central nervous system
Source: Data gathered from the Third International Workshop on Chromosomes in Leukemia (1981 and 1983) and other references cited in the text.

Table 2 Cytogenetic Abnormalities in Acute Nonlymphocytic Leukemia (ANLL)

Karyotype	Med. age	Med. surv.	% total	Most freq. FAB class.	Clinical comments
Normal	49 y	10 mo	45%	M2, M4, less M3	Auer rods common
del(3)(q21 or q26) t(3;5)(q21;q25 or p31-34)			3.6%	M2, M4, less M1, M6	Thrombocytopenia, generally assoc. with pancytopenia
t(4;11)(q21;q23)				M1	TdT+, both myeloid & lymph. (B-cell) lineages, young age, poor prognosis
del(5)(q12q33 or q15q33)			4%	M2, less M4, M6	Assoc. with MDS, secondary to toxic exposure; additional chrom. abn. signal ANLL
−5, 5q−, −7, and 7q−	39-59 y	3-4 mo	8.6%		Common in secondary leukemia, poor prognosis
del(6)(q23)					Hairy cell leukemia, lymphoblastic lymphoma/leukemia
t(6;9)(p23;q34) del(6)(p23)	41 y	5 mo		M2, M3, M4	Basophilia, poor response
Monosomy 7			6.5%	M2, M4, M6 (never M5)	Refractory anemia, thrombocytopenia, recurrent infections, poor response, short survival
t(8;21)(q22;q22) or complex trans.		9.5 mo	7%	M2	High remiss. rate, long surv.; poor prognosis when assoc. with loss of sex chromosomes
+8	47 y	6 mo	5.4%	M4, M2, M5	Elevated neuraminidase (75% patients)
9q−			1.2%	M2, M1, M4	MPD, rarely sole abnormality
t(9;22)(q34;q11)			9.9%	M1, M2	Assoc. with −7, +Ph[1], +8, i(17q) survival: 31 mo in M1, 59 mo in M2

11q⁻	49 y	8 mo	5%	M5, less M4, M2	Hepatosplenomegaly, enlarg. lymph node bleeding, refractory to therapy Transloc. to chrom: 10, 13, 19, 1, 6, 17, 8, 11, 12, 22, X (order of freq.)
del(12)(p12)	59 y	2 mo	2.5%	M1-6, except M3	
+13					Myelofibrosis with myeloid metaplasia, short survival
14q⁻					Hairy cell leukemia, lymphoblastic lymphoma/ leukemia
t(15;17)(q25;q22)	25 y	3 mo	6.5%	M3, M3V	Variable geographic distribution
inv(16)(p13q22)	35 y		2%	M4, M4Eo, less M2Eo, M5Eo	All patients: Auer rods, hepatomegaly, elevated serum neuraminidase, esoinophils, favorable prognosis
del(20)(q1104q1109)		2 mo		M6, M1, M2	Cytopenia, relatively older age
+21				M7	
Missing Y					Freq. (82.3%) assoc. with t(8;21) in M2
Marked hypodiploidy					Rare
Near tetraploidy					Rare, unfavorable prognosis
Polyploidy, chromosomal breakage, rings, other structural abnormalities				M6	

TdT = terminal deoxyribonucleotidyl transferase
MPD = myeloproliferative disorder
Source: Data gathered from references cited in the text.

The structural and numerical changes seen in ANLL and their relationship to clinical findings, prognosis, and survival are listed, by specific subgroup, in Table 2.

C. Heterochromatin, DMs, and HSRs

Several chromosomes show genetic variability of heterochromatin patterns and some investigators (Atkin, 1977; Shabtai and Halbreit, 1979) have proposed that variant patterns are associated with an increased risk for malignancy; other investigators, however, have observed no such relationship (Berger et al., 1983).

DMs and HSRs are usually associated with resistance to antimetabolic drugs; they have also been seen in a variety of malignancies prior to treatment but have rarely been observed in acute leukemia. Their significance in such cases remains unknown.

Fragile Sites and Oncogenes

A high incidence of cancer is seen in individuals with constitutional chromsome abnormalities or inherited chromosome instability syndromes. Development of malignancy in these individuals may be due to chromosome breakage at specific sites, causing chromosomal rearrangements which result in alterations of gene dosage, or activation of oncogenes, leading to malignant transformation.

Several studies have been made investigating the location of fragile sites (sites of frequent breakage) and comparing them to known oncogene locations. Yunis and Soreng (1984) demonstrated 51 chromosome fragile sites and noted that 7 of the 17 known oncogenes mapped at or near constitutive fragile sites (c-fra), and in four instances, both heritable (h-fra) and constitutive fragile sites were mapped to the same location. They also observed that 20 of the 51 c-fra and 6 of the 16 h-fra sites were located at or close to breakpoints found in 26 of the 31 specific structural abnormalities described in leukemia, lymphoma, and solid tumors. In a study of fragile sites in normal individuals (Whang-Peng et al., 1985b), the four most common were located at breakpoints associated with specific malignancies: 3p14.2 in small cell lung cancer, 1q21.3 in pre-B-ALL, 7q32.3 in ANLL, and 11q13.3 [location of bcl-1 oncogene and t(11;14) in non-Hodgkin's lymphoma]. Although the mechanism involved in chromosome breakage is unknown, many agents known to produce it are also implicated in carcinogenesis, e.g., certain chemicals, ionizing radiation, viruses, and spontaneous mutations. In order to understand the actual process of malignant transformation, it will be necessary to continue research into the basic mechanisms triggering chromosome translocation and oncogene activation.

REFERENCES

Abe, R., Ryan, D., Cecalu, P. O., Cohen, H., and Sandberg, A. A. (1983). Cytogenetic findings in congenital leukemia: case report and review of the literature. *Cancer Genet. Cytogenet.* 9: 139-144.

Abe, S., Golomb, H. M., Rowley, J. D., Mitelman, F., and Sandberg, A. A. (1980). Chromosomes and causation of human cancer and leukemia. XXXV. The missing Y in acute non-lymphocytic leukemia (ANLL). *Cancer* 45: 84-90.

Abe, S., Kohno, S., Kubonishi, I., Minowada, J., and Sandberg, A. A. (1979). Chromosomes and causation of human cancer and leukemia. XXXIII. 5q− in a case of acute lymphoblastic leukemia (ALL). *Am. J. Hematol.* 6: 259-266.

Arthur, D. C., and Bloomfield, C. D. (1983). Partial deletion of the long arm of chromosome 16 and bone marrow eosinophilia in acute nonlymphocytic leukemia: A new association. *Blood* 61: 994-998.

Atkin, N. B. (1977). Chromosome 1 heteromorphism in patients with malignant disease: A constitutional marker for a high-risk group? *Br. Med. J.* 1: 358.

Berger, R., Bernheim, A., Mitelman, F., and Rydholm, A. (1983). C-band pattern in lymphocytes of patients with soft tissue sarcomas. *Cancer Genet. Cytogenet.* 9: 145-150.

Berger, R., Bernheim, A., Valensi, F., and Flandrin, G. (1985). 14q− in two hairy cell leukemia patients. *Cancer Genet. Cytogenet.* 16: 91-93.

Bernstein, R., Pinto, M. R., Morcom, G., Macdougall, L. G., Bezwoda, W., Dukes, I., Penfold, G., and Mendelow, B. (1982). Karyotype analysis in acute nonlymphocytic leukemia (ANLL): Comparison with ethnic group, age, morphology, and survival. *Cancer Genet. Cytogenet.* 6: 187-199.

Bitter, M. A., Neilly, M. E., Le Beau, M. M., Pearson, M. G., and Rowley, J. D. (1985). Rearrangements of chromosome 3 involving bands 3q21 and 3q26 are associated with normal or elevated platelet counts in acute non-lymphocytic leukemia. *Blood* 66: 1362-1370.

Bloomfield, C. D., Brunning, R. S., Smith, K. A., and Nesbit, M. E. (1980). Prognostic significance of the Philadelphia chromosome in acute lymphocytic leukemia. *Cancer Genet. Cytogenet.* 1: 229-238.

Borgstrom, G. H., Vuopio, P., and de la Chapelle, A. (1976). Polyploidy of the bone marrow. *Scand. J. Haematol.* 17: 123-131.

Boveri, T. (1902). Uber mehrpolige Mitosen als Mittel zur Analyse des Zellkerns. *Verh. Phys. Med. Ges.* 35: 67-88.

Cabrol, C., Werner-Favre, C., Wyss, M., Pitmon, D., and Engel, E. (1983). Acute lymphoblastic leukemia in two children with a congenital chromosome anomaly: Familial inv(11)(15q13) in one and ring chromosome no.21 in the other. *Cancer Genet. Cytogenet.* 8: 67-74.

Carroll, A. J., Crist, W. M., Parmley, R. T., Roper, M., Cooper, M. D., and Finley, W. H. (1984). Pre-B cell leukemia associated with chromosome translocation. *Blood* 63: 721-724.

Caspersson, T., Farber, S., Foley, G. E., Kudynowski, J., Modest, E. J., Simonsson, E., Wagh, U., and Zech, L. (1968). Chemical differentiation along metaphase chromosomes. *Exp. Cell Res.* 49: 219-222.

Chaganti, R. S. K., Jhanwar, S. C., Arlin, Z., Koziner, B., Ambati, A., Andreeff, M., and Clarkson, B. D. (1983). Non-T, Non-B acute lymphoblastic leukemia (L3) with t(8;22) and two 14q+ chromosomes. *Cancer Genet. Cytogenet.* 10: 95-103.

Chaganti, R. S. K., Miller, D. R., Meyers, P. A., and German, J. (1979). Cytogenetic evidence of the intrauterine origin of acute leukemia in monozygotic twins. *N. Eng. J. Med.* 300: 1033-1034.

Chan, W. C., Brynes, R. K., Kim, T. H., Verras, A., Schick, C., Green, R. J., and Ragab, A. H. (1983). Acute megakaryoblastic leukemia in early childhood. *Blood* 62: 92-98.

Chitambar, C., Robinson, W., and Glode, L. (1983). Familial leukemia and aplastic anemia associated with monosomy 7. *Am. J. Med.* 75: 756-762.

Clare, N., Boldt, D., Messerschmidt, G., Zelter, P., Hansen, K., and Manhoff, L. (1986). Lymphocyte malignancy and chromosome 14: structural aberrations involving band q11. *Blood* 67:704-709.

Como, R., Sarna, G., and Sparkes, R. S. (1979). Marked hypodiploidy in a case of acute undifferentiated leukemia. *Am. J. Hematol.* 6: 143-147.

Conjalka, M. S., Cuttner, J., Wisniewski, L., Goldberg, J. D., Reisman, A., Elliott, R., Desnick, R., Holland, J. F., and Berk, P. D. (1983). Pretreatment marrow cytogenetic status: a predictor of response to remission induction therapy in acute myelogenous leukemia. *Mt. Sinai J. Med.* 50: 201-207.

Croce, C., Isobe, M., Palumbo, A., Puck, J., Ming, J., Tweardy, D., Erikson, J., Davis, M., and Rovera, G. (1985). Gene for *a* chain of human T-cell receptor: Location on chromosome 14 region involved in T-cell neoplasms. *Science* 227: 1044-1047.

Cuttner, J., Seremetis, S., Najfeld, V., Dimitrui-Bona, A., and Winchester, R. A. (1984). TdT-positive acute leukemia with monocytoid characteristics: Clinical, cytochemical, cytogenetic, and immunologic findings. *Blood* 64: 237-243.

Daeschner, C., Elder, F., Carpentieri, U., and Haggard, M. E. (1985). Leukemia with a novel 4q11q rearrangement. *Cancer Genet. Cytogenet.* 16: 245-250.

Davis, M. P., Dewald, G. W., Pierre, R. V., and Hoagland, H. C. (1984). Hematologic manifestations associated with deletions of the long arm of chromosome 20. *Cancer Genet. Cytogenet.* 12: 63-71.

De Braekeleer, M., Poon, M. C., Russell, J., and Lin, C. C. (1985). A case of acute lymphoblastic leukemia with t(10;19)(q26;q13). *Cancer Genet. Cytogenet.* 16: 369-372.

Debiec-Rychter, M., Kaluzewski, B., Bugala, I., and Zajazkowska, D. (1985). Isochromosome X in acute myeloblastic leukemia. *Cancer Genet. Cytogenet.* 15: 137-141.

Diaz, M. O., Le Beau, M. M., Rowley, J. D., Drabkin, H. A., and Patterson, D. (1985). The role of the c-*mos* gene in the 8;21 translocation in human acute myeloblastic leukemia. *Science* 229: 767-769.

Douglass, E. C., and Freeman, D. L. (1983). Hypotetraploidy in erythroleukemia. *Cancer Genet. Cytogenet.* 8:231-234.

Esseltine, D. W., Vekemans, M., Seemayer, T., Reece, E., Gordon, J., and Whitehead, V. M. (1982). Significance of a (4;11) translocation in acute lymphoblastic leukemia. *Cancer* 50: 503-506.

Fleischman, E. W., Prigogina, E. L., Iljinskaja, G. W., Konstantinova, L. N., Puchkova, G. P., Volkova, M. A., Frenkel, M. A., and Balakirev, S. A. (1983). Chromosomal rearrangements with a common breakpoint at 6p23 in five cases of myeloid leukemia. *Hum. Genet.* 64: 254-256.

Fourth International Workshop in Chromosomes in Leukemia, 1982. (1984). A prospective study of acute nonlymphocytic leukemia. *Cancer Genet. Cytogenet.* 11: 249-360.

Freireich, E. J., Whang, J., Tjio, J. H., Levin, R. H., Brittin, G. M., and Frei, E. (1964). III: Refractory anemia, granulocytic hyperplasia of bone marrow, and a missing chromosome in marrow cells. A new clinical syndrome? *Clin. Res.* 12: 284 (abstract).

Gibas, Z., Becher, R., and Sandberg, A. A. (1983). Chromosomes and causation of human cancer and leukemia. LIII. Comprehensive cytogenetic analysis of an erythroleukemia. *Cancer Genet. Cytogenet.* 10: 241-253.

Golomb, H. M., Vardiman, J., and Rowley, J. D. (1976). Acute nonlymphocytic leukemia in adults: Correlations with Q-banded chromosomes. *Blood* 48: 9-21.

Golomb, H. M., Lindgren, V., and Rowley, J. D. (1978). Chromosome abnormalities in patients with hairy cell leukaemia. *Cancer* 41: 1374-1380.

Gralnick, H., Galton, D. A. G., Catovsky, D., Sultan, C., and Bennett, J. M. (1977). Classification of acute leukemia. *Ann. Int. Med.* 87: 740-753.

Gyger, M., Bonny, Y., and Forest, L. (1982). Childhood monosomy 7 syndrome. *Am. J. Hematol.* 13: 329-334.

Haas, O. A., Bettelheim, P., Schmidmeier, W., Gadner, H., Ludwig, H., Majdic, O., and Schulz, U. (1985). 5q− chromosome in acute leukemia with lymphoid morphology and expression of myeloid membrane determinants. *Blood* 65: 1342-1348.

Hartley, S. E., and Toolis, F. (1980). Double minute chromosomes in a case of acute myeloblastic leukemia. *Cancer Genet. Cytogenet.* 2: 275-280.

Hecht, F., Hecht, B. K., Berger, C., Morgan, R., Jarzabek, V., Vyvial, T., Isaacs, J., and Epstein, A. (1983). Position effect in translocation (2;8) in acute lymphocytic leukemia with kappa light chain immunoglobulin expression. *Cancer Genet. Cytogenet.* 10: 255-259.

Hogge, D. E., Misawa, S., Parsa, N. Z., Pollak, A., and Testa, J. R. (1984). Abnormalities of chromosome 16 in association with acute myelomonocytic leukemia and dysplastic bone marrow eosinophils. *J. Clin. Oncol.* 2: 550-557.

Hsu, L. Y. F., Greenberg, M. L., Kohan, S., and Wittman, R. (1979). Trisomy 13 in bone marrow cells in acute myelocytic leukemia and myelofibrosis. *Clin. Genet.* 15: 327-331.

ISCN (1985): An International System for Human Cytogenetic Nomenclature, Harnden, D. G., and Klinger, H. P. (Eds): published in collaboration with *Cytogenet. Cell Genet.* (Karger, Basel 1985), 117 pp.

Juliusson, G., Robert, K. H., Ost, A., Friberg, K., Biberfeld, P., Zech, L., and Gahrton, G. (1985). Del(3)(p13) in B-prolymphocytic leukemia—A new nonrandom chromosomal aberration possibly related to the *c-ras* oncogene. *Cancer Genet. Cytogenet.* 14: 191-195.

Kamada, N., Dohy, H., Okada, K., Oguma, N., Kuramoto, A., Tanaka, K., and Uchino, H. (1981). In vivo and in vitro activity of neutrophil alkaline phosphatase in acute myelocytic leukemia with 8;21 translocation. *Blood* 58: 1213-1217.

Kaneko, Y., Kimpara, H., Kawai, S., and Fujimoto, T. (1983). 8;21 chromosome translocation in eosinophilic leukemia. *Cancer Genet. Cytogenet.* 9: 181-183.

Kao, Y. S., Reine, G. A., and Miletello, G. P. (1984). Translocation (6;9)(p.23; p34) in acute myeloblastic leukemia (M2) with bone marrow eosinophilia. *Am. J. Human Genet.* 36: 31S (Abstract).

Khalid, G., Li, Y. S., Flemans, R. J., and Hayhoe, F. G. J. (1981). Chromosomal abnormalities in a case of hairy cell leukaemia. *Leukemia Res.* 5: 431-435.

Knuutila, S., Rajantie, J., Leskinen, R., Rapola, J., and de la Chapelle, A. (1985). t(11;19)(q23;p11) in a child with acute T-cell leukemia. *Cancer Genet. Cytogenet.* 15: 181-186.

Kocova, M., Kowalczyk, J. R., and Sandberg, A. A. (1985). Translocation 4;11 acute leukemia: Three case reports and review of the literature. *Cancer Genet. Cytogenet.* 16: 21-32.

Kowalczyk, J. P., Grossi, M., and Sandberg, A. A. (1984). A case of ALL with 4q trisomy. *Cancer Genet. Cytogenet.* 11: 31-36.

Kowalczyk, J., and Sandberg, A. A. (1983). A possible subgroup of ALL with 9p. *Cancer Genet. Cytogenet.* 9: 383-385.

Larson, R. A., Le Beau, M. M., Vardiman, J. W., Testa, J. R., Golomb, H. M., and Rowley, J. D. (1983). The predictive value of initial cytogenetic studies in 148 adults with acute nonlymphocytic leukemia: a 12-year study (1970-1982). *Cancer Genet. Cytogenet.* 10: 219-236.

Le Beau, M. M., Larson, R. A., Bitter, M. A., Vardiman, J. W., Golomb, H. M., and Rowley, J. D. (1983). Association of an inversion of chromosome 16 with abnormal marrow eosinophils in acute myelomonocytic leukemia. *N. Eng. J. Med.* 309: 630-636.

Levan, G., and Mitelman, F. (1979). Absence of late-replicating X-chromosome in a female patient with acute myeloid leukemia and the 8;21 translocation. *J. Nat'l. Cancer Inst.* 62: 273-275.

Li, F., Hecht, F., Kaiser-McCaw, B., Baranko, P. V., and Potter, N. (1981). Ataxia-pancytopenia: syndrome of cerebellar ataxia, hypoplastic anemia, monosomy 7, and acute myelogenous leukemia. *Cancer Genet. Cytogenet.* 4: 189-196.

Li, Y. S., Khalid, G., Matthews, J. G., and Hayhoe, F. G. J. (1983). A case of erythroleukaemia with homogeneously staining regions on chromosomes. *Leukemia Res.* 7: 755-759.

Lonnqvist, B., Gahrton, G., Eriksson, P., Friberg, K., and Zech, L. (1979). Isochromosome 17 in a patient with a myeloproliferative disorder terminating in eosinophilic leukemia. *Acta Med. Scand.* 206: 321-325.

Louwagie, A., Criel, A., Verfaillie, C. M., Valcke, Y. J., Lamberts, H., Hidafat, M., Mecucci, C., and Van Den Berghe, H. (1985). Philadelphia positive T-acute lymphoblastic leukemia. *Cancer Genet. Cytogenet.* 16: 297-300.

Macdougall, L. G., Brown, J. A., Cohen, M. M., and Judisch, J. M. (1974). C-monosomy myeloproliferative syndrome: a case of 7-monosomy. *J. Pediatr.* 84: 256-259.

Mandel, E. M., Shabtai, F., Gafter, U., Klein, B., Halbrecht, I., and Djaldetti, M. (1977). Ph^1 positive acute lymphocytic leukemia with chromosome 7 abnormalities. *Blood* 49: 281-287.

Mecucci, C., Vermaelen, K., Kulling, G., Michaux, J. L., Noens, L., Van Hove, W., Tricot, G., Louwagie, A., and Van Den Gerghe, H. (1984). Interstitital 9q- deletions in hematologic malignancies. *Cancer Genet. Cytogenet.* 12: 309-319.

Michael, P. M., Garson, O. M., and Callen, D. F. (1985). A review of the t(1;19) breakpoints in acute lymphocytic leukemia. *Cancer Genet. Cytogenet.* 17: 79-80.

Michael, P. M., Levin, M. D., and Garson, O. M. (1984). Translocation 1;19–a new cytogenetic abnormality in acute lymphocytic leukemia. *Cancer Genet. Cytogenet.* 12: 333-341.

Mirro, J., Kitchingman, G., Williams, D., Lauzon, G. J., Lin, C. C., Callihan, T., and Zipf, T. (1986). Clinical and laboratory characteristics of acute leukemia with the 4;11 translocation. *Blood* 67: 689-697.

Mitelman, F., Brandt, L., and Nilsson, P. G. (1978). Relation among occupational exposure to potential mutogenic/carcinogenic agents, clinical findings, and bone marrow chromosomes in acute nonlymphocytic leukemia. *Blood* 52: 1229-1237.

Mitelman, F. (1985). *Catalog of Chromosome Aberrations in Cancer, Second Edition*. Alan R. Liss, New York.

Miyamoto, K., Tomita, N., Ishii, A., Nonaka, H., Kondo, T., Tanaka, T., and Kitajima, K. (1984). Chromosome abnormalities of leukemia cells in adult patients with T-cell leukemia. *J. Natl. Cancer Inst.* 73: 353-362.

Mufti, G. J., Hamblin, T. J., Oscier, D. G., and Johnson, S. (1983). Common ALL with pre-B-cell features showing (8;14) and (14;18) chromosone translocations. *Blood* 62:1142-1146.

Neame, P. B., Soamboonsrup, P., Browman, G., Barr, R. D., Saeed, N., Chan, B., Pai, M., Benger, A., Wilson, W. E. C., Walker, I. R., and McBride, J. A. (1985). Simultaneous or sequential expression of lymphoid and myeloid phenotypes in acute leukemia. *Blood* 65: 142-148.

Newburger, P. E., Latt, S. A., Pesando, J. M., Gustashaw, K., Powers, M., Chaganti, R. S. K., and O'Reilly, R. J. (1981). Leukemia relapse in donor cells after allogeneic bone-marrow transplantation. *N. Eng. J. Med.* 304: 712-714.

Nowell, P. C., and Hungerford, D. A. (1960). A minute chromosome in human chronic granulocytic leukemia. *Science* 132: 1497.

Ohyashiki, K., Oshimura, M., Uchida, H., Nomoto, S., Sakai, N., Tonomura, A., and Ito, H. (1985). Cytogenetic and ultrastructural studies on ten patients with acute promyelocytic leukemia, including one case with a complex translocation. *Cancer Genet. Cytogenet.* 14: 247-255.

Oshimura, M., Freeman, A. I., and Sandberg, A. A. (1977). Chromosomes and causation of human cancer and leukemia. XXIII. Near-haploidy in acute leukemia. *Cancer* 40: 1143-1148.

Parkin, J. L., Arthur, D. C., Abramson, C. S., McKenna, R. W., Kersey, J. H., Heideman, R. L., and Brunning, R. D. (1982). Acute leukemia associated with the t(4;11) chromosome rearrangement: Ultrastructural and immunologic characteristics. *Blood* 60: 1321-1331.

Pasquali, F., and Casalone, R. (1981). Rearrangement of three chromosomes (Nos. 2, 8, and 21) in acute myeloblastic leukemia. Evidnece for more than one specific event. *Cancer Genet. Cytogenet.* 3: 335-339.

Pasquali, F., Bernasconi, P., Casalone, R., Fraccaro, M., Bernasconi, C., Lazzarino, M., Morra, E., Alessandrino, E. P., Marchi, M. A., and Sanger, R. (1982). Pathogenetic significance of "pure" monosomy 7 in myeloproliferative disorders. Analysis of 14 cases. *Hum. Genet.* 62: 40-51.

Pierre, R. V., and Hoagland, H. C. (1972). Age-associated aneuploidy: Loss of Y chromosome from human bone marrow cells with aging. *Cancer* 30: 889-894.

Pittman, S., and Catovsky, D. (1983). Chromosome abnormalities in B-cell prolymphocytic leukemia: A study of nine cases. *Cancer Genet. Cytogenet.* 9: 355-365.

Priest, J. R., Robison, L. L., McKenna, R. W., Lindquist, L. L., Warkentin, P. I., LeBien, T. W., Woods, W. G., Kersey, J. H., Coccia, P. I., and Nesbit, M. E. (1980). Philadelphia chromosome positive childhood acute lymphoblastic leukemia. *Blood* 56: 15-22.

Pui, C. H., Williams, K. L., Kalwinsky, D. K., Look, T. A., Melvin, S. L., Dodge, R. K., Rivera, G., Murphy, S. B., and Dahl, G. V. (1986). Cytogenetic features and serum lactic dehydrogenase level predict a poor treatment outcome for children with pre-B-cell leukemia. *Blood* 67: 1688-1692.

Pui, C. H., Williams, D. L., Scarborough, V., Jackson, C. W., Price, R., and Murphy, S. (1982). Acute megakaryoblastic leukaemia associated with intrinsic platelet dysfunction and constitutional ring 21 chromosome in a young boy. *Br. J. Haematol.* 50: 191-200.

Rowley, J. (1982). Chromosome abnormalities in human acute nonlymphocytic leukemia: relationship to age, sex, and exposure to mutagens. *Natl. Cancer Inst. Monogr.* 60: 17-23.

Rowley, J. D., and Potter, D. (1976). Chromosomal banding patterns in acute nonlymphocytic leukemia. *Blood* 47: 705-721.

Rowley, J. D., Golomb, H. M., and Doughery, C. (1977). Translocation, a consistent chromosome change in acute promyelocytic leukaemia. *Lancet* 1: 549-550.

Russell, M. H., Miller, P., and Killam, A. (1982). Familial pericentric inversion of chromosome 11 detected prenatally. *J. Med. Genet.* 19: 151-152.

Sadamori, N., Han, T., Kakati, S., and Sandberg, A. A. (1983a). Chromosomes and causation of human cancer and leukemia. LI. A hairy cell leukemia case with 14q+ and ring chromosomes: Significance of ring chromosomes in blood disorders. *Cancer Genet. Cytogenet.* 10: 67-77.

Sadamori, N., Han, T., Minowada, J., Bloom, M. L., Henderson, E. S., and Sandberg, A. A. (1983b). Possible specific chromosome change in prolymphocytic leukemia. *Blood* 62: 729-736.

Sakurai, M., Kaneko, Y., and Abe, R. (1982). Further characterization of acute myelogenous leukemia with t(8;21) chromosome translocation. *Cancer Genet. Cytogenet.* 6: 143-152.

Sandberg, A. A. (1980). *The Chromosomes in Human Cancer and Leukemia.* Elsevier-North Holland, New York.

Sandberg, A. A., Kohno, S., Wake, N., and Minowada, J. (1980). Chromosomes and causation of human cancer and leukemia. XLII. Ph[1]-positive ALL: An entity within myeloproliferative disorders? *Cancer Genet. Cytogenet.* 2: 145-174.

Sandberg, A. A., Wake, N., and Kohno, S. (1982). Chromosomes and causation of human cancer and leukemia. XLVII. Severe hypodiploidy and chromosome conglomerations in ALL. *Cancer Genet. Cytogenet.* 5: 293-307.

Sandberg, A. A., Abe, S., Kowalczyk, J. R., Zedgenidze, A., Takeuchi, J., and Kakati, S. (1982). Chromosomes and causation of human cancer and leukemia. L. Cytogenetics of leukemias complicating other diseases. *Cancer Genet. Cytogenet.* 7: 95-136.

Sandberg, A. A., Morgan, R., McCallister, J. A., Kaiser-McCaw, B., and Hecht, F. (1983). Acute myeloblastic leukemia (AML) with t(6;9)(p23;q34): A specific subgroup of AML? *Cancer Genet. Cytogenet.* 10: 139-142.

Sariban, E., Oliver, C., Corash, L., Cossman, J., Whang-Peng, J., Jaffe, E. S., Gralnick, H. R., and Poplack, D. G. (1984). Acute megakaryoblastic leukemia in childhood. *Cancer* 54: 1423-1428.

Sasaki, M., Kondo, K., and Tomiyasu, T. (1983). Cytogenetic characterization of ten cases of Ph[1]-positive acute myelogenous leukemia. *Cancer Genet. Cytogenet.* 9: 119-128.

Schwartz, S., Jiji, R., Kerman, S., Meekins, J., and Cohen, M. M. (1983). Translocation (6;9)(p23;q34) in acute nonlymphocytic leukemia. *Cancer Genet. Cytogenet.* 10: 133-138.

Seabright, M. A. (1971). A rapid banding technique for human chromosomes. *Lancet* 2: 971-972.

Second International Workshop on Chromosomes in Leukemia, 1979 (1980). Chromosomes in preleukemia. *Cancer Genet. Cytogenet.* 2: 108-113.

Shabtai, F., and Halbrecht, I. (1979). Risk of malignancy and chromosomal polymorphism: a possible mechanism of association. *Clin. Genet.* 15: 73-77.

Shiraishi, Y., Taguchi, H., Niiya, K., Shiomi, F., Kikukawa, K., Kubonishi, S., Ohmura, T., Hamawaki, M., and Ueda, N. (1982). Diagnostic and prognostic significance of chromosome abnormalities in marrow and mitogen response of lymphocytes of acute nonlymphocytic leukemia. *Cancer Genet. Cytogenet.* 5: 1-24.

Stivrins, T. J., Davis, R. B., Sanger, W., Fritz, J., and Purtilo, D. T. (1984). Transformation of Fanconi's anemia to acute nonlymphocytic leukemia associated with emergence of monosomy 7. *Blood* 64: 173-176.

Stricker, R. B., and Linker, C. A. (1983). Acute lymphoblastic leukemia with monosomy 7 in a Hiroshima survivor 37 years after the bomb. *J. Am. Med. Asso.* 250: 640-641.

Sweet, D. L., Golomb, H. M., Rowley, J. D., and Vardiman, J. M. (1979). Acute myelogenous leukemia and thrombocythemia associated with an abnormality of chromosome no. 3. *Cancer Genet. Cytogenet.* 1: 33-37.

Talpaz, M., Kantarjian, H. M., McCredie, K., Trujillo, J. M., Keating, M. J., and Gutterman, J. U. (1986). Hematologic remission and cytogenetic improvement induced by recombinant human interferon $alpha_A$ in chronic myelogeneous leukemia. *N. Engl. J. Med.* 314: 1065-1069.

Testa, J. R., Oguma, N., Pollak, A., and Wiernik, P. H. (1983). Near-tetraploid clones in acute leukemia. *Blood* 61: 71-78.

Testa, J. R., and Rowley, J. D. (1980). Chromosomal banding patterns in patients with acute nonlymphocytic leukemia. *Cancer Genet. Cytogenet.* 1: 239-247.

Third International Workshop on Chromosomes in Leukemia, 1980 (1981). Chromosomal abnormalities in acute lymphoblastic leukemia. *Cancer Genet. Cytogenet.* 4: 95-137.

Third International Workshop on Chromosomes in Leukemia. (1983). Chromosomal abnormalities and their clinical significance in acute lymphoblastic leukemia. *Cancer Res.* 43: 868-873.

Trent, J. M., Durie, B. G. M., Davis, J. R., and Veomett, I. (1983). Cytogenetic and clinical assessment of six patients with erythroleukemia. *Anticancer Res.* 3: 111-116.

Trujillo, J. M., Cork, A., Drewinko, B., Hart, J. S., and Freireich, E. J. (1971). Case Report: Tetraploid Leukemia. *Blood* 38: 632-637.

Van Den Berghe, H., Cassiman, J-J., David, G., Fryns, J-P., Michaux, J-L., and Sokal, G. (1974). Distinct haematological disorder with deletion of long arm of no. 5 chromosome. *Nature* 251: 437-438.

Van Den Berghe, H. (1977). The 5q− anomaly: a short synopsis. *Internatl. Confer.*, Helsinki (Abstract).

Vermaelen, K., Barbieri, D., Michaux, J., Tricot, G., Casteels-Van Daele, M., Noens, L., Van Hove, W., Drochmans, A., Louwagie, A., and Van Den Berghe, H. (1983a). Anomalies of the long arm of chromosome 11 in human myelo- and lymphoproliferative disorders. I. Acute nonlymphocytic leukemia. *Cancer Genet. Cytogenet.* 10: 105-116.

Vermaelen, K., Michaux, J. L., Louwagie, A., and Van Den Berghe, H. (1983b). Reciprocal translocation t(6;9)(p21;q33): A new characteristic chromosome anomaly in myeloid leukemias. *Cancer Genet. Cytogenet.* 10: 125-131.

Webber, L. W., and Garson, O. M. (1983). Fluorodeoxyuridine synchronization of bone marrow cultures. *Cancer Genet. Cytogenet.* 8: 123-132.

Werner-Favre, C., Cabrol, C., Beris, P., and Engel, E. (1983). Isochromosome 21 and other chromosomal abnormalities in a patient with erythroleukemia. *Ann Genet.* 26: 240-242.

Werner-Favre, C., Engel, E., and Beris, P. (1985). Translocation t(3;5) in ANLL. *Cancer Genet. Cytogenet.* 16: 279.

Whang-Peng, J., Knutsen, T., Ziegler, J., and Leventhal, B. (1976). Cytogenetic studies in acute lymphocytic leukemia: Special emphasis in long-term survival. *Med. Ped. Oncol.* 2:333-351.

Whang-Peng, J., Knutsen, T., O'Donnell, J. F., and Brereton, H. D. (1979). Acute non-lymphocytic leukemia and myeloproliferative syndrome following radiation therapy for non-Hodgkin's lymphoma and chronic lymphocytic leukemia. *Cancer* 44: 1592-1600.

Whang-Peng, J., Bunn, P. A., Knutsen, T., Kao-Shan, C. S., Broder, S., Jaffe, E. S., Gelmann, E., Blattner, W., Lofters, W., Young, R. C., and Gallo, R. C. (1985a). Cytogenetic studies in human T-cell lymphoma virus (HTLV)-positive leukemia-lymphoma in the United States. *J. Natl. Cancer Inst.* 74: 357-369.

Whang-Peng, J., Lee, E., Kao-Shan, C. S., Boccia, R., and Knutsen, T. (1985b). Genes, fragile sites, chromosomal translocations, and cancer in aging. In *Interrelationship Among Aging, Cancer And Differentiation*, B. Pullman, P. O. P. Ts'o, and E. L. Schneider (eds.). D. Reidel Publ. Co., Dordrecht, Netherlands, pp 233-243.

Whang-Peng, J., Triche, T. J., Knutsen, T., Miser, J., Kao-Shan, S., Tsai, S., and Israel, M. A. (1986). Cytogenetic characterization of selected small round cell tumors of childhood. *Cancer Genet. Cytogenet.* 21: 185-208.

Williams, D. L., Tsiatis, A., Brodeur, G. M., Look, A. T., Melvin, S. L., Bowman, W. P., Kalwinsky, D. K., Rivera, G., and Dahl, G. V. (1982). Prognostic importance of chromosome number in 136 untreated children with acute lymphoblastic leukemia. *Blood* 60: 864-871.

Williams, D. L., Look, A. T., Melvin, S. L., Roberson, P. K., Dahl, G., Flake, T., Stass, S. (1984). New chromosomal translocations correlate with specific immunophenotypes of choldhood acute lymphoblastic leukemia. *Cell* 36: 101-109.

Williams, D. L., Harber, J., Murphy, S. B., Look, A. T., Kalwinsky, D. K., Rivera, G., Melvin, S. L., Stass, S., and Dahl, G. V. (1986). Chromosomal translocations play a unique role in influencing prognosis in childhood acute lymphoblastic leukemia. *Blood* 68: 205-212.

Wisniewski, L. P., and Hirschhorn, K. (1983). Acquired partial deletions of the long arm of chromosome 5 in hematologic disorders. *Am. J. Hematol.* 15: 295-310.

Yamada, K., Sugimoto, E., Amano, M., Inamura, Y., Kubnota, T., and Matsumoto, Y. (1983). Two cases of acute promyelocytic leukemia with variant translocations: The importance of chromosome no. 17 abnormality. *Cancer Genet. Cytogenet.* 9: 93-99.

Yoo, T. J., Orman, S. V., Patil, S. R., Drominey, C., Needleman, S., Rajtora, D., Graves, N., Ackerman, L., and Taylor, W. W. (1984). Evolution to eosinophilic leukemia with a t(5;11) translocation in a patient with idiopathic hypereosinophilic syndrome. *Cancer Genet. Cytogenet.* 11: 389-394.

Yunis, J. J. (1976). High resolution of human chromosomes. *Science* 191: 1268-1270.

Yunis, J. J. (1984). Recurrent chromosomal defects are found in most patients with acute nonlymphocytic leukemia. *Cancer Genet. Cytogenet.* 11: 125-137.

Yunis, J. J., Bloomfield, C. D., and Ensrud, K. (1981). All cases of acute nonlymphocytic leukemia may have a chromosomal defect. *N. Eng. J. Med.* 305: 135-139.

Yunis, J. J., Brunning, R. D., Howe, R. B., and Lobell, M. (1984). High-resolution chromosomes as an independent prognostic indicator in adult acute nonlymphocytic leukemia. *N. Eng. J. Med.* 311: 812-818.

Yunis, J. J., and Soreng, A. L. (1984). Constitutive fragile sites and cancer. *Science* 226: 1199-1205.

6

Nucleic Acid Flow Cytometry

An Aid to Diagnosis and Prognosis in Acute Leukemia in Adults

RONALD S. WALTERS, DENNIS A. JOHNSTON, DENNIS O. DIXON, SANFORD A. STASS, MICHAEL J. KEATING, JOSE M. TRUJILLO, KENNETH B. McCREDIE, and BART BARLOGIE *The University of Texas System Cancer Center, M. D. Anderson Hospital and Tumor Institute, Houston, Texas*

I. INTRODUCTION

Acute leukemia is a varied group of disorders arising in the bone marrow and causing clinical symptoms by way of quantitative or functional defects in hemopoiesis and as a result of tumor bulk from organomegaly or high white blood cell count with leukostasis. The diagnosis of acute leukemia relies mainly on morphologic criteria, which have been refined in recent years using the French-American-British (FAB) classification (1), the reproducibility of which, however, remains imperfect (2). With the use of immunologic means, cell lineage and stage of differentiation can now be better defined, leading to the recent recognition of mixed-lineage leukemias (3,4). While a difference in prognosis between lymphoblastic and myeloblastic leukemias has long been recognized in children (5,6), this has only recently been suggested in adults, where some studies have demonstrated a superior prognosis in acute lymphocytic leukemia (ALL) compared to acute myelogenous leukemia (AML) (7,8). Adult AML encompasses a wide spectrum of clinical disease manifestation and prognosis, where traditional morphology offers little discrimination. The only pretreatment variable recognized to favorably affect prognosis is younger age (9); the FAB classification has been insensitive to both remission induction and survival (10). In recent years, with the systematic application of modern banding technology, cytogenetics has emerged as a dominant disease feature affecting both initial drug sensitivity and long-term survival (11, 12).

Supported by CA 28153 and CA 16672 from the National Cancer Institute, National Institutes of Health, Bethesda, Maryland.

We have applied quantitative cytology to the study of leukemias and other hematologic malignancies to determine whether examination of cellular DNA and RNA content, which are sensitive to genomic abnormalities, cell proliferation and differentiation (13,14), may be associated with drug responsiveness and prognosis. Nucleic acid content can be conveniently assessed objectively and quantitatively by means of appropriate fluorochromes used in conjunction with flow cytometry (15,16). Employing the metachromatic dye acridine orange (AO) for correlated DNA and RNA analysis (17), we have systematically evaluated the diagnostic and prognostic usefulness of DNA-derived ploidy and cell cycle compartment distribution as well as the usefulness of RNA content as a measure of differentiation and proliferation in various forms of leukemia in adults (18).

II. MATERIALS AND METHODS

A. Patients

Between 1979 and 1986, bone marrow aspirates and biopsies from 411 patients with various forms of leukemia–AML; ALL; chronic myelogenous leukemia (CML); chronic lymphocytic leukemia (CLL); and myelodysplastic syndromes (MDS)–were evaluated by acridine orange flow cytometry (AO FCM). During the same time period, 49 normal volunteers or patients with solid tumors without bone marrow involvement and without prior chemotherapy were also studied.

B. Cell Preparation

Bone marrow aspirates and biopsies were obtained from the iliac crest under local anesthesia and promptly transferred into heparin-containing RPMI 1640 medium. Marrow biopsies were subjected to mechanical dispersion with surgical blades and subsequent syringing through progressively smaller gauge size needles (19). In the case of marrow aspirates, Hypaque-Ficoll gradient separation was applied, and interphase cells were collected for further analysis (20). Single-cell suspensions from biopsies and aspirates were stained with acridine orange for correlated analysis of DNA and RNA content, which was carried out with a mercury arc ICP 22 flow cytometer (21). Excess sample was fixed in 70% ethanol and was available for high-resolution DNA analysis with a dye combination of ethidium bromide and mithramycin (22).

C. Derived Parameters

Routinely, 10,000 cells were analyzed per sample into a 64 by 64 DNA-RNA histogram, and "boxogram" gaiting procedures were applied to biparametric DNA-RNA distributions to derive 3 major variables (18) (Figure 1):

The DNA index (DI) as a measure of ploidy was defined as the ratio of relative $G_{1/0}$ DNA contents of test sample and normal blood lymphocytes (20,23).

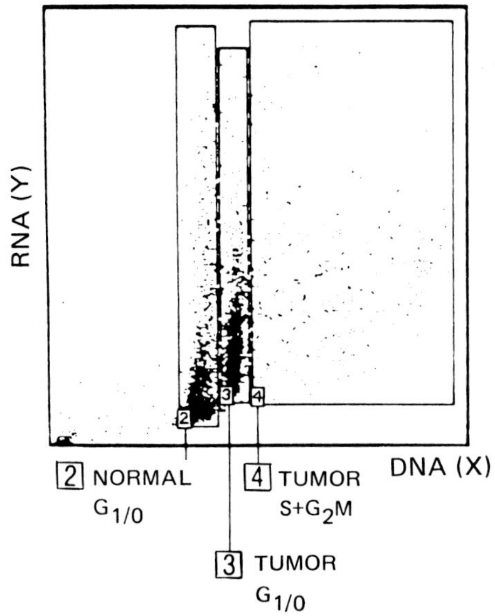

$$\text{DNA INDEX} = \frac{X_3}{X_2}$$

$$\text{RNA INDEX} = \frac{Y_3}{Y_2}$$

$$(S+G_2M)\ \% = \frac{\#4}{\#(3+4)} \times 100$$

Figure 1 Acridine-orange-derived DNA-RNA distribution in a case of hyperdiploid ALL. Derivation of standard acridine orange flow cytometry (AO FCM) parameters: DNA and RNA index; (%S+G_2M).

The percentage of cells in (S+G_2M) was defined by separating the acridine-orange-derived DNA-RNA distributions along the $G_{1/0}$ boundary from low to high RNA content (18).

The RNA index (RI) of $G_{1/0}$ cells was derived from the ratio of mean RNA fluorescence in $G_{1/0}$ and the median fluorescence of peripheral blood lymphocyte $G_{1/0}$ cells (13,14).

In addition to these 3 variables, 19 others were applied to better define the full complexity of AO distribution patterns (Table 1). Parameters 1-6 and 17 were calculated from the RNA histogram of the $G_{1/0}$-phase. P (G_1, 25), P (G_1, 50), P (G_1, 75), and P (G_1, 100) are the channels where 25%, 50%, 75% and 100% of the cells, respectively, exceed the RNA channel in G_1; that is, the third quartile, median, first quartile, and minimum channel, respectively. The percentile ratios defined as parameters 1-3 are measures of dispersion of the RNA histogram. Other measures are the standard deviation (S) (parameter 5), skewness (g_1) (parameter 17), and kurtosis (g_2) (parameter 6). If f (G_1, x) denotes the RNA histogram cell count of G_1, at channel x, where $0 \leqslant x \leqslant 63$, then the sample mean

Table 1 Classification and Clustering Parameters

Parameter	Description
1. $P(G_1, 50) / P(G_1, 25)$	G_1-RNA ratio of median to upper 25% cutoff
2. $P(G_1, 75) / P(G_1, 25)$	G_1-RNA ratio of lower 75% to upper 25% cutoff
3. $P(G_1, 100) / P(G_1, 25)$	G_1-RNA ratio of minimum RNA to upper 25% cutoff
4. $SKEW(G_1)$	G_1-RNA skewness from median
5. $s^2 G_1$	G_1-RNA variance
6. $g_2(G_1)$	G_1-RNA kurtosis
7. P (S, 50) / P (S, 25)	S-RNA ratio of median to upper 25% cutoff
8. P (S, 75) / P (S, 25)	S-RNA ratio of lower 75% to upper 25% cutoff
9. P (S, 100) / P (S, 25)	S-RNA ratio of minimum RNA to upper 25% cutoff
10. SKEW(S)	S-RNA skewness from median
11. $s^2 S$	S-RNA variance
12. g_2 (S)	S-RNA kurtosis
13. $P(S, 25) / P(G_1, 25)$	Ratio of S-RNA 25% to G_1-RNA 25%
14. $P(S, 50) / P(G_1, 50)$	Ratio of S-RNA median to G_1-RNA median
15. $P(S, 75) / P(G_1, 75)$	Ratio of S-RNA 75% to G_1-RNA 75%
16. $P(S, 100) / P(G_1, 100)$	Ratio of S-RNA minimum to G_1-RNA minimum
17. $g_1(G_1)$	G_1-RNA skewness
18. g_1 (S)	S-RNA skewness
19. $\bar{x} G_1 / P(G_1, 50)$	G_1-RNA Index (mean/median)
20. G_1%	percentage of cells in G_1
21. $(S+G_2M)$%	percentage of cells in $(S+G_2M)$
22. DNA index	ratio of abnormal to normal G_1 location

$$\overline{x}_{G_1} = \Sigma_{x=0}^{63} f(G_1, x)\frac{x}{F}$$

the sample variance

$$S^2{}_{G_1} = \Sigma_{x=0}^{63} f(G_1, x)\frac{(x-\overline{x}_{G_1})^2}{63F}$$

the sample third moment

$$k_3 = 64\,\Sigma_{x=0}^{63} f(G_1,x)\,\frac{(x-\overline{x}_{G_1})^3}{63{\bullet}62\,F}$$

and sample fourth moment

$$k_4 = \frac{\Sigma_{x=0}^{63} f(F,x)\,(x-\overline{x}_{G_1})^2\,64{\bullet}65\,/\,63F - 3[63S^2{}_{G_1}]^2}{62{\bullet}61}$$

where

$$F = \Sigma_{x=0}^{63} f(G_1,x)$$

Customarily, k_3 and k_4 are made dimensionless by calculating the skewness

$$g_1\,(G_1) = \frac{k_3}{S^3{}_{G_1}}$$

and kurtosis

$$g_2\,(G_1) = \frac{k_4}{S^4 G_1} - 3$$

which are the 17th and 5th parameters, respectively (24). A measure of skewness based upon the difference in the mean and mode

$$\mathrm{SKEW}(G_1) = \frac{\overline{x}_{G_1} - x_{MODE}}{S_{G_1}}$$

can be calculated as

$$\mathrm{SKEW}(G_1) = \frac{g_1\,(g_2 + 6)}{2(5g_2 - 6g_1^2 + 6)}$$

(parameter 4) (25). Corresponding parameters are calculated for S-phase. Ratios of percentiles (parameters 13-16) were also included.

D. Methods of Classification and Clustering

As described in the previous section, 22 parameters were calculated from each AO histogram. There were six populations, π_i; i = 1, . . ., 6 (AML, ALL, normal, CML, CLL, MDS) with differing numbers of observations, η_i, i = 1, . . ., 6 (260, 90, 49, 25, 18, 18, respectively) in each. The data for patient/control j in population i can be denoted by the vector $Y_{ij} = (y_{ij1}, \ldots, y_{ij22})$. Means

$$\overline{Y}_i = \Sigma_{j=1}^{\eta_i} \frac{Y_{ij}}{\eta_i}$$

$$= (\Sigma\frac{y_{ij1}}{\eta_i}, \ldots, \Sigma\frac{y_{ij22}}{\eta_i})$$

$$= (\overline{y}_{i1}, \ldots, \overline{y}_{i22})$$

and variance-covariance matrix

$$S_i = \Sigma_{j=1}^{\eta_i} \frac{(Y_{ij} - \overline{Y}_i)(Y_{ij} - \overline{Y}_i)^2}{\eta_i - 1}$$

$$= \frac{1}{\eta_i - 1} \begin{Bmatrix} \Sigma (y_{ij1} - \overline{y}_{i1})^2 & \cdots & \Sigma (y_{ij1} - y_{\circ,})(y_{ij22} - \overline{y}_{i22}) \\ \vdots & & \vdots \\ \Sigma (y_{ij22} - \overline{y}_{i22})(y_{ij1} - \overline{y}_{i1}) & \cdots & \Sigma (y_{ij22} - \overline{y}_{i22})^2 \end{Bmatrix}$$

are calculated. A pooled variance-covariance matrix can be calculated

$$S_p = \frac{\Sigma_{i=1}^{6} (\eta_i - 1) S_i}{\Sigma_{i=1}^{6} (\eta_i - 1)}$$

Two different types of population characterization were used on these data, classification and clustering.

Classification

The classification was accomplished using two related techniques: maximum likelihood normal discrimination techniques and the linear discriminant function (26).

Briefly, the natural logarithms of the likelihood functions are

$$1n\ L_i = Q_i - .5|\ S_i| - .5(Y - \overline{Y}_i)^T S_i^{-1} (Y - \overline{Y}_i)$$

where Q_i is the risk constant, "| |" denotes matrix determinant, "T" denotes matrix transpose, and "$^{-1}$" denotes matrix inverse. The maximum likelihood classification of the unknown data vector Y into a population π_i, i=1, . . . , 6 is the population, say k, which maximizes 1n L_i, i=1 . . . , 6; or

$$\ln L_k = \max_{1 \leqslant i \leqslant 6} \ln L_i$$

and we would decide that Y came from population k. This is often referred to as the *maximum likelihood classification*. The classification process can be simplified if the variance-covariance matrices can be assumed to be approximately equal, in which case, S_p is substituted for S_i. Since $|S_p|$ is the same in each equation, the maximum likelihood equation can be reduced to

$$C_i = Q_i - .5(Y-\overline{Y}_i)^T S_p^{-1} (Y-\overline{Y}_i)$$

which has a maximum over i=1, . . ., 6 when

$$C_i' = Q_i + Y^T S_p^{-1} \overline{Y}_i - .5\overline{Y}_i^T S_p^{-1} \overline{Y}_i$$

has a maximum. C_i' is called the *linear discriminant function*. The elements of the vector $b_i = S_p^{-1}\overline{Y}_i$ are referred to as the discrimination coefficients while

$$a_i = Q_i - .5\overline{Y}^T{}_i S_p^{-1} \overline{Y}_i$$

is the constant term. On comparing two populations, say π_1 and π_2, we can calculate

$$\begin{aligned} V &= C_1' - C_2' \\ &= Q_1 - Q_2 + Y^T S_p^{-1} (\overline{Y}_1 - \overline{Y}_2) - .5(\overline{Y}_1 + \overline{Y}_2)^T S_p^{-1} (\overline{Y}_1 - \overline{Y}_2) \end{aligned}$$

for which the second term is also called the linear discriminant function. Using the linear discriminant function, we will decide that Y came from population k if

$$C'_k = \max_i C_i'$$

Clustering

The clustering was accomplished using a variation of Ball and Hall (27). The procedure is iterative of the form:

Loop:

1. Choose some initial values for the means of m clusters, say $y_1, \ldots, y_m$.
2. Classify the $\Sigma\, n_i$ samples into the m clusters by minimum distance.
3. Recalculate the means using the new cluster members.

Then either even loop:

4. If any cluster has too large a standard deviation (>.84, normalized) in any parameter, split the cluster into two clusters by adding and subtracting a

constant to that mean and return to step 2 (e.g., if if two clusters are split, there will now be m + 2 cluster means).

Or odd loop:

5. Compute the distance between clusters; if too close, combine the clusters into one cluster by averaging the means and return to step 2 (e.g., if two clusters are combined, there will now be m − 1 cluster means).

The interaction stops when there are no more changes in the means or when there is a maximum number of loops.

The fundamental question to be answered by the discriminant analysis is "Can flow cytometric DNA/RNA parameters discriminate between leukemic and normal bone marrow?" Subsidiary questions of whether the DNA/RNA parameters can subdiagnose the type of leukemia, which parameters are critical in the diagnosis, and whether there are sufficient data in this collection to yield stable results, are equally important. The question of subdiagnosis will be answered in the discrimination of leukemic and normal individuals; the critical parameters will be analyzed by a forward parameter selection procedure, and the sample size will be tested by repeated subsampling—the holdout method (28,29)—using a random number generator and comparing the subsampling runs.

An alternative formulation of the question might be "Into what groups can we subdivide the data set so that the membership in the group is consistent?," and subsequently, "Do the traditional groupings of diagnosis follow these data clusters?" This will be accomplished by using cluster analysis to cluster the data into homogeneous subsets.

III. RESULTS

A. Acridine Orange as a Tool in the Diagnosis of Acute Leukemia (13,14,18,30)

General Description

Figure 2 illustrates representative three-dimensional DNA-RNA displays of normal bone marrow, AML, CML benign phase and lymphoid blast crisis, ALL and Burkitt's lymphoma; CLL and hairy cell leukemia (HCL). The major differences between these conditions can be summarized as follows. Normal bone marrow is characterized by a relatively uniform RNA content in the $G_{1/0}$ compartment with a rapid trailing towards higher RNA values, whereas there is a more gradual decline in the relative frequency of cells with higher RNA content in $(S+G_2M)$. The percentage of cells in $(S+G_2M)$ is typically high with an average of about 20%. CML in benign phase has a distribution pattern quite similar to normal bone marrow, the main difference being a more protracted decline in the incidence of cells with high RNA especially in $G_{1/0}$, resulting in a more obvious trailing. Numeric indices of DI, RI and $\%(S+G_2M)$ are almost identical to those of normal

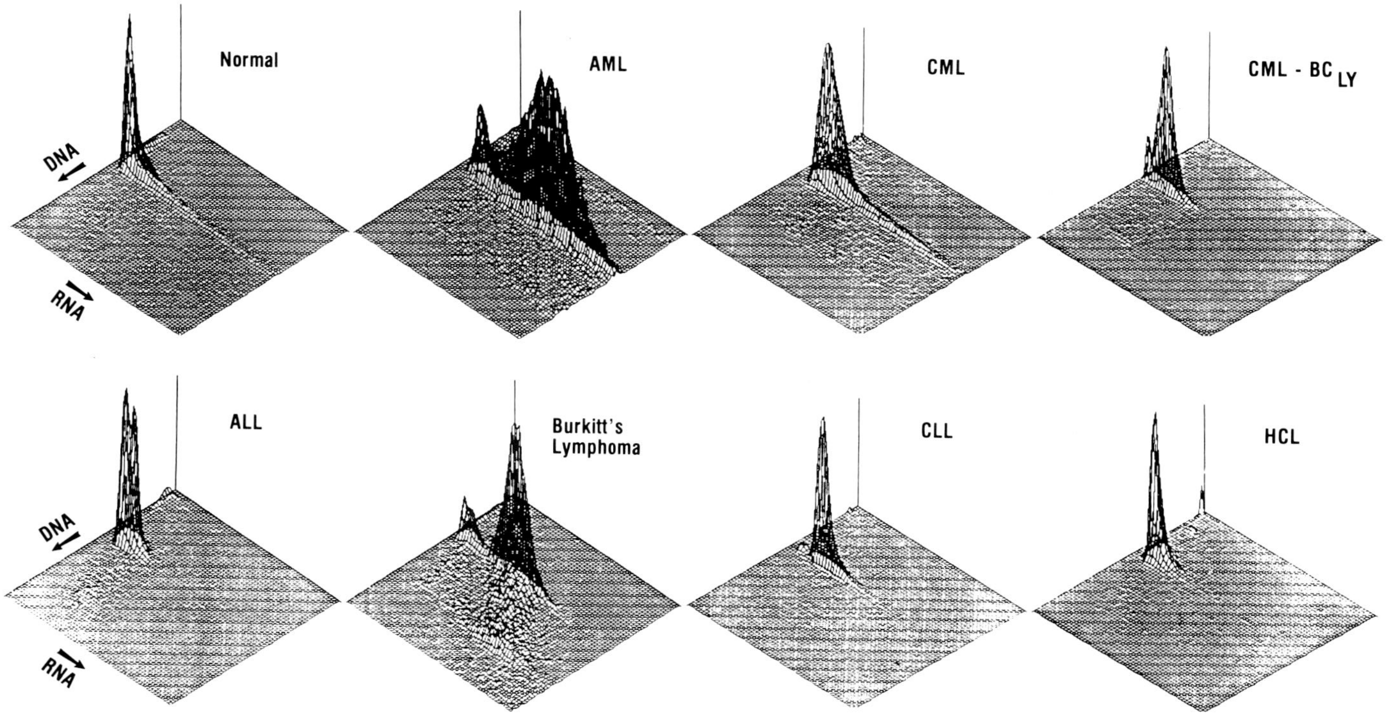

Figure 2 Representative DNA-RNA histograms of bone marrow cells obtained from a normal volunteer and patients with different leukemic conditions (for details, see text).

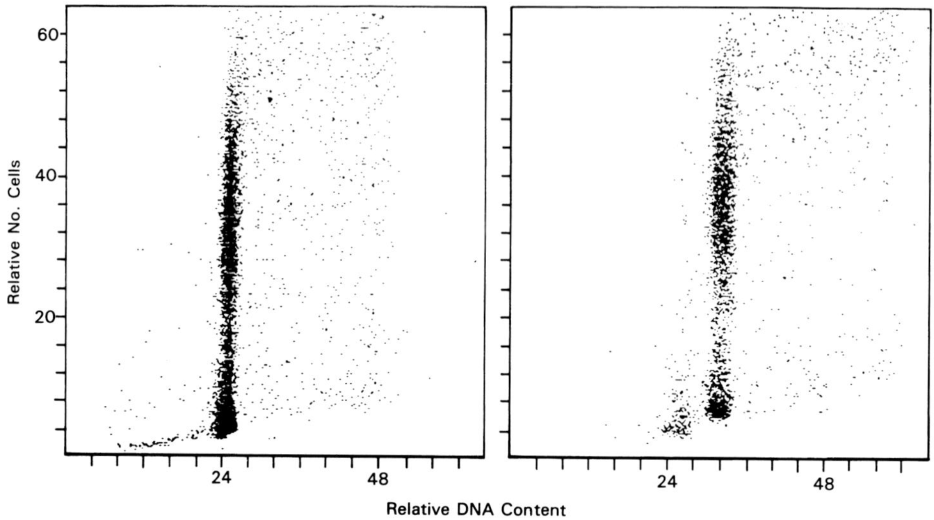

(a)

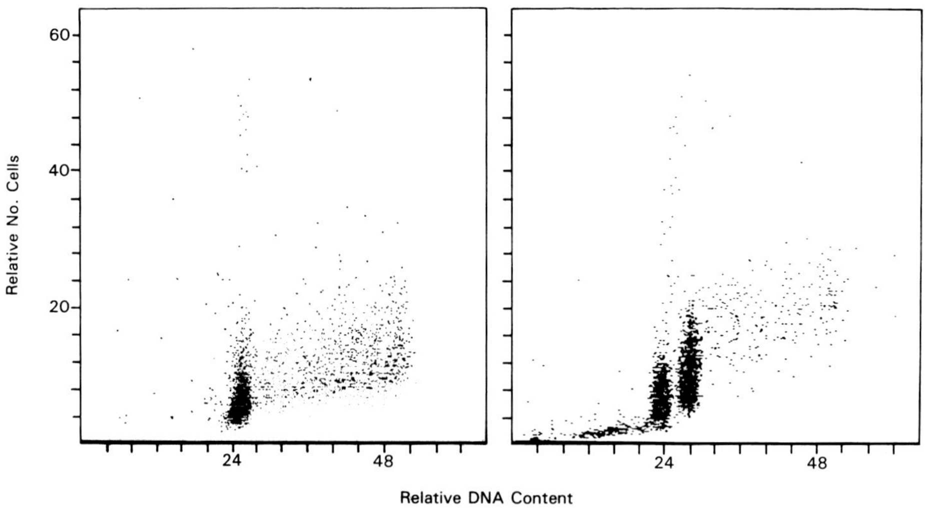

(b)

Figure 3 DNA-RNA histograms in diploid and hyperdiploid AML (a) and ALL (b).

bone marrow. In CLL and HCL, the most striking finding is one of uniformity, where typically 90-95% of all cells are found in the $G_{1/0}$ compartment with a low RNA and uniformly diploid DNA content. Compared to CLL, ALL is characterized by more RNA dispersion and higher %(S+G_2M) values (particularly in L3-ALL), also displaying aneuploidy in about 25% of cases. While numeric indices of RI and %(S+G_2M) are frequently similar to those of normal marrow, ALL generally has a Gaussian rather than a log-normal RNA distribution, usually also with a slightly higher RNA index. AML is readily distinguished by higher RI values, often with bimodal RNA distributions, reflecting residual normal hemopoiesis and myeloid blasts, respectively (14,18). This can be gleaned from aneuploid cases permitting separate analysis of residual normal diploid cells with low and aneuploid cells with high RNA content (Figure 3). The proliferative compartment varies widely as in ALL. Particularly in AML, there is a marked heterogeneity in DNA-RNA distribution patterns even within specific morphologic or cytogenetic groups, reflecting varying degrees of blast maturation and of marrow involvement, all contributing to more or less RNA trailing mainly in $G_{1/0}$. Another pattern commonly encountered in the followup of patients with acute leukemia is that of treatment-induced marrow hypoplasia with uniformly low RNA content in $G_{1/0}$ and low %(S+G_2M), yet discernibly greater dispersion than in CLL/HCL.

DNA Ploidy (31,32)

Aneuploidy is typically absent in normal marrow, CLL, HCL (not shown) and benign phase CML, but is present in about 10% of myelodysplastic syndromes

Table 2 Acridine Orange Flow Cytometry in Leukemia

Diagnosis	N	% Aneuploidy	%(S+G_2M) Mean (SD)	RNA index Mean (SD)
Normal	49	0	18 (4.6)	0.98 (.19)
AML[a]	260	25	13 (5.3)	1.99 (.83)
ALL[b]	90	26	13 (8.2)	1.50 (.55)
CML[c]	25	0	13 (6.2)	1.18 (.49)
CLL[d]	18	0	5 (3.9)	0.94 (.21)
MDS[e]	18	11	17 (10.1)	1.22 (.29)

[a]AML = Acute myelogenous leukemia.
[b]ALL = Acute lymphocytic leukemia.
[c]CML = Chronic myelogenous leukemia.
[d]CLL = Chronic lymphocytic leukemia.
[e]MDS = Myelodysplastic syndromes.

(more frequently in refractory anemia with excess blasts (RAEB) and refractory anemia with excess blasts in transformation (RAEB-IT); in 25% of AML; 26% of ALL; and in half of usually myeloid blast crisis of CML (Table 2). Analysis of DNA-ploidy in relationship to cytogenetics in AML and ALL revealed absence of DNA abnormalities in Philadelphia chromosome-positive (Ph^+) disease and a high incidence of DNA aneuploidy (>40%) in patients with karyotypic instability, hyperdiploidy and certain translocations (Tables 3 and 4). Among the 44 patients with AML exhibiting balanced translocations t(15;17), t(8;21) and inv 16, 36% had hyperdiploid DNA stemlines of the low-degree variety (DNA index ⩽1.15), and none showed DNA index values greater than 1.15. In contrast, the karyotype instability and hyperdiploidy groups contained 22% and 12% of patients, respectively, with more marked DNA excess (Table 3). In ALL, such high-degree DNA hyperdiploid abnormalities were 4 times more common than in AML and were particularly prevelant among patients with insufficient metaphases (Table 4). Twenty percent of patients with both diploid AML and ALL had an aneuploid DNA stemline.

Table 3 Cytogenetics and DNA-Ploidy in Acute Myelogenous Leukemia

			Percent patients with DNA index			
Karyotype	N	Percent DNA-aneuploid	<1.0	1.0	1.01-1.15	>1.15
Diploid	101	20	3	80	17	0
Hyperdiploid	26	54	0	46	42	12
Hypodiploid	21	28	14	72	14	0
Pseudodiploid	13	8	0	92	8	0
t(15;17)	15	47	0	53	47	0
t(8;21)	15	26	0	74	26	0
inversion 16	14	36	0	64	36	0
t(9;22)	4	0	0	100	0	0
11q−	2	0	0	100	0	0
Karyotype instability	14	43	7	57	14	22
Insufficient metaphases	15	20	0	80	13	7
Constitutional abnormality	1	0	0	100	0	0
Missing	2	0	0	100	0	0
Total	243	27	3	73	21	3

Table 4 Cytogenetics and DNA-Ploidy in Acute Lymphocytic Leukemia

Karyotype	N	Percent DNA-aneuploid	Percent patients with DNA index <1.0	1.0	1.01-1.15	>1.15
Diploid	25	20	0	80	12	8
Hyperdiploid	5	40	0	60	20	20
Hypodiploid	3	0	0	100	0	0
Pseudodiploid	6	0	0	100	0	0
t(9;22)	11	0	0	100	0	0
14q+	3	67	0	33	33	33
Karyotype instability	5	60	40	40	20	0
Insufficient metaphases	17	42	6	59	6	29
Total	75	25	4	75	9	12

Table 5 relates the quantitative abnormalities in DNA content to modal chromosome number. Five of nine patients with a hypodiploid DNA stemline (DI <1) had a concordant hypodiploid karyotype, and the only one with hyperdiploid chromosomal aberrations had a second DNA stemline with a DNA index of 2.0. Similarly, 7 of 9 patients with a marked DNA excess greater than 15% (DI >1.15) had hyperdiploid metaphases, mostly with more than 50 chromosomes. One-third

Table 5 Comparison of DNA-Ploidy and Cytogenetics

DNA index	N	Number of patients with modal chromosome number <46	46P[a]	46N[b]	47-50	>50
<0.95	7	4	0	3	0	0
0.95-1.05	229	43	55	109	22	0
1.06-1.1	18	0	6	4	8	0
1.11-1.2	22	3	2	9	7	1
>1.2	9	0	0	1	1	7
Total	285	50	63	126	38	8

[a]46 P = pseudodiploid including translocations.
[b]46 N = normal diploid.

of patients with distinct DNA abnormalities exhibited a normal diploid karyotype, however. Conversely, among patients with a normal diploid DNA complement, half had an abnormal karyotype including both hypodiploid (19%) and hyperdiploid aberrations (9%). Thus, while there was a general correspondence between DI and modal chromosome number in terms of a progressive shift toward a higher degree of hyperdiploid abnormality with increasing DNA index, many exceptions were noted and perhaps not unexpected, as individual human chromosomes vary by almost 5-fold in DNA content (33).

While inferior to cytogenetics for the detection of genomic aberrations, DNA flow cytometry (FCM) increased the overall aneuploidy rate by 9% in AML and 16% in ALL by virtue of ploidy abnormalities among patients with diploid metaphases and insufficient mitoses (Table 6). Compared to more recent cytogenetic studies reporting almost universal occurrence of clonal karyotype aberrations in acute leukemia (12,34), our observation of DNA aneuploidy indicating numeric genetic abnormalities in 20% of patients with normal diploid mitoses (44% of total population) was indeed expected. The discrepancy between numeric genomic abnormalities detected by DNA FCM and diploid karyotype or structural chromosomal aberrations on cytogenetic examination was previously attributed to differences in target cells examined, i.e., $G_{1/0}$ cells for DNA index analysis and mitotic cells in the case of chromosomal analysis (16,20). It is conceivable and has been reported in heterogeneous tissue such as leukemic bone marrow that residual diploid cells preferentially traverse to mitosis, whereas cells with a lower proliferative activity account for the DNA abnormality.

Table 6 Aneuploidy, by Cytogenetics and DNA Flow Cytometry

	Acute myelogenous leukemia (AML)	Acute lymphocytic leukemia (ALL)
Number of patients	241	75
Abnormal karyotype		
Overall	52%	44%
DNA-aneuploid	34%	21%
Normal karyotype		
Overall	42%	33%
DNA-aneuploid	20%	20%
Insufficient metaphases		
Overall	6%	23%
DNA-aneuploid	20%	42%
Aneuploid by either method	61%	60%

RNA Index and Proliferative Activity

The proportion of cells in ($S+G_2M$) was typically low in CLL and HCL (latter not shown), intermediate in AML, ALL, and CML with a wide range of values; and highest in MDS and morphologically normal bone marrow (see Table 2). RI values of about 1.0 were typical for normal marrow and CLL, HCL, CML benign phase and MDS; intermediate values of approximately 1.5 were observed in ALL; and highest values were found in AML. Relevant to the distinction of AML from ALL, including FAB categories, Table 7 illustrates a strong association of high RNA index values >1.5 with AML (88% vs 12% ALL); by contrast, among the acute leukemias with RNA index values ⩽1.5, 46% were ALL and 54% AML. There was too much heterogeneity in RNA index within FAB categories for this FCM parameter to be useful in distinguishing morphologic subtypes of AML or ALL.

In order to examine the combined role of RNA index and proliferative activity, "RNA-proliferation maps" were constructed for the various myelodysplastic syndromes as well as for FAB and cytogenetic categories in AML. With the transition from minimal myelodysplasia to overt AML, a progressive decrease in proliferative activity and a corresponding increase in RNA index was noted; however, there was considerable overlap among the different categories (Figure 4). Such overlap was also observed among FAB (Figure 5) and cytogenetic categories of AML (Figure 6). Table 8 portrays the significant difference in proliferative activity

Table 7 RNA Index and FAB Classification

		Percent Patients with FAB Category								
RNA index	N	M1	M2	M3	M4	M5	M6	L1	L2	L3
<1.0	27	11	19	4	7	4	0	11	41	4
1.0-1.5	87	23	16	2	12	3	0	12	32	0
1.6-2.0	82	20	24	7	24	7	0	1	15	1
2.1-2.5	42	12	29	12	36	0	0	0	7	5
2.6-3.0	22	14	9	23	36	9	0	0	5	5
>3.0	21	14	29	10	10	33	5	0	0	0
⩽1.5	114	20	17	3	11	4	0	11	34	1
					54%				46%	
>1.5	167	16	24	11	27	9	1	1	9	2
					88%				12%	

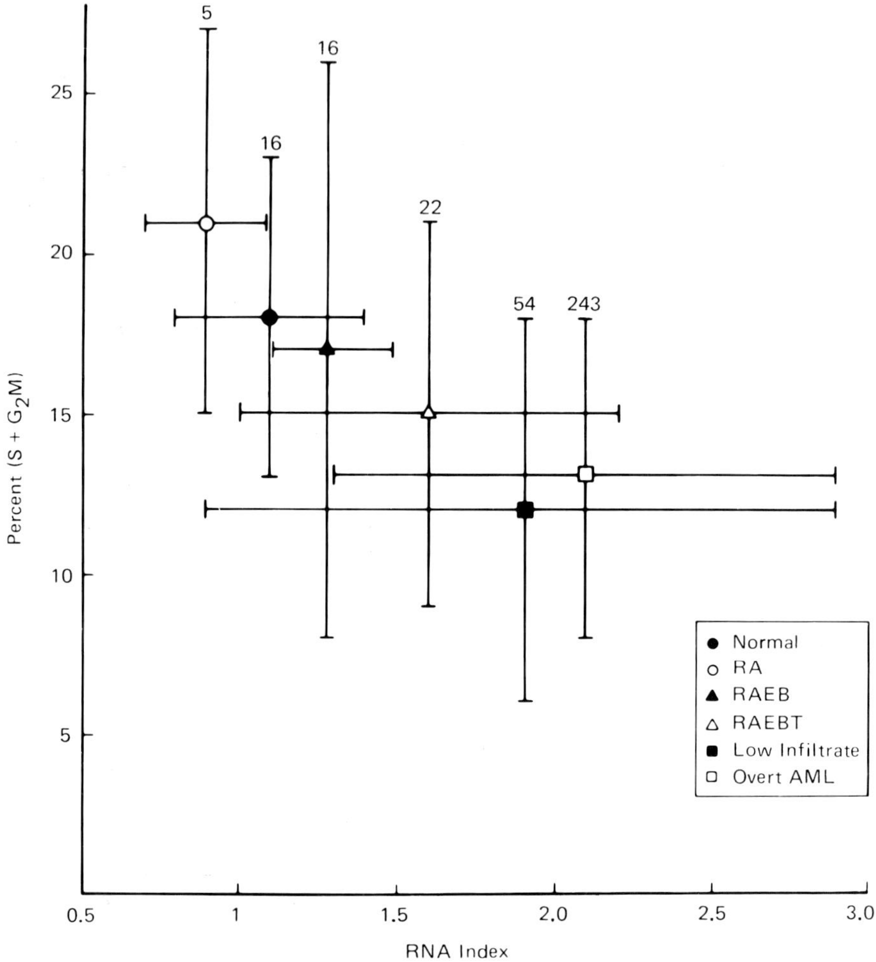

Figure 4 "RNA-proliferation maps" for normal bone marrow; myelodysplastic syndromes (RA = refractory anemia; RAEB = refractory anemia with excess blasts; RAEB-IT = refractory anemia with excess blasts in transformation; CMML = chronic myelomonocytic leukemia) and for AML (low infiltrate and overt). Note the progressive decrease in proliferative activity and increase in RNA index with increasing "leukemicness."

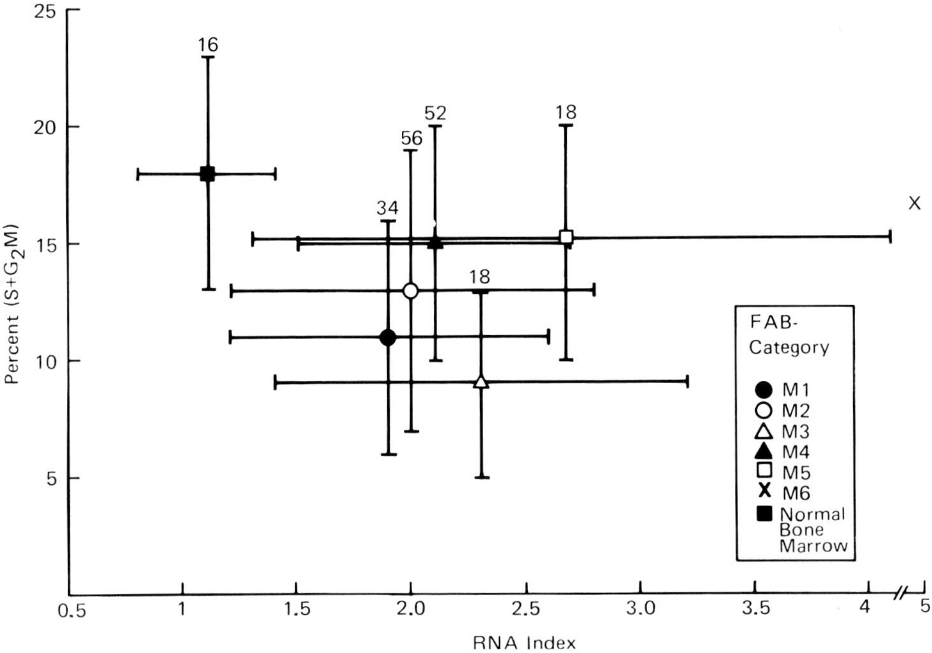

Figure 5 "RNA-proliferation maps" as related to FAB classification. Note the considerable overlap between morphologic groups.

among individual cytogenetic groups in AML, using a mean rank test. Average values of $(S+G_2M)\%$ were noted for diploid karyotypes, whereas very low values were associated with t(15;17) translocations and insufficient metaphases, and highest values were observed in patients with numeric chromosomal aberrations (both hypo- and hyperdiploidy) and those with the Philadelphia translocation. There was no significant difference in RI values although, as a group, structural aberrations displayed the highest RI values (p=0.09). Thus, we recognized differences in RI and $(S+G_2M)$ values among subgroups of AML and ALL, however, without affording sufficient separation of these 2 major disease categories.

AO FCM Visual Patterns

A number of additional features were recognized to distinguish a variety of hematologic diseases in the bone marrow (see Figure 2). Over the past 3 years, these visual FCM patterns have been assigned to a variety of diagnoses (Table 9). Concordance with morphologic diagnosis was achieved in almost 80% of AML cases, 70% of ALL patients, 80% of those with CML and more than 95% of

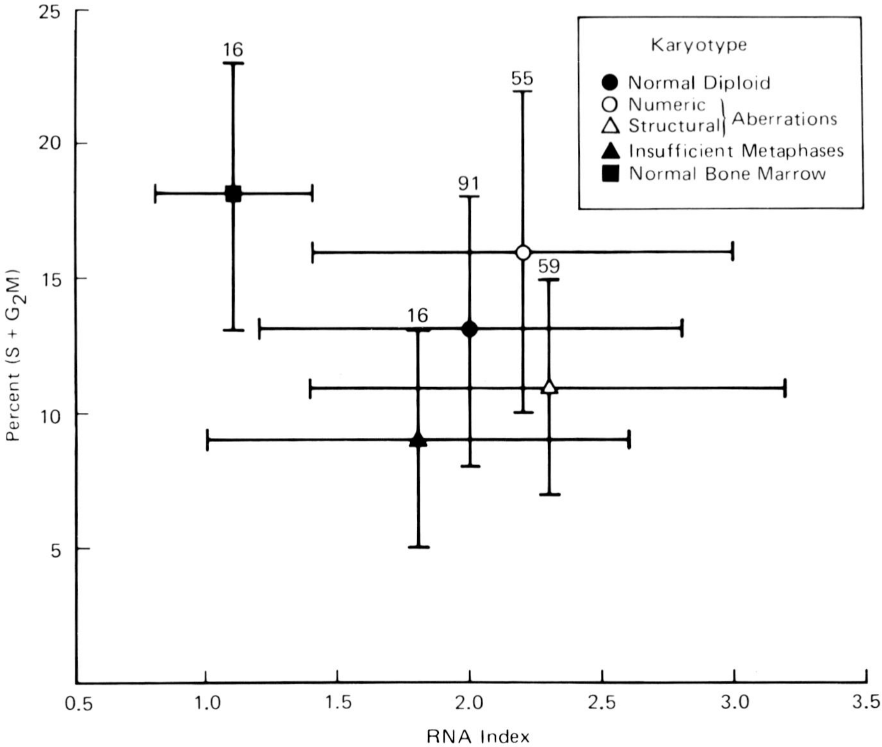

Figure 6 "RNA-proliferation maps" related to cytogenetic categories in acute myelogenous leukemia (AML). Note the considerable overlap. Structural chromosomal aberrations were characterized by higher RNA and lower $S+G_2M$ values compared to AML with numeric anomalies.

individuals with CLL or HCL. Hence, the visual FCM pattern recognition, principally employing the considerations mentioned earlier in Figure 2, provided considerably better discrimination of bone marrow disorders than was possible on the basis of the 3 main FCM variables, DI, RI and $\%(S+G_2M)$.

Discriminant Analysis

In order to account for the above visual FCM patterns objectively, additional quantitative parameters were derived, as summarized in Table 1. Table 10 provides a summary of mean statistics for each of these 22 parameters among the 6 diagnostic categories along with their relative rank in univariate disease classification. Surprisingly, none of the 3 main FCM variables (DNA index, RNA index, $\%(S+G_2M)$) ranked among the first 7 parameters found to be important in a

Table 8 Cytogenetics and Acridine Orange Flow Cytometry in Acute Myelogenous Leukemia[a]

Karyotype	No. of patients	$\%(S+G_2M)$ mean rank[b]	RNA index mean rank[c]
Diploid	104	127	116
Ph^+	7	152	148
Hyperdiploid	24	166	137
Hypodiploid	19	160	127
Pseudodiploid	17	123	121
t(8;21)	15	109	159
t(15;17)	16	79	169
inv 16	13	127	147
Karyotypic instability	16	148	114
Insufficient metaphases	21	73	105

[a]n = 260.
[b]p = .001.
[c]p = .085.

Table 9 Acridine Orange Flow Cytometry "Pattern" and Morphologic Diagnosis of Leukemia

Morphologic diagnosis	N	Percent Patients with FCM Pattern AML	ALL	CML	CLL	Other
Acute myelogenous leukemia (AML)	260	77	15			8
Acute lymphocytic leukemia (ALL)	90	21	67			12
Chronic myelogenous leukemia (CML)	25			83		17
Chronic lymphocytic leukemia (CLL)	18				98	2

Table 10 Mean and Standard Deviation for all Parameters for Each Diagnosis Group

Parameter	AML[a]	ALL[b]	Normal	CML[c]	CLL[d]	MDS[e]	Rank of single classification
1	.659[f] (.125)[g]	.752 (.084)	.650 (.106)	.662 (.147)	.806 (.063)	.566 (.106)	1
2	.427 (.130)	.553 (.130)	.505 (.111)	.537 (.149)	.677 (.075)	.388 (.107)	2
3	.180 (.081)	.267 (.101)	.291 (.090)	.325 (.122)	.408 (.064)	.210 (.097)	3
4	4.30 (3.66)	6.99 (5.64)	10.3 (2.70)	11.0 (4.16)	17.0 (4.94)	7.41 (2.98)	17
5	9.79 (3.10)	6.02 (2.77)	8.46 (2.12)	7.99 (2.59)	4.09 (1.25)	9.51 (2.43)	15
6	2.80 (6.57)	11.2 (19.0)	9.69 (4.50)	11.9 (11.1)	32.5 (16.85)	5.34 (5.23)	22
7	.655 (.361)	.628 (.395)	.596 (137)	.637 (.352)	.109 (.211)	.576 (.245)	6
8	.411 (.249)	.474 (.302)	.411 (.112)	.456 (.356)	.089 (.174)	.367 (.196)	5
9	.206 (.146)	.251 (.185)	.220 (.072)	.277 (.286)	.058 (.117)	.177 (.126)	4
10	1.02 (2.35)	3.11 (4.74)	2.04 (.624)	2.16 (2.28)	13.3 (8.28)	2.34 (3.21)	16
11	11.5 (5.23)	7.12 (4.82)	12.82 (2.61)	12.75 (3.89)	3.16 (5.29)	12.6 (5.18)	19

12	.861 (3.25)	4.36 (7.62)	1.99 (1.34)	2.51 (4.84)	2.24 (4.42)	.871 (2.18)	18
13	1.49 (.782)	1.34 (.865)	2.89 (1.03)	2.98 (1.40)	.607 (1.26)	1.88 (.798)	9
14	1.79 (.933)	1.47 (.913)	2.67 (.684)	2.90 (1.37)	.538 (.926)	2.24 (1.06)	10
15	1.88 (.982)	1.60 (1.05)	2.37 (.573)	2.36 (1.03)	.535 (.921)	2.05 (.921)	11
16	2.07 (1.18)	1.80 (1.31)	2.21 (.574)	2.18 (.816)	.579 (.966)	1.74 (.824)	14
17	1.16 (.985)	1.87 (1.52)	2.89 (.754)	3.02 (1.14)	4.38 (1.26)	2.05 (.835)	13
18	.355 (.955)	.873 (1.27)	1.52 (.417)	1.48 (1.05)	.746 (1.30)	.884 (.815)	12
19	1.99 (.826)	1.50 (.545)	.98 (.189)	1.18 (.487)	.944 (.206)	1.22 (.290)	8
20	87.0 (7.16)	87.1 (8.29)	81.7 (4.64)	84.5 (13.6)	95.5 (3.94)	83.4 (10.1)	21
21	12.6 (5.27)	12.7 (8.23)	18.3 (4.64)	13.2 (6.16)	4.50 (3.94)	16.6 (10.1)	20
22	1.02 (.084)	1.04 (.144)	1.0 (0.00)	1.0 (0.00)	1.0 (0.00)	1.01 (.029)	7

[a]AML = Acute myelogenous leukemia.
[b]ALL = Acute lymphocytic leukemia.
[c]CML = Chronic myelogenous leukemia.
[d]CLL = Chronic lymphocytic leukemia.
[e]MDS = Myelodysplastic syndromes.
[f]Mean.
[g]Standard deviation.

univariate classification analysis. Rather, the 6 parameters sensitive to RNA skewness and dispersion in both $G_{1/0}$ and $(S+G_2M)$ compartments (Numbers 1-3 and 7-9, see Table 1) were most important in distinguishing the 6 diagnostic groups under consideration.

To determine which of the parameters in combination were the most discriminatory, a stepwise procedure was employed: each parameter was entered singly as a discriminator of AML, ALL and normal. CML, CLL and MDS were not used because of small numbers of patients. Table 10 lists the ranking of log likelihoods when each parameter was entered singly. Parameter 1 ($P(G_1,50)/P(G_1,25)$; see Table 1) was the most significant. Parameter 1 was retained in the discriminator while the remaining 21 parameters were added, one at a time, to find the pair of discriminators with the maximum likelihood. Parameter 3 was this parameter. This procedure was continued. The first 14 parameters, entered in order of significance in discrimination, were 1,3,22,9,8,7,19,13 14 15,2,18,17, and 5. These are 13 of the 14 singly most discriminatory, only differing in the 14th most significant which was not chosen favoring parameter 5, the 15th most significant singly. This indicates a surprising degree of independency among these parameters.

Using a linear discriminant function with all 22 parameters, a decision matrix was constructed (Table 11). The overall correct classification into 6 groups was 62.8%; misclassification was high in AML (16.5% as ALL and 15.4% as MDS) and in CML (25.7% as normal). However, when the table was reduced to 2 categories, i.e., normal and abnormal (among all 6 diagnostic groups), the overall correct classification was 93%, with sensitivity to the diagnosis of leukemia of 95% and specificity of 80%. When the analysis was restricted to the 3 main diagnostic groups of AML, ALL and normal, sensitivity and specificity of diagnosing leukemia vs normal increased further to 94.4% and 91.8%, respectively.

There was a remarkable consistency in disease classification as evidenced by small standard deviations when 12 classifications were performed in AML, ALL and normal groups, using 50% of samples randomly. We also examined the effect of leukemic blast percentage on disease classification by AO FCM and noted that, down to 30% blasts on marrow differential, sensitivity and specificity of distinguishing between leukemia and normal marrow were not affected.

Because all normal, CML, and CLL categories were diploid, the variance-covariance matrices including parameter 22 were singular for these diagnoses, and the maximum likelihood classification could not be calculated. Also, $G_{1/0}$ and S% are linearly dependent, so that calculation of inverse variance-covariance matrices could not be performed. To compare linear discriminant and maximum likelihood analysis, classifications were performed without DNA index and $\%(S+G_2M)$ (parameters 22 and 21) on AML, ALL, and normal categories only. The maximum likelihood method was superior to the linear discriminant analysis

Table 11 Linear Discriminant Function Decision Matrix with 22 Parameters

A. Classification with 6 Diagnostic Categories

Decision	True Diagnosis: AML	ALL	Normal	CML	CLL	MDS	Total
AML	153 (58.9)[a]	14 (15.6)	0 (0.0)	1 (2.9)	0 (0.0)	2 (11.1)	170
ALL	43 (16.5)	58 (64.4)	1 (2.0)	1 (2.9)	1 (5.6)	2 (11.1)	106
Normal	9 (3.5)	2 (2.2)	39 (79.6)	9 (25.7)	1 (5.6)	2 (11.1)	62
CML	12 (4.6)	2 (2.2)	4 (8.2)	20 (57.1)	1 (5.6)	1 (5.6)	40
CLL	3 (1.2)	10 (11.1)	0 (10.2)	2 (5.7)	15 (83.3)	1 (5.6)	31
MDS	40 (15.4)	4 (4.4)	5 (10.2)	2 (5.7)	0 (0.0)	10 (55.6)	61
Total	260	90	49	35	18	18	470

$$\text{Overall Correct Classification} = \frac{153 + 58 + 39 + 20 + 15 + 10}{470} = 62.8\%$$

B. Classification into Normal or Abnormal

Decision	True Diagnosis: Normal	Abnormal	Total
Normal	39	23	62
Abnormal	10	398	408
Total	49	421	470

$$\text{Overall Correct Classification} = \frac{39 + 398}{470} = 93\%$$

[a]Percent of actual in parentheses.

Table 12 Classification of Acute Myelogenous Leukemia (AML), Acute Lymphocytic Leukemia (ALL), and Normal Bone Marrow (20 Parameters)

A. Using Maximum Likelihood

	Actual Diagnosis		
Decision	AML	ALL	Normal
AML	220 (84.62)[a]	27 (30.00)	0 (0.00)
ALL	28 (10.77)	62 (68.89)	0 (0.00)
Normal	12 (4.62)	1 (1.11)	49 (100.00)
Total	260	90	49

B. Using Linear Discrimination

	Actual Diagnosis		
Decision	AML	ALL	Normal
AML	195 (75.00)[a]	14 (15.56)	0 (0.00)
ALL	49 (18.85)	70 (77.78)	1 (2.04)
Normal	16 (6.15)	6 (6.67)	48 (97.96)
Total	260	90	49

[a]Percent of actual in parentheses.

in distinguishing the 3 subgroups tested, with correct classifications of 97% vs 94% ($p=0.006$) (Table 12).

Having established a set of new quantitative parameters that is sensitive to objective disease classification (particularly normal vs AML vs ALL), we examined their relationship to FAB categories and to cytogenetics. Out of 22 FCM parameters tested, 15 showed significant differences between FAB groups; 12 completely separated L1-L2 from M1-M5, and 4 of the 12 separated L1 and L2 as well (Table 13; one-way analysis of variance). Similarly, among 22 FCM parameters tested in relationship to cytogenetics, 14 revealed significant differences (Table 14).

Table 13 Relationship of FAB Categories to FCM Classification

FCM parameter	P-value	FAB categories[a] (order, if p <.05)
1	<.001	M2 M5 M4 M3 M1 L2 L1
2	<.001	M2 M3 M5 M4 M1 L2 L1
3	<.001	M3 M2 M5 M4 M1 L2 L1
4	<.001	M3 M5 M4 M2 M1 L2 L1
5	<.001	L1 L2 M1 M4 M3 M2 M5
6	<.001	M3 M4 M2 M5 M1 L2 L1
7	.48	
8	.30	
9	.17	
10	<.001	M5 M4 M3 M2 M1 L2 L1
11	<.001	L1 L2 M1 M3 M4 M2 M5
12	<.001	M3 M4 M5 M2 M1 L1 L2
13	.005	
14	<.001	L1 M1 M3 L2 M4 M2 M5
15	<.001	L1 M1 L2 M3 M4 M2 M5
16	.21	
17	<.001	M3 M5 M4 M2 M1 L2 L1
18	<.001	M5 M3 M4 M2 M1 L2 L1
19	<.001	L1 L2 M1 M2 M4 M3 M5
20	.51	
21	.015	M3 M1 L2 L1 M2 M5 M4
22	.76	

[a]Order of means from smallest to largest; Underline indicates means not statistically different at p = .05 using the Student-Newman-Kurls mean ranking procedure; M6 was excluded for having only one observation.

Table 14 Relationship of Cytogenetics to FCM Classification Parameters in Acute Myelogenous Leukemia (AML)

Flow cytometry parameter	P-value	Cytogenetics code[a] (order, if $p < .05$)
1	.027	9 4 2 8 5 3 7 1 6 10[b]
2	<.001	9 6 7 4 1 5 2 3 8 10
3	<.001	6 9 7 4 5 1 3 2 8 10
4	.003	7 6 9 3 4 1 5 10 2 8
5	<.001	10 8 5 2 1 3 4 7 9 6
6	.25	
7	.56	
8	.52	
9	.31	
10	.014	6 7 9 4 3 8 1 2 5 10
11	<.001	10 7 5 1 8 3 2 4 9 6
12	.51	
13	.01	10 7 6 9 5 3 1 4 2 8
14	.009	10 7 6 5 1 3 9 4 8 2
15	.015	10 7 5 3 1 9 8 4 2 6
16	.04	10 9 1 2 5 7 3 8 6 4
17	.003	7 6 9 3 4 1 5 10 2 8
18	.44	
19	.003	10 2 5 1 8 3 4 9 7 6
20	.30	
21	<.001	7 10 6 9 5 1 8 4 3 2
22	.14	

[a]Key to code: 1 = diploid; 2 = Ph$^+$; 3 = hyperdiploid; 4 = hypodiploid; 5 = pseudodiploid; 6 = t(8;21); 7 = t(15;17); 8 = inv 16; 9 = karyotypic instability; 10 = insufficient metaphases.

[b]Order of means from smallest to largest; Underline indicates means not statistically different at p = .05 using the Student-Newman-Kurls mean ranking procedure.

Cluster Analysis

To examine for the presence of "natural" clusters in the data without regard to diagnosis, the Isodata clustering procedure was utilized. Three criteria control the Isodata procedure after each parameter is standardized by dividing by the standard deviation of that parameter: (a) The criterion for splitting, which occurs if the standard deviation of a parameter is greater than the splitting criterion level; (b) the criterion for combining clusters, which occurs if the root mean square distance between cluster means falls below the criterion; and (c) the amount added and subtracted in the parameter which caused a cluster to split used to establish two new cluster centers for classification of clusters in the next iteration. Table 15 gives the resultant clusters for criteria 1.65, 2.00, and 1.00 respectively. Cluster

Table 15 Cluster Analysis of Six Diagnoses with Normalized Distance

Cluster number	Actual Diagnosis					
	AML[a]	ALL[b]	Normal	CML[c]	CLL[d]	MDS[e]
1	67 (25.8)	6 (6.7)	0 (0.0)	0 (0.0)	0 (0.0)	0 (0.0)
2	33 (12.7)	11 (12.2)	1 (2.0)	0 (0.0)	0 (0.0)	1 (5.6)
3	8 (3.1)	4 (4.4)	37 (75.5)	14 (40.0)	1 (5.6)	4 (22.2)
4	32 (12.3)	31 (34.4)	1 (2.0)	1 (2.9)	0 (10.0)	1 (5.6)
5	4 (1.5)	11 (12.2)	0 (0.0)	2 (5.7)	13 (72.2)	1 (5.6)
6	93 (35.8)	9 (10.0)	3 (6.1)	8 (22.9)	0 (0.0)	10 (55.6)
7	5 (1.9)	4 (4.4)	0 (0.0)	2 (5.7)	1 (5.6)	0 (0.0)
8	16 (6.2)	10 (11.1)	7 (14.3)	7 (20.0)	3 (16.7)	1 (5.6)
9	2 (0.7)	4 (4.4)	0 (0.0)	1 (2.9)	0 (0.0)	0 (0.0)
Total	290	90	49	35	18	18

[a]AML = acute myelogenous leukemia.
[b]ALL = acute lymphocytic leukemia.
[c]CML = chronic myelogenous leukemia.
[d]CLL = chronic lymphocytic leukemia.
[e]MDS = myelodysplastic syndromes.

1 consists mostly of AML; cluster 3 consists mostly of normal; 72.2% of CLL is in cluster 5. Cluster 4 contains 34.4% of ALL but also 12.3% of AML. Cluster 3 also contains 40% of CML. Cluster 6 is also interesting: it contains 35.8% of AML but 55.6% of MDS; it also contains the highest percentage of CML (22.9%) not in the normal cluster, cluster 3.

FCM and Prognosis in Acute Leukemia: Standard FCM Parameters

We examined the relationship of DNA ploidy, RNA index and %(S+G_2M) to remission induction, remission duration, and survival. This was carried out in 243 patients with AML and in 75 patients with ALL entered since 1979 on 2 major treatment protocols with adriamycin or m-AMSA combined with vincristine, cytosine arabinoside and prednisone (OAP) or with high dose Ara-C. Prognosis, particularly survival, for 3 different time segments has remained similar, thus justifying pooling different treatment groups for this analysis.

While the presence of DNA aneuploidy did not affect remission induction, response duration, or survival (Table 16), both hypodiploid and low-degree hyperdiploid DNA index values were associated with a short median survival in ALL, whereas in AML high-degree hyperdiploid abnormalities identified a small subgroup with especially short survival (Figure 7). Pretreatment cell cycle kinetics or RNA index did not affect outcome in either ALL or AML (Tables 17 and 18). However, a significant impact of cytogenetics was observed in AML for both remission induction and survival (Table 19).

Appreciating the prognostic importance of chromosomal patterns in AML, FCM variables were reexamined within defined cytogenetic categories. In patients with structural aberrations, the presence of DNA-aneuploidy, namely hyperdiploidy

Table 16 Outcome of Adults with Acute Leukemia, According to DNA-Ploidy

Diagnosis	DNA index	N	%CR	Median CR duration (weeks)	Median survival[a] (weeks)
Acute myelogenous leukemia (AML)	<1.0	7	50	234+	71
	1.0	177	71	57	52
	1.01-1.15	50	67	81	60
	>1.15	9	44	177	7
Acute lymphocytic leukemia (ALL)	<1.0	3	0	–	4
	1.0	56	55	40	39
	1.01-1.15	7	57	42	15
	>1.15	9	60	29	31

[a]Survival in ALL $P < .001$.

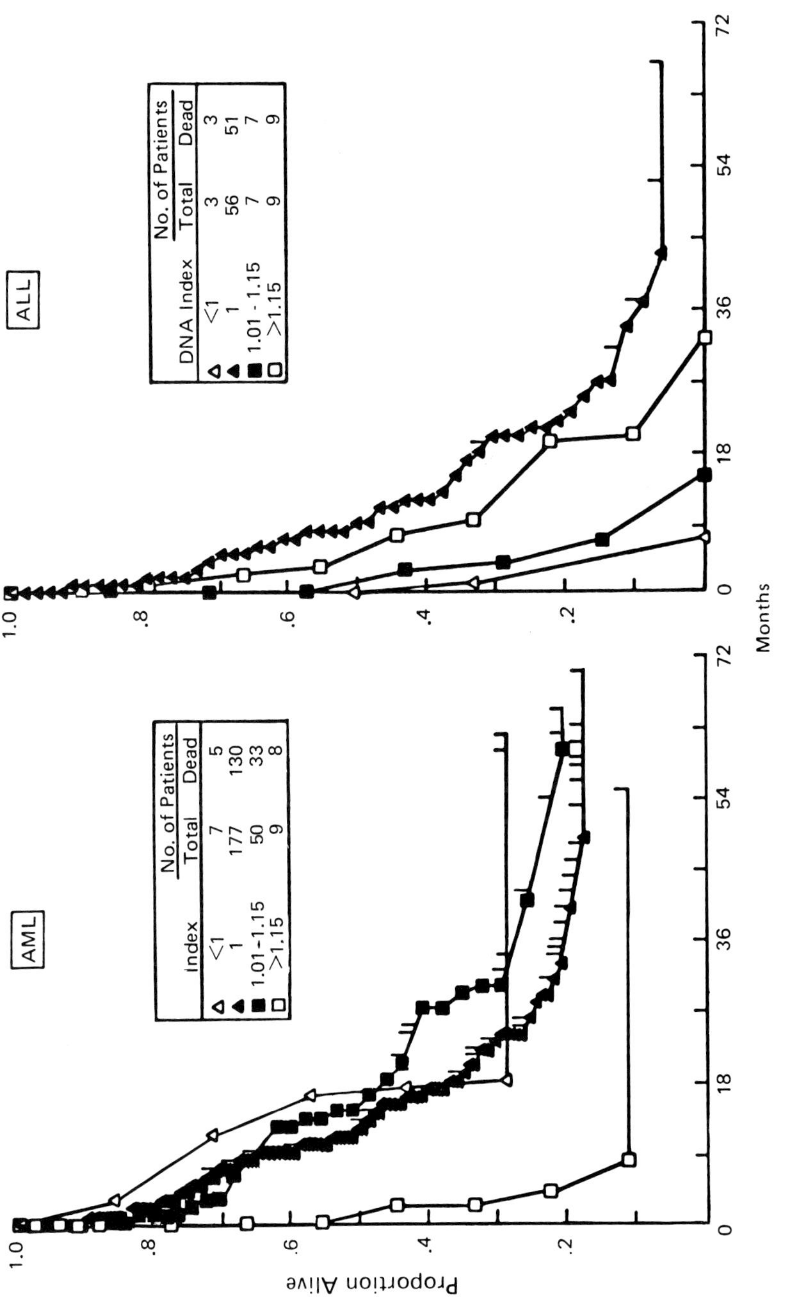

Figure 7 Survival in acute myelogenous leukemia (AML) and acute lymphocytic leukemia (ALL) according to DNA ploidy. Note the unfavorable effect of hypodiploid and low-degree hyperdiploid DNA index in ALL, whereas in AML high-degree hyperdiploid abnormalities identified the highest risk group.

Table 17 Outcome of Adults with Acute Leukemia According to Cytokinetics

Diagnosis	$(S+G_2M)\%$	N	%CR	Median CR duration (weeks)	Median survival (weeks)
Acute myelogenous	<10	59	76	63	49
leukemia	10-15	98	68	63	59
	>15	69	68	57	60
Acute lymphocytic	<10	20	40	27	36
leukemia	10-15	21	48	24	20
	>15	21	62	39	46

Table 18 Outcome of Adults with Acute Leukemia According to RNA Content

Diagnosis	RNA index	N	%CR	Median CR duration (weeks)	Median survival (weeks)
Acute myelogenous	<1.5	42	64	57	45
leukemia	1.5-2.0	83	70	54	57
	>2.0	98	71	81	52
Acute lymphocytic	<1.3	17	65	27	33
leukemia	1.3-1.5	20	55	42	65
	>1.5	26	39	73	30

Table 19 Outcome of Adults with Acute Myelogenous Leukemia According to Cytogenetics

Karyotype	N	Median age (yrs)	%CR[a]	Median CR duration[b] (weeks)	Median survival[c] (weeks)
Normal diploid	101	52	79	57	69
Structural aberrations	66	34	71	87	70
Numeric aberrations	60	54	48	34	23
Insufficient metaphases	16	52	63	84	50

[a] $p < 0.001$.
[b] $p = .09$.
[c] $p = .002$.

Table 20 Outcome for Adults with Acute Myelogenous Leukemia with Structural Aberrations According to DNA/RNA Parameters

Parameter	N	Median age (yrs)	%CR	Median CR duration (weeks)	Median survival (weeks)
DNA index					
Diploid	47	35	68	62	45
Aneuploid	19	32	79	276+[a]	280+[b]
$(S+G_2M)\%$					
$\leqslant 12$	38	34	71	80	52
> 12	23	34	78	79	210
RNA index					
< 2.0	27	46	67	86	70
> 2.0	33	30	76	97	88

[a]P = .05.
[b]P = 0.001.

of the low-degree type, was associated with superior remission duration and survival (Table 20), but not in other chromosomal categories.

We had previously noted a strong relationship between age and likelihood of complete remission, with a dramatic decline beyond the fifth decade (80% vs 52%, $p<0.001$). We therefore reanalyzed FCM parameters separately in young and older patients according to cytogenetic categories. The importance of age for remission induction was only evident among patients with abnormal karyotypes and $\%(S+G_2M) \geqslant 10\%$ (Table 21). Conversely, high $\%(S+G_2M)$ values implied drug sensitivity in young and resistance in older patients.

Table 21 Remission Induction in Adult Acute Myelogenous Leukemia Related to Age, Cytogenetics and Cytokinetics

			% Complete Remission		
Karyotype	$(S+G_2M)\%$	N	<50 yrs	>50 yrs	P value
Normal diploid	<10	23	100	67	0.1
	10-15	38	80	74	n.s.
	>15	33	89	80	n.s.
Aneuploid	<10	28	78	60	n.s.
	10-15	53	81	29	<0.001
	>15	35	93	25	<0.001

Having established a three-way interrelationship between age, cytogenetics, and cytokinetics for complete remission, the three clinical endpoints of remission, remission duration, and survival were reanalyzed in the context of the three cytogenetic categories of diploidy, numeric, and structural aberrations, and separately for young and old patients. We noted discordant effects of DNA-aneuploidy and of pretreatment %(S+G_2M) in different cytogenetic groups in young and old patients (Tables 22 and 23). Specifically, DNA aneuploidy and high %(S+G_2M) were good risk features in young patients and adversely affected older individuals with structural aberrations.

Table 22 Relative Death Rates by Age, Ploidy, and Cytogenetics in Adult Acute Myelogenous Leukemia

		Relative Death Rates		
Karyotype	DNA index	Age ≤60	Age >60	Ratio[a]
Normal	Diploid	1.00 (56)[b]	2.16 (25)	2.16
	Aneuploid	1.36 (12)	0.97 (8)	0.71
Numeric abnormalities	Diploid	1.56 (20)	5.85 (15)	3.74
	Aneuploid	2.56 (18)	1.92 (8)	0.75
Structural abnormalities	Diploid	1.27 (35)	4.87 (12)	3.85
	Aneuploid	0.24 (17)	24.43 (2)	103.40

[a]P = 0.002.
[b]( ), number of patients.

Table 23 Relative Death Rates by Age, Cytokinetics, and Cytogenetics in Adult Acute Myelogenous Leukemia

		Relative Death Rates		
Karyotype	(S+G_2M)%	Age ≤60	Age >60	Ratio[a]
Normal	<10	1.00 (14)[b]	1.87 (8)	1.87
	10-15	0.96 (23)	1.64 (15)	1.70
	>15	0.93 (26)	1.44 (7)	1.55
Numeric abnormalities	<10	1.65 (6)	1.83 (4)	1.11
	10-15	1.83 (15)	2.82 (6)	1.54
	>15	2.04 (15)	4.33 (10)	2.12
Structural abnormalities	<10	1.65 (14)	3.07 (5)	1.86
	10-15	0.62 (27)	5.97 (6)	9.66
	>15	0.23 (6)	11.61 (3)	50.09

[a]P = 0.03.
[b]( ), number of patients.

Table 24 Prognostic Importance of Acridine Orange Flow Cytometry Parameters in AML and ALL (Stepwise Proportional Hazards Regression Analysis)

	Survival				Length of Remission			
	AML		ALL		AML		ALL	
Parameter	P-value	Order	P-value	Order	P-value	Order	P-value	Order
1	.95		.25		.79		.23	
2	.17		.31		.04		.25	
3	.03		.53		.18		.61	3–
4	.05		.36		.49		.60	
5	.01	1+	.05		.01	1+	.75	
6	.33		.36		.99		.95	
7	.03		.03		.90		.04	
8	.24		.12	4+	.36		.03	
9	.90		.30		.24		.04	
10	.13		.09	3–	.51		.26	
11	.02		.02		.18		.87	
12	.67	2+	.72		.92	2+	.02	1–
13	.63		.06		.52		.29	
14	.29		.005	1–	.78		.14	
15	.18		.005		.58		.09	
16	.24		.05		.46	3–	.05	
17	.04	3–	.35		.49		.59	
18	.42		.49		.76		.25	
19	.61	4–	.02	2–	.17		.11	2–
20	.50		.02		.20		.06	
21	.23		.30		.71		.06	

AML = acute myelogenous leukemia; ALL = acute lymphocytic leukemia.

FCM and Prognosis in Acute Leukemia: All 22 Parameters

Recognizing the accuracy of objective disease classification by means of refined FCM variables, their prognostic role was also examined separately in AML and ALL, using continuous variables. The results of stepwise proportional hazards regression analyses for both remission time and survival are summarized in Table 24. The p values listed pertain to the parameters entered singly into the model. The order of entry of each parameter is also given until the significance of the entering parameter exceeded 0.1. The order of entry was not the order of significance on the single regression indicating relationships among variables. For example, concerning survival in AML, parameters 3 and 4 changed from .03 and .05 to .51 and .48, respectively, after parameter 5 had been entered, whereas parameter 12 changed from .67 to .03. The first 4 parameters entered for survival in AML were 5 (the variance of G_1), 12 (the kurtosis of S), 17 (the skewness of RNA in G_1) and 19 (the G_1 RNA index). The "plus" or "minus" after the order of entry indicate whether the parameter was a positive or negative factor for survival or remission duration. For AML, parameters 5 and 12 were significant positive factors for both survival and remission time. As measures of RNA variance in G_1 and of RNA "flatness" in S, these parameters relate to RNA heterogeneity, and higher values may indicate increasing leukemic cell differentiation. It is interesting that, for ALL remission duration, parameter 12 was a negative factor, and parameter 3 (measuring the width of the G_1-RNA histogram) was also negative. For ALL, a high ratio of median RNA in S vs G_1 (parameter 14) was the most significant variable adversely affecting survival. The standard RNA index in G_1 (parameter 19, as a continuous variable) adversely affected remission and survival times in ALL and only survival in AML. Except for this parameter, different variables were associated with remission duration and survival in AML and ALL.

IV. SUMMARY AND PERSPECTIVE

Attempts to capture the well-known clinical heterogeneity of acute leukemias as revealed under current practice of cytotoxic therapy have led to the recognition of favorable and adverse chromosomal patterns as a dominant disease-related feature associated with initial response and response duration and survival in AML (11,12). While some of these cytogenetic categories are associated with distinct clinical entities (35,36,37), morphologic subcategories of adult AML and ALL have been of little relevance clinically (10).

In view of the established importance of cytogenetics, cytokinetics, and tumor cell differentiation for disease progression and drug sensitivity, AO FCM was expected, as in lymphoma and myeloma (38,39), to provide an objective classification of leukemia based on biologically relevant parameters. Thus, it was perhaps not surprising to find a tremendous overlap in the three main FCM parameters

(DNA and RNA index, $(S+G_2M)\%$) among morphologic disease categories, which by themselves had limited prognostic implications. We did note, however, significant differences in proliferative activity and also in RNA and DNA index among cytogenetic groups in AML.

When analyzed for their clinical role, the 3 standard FCM features had only supplementary prognostic importance, pertaining to relatively small groups of patients. Unlike the situation in children, where high-degree DNA-hyperdiploid abnormalities corresponding to >50 chromosomes readily identifed a major favorable subgroup of ALL (40), the dominant DNA stemline in adults was diploid, and aneuploidy present in about a quarter of patients typically was of a lower degree, rendering some favorable attributes to AML with chromosomal translocations. In addition, the rare occurrence of hypodiploidy in ALL and high-degree hyperdiploidy in AML were associated with very short survival (41a). The notion of DNA-aneuploid stemlines in patients with diploid disease or only structural chromosomal aberrations was attributed to differences in target cells examined: i.e., $G_{1/0}$ cells for DNA index analysis and mitotic cells in the case of chromosomal analysis. DNA-ploidy analysis is independent of proliferative activity and has been shown by the premature chromosome condensation technique to recognize chromosomal abnormalities present in $G_{1/0}$ cells when mitoses were diploid (20).

There were interesting 3-way interactions between FCM variables, cytogenetics and age, where opposite prognostic directions of cytokinetic and DNA-ploidy variables were observed in different age and cytogenetic groups (41a). We have previously reasoned that the drug resistance associated with high $\%(S+G_2M)$ in older patients may imply a biologically different condition from that in younger patients experiencing high remission rates; perhaps long cycle times in old and high growth fraction disease in the younger population (41). This issue can now be readily examined by measuring cell cycle times using in vivo or in vitro BUdR monoclonal antibody technology (Figure 8) (42). Thus, correlated DNA-BUdR analysis should provide information on the heterogeneity of cell cycle time parameters which may be more important than cell cycle compartment distribution to consideration of lethal drug effects (43).

Appreciating the limited diagnostic and prognostic usefulness of the three standard FCM variables and realizing that FCM visual patterns correlated well with morphologic diagnoses, efforts were undertaken to account more adequately for the great complexity of DNA-RNA distributions in normal and leukemic bone marrows. Introduction of 19 more objective parameters for a total of 22 provided the sensitivity and specificity required for a clinically potentially useful distinction of normal and leukemic conditions. There was a high degree of consistency in disease classification, which was minimally affected by the degree of leukemic cell infiltration down to 30%. Thus, mainly by way of RNA dispersion in $G_{1/0}$ and $(S+G_2M)$ compartments it was possible to distinguish between normal

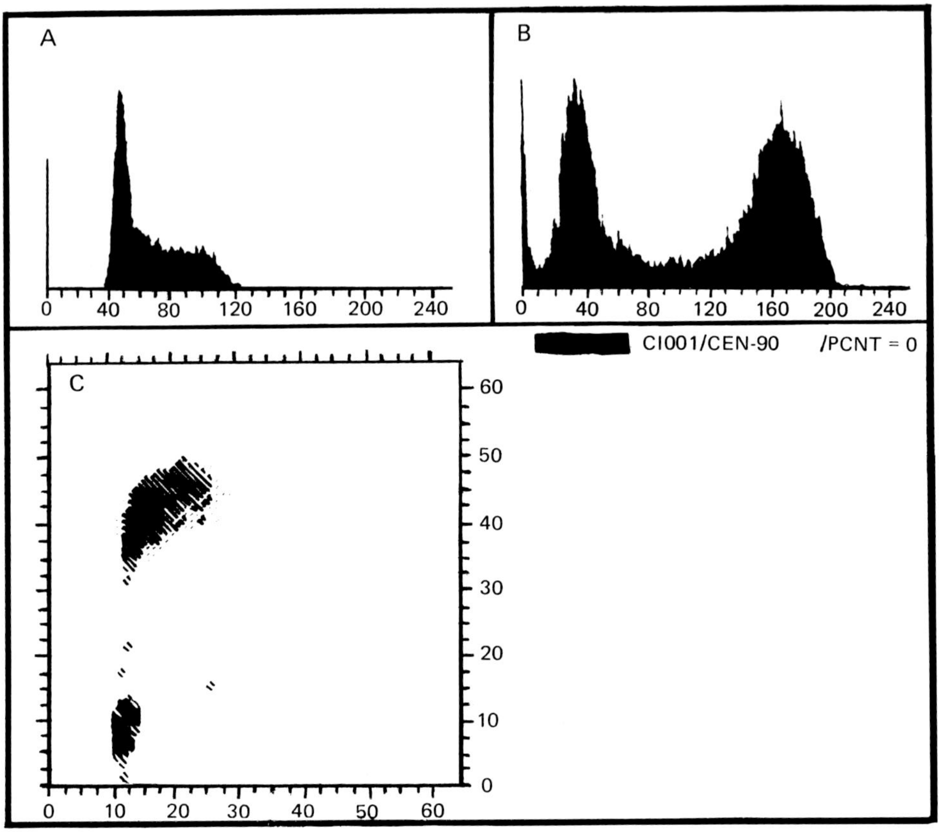

Figure 8 DNA-anti-BUdR monoclonal antibody distribution in ARH 77 human myeloma cells. Note the marked increase in bromodeoxyuridine (BUdR)-related fluorescence with the transition from G_1 into S. This method allows more objective analysis of cell cycle compartments and provides information on relative DNA synthetic rates, thus potentially recognizing ineffective DNA synthesis and S_0 cells (see text).

and leukemic states and also between AML and ALL with a high degree of accuracy. As was evident from a stepwise procedure, most of the singly important variables retained their importance when used in combination, emphasizing their relatively independent contributions. Given the problems in reproducibly applying the FAB classification, a perfect correlation between AO FCM and morphologic diagnoses was not observed and also not expected. Many of the 22 FCM parameters, however, did show significant differences between FAB and cytogenetic categories. The reproducibility and discriminatory capacity afforded by one cytochemical stain (acridine orange–AO) warrants further exploration of

AO FCM parameters for objective and quantitative classification of leukemic bone marrows. Similarly, the "natural clustering" irrespective of morphologic diagnosis needs to be further investigated for prognostic implications.

Preliminary analysis suggests that several of the newly introduced FCM parameters relating to RNA heterogeneity affect remission and survival times in both AML and ALL. Interestingly, different variables pertained to AML and ALL, and RNA heterogeneity was usually favorable for AML ("plus" in Table 24) but often unfavorable ("minus") in ALL. Thus, utilization of the full complexity of AO FCM provided parameters that were not only useful in objective disease classification but also in assessing prognosis.

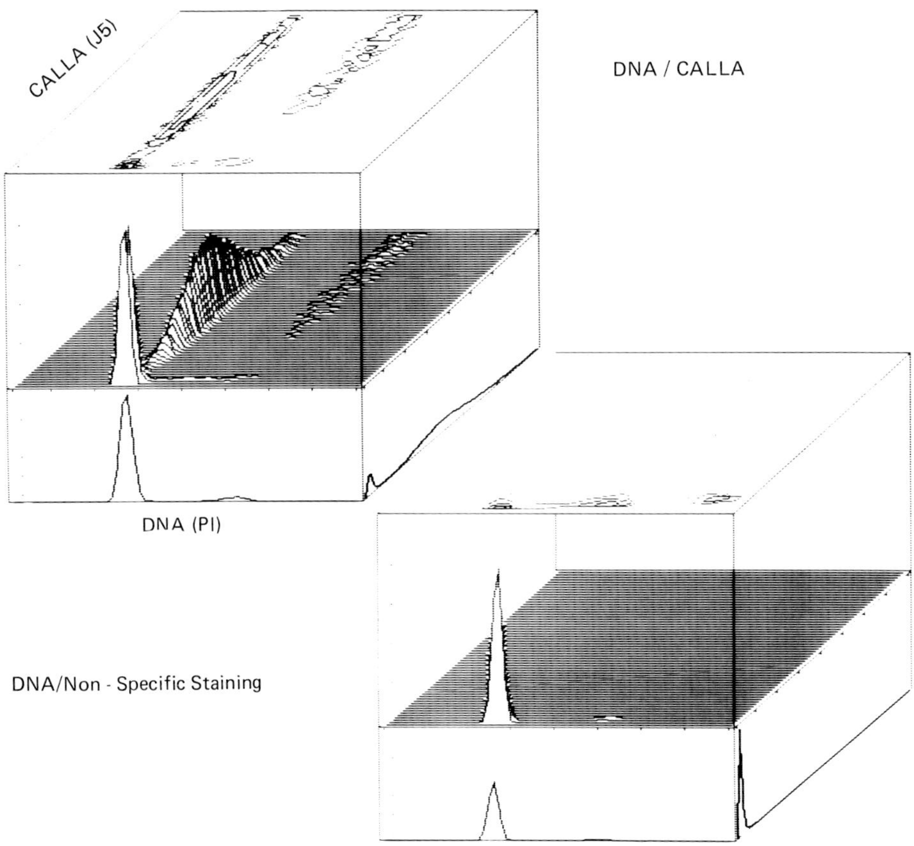

Figure 9 DNA-CALLA antigen analysis in ALL. Note that CALLA expression is restricted to the hyperdiploid DNA stemline.

Several laboratories are currently examining the quantitative expression of various myeloid and lymphoid antigens. When coupled with the analysis of DNA content, such studies permit investigation into leukemia-specific phenotypes in cases with DNA stemline abnormalities (44) (Figure 9) and into the cell-cycle-related expression of these cell surface antigens. Of great biological and practical importance is the recognition of biphenotypic leukemias (45). The concurrent expression of myeloid and lymphoid or T and B markers in the same cell suggests either aberrant expression or expansion of an early progenitor compartment consistent with stem cell disease. Studies by Mirro et al. suggest that most biphenotypic leukemias have a subpopulation of cells sharing the 2 different phenotypes (46). Other investigators have noted, using DNA FCM, the presence of "bigenotypic" and/or "biphenotype" abnormalities, dependent upon whether different levels of RNA content were associated with the same or different DNA stemlines (47).

Recognizing the dominant role of chromosomal patterns for the clinical course of adults with AML, the role of cellular oncogenes located at or near chromosomal breakpoints is subject of intense investigation (48,49). FCM is ideally suited to study, on a cell-by-cell basis, the heterogeneity of abnormal gene expression in terms of m-RNA and protein expression using in situ hybridization with biotin-labeled DNA probes or with monoclonal antibodies (50,51). Thus, the role of oncogenes for cell proliferation and differentiation in human leukemias can be evaluated. When performed along with DNA content analysis in DNA-aneuploid disease, such studies can shed light on neoplasia-specific and cell cycle-related oncogene expression.

FCM also lends itself to studying therapeutic interventions in terms of interference with surface antigen expression or with cell cycle compartment distribution. Several antitumor agents, most notably anthracyclines, are authentically fluorescent and can therefore be readily traced at the cellular level (52,53). Other DNA-reactive compounds, such as amsidines, can be detected by means of competing fluorescent compounds such as Hoechst 33342 (54). FCM studies have recently been extended to Ara-C cellular pharmacology utilizing monoclonal antibody against Ara-C incorporated into DNA (55). Similarly, dihydrofolate reductase as the target enzyme for methotrexate has become amenable to FCM analysis through the use of appropriate monoclonal antibodies (56). With increasing interest in the role of lymphokines and their receptors for the regulation of normal and leukemic hemopoiesis, FCM analysis can be expected to provide insight into the heterogeneity and modulation under therapy of receptor expression. We have already demonstrated the feasibility of performing hormone receptor analysis by FCM using fluorescently labelled estradiol and cortisol probes (57).

In summary, FCM is an ideal tool to examine the cellular heterogeneity of acute leukemias and other neoplasms which, when combined with cell sorting, permits further morphologic, cytogenetic or biochemical analysis of desired cell subpopulations. An ever-increasing variety of cellular and membrane constituents has been recognized to be of biologic and clinical interest in studying acute leukemia. Nucleic acid AO FCM, in its refined form, with many parameters reflecting RNA heterogeneity and dispersion, affords objective discrimination between normal and leukemic bone marrow and identifies quantitative differences among different leukemias, the prognostic value of which needs to be further investigated. Studies are currently underway in several laboratories to determine whether FCM variables relevant to cellular and molecular genetics and to drug resistance may be useful for the management of patients with leukemia.

ACKNOWLEDGMENT

The authors gratefully acknowledge the collaboration of the members of the Department of Hematology of the M. D. Anderson Hospital and Tumor Institute in providing samples to the Cytometry Laboratory. We are grateful to Leslie Smallwood and Quang Tang for performing many aspects of the laboratory procedures and statistical analyses. Eva Menefee did an excellent job in typing the manuscript.

REFERENCES

1. Bennett, J. M., Catovsky, D., Daniel, M. T., Flandrin, G., Galton, D. A. G., Gralnick, H. R., and Sultan, C. (1976). Proposals for the classification of the acute leukemias (FAB cooperative group). *Brit. J. Haem.* 33:451-458.
2. Childs, C., and Stass, S. (1987). Acute leukemia: Characterization and diagnosis. In: *Practical Application of Laboratory Studies in the Differential Diagnosis of Acute Leukemia*, in press.
3. Foon, K. A., and Todd, R. F. (1986). Review: Immunologic classification of leukemia and lymphoma. *Blood* 68:1-31.
4. Greaves, M. F., Chan, L. C., Furley, A. J. W., Watt, S. M., and Molgaard, H. V. (1986). Review: Lineage promiscuity in hemopoietic differentiation and leukemia. *Blood* 67:1-11.
5. Riehm, H. (1984). Therapie der akuten lymphoblastischen Leukaemie des Kindes. In *Therapie der Akuten Leukaemien*, T. Buechner, D. Urbanitz, and J. van de Loo (eds.). Springer-Verlag, Berlin, pp. 51-58.
6. Schellong, G., Creutzig, U., and Ritter, J. (1984). Therapie der akuten myeloischen leukamie bei kindern. In *Therapie der Akuten Leukaemien*, T. Buchner, D. Urbanitz, and J. van de Loo (eds.). Springer-Verlag, Berlin, pp. 73-85.
7. Clarkson, B., Gee, T., Arlin, Z., Mertelsmann, R., Kempin, S., Dinsmore, R., O'Reilly, R., Andreeff, M., Berman, E., Higgins, C., Little, C., Cirrincoine, C., and Ellis, S. (1984). Current status of treatment of acute leukemia in adults: An overview. In *Therapie der Akuten Leukaemien*. T. Buchner, D. Urbanitz, and J. van de Loo (eds.). Springer-Verlag, Berlin, pp. 1-32.

8. Hoelzer, D., Thiel, E., Loeffler, H., Bodenstein, H., Plaumann, L., Buchner, T., Urbanitz, D., Koch, P., Heimpel, H., Engelhardt, R., Mueller, U., Wendt, F.-C., Sodomann, H., Ruehl, H., Herrmann, F., Kaboth, W., Dietzfelbinger, H., Pralle, H., Lunschken, Ch., Hellriegel, K.-P., Spors, S., Nowrousian, R. M., Fischer, J., Fulle, H., Mitrou, P. S., Pfreundschuh, M., Gorg, Ch., Emmerich, B., Queisser, W., Meyer, P., Labedzki, L., Essers, U., Konig, H., Mainzer, K., Herrmann, R., Messerer, D., and Zwingers, T. (1984). Intensified therapy in acute lymphoblastic and acute undifferentiated leukemia in adults. *Blood* 64:38-47.
9. Keating, M., McCredie, K., Bodey, G., Smith, T., Gehan, E., and Freireich, E. (1982). Improved prospects for long-term survival in adults with acute myelogenous leukemia. *JAMA* 248:2481-2486.
10. Kalwinsky, K. D., Roberson, P., Dahl, G., Harber, J., Rivera, G., Bowman, W., Pui, C.-H., Ochs, J., Abromwitch, M., Costlow, M. E., Melvin, S., Stass, S., Williams, D., and Murphy, S. (1985). Clinical relevance of lymphoblastic biological features in children with acute lymphoblastic leukemia. *J. Clin. Oncol.* 3:477-484.
11. Rowley, J. D. (1981). Association of specific chromosome abnormalities with type of acute leukemia and with patient's age. *Cancer Res.* 41:3407-3410.
12. Yunis, J. J., Bloomfield, C., and Ensrud, K. (1983). All patients with acute non-lymphocytic leukemia may have a chromosomal defect. *New Engl. J. Med.* 305:135-139.
13. Andreeff, M., Darzynkiewicz, Z., Sharpless, T., Clarkson, B., and Melamed, M. (1980). Discrimination of human leukemia subtypes by flow cytometric analysis of cellular DNA and RNA. *Blood* 55:282-293.
14. Barlogie, B., Latreille, J., Freireich, E., Fu, C., Mellard, D., Meistrich, M., and Andreeff, M. (1980). Characterization of hematologic malignancies by flow cytometry. *Blood Cells* 6:719-744.
15. Buechner, T., Barlogie, B., Hiddemann, W., Kamanabroo, D., and Goehde, W. (1974). Accumulation of S-phase cells in the bone marrow of patients with acute leukemia by cytosine arabinoside. *Blut* 28:299.
16. Barlogie, B., Raber, M., Schumann, J., Johnson, T., Drewinko, B., Swartzendruber, D., Gohde, W., Andreeff, M., and Freireich, E. (1983). Perspectives in cancer research: Flow cytometry in clinical cancer research. *Cancer Res.* 43:3982-3997.
17. Traganos, F., Darzynkiewicz, Z., Sharpless, T., and Melamed, M. (1977). Simultaneous staining of ribonucleic and dexynucleic acid in unfixed cells using acridine in a flow cytofluorometric system. *J. Histochem. Cytochem.* 25:46-56.
18. Barlogie, B., Maddox, A., Johnston, D., Raber, M., Drewinko, B., Keating, M., and Freireich, E. (1983). Quantitative cytology in leukemia research. *Blood Cells* 9:35-55.
19. Dosik, G., Barlogie, B., Goehde, W., Johnston, D., Tekell, J., and Drewinko, B. (1980). Flow cytometry of DNA content in human bone marrow: A critical re-appraisal. *Blood* 55:734-740.

20. Barlogie, B., Hittelman, W., Spitzer, G., Hart, J., Trujillo, J., Smallwood, L., and Drewinko, B. (1977). Correlation of DNA distribution abnormalities with cytogenetic findings in human adult leukemia and lymphoma. *Cancer Res.* 37:4400-4407.
21. Goehde, W., and Dittrich, W. (1971). Implusfluorometrie–Ein neuartiges Durchflussverfahren zur ultraschnellen Mengenbestimmung von Zellinhaltsstoffen. *Acta Histochem.* (Suppl.) 10:429-437.
22. Barlogie, B., Spitzer, G., Hart, J., Johnston, D., Buechner, T., Schumann, J., and Drewinko, B. (1976). DNA-histogram analysis of human hemopoietic cells. *Blood* 48:245-258.
23. Hiddemann, W., Schumann, J., Andreeff, M., Barlogie, B., Herman, C., Leif, R., Mayall, B., Murphy, R., and Sandberg, A. (1984). Special report: Convention on nonmenclature for DNA cytometry. *Cytometry* 5:445-446.
24. Zar, T. H. (1984). *Biostatistical Analysis*, 2nd Ed. Prentice-Hall, Englewood Cliffs, N.J.
25. Cramer, H. (1946). *Mathematical Methods of Statistics*. Princeton University Press, Princeton, N.J.
26. Lachenbruch, P. A., and Mickey, M. R. (1968). Estimation of error rates in discriminant analysis. *Technometrics* 10:1-11.
27. Ball, G. H., and Hall, D. J. (1967). A clustering technique for summarizing multivariante data. *Behavioral Science* 12:153-155.
28. Lachenbruch, P. A. (1975). *Discriminant Analysis*. Hafner, New York.
29. Efron, B., and Tibshirani, R. (1986). Bootstrap methods for standard errors, confidence intervals, and other measures of statistical accuracy. *Statistical Science* 1:54-77.
30. Darzynkiewicz, Z., Traganos, F., and Melamed, M. (1980). New cell cycle compartments identified by multi-parameter flow cytometry. *Cytometry* 1:98-108.
31. Barlogie, B., Drewinko, B., Schumann, J., Gohde, W., Dosik, G., Johnston, D., and Freireich, E. (1980). Cellular DNA content as a marker of neoplasia in man. *Am. J. Med.* 79:195-203.
32. Buechner, T., Bloomfield, C., Hiddemann, W., Hossfeld, K. D., and Schumann, J. (1985). *Tumor Aneuploidy*. Springer-Verlag, Berlin, Heidelberg.
33. Carrano, A. V., Gray, J., Langlois, R. G., Burkhart-Schultz, K. J., and Van Dilla, M. A. (1979). Measurement and purification of human chromosomes by flow cytometry and sorting. *PNAS* 76:1382.
34. Williams, D., Harber, J., Murphy, S., Look, A., Kalwinsky, D., Rivera, G., Melvin, S., Stass, S., and Dahl, G. (1986). Chromosomal translocations play a unique role in influencing prognosis in childhood acute lymphoblastic leukemia. *Blood* 68:205-212.
35. Trujillo, J., Cork, A., Ahearn, M., Yunis, E., and McCredie, K. (1979). Hematologic and cytologic characterization of the 8/21 translocation in acute granulocytic leukemia. *Blood* 53:695-706.
36. Van den Berghe, H., Louwafie, A., Broekaert-van Orshoven, A., David, G., Verwilghen, R., Michaux, J. L., and Sokal, G. (1979). Chromosome abnormalities in acute promyelocytic leukemia (APL). *Cancer* 43:558-562.

37. Arthur, D. C., and Bloomfield, C. (1983). Partial deletion of the long arm of chromosome 16 and bone marrow eosinophilia in acute non-lymphocytic leukemia: A new association. *Blood* 61:994-998.
38. Srigley, J., Barlogie, B., Butler, J., Osborne, B., Blick, M., Johnston, D., Kantarjian, H., Reuben, J., Batsakis, J., and Freireich, E. (1985). Heterogeneity of non-Hodgkin's lymphoma probed by nucleic acid cytometry. *Blood* 65:1090-1098.
39. Barlogie, B., Alexanian, R., Smith, L., Dixon, D., Smallwood, L., and Delasalle, K. (1985). Prognostic implications of tumor cell DNA and RNA content in multiple myeloma. *Blood* 66:338-341.
40. Look, A., Roberson, P. K., Williams, D. L., Rivera, G., Bowman, W. P., Pui, C.-H., Ochs, J., Abromowitch, M., Kalwinsky, D., Dahl, G., George, S., and Murphy, S. (1985). Prognostic importance of blast cell DNA content in childhood acute lymphoblastic leukemia. *Blood* 65:1079-1086.
41a. Barlogie, B., Stass, S., Dixon, D., Keating, M., Cork, A., Trujillo, J. M., McCredie, K. B., and Freireich, E. J. (1987). DNA-aneuploidy in adult acute leukemia. *Cancer Genet. and Cytogenet.*, in press.
41. Kantarjian, H., Barlogie, B., Keating, M., Hall, R., Smith, T., McCredie, K., and Freireich, E. (1985). Pretreatment cytokinetics in acute myelogenous leukemia: Age-related prognostic implications. *JCI* 76:319-324.
42. Gratzner, H. G. (1982). Monoclonal antibody to 5-bromo- and 5-iodo-deoxyuridine: A new sensitivity of chromatin to acid denaturation in quiescent and cycling cells revealed by flow cytometry. *J. Histochem. Cytochem.* 27: 478-485.
43. Teodori, L., Barlogie, B., Drewinko, B., Swartzendruber, D., and Mauro, F. (1981). Reduction of 1-β-D-arabinofuranosylcytosine and adriamycin cytotoxicity following cell cycle arrest by anguidine. *Cancer Res.* 41:1263-1270.
44. Look, A., Melvin, S. L., Williams, D., Brodeur, G., Dahl, C., Kalwinsky, D., Murphy, S., and Mauer, A. (1982). Aneuploidy and percentage of S-phase cells determined by flow cytometry correlate with cell phenotype in childhood acute leukemia. *Blood* 60:959-967.
45. Smith, L., Curtis, J., Messner, H., Senn, J., Furthmayr, H., and McCullough, E. (1982). Lineage infidelity in acute leukemia. *Blood* 61:1138-1145.
46. Mirro, J., Zipf, T., Pui, C.-H., Kitchingman, F., Williams, D., Melvin, S., Murphy, S., and Stass, S. (1985). Acute mixed lineage leukemia: Clinicopathologic correlations and prognostic significance. *Blood* 66:1115-1123.
47. Andreeff, M., Redner, A., Thongprasert, S., Eagle, B., Steinherz, P., Miller, D., and Melamed, M. (1985). Multiparameter flow cytometry for determination of ploidy, proliferation and differentiation in acute leukemia: Treatment effects and prognostic value. In *Tumor Aneuploidy*. T. Buchner, C. Bloomfield, W. Hiddemann, D. Hossfeld and J. Schumann (eds.). Springer-Verlag, Berlin, pp. 81-106.
48. Dalla-Favera, R., Bregni, M., Erikson, J., Patterson, D., Gallo, R., and Croce, C. (1982). Human c-myc onc gene is located on the region of chromosome 8 that is translocated in Burkitt lymphoma cells. *PNAS* 79:7824-7827.

49. Tsujimoto, Y., Yunis, J., Onorato-Showe, L., Erikson, J., Nowell, P., and Croce, C. (1984). Molecular cloning of the chromosomal breakpoint of B-cell lymphomas and leukemias with the t(11;14) chromosome translocation. *Science* 224:1403-1406.
50. Shaw, G., Harper, M., Hahn, B., Epstein, L., Gajdusek, D., Price, R., Navia, B., Petito, C., O'Hara, C., Groopman, J., Cho, E.-S., Oleske, J., Wong-Staal, F., and Gallo, R. (1985). HTLV-III infection in brains of children and adults with AIDS encephalopathy. *Science* 227:177-182.
51. Andreeff, M., Slater, D., Bressler, J., and Furth, M. Cellular ras oncogene expression and cell cycle measured by flow cytometry in hematopoietic cell lines. *Blood* 67:676-681.
52. Krishan, A., and Ganapathis, R. (1980). Laser flow cytometric studies on the intracellular fluorescence of anthracycles. *Cancer Res.* 48:3895-3900.
53. Sonneveld, P., and van den Engh, G. (1981). Differences in uptake of adriamycin and daunorubicin by normal BM cells and acute leukemia cells determined by flow cytometry. *Leukemia Res.* 5:251-257.
54. Andersson, B., Geran, M., Barlogie, B., Van, N. T., and McCredie, K. (1986). Analysis of nuclear m-AMSA content by DNA fluorochrome competition. *Eur. J. Cancer Clin. Oncol.* 22:883-889.
55. Gray, J. Unpublished.
56. Kaufman, R. J., Bertino, J. R., and Schimke, R. K. (1978). Quantitation of dihydrofolate reductase in individual parental and methotrexate-resistant murine cells: Use of a fluorescence activated cell sorter. *J. Biol. Chem.* 253: 5852.
57. Van, N. T., Raber, M., Barrows, G., and Barlogie, B. (1984). Estrogen receptor analysis by flow cytometry. *Science* 224:876-879.

7

Immunophenotype in the Characterization and Diagnosis of Acute Leukemia
Lymphoid Markers

JEFFREY COSSMAN and STEFANIA PITTALUGA *National Cancer Institute, National Institutes of Health, Bethesda, Maryland*

I. INTRODUCTION

The application of laboratory marker techniques to acute lymphoblastic leukemias has established a solid foundation for precise diagnosis and classification. Diagnostic marker analysis is based on the conceptual framework, derived from multiple independent lines of evidence, that lymphoblastic neoplasms are clonal expansions of malignantly transformed cells whose differentiation has been interrupted and arrested early in lymphocyte development. By comparing certain differentiated features of normal early lymphocytes with those of lymphoblastic neoplasms, it is clear that normal and neoplastic cells generally share sufficient key characteristics to allow the determination of both cellular lineage and stage of differentiation of a neoplasm. Armed with this information, one can accurately deduce if a leukemia is lymphoid, whether it is of immature (lymphoblastic) or mature (lymphocytic) differentiation, and, finally, if it is derived from T- or B-cell lineage.

Although the event(s) mediating malignant transformation and differentiation arrest are not yet defined, the lineage, differentiation stage, and clonality of lymphoblastic neoplasms can be directly addressed on most clinical samples. To accomplish this, a select battery of antibody probes is used to identify immunoreactive molecules known to be associated with lineage (B or T cells) or differentiation stage (Greaves et al., 1977; Reinherz et al., 1980; Bernard et al., 1981; Cossman et al., 1983a; Nadler et al., 1984). To determine clonality and corroborate the lineage determined by phenotype, leukemia cell DNA can be subjected to restriction fragment (Southern blot) analysis to detect gene rearrangements (Korsmeyer et al., 1983; Bertness et al., 1985; Flug et al., 1985; Rabbitts et al., 1985; Waldmann et al., 1985). The two techniques, phenotyping and genotyping, are complementary approaches which together have generated a powerful diagnostic technology for the detection and classification of lymphoblastic leukemia and lymphoma. Here we summarize the application of the laboratory techniques which have proven to be most informative in lymphoblastic neoplasia.

II. NORMAL LYMPHOID DEVELOPMENT

To gain a more complete understanding of the rationale and interpretation of diagnostic markers, we will first briefly review the salient points of normal lymphocyte development that directly pertain to lymphoblastic neoplasms. By recognizing the distinguishing phenotypic and genetic attributes of normal immature B and T cells, we can establish a useful marker profile for characterizing corresponding neoplasms.

A. Pre-B-Cell Differentiation

Stem cells which ultimately develop into B cells arise in the bone marrow and liver of mammals (reviewed in Lipford and Cossman, 1986). Early B-cell differentiation involves a programmed cascade of events whose aim is to produce B cells capable of secreting antibody with an antigen-binding moiety is capable of binding a specific antigen. Like most differentiating cells, the cell destined to become a B cell undergoes a remarkable series of changes. During this process, the developing B-cell precursor expresses a complex and changing array of surface membrane-bound macromolecules. These surface structures are usually proteins and glycoproteins which may function either as receptors for growth factors or as regulators of differentiation. However, for most of these surface membrane molecules, the function is not yet known. The patterned expression of these cell surface markers can be traced by analysis with monoclonal antibodies, and the sequence of their expression is shown in Figure 1 (right).

The earliest identifiable surface markers of B-cell precursors are Ia, the major histocompatibility class II antigens, and the B-cell-associated surface antigen detected by monoclonal antibody B4 (Nadler et al., 1983). Next, precursors of B cells rearrange their immunoglobulin genes in preparation for antibody synthesis (Tonegawa, 1983; Nadler et al., 1984). The details of this process will be outlined below. Once successful rearrangements have occurred, small amounts of intracytoplasmic immunoglobulin μ heavy chain appear and are detectable by the use of sensitive indirect immunostaining techniques (Gathings, Lawton, and Cooper, 1977). Concomitantly, the cell surface expresses the so-called common acute lymphoblastic leukemia antigen (CALLA), which is a 95,000 to 100,000 dalton surface membrane glycoprotein detectable with either heteroantiserum (Greaves et al., 1975) or monoclonal antibodies such as J5 (Ritz et al., 1980). CALLA persists throughout early B-cell differentiation and disappears from most normal B cells and plasma cells (Ritz et al., 1981). The B-cell-associated antigen B1 is expressed later during pre-B-cell differentiation and persists throughout all of

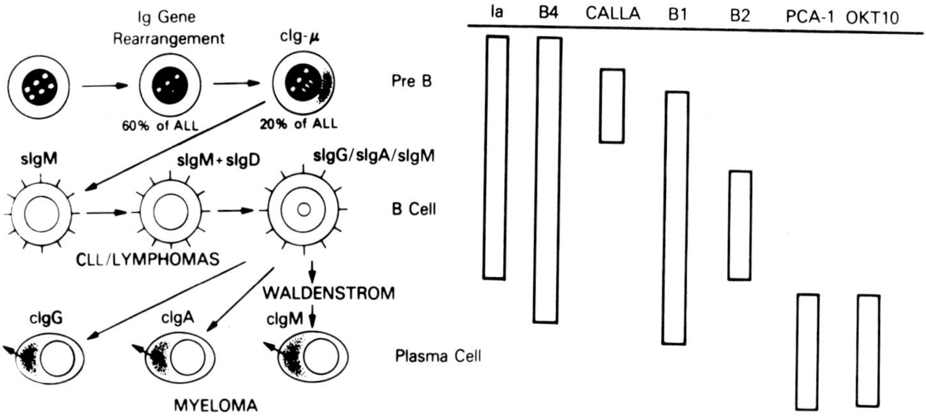

Figure 1 Human B-cell development. During their differentiation, human B cells pass through three developmental stages: pre B-cell, B cell, and plasma cell. The lymphoblastic neoplasms of B-cell lineage correspond to stages of pre B-cell development. Normally, during the pre-B cell stage, immunoglobulin genes undergo rearrangement in order to encode functional immunoglobulin protein. Gene rearrangements occur prior to the production and accumulation of cytoplasmic immunoglobulin μ heavy chains. Coordinate with the rearrangement and expression of the immunoglobulin genes is the expression of a variety of cell surface markers shown at right.

mature B-cell stages, but disappears at the secretory plasma cell stage (Stashenko et al., 1980). Other cell markers such as B2 (Nadler et al., 1981) and PCA-1 (Anderson et al., 1983) appear later during more mature stages of B-cell differentiation and are generally not useful as markers to define early stages of pre-B-cell differentiation associated with the acute lymphoblastic leukemias (ALL) and lymphomas.

As mentioned, during the early developmental pathway of B cells, the genes encoding immunoglobulin rearrange, bringing together in a continuous open reading frame genetic information encoding the variable regions of the immunoglobulin heavy and light chain genes (Tonegawa, 1983). Successful (productive) rearrangements must occur for the B cell to produce fully assembled immunoglobulin molecules. The rearrangements of the immunoglobulin heavy chain gene and the two immunoglobulin light chain gene loci, κ and λ, occur in an ordered, hierarchical manner (Hieter et al., 1981; Korsmeyer et al., 1981; Siminovitch et al., 1985). First, one immunoglobulin heavy chain gene rearranges and, if unsuccessful, the second heavy chain gene allele undergoes rearrangement. Following this, the κ alleles undergo rearrangement, and if these are unsuccessful the κ genes may be deleted, a process mediated by a genetic fragment within the κ locus called the

κ-deleting element (Ritchie et al., 1984; Siminovitch et al., 1985). λ genes rearrange only after both κ alleles have either been rearranged or deleted (Hieter et al., 1981; Korsmeyer et al., 1981; Siminovitch et al., 1985). As will be seen, this ordered hierarchy is recapitulated in the precursor B-cell neoplasms (Korsmeyer et al., 1981). Once successful rearrangements have occurred, the cell traverses into the mature B-cell compartment and can then express the immunoglobulin on the cell surface. Subsequent to this, the immunoglobulin may undergo heavy chain class switching through a genetic reorganizational event and, finally, the cell differentiates into an immunoglobulin-secreting plasma cell, the terminal stage of B-cell differentiation.

During pre-B-cell differentiation, cells contain the intranuclear enzyme terminal deoxynucleotidyl transferase (TdT), which is also present during early T-cell differentiation (Bollum, 1979). This enzyme disappears from cells as they mature. TdT is thought to function as a catalyst for the insertion of nucleotides at the joins during variable gene rearrangement (Alt and Baltimore, 1982). By inserting nucleotides between variable region coding segments, such as between the variable (V) and diversity (D) genes or between the V and joining (J) genes, coding information can be altered. This nucleotide insertional event generates what has become known as N-region diversity, a mechanism utilized by precursor B cells to expand the diversity of specificities of antibody molecules encoded by the immunoglobulin genes (Tonegawa, 1983).

B. Pre-T-Cell Differentiation

T-cell precursors presumably also arise in the bone marrow but diverge from B cells by entering the thymus where they undergo the developmental pathway leading to mature T-cell function. Here, T-cell precursors acquire their own sequential array of cell surface proteins which serve as markers of their differentiation status. These cell surface molecules, like those of B cells, are detected by a battery of monoclonal antibodies which were developed by the immunization of mice with T-cells (see Bernard et al., 1984; Reinherz et al., 1980, 1986). A wide variety of cell surface markers have been described in the developing thymocyte, and the markers most relevant to the discussion presented here are shown in Figure 2. As seen in Figure 2, the earliest identifiable stages of T-cell differentiation are seen in the thymic cortex, where early precursor T cells express cell surface markers such as T1, T11, and 3A1. These markers, as well as others, are also designated by a universal terminology for "cluster differentiation" in which comparable monoclonal antibodies which appear to detect the same antigen are given a single name (Bernard et al., 1984). For example, T1 is known as CD5, T11 is CD2, and 3A1 is CD7 (Bernard et al., 1984). T1 and T11 are also considered pan T markers since virtually all mature T cells express these two cell surface markers. Indeed, all three markers, T1, T11 (Reinherz et al., 1980), and 3A1 (Haynes et al., 1980), are seen not only in very early stages of thymocyte differentiation but

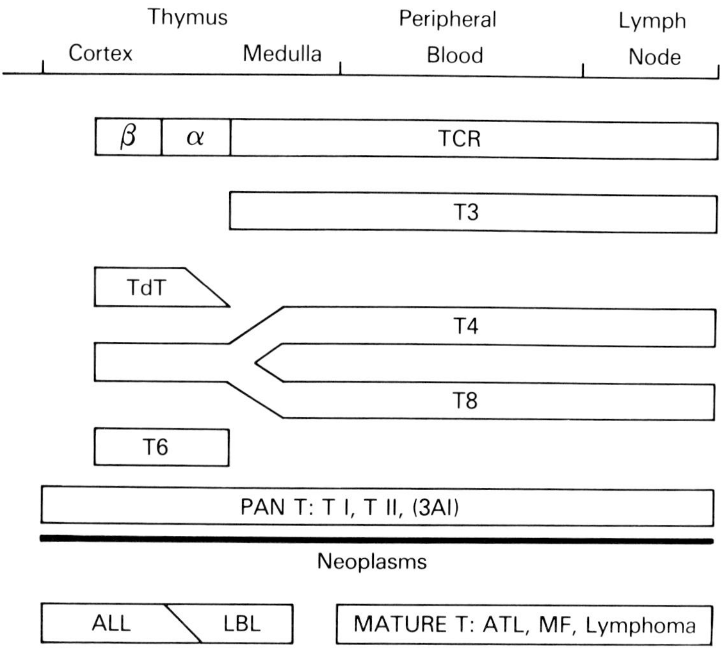

Figure 2 Human T-cell development. The developmental pathway of T cells is characterized by the acquisition and loss of a variety of cellular markers. Human T-cell neoplasms correspond to discrete stages within this developmental pathway. The top bar, T-cell receptor (TCR), indicates transcription of the β subunit prior to that of a and subsequently the translation and surface expression of the T-cell receptor complex (TCR). Concomitantly, surface membrane T3 molecules appear with surface TCR in a noncovalently linked, multichain, molecular complex. Abbreviations: ALL, acute lymphoblastic leukemia; LBL, lymphoblastic lymphoma; ATL, adult T-cell leukemia/lymphoma; MF, mycosis fungoides.

persist throughout T-cell development and occur on mature cells of the peripheral blood in lymph nodes.

Somewhat later in cortical thymocyte differentiation, cells begin to express the so-called cortical thymocyte marker T6 (CD1) (Reinherz et al., 1980), which disappears as cells enter the thymic medulla and develop a more mature T-cell phenotype. Simultaneously during cortical thymocyte development, cells coexpress the cell surface molecules T4 (CD4) and T8 (CD8) (Reinherz et al., 1980), which are associated with helper and suppressor function, respectively, in mature T cells. These two cell surface markers appear to be coexpressed only during this brief period of intrathymic differentiation as they are mutually exclusive in mature T cells. Concurrently, thymocytes contain the intranuclear enzyme TdT

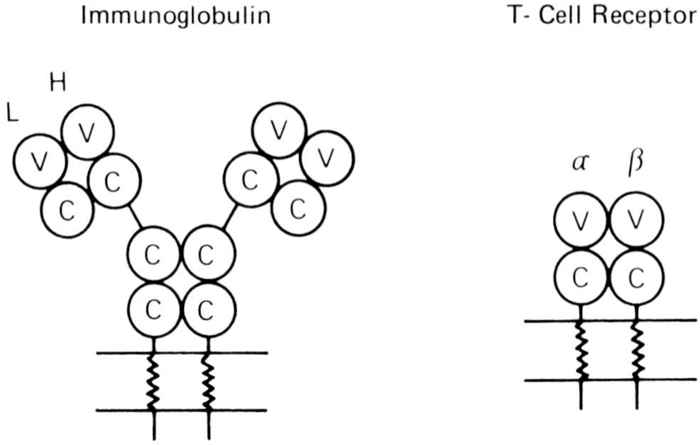

Figure 3 Configuration of the antigen receptors of lymphocytes. B cells express immunoglobulin, a four-chain complex composed of two identical heavy and two identical light chains with their variable (V) regions exposed to the external environment and invariant or constant (C) regions, which include a segment linking the receptor into the cell membrane. The general organization of the T-cell receptor is similar to that of immunoglobulin and is composed of a heterodimer with α and β subunits, which each consist of a variable (V) and a constant (C) region. The two chains are linked by a disulfide bond and together are carried in the cell surface membrane.

(Bollum, 1979), and it should be emphasized that TdT is not a specific marker of T cells since it also appears in precursor B cells.

By analogy to B cells, human T cells also express receptors for antigen quite similar to those of immunoglobulin (Meuer et al., 1983). Unlike immunoglobulin, these T-cell antigen receptors are not secreted but remain bound to the cell surface membrane. The T-cell antigen receptor is a heterodimer composed of one α and one β chain (Figure 3), each of which contains variable and constant region domains (Meuer et al., 1983; Hannum et al., 1984; Sim et al., 1984; Siu et al., 1984; Yanagi et al., 1984, 1985). The variable region is exposed to the external environment, much like that of the immunoglobulin on the surface of B cells. The protein has a transmembrane component and an intracytoplasmic domain, and presumably functions as a receptor in mature T cells (Hannum et al., 1984; Sim et al., 1984; Siu et al., 1984; Yanagi et al., 1984, 1985). To produce a T-cell receptor, the T-cell precursor must successfully rearrange its T-cell receptor α and β genes by joining together their variable region coding information as occurs in the immunoglobulin genes of precursor B cells (Figure 4) (Hannum et al., 1984; Sim et al., 1984; Siu et al., 1984; Yanagi et al., 1984, 1985). An ordered hierarchy of gene expression occurs for the T-cell receptor chains in which the β gene is

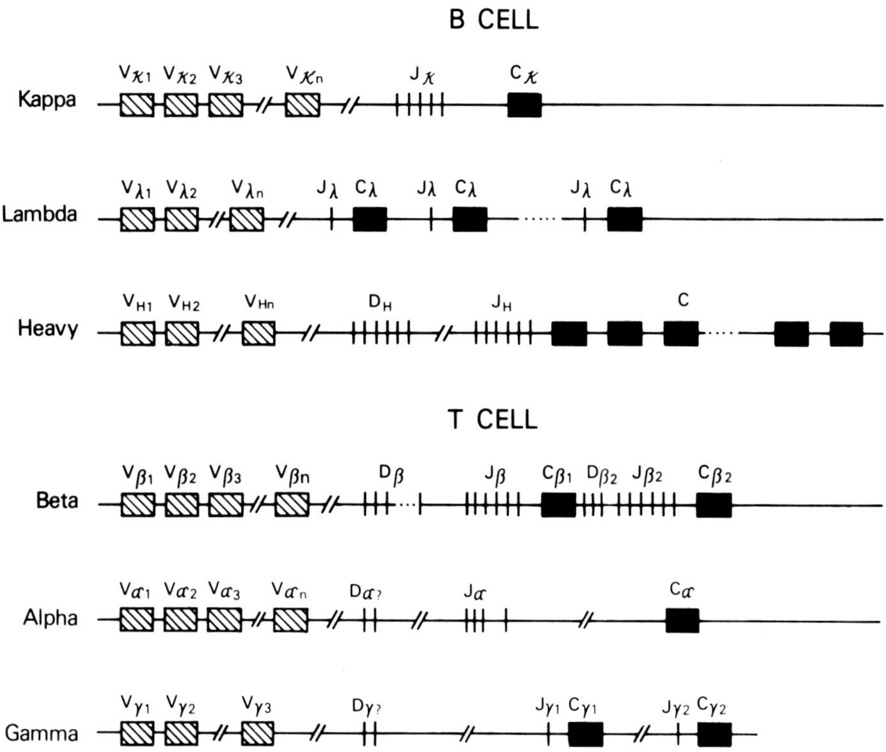

Figure 4 Immunoglobulin and T-cell receptor genes κ, λ, and heavy and the T-cell receptor genes β, a, and γ show a similar overall genetic organization which features multiple variable (V) regions linked to constant domains. Rearrangements of variable region genes allow the joining of the V gene to joining (J) genes and, where present, diversity (D) genes are included to form a continuous V/D/J segment. It is not yet evident whether D genes exist for the a and γ families.

transcribed prior to a in developing thymocytes (Figure 2) (Collins et al., 1985; Raulet et al., 1985; Royer et al., 1985). However, it is not yet known for certain what the order of rearrangement is for these two genes since it is quite difficult to detect rearrangement of the a gene due to an exceedingly large J region composed of approximately 35 separate Ja genes spanning a region of approximately 50,000 bases (Hayday et al., 1985a; Yoshikai et al., 1985).

A third rearranging gene of T cells, the γ gene, has a genetic organization similar to that of the T-cell receptor genes and immunoglobulin genes (Saito et al., 1984; Hayday et al., 1985b). It, too, rearranges during early T-cell development but appears to be transcribed for only a very brief period of time during fetal thymic ontogeny (Raulet et al., 1985; Snodgrass et al., 1985). The function of this enigmatic gene product is not known, although it is expressed in cytotoxic T cells and may be involved either in recognition of major histocompatibility complex (MHC) antigens or in the function of cell killing (Kranz et al., 1985).

Antibodies to detect T-cell receptors include WT31 (Spits et al., 1985), and one can determine whether the T-cell receptor is expressed by the use of antibodies detecting the T3 (CD3) molecular complex. T3 is a protein complex consisting of at least three chains, δ, γ, and ϵ, which are noncovalently linked to the T-cell receptor (Borst et al., 1983, 1985; van den Elsen et al., 1984), presumably via a bond between the T-cell receptor and one chain of the T3 complex. T3 is thought to stabilize the T-cell receptor in the cell membrane and provide a pathway for calcium flux during antigen receptor-mediated cell activation (Weiss and Stobo, 1984; Brenner et al., 1985).

From studies of mutants of the Jurkat T-cell ALL cell line, it has been shown that the T3 molecular complex and T-cell receptor are obligatorily coexpressed (Imboden and Stobo, 1985; Ohashi et al., 1985). That is, cell surface T3 cannot be expressed unless a complete T-cell receptor heterodimer is present, since lack of the β subunit is sufficient to prevent expression of both T-cell receptors and T3 on the cell surface (Ohashi et al., 1985). Reconstitution of a translatable β gene transcript in these mutants allows the cell to produce a cell surface T-cell receptor/T3 complex (Ohashi et al., 1985). The T-cell receptor and T3 are therefore expressed simultaneously during the more mature stages of medullary thymocyte differentiation and persist throughout the life span of the T cell as it circulates in the peripheral blood and enters lymph nodes (Figure 3).

III. PRE-B-CELL NEOPLASMS

Since the discovery of Korsmeyer and colleagues (1983), it has become evident that the majority of ALL cases are clonal expansions of precursor B cells. Prior to the molecular genetic studies performed by these investigators, most cases of ALL were considered non-T, non-B or common ALL, which did not express markers of either B or T lineage but did express the so-called CALLA marker (Greaves et al., 1977). By analyzing immunoglobulin gene rearrangements, Korsmeyer reported that all cases of common ALL contained one or more immunoglobulin gene rearrangements (Korsmeyer et al., 1981, 1983). T-cell ALLs, except in isolated instances (Ha et al., 1984; Kitchingman et al., 1985), lacked immunoglobulin gene rearrangements and, therefore, immunoglobulin gene rearrangement appeared to be a relatively specific marker of lineage among cases of ALL (Korsmeyer et al., 1983). Furthermore, gene rearrangement studies identified the cases of common ALL as precursor B-cell type since they contained rearranged immunoglobulin genes, but the immunoglobulin genes were either not expressed, i.e., no immunoglobulin was present, or only μ heavy chain of immunoglobulin was detectable (Vogler et al., 1978; Korsmeyer et al., 1983). A hierarchy of gene rearrangements in which heavy chain gene rearrangements preceded those of κ which, in turn, preceded λ light chain gene rearrangements was seen in the human precursor B-cell neoplasms (Korsmeyer et al., 1981).

Two other lines of evidence complemented these findings and helped establish the precursor B-cell lineage of common ALL. First, it was shown that, although the neoplastic cells of common ALL in most cases do not contain detectable immunoglobulin, these cells can be induced by exposure to phorbol ester, tetradecanoyl-phorbol-acetate (TPA), to rapidly synthesize both cytoplasmic and surface immunoglobulin heavy and light chains (Cossman et al., 1982; Nadler et al., 1982). Thus, although the leukemia cells were frozen at a precursor B-cell stage of differentiation, they could be induced to differentiate to more mature stages and express their rearranged immunoglobulin genes. These experiments further documented that the immunoglobulin genes of precursor B-cell neoplasms were not aberrantly rearranged in a nonproductive manner but were rearranged in a configuration encoding translatable mRNAs. Therefore, the lack of immunoglobulin production by common ALL cells must be caused by a mechanism other than aberrant immunoglobulin gene rearrangements.

A second line of evidence indicating the B-cell nature of so-called "non-T, non-B" common ALL cases was the advent of antibodies which detected very early stages of B-cell differentiation. Foremost among these is antibody B4 (CD19), which detects a 95 kilodalton protein as reported by Nadler et al. (1983). This antigen is found on most mature B cells in the peripheral blood, spleen, lymph node, and tonsils, and also on early B cells in the bone marrow. It is not seen on T cells regardless of the stage of differentiation (Nadler et al., 1983). Importantly, it is found on greater than 90% of cases of non-T ALL and correlates precisely with the detection of immunoglobulin gene rearrangements in these precursor B-cell neoplasms (Nadler et al., 1983, 1984). Thus, B4 antibody identifies precursor B-cell neoplasms regardless of their ability to produce immunoglobulin and provides further evidence for the B-cell nature of common ALL. The earliest identifiable normal and neoplastic B-cell precursors express B4 and Ia antigens and have undergone immunoglobulin gene rearrangements (Nadler et al., 1984).

Upon its initial discovery, CALLA (CD10) was thought to represent a relatively specific marker for common ALL and, thus, antibodies against CALLA were considered to be potentially useful for specific diagnosis and serotherapy (Greaves et al., 1975; Ritz et al., 1980). However, following the early reports it was discovered that CALLA is expressed on a wide range of cells outside of common ALL. CALLA was detected on epithelial cells, including normal renal tubular and glomerular epithelium, fetal small intestine, and breast myoepithelium (Metzgar et al., 1981). We, and others, identified CALLA on the cell surface of normal human neutrophils (Figure 5) (Braun et al., 1983; Cossman et al., 1983b). Among

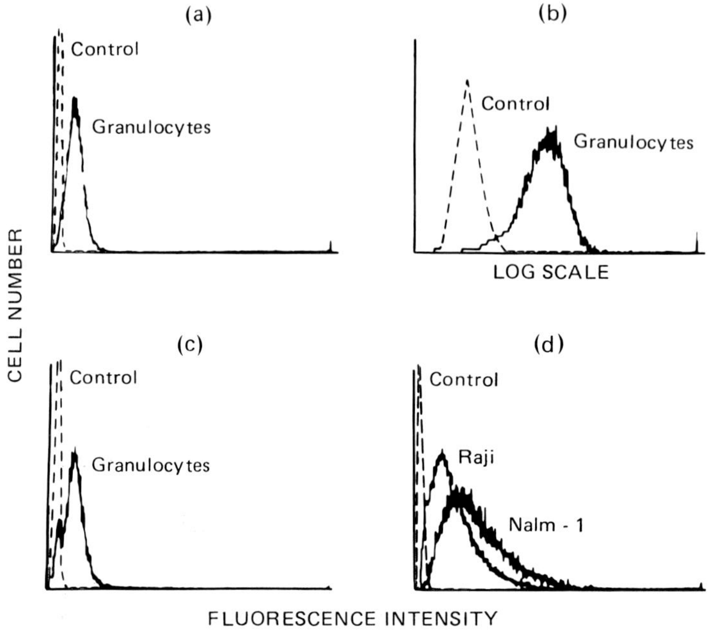

Figure 5 CALLA is expressed by normal human granulocytes. Flow cytometric analysis of cells stained by the anti-CALLA monoclonal antibody J5 shows faint but clearly positive reactivity with granulocytes from normal individuals (a), (b), and (c). The control consists of a nonimmune murine IgG2a, and in (c) granulocytes were preincubated with a human IgG1 myeloma protein to saturate Fc receptors. Persistent positive reactivity of granulocytes with J5 antibody in this experiment indicates the specificity of the antibody for granulocytes. As seen in (d), pre B-cell ALL cells (NALM-1) and Burkitt's lymphoma (Raji) both express CALLA.

hematopoietic neoplasms, CALLA occurs in Burkitt's lymphoma (Figure 5), follicular lymphoma, and in 25% of cases of T-cell ALL (Ritz et al., 1981). Whether CALLA is present on any mature B cells, either in the circulation or in the follicles of lymphoid tissue, has not yet been determined with certainty.

CALLA is found in greater than 70% of cases of common ALL and seems to be a differentiation-associated cell surface marker which appears somewhat after the presentation of Ia and B4 (Nadler et al., 1984; Hokland et al., 1983). Despite its broad range of reactivity, CALLA is still a useful marker as an aid in the diagnosis of ALL, follicular lymphoma, and Burkitt's lymphoma, since it is not generally expressed by circulating or tissue-fixed normal B cells.

Approximately 20% of cases of common ALL contain intracytoplasmic immunoglobulin, usually in the form of μ heavy chains. The amount of immunoglobulin present is often quite sparse and requires sensitive indirect immunodetection techniques, such as those employing avidin and biotin. When immunoglobulin is present, cells are referred to as pre-B cells (Vogler et al., 1978). Virtually all cases of precursor B-cell neoplasms contain the enzyme TdT (Bollum, 1979).

Although the vast majority of precursor B-cell neoplasms present as acute leukemias, in some instances neoplasms with identical phenotypes present as lymphomas (Cossman et al., 1983a). These lymphomas are morphologically indistinguishable from the more typical T-cell type of lymphoblastic lymphoma and may even have covoluted nuclear membranes (Cossman et al., 1983a) (Figure 6),

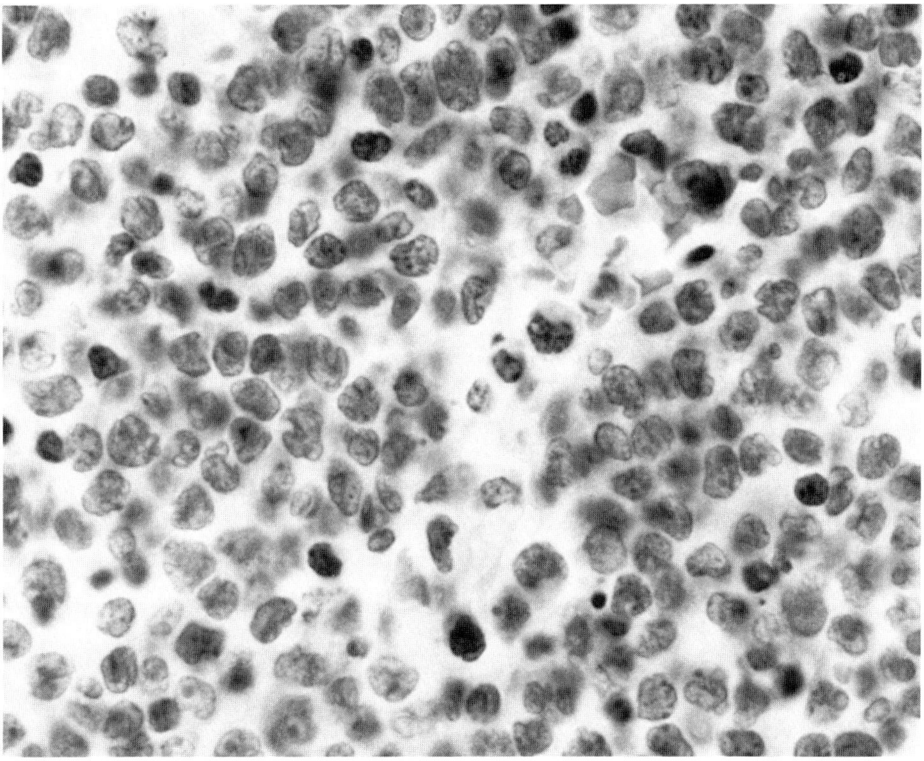

Figure 6 Convoluted lymphoblastic lymphoma with a pre B-cell phenotype. Morphologically, this lymphoblastic lymphoma has the typical fine chromatin and nuclear convolutions characteristic of lymphoblastic lymphoma. These features were previously considered to be pathognomonic of T-cell derivation, but this cell expressed B-cell antigens, contained intracytoplasmic immunoglobulin, and had no T-cell markers. Thus, the morphological findings are not specific for a given immunological type.

a feature once thought to be a hallmark of T-cell lymphoblastic neoplasms (Barcos and Lukes, 1975). Clinically, precursor B-cell lymphomas appear to have a relatively favorable prognosis and have responded to therapeutic intervention.

IV. PRE-T-CELL NEOPLASMS

Approximately 20% of ALL (Greaves et al., 1977) and 80% of lymphoblastic lymphomas (Cossman et al., 1983a) have a T-cell phenotype. Although phenotypes are heterogeneous, the corresponding differentiation stages are limited to the immature phase of T-cell differentiation associated with intrathymic T-cell development. In this regard, the T-cell lymphoblastic neoplasms can be considered precursor T-cells as evidenced by their thymocyte-like phenotype characterized by expression of TdT (Bollum, 1979; Braziel et al., 1983) (Figure 7), frequent expression of the thymocyte marker T6 (CD1), and coexpression of T4 (CD4) and T8 (CD8) (Greaves et al., 1977; Reinherz et al., 1980; Bernard et al., 1981; Cossman et al., 1983a). Unlike mature T cells, approximately 25% of cases of T-cell lymphoblastic neoplasms express CALLA (Greaves et al., 1983) and, thus, CALLA can be a useful marker in the diagnosis of T lymphoblastic neoplasms.

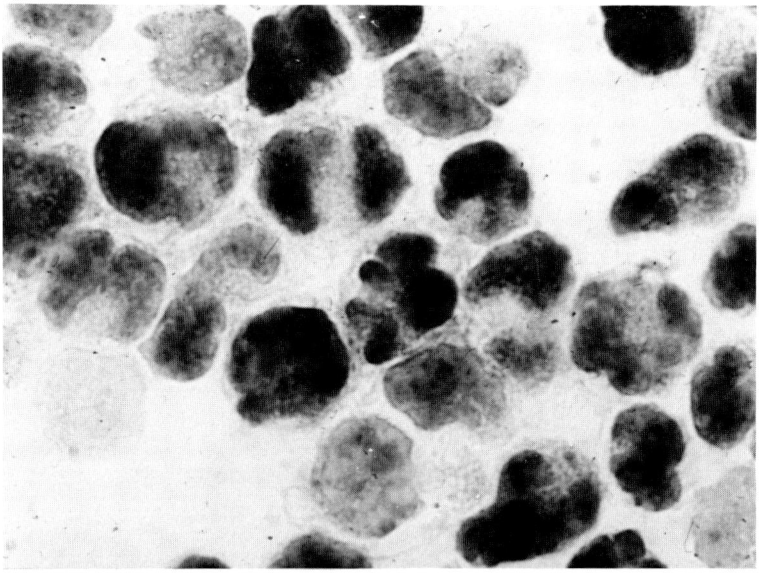

Figure 7 TdT in T-cell ALL. A cytocentrifuge preparation of the human T-cell ALL cell line, MOLT-4, was stained with a rabbit anti-serum to TdT (Bethesda Research Laboratories, Gaithersburg, MD) and developed by an avidin-biotin peroxidase complex. Intense staining is present in the nuclei. (X1,000)

The distinction between lymphoblastic lymphoma and lymphoblastic leukemia is somewhat arbitrary; criteria used to distinguish them have varied. In general, cases presenting predominantly as leukemia have an overall less mature phenotype in that they appear to express more abundant TdT and simultaneously co-express T4 and T8, as compared to the T-cell lymphoblastic lymphomas, which show fainter TdT and have often already committed to selective expression of either the T4 or T8 type (Greaves et al., 1977; Reinherz et al., 1980; Bernard et al., 1981; Cossman et al., 1983). All lymphoblastic neoplasms, regardless of their presentation as leukemia or lymphoma, T-cell or B-cell nature, express TdT and thus this is the single unifying marker for distinction between lymphoblastic (immature) and lymphocytic (mature) neoplasms (Bollum, 1979; Braziel et al., 1983).

Phenotypic heterogeneity among the T-cell lymphoblastic neoplasms can be accounted for in large measure by differences in the arrested stage of differentiation. As seen in Figure 2, intrathymic T-cell differentiation encompasses a broad range of phenotypes, and the corresponding T-cell neoplasms reflect this phenotypic diversity. The cellular markers which appear earliest in T-cell differentiation are those which also are expressed in the majority of T-cell neoplasms, 3A1 (CD7), T1 (CD5), and T11 (CD2) (Greaves et al., 1977; Reinherz et al., 1980; Bernard et al., 1981; Cossman et al., 1983a; Chan et al., 1985; Pittaluga et al., 1986). It is now evident from work performed independently by several laboratories that the CD7 determinant detected by antibodies 3A1 (Haynes et al., 1980) or Leu9 (Link et al., 1983) is expressed by all T lymphoblastic neoplasms, whereas the T1 (CD5) and T11 (CD2) markers are present on the majority of, but not all, cases of T-cell lymphoblastic leukemias and lymphomas (Greaves et al., 1977; Reinherz et al., 1980; Bernard et al., 1981; Cossman et al., 1983a; Link et al., 1983; Lopez et al., 1985; Pittaluga et al., 1986). Thus, for purposes of diagnosis and classification of a lymphoblastic neoplasm as T cell, CD7 (3A1 or Leu9) is the single most useful marker. Moreover, CD7 is *not* expressed by any precursor B-cell neoplasms (Korsmeyer et al., 1983) and therefore provides a highly specific lineage marker for lymphoblastic neoplasia. Markers T1 and T11 are expressed on the majority (60-75%) of cases of T lymphoblastic neoplasms and are not seen in precursor B-cell neoplasms (Greaves et al., 1977; Reinherz et al., 1980; Bernard et al., 1981; Cossman et al., 1983a; Lopez et al., 1985; Pittaluga et al., 1986). In contrast to the T1 and T11 markers, the CD7 determinant is not present on all mature normal T cells, since approximately 15% of peripheral blood T cells lack this marker (Haynes et al., 1980).

Although the function of the CD7 determinant is not known, it is interesting that it is expressed by all cases of T lymphoblastic neoplasms, including those which have not yet undergone rearrangement of their T-cell receptor β chain genes (Pittaluga et al., 1986). Virtually all cases of T lymphoblastic neoplasms contain one or more rearranged T-cell receptor genes, including both the β and γ genes (Bertness et al., 1985; Flug et al., 1985; Rabbitts et al., 1985; Waldmann et al., 1985; Pittaluga et al., 1986). Rearrangements of α chain genes are difficult to detect due to the unusually large size of the J_α region (Siu et al., 1984; Yanagi et al., 1985), as mentioned previously. Despite frequent rearrangement of the T-cell receptor genes in lymphoblastic neoplasms, rare cases retain these genes in their germline configuration (Pittaluga et al., 1986), presumably due to arrest at very early stages of pre-T-cell development. Despite this, these cases still express the CD7 surface marker and, in two cases studied in our laboratory, these cells did not express in one instance the T1 (CD5) and in the other case the T11 (CD2) surface markers (Pittaluga et al., 1986). Thus, 3A1 is a very early surface molecule appearing during pre-T development (Lobach et al., 1985), and one might speculate that it could be involved in the regulatory pathway leading to the rearrangement and expression of T-cell receptor genes.

Rearrangement of T-cell receptor genes in lymphoblastic neoplasms is a useful marker of clonality since rearrangement is evidence of clonal proliferation (Bertness et al., 1985; Flug et al., 1985; Rabbitts et al., 1985; Waldmann et al., 1985). A single restriction fragment size indicates a uniform variable gene rearrangement which must be due to clonal expansion of a single precursor cell. Since no phenotypic marker of clonality is readily available for T-cell neoplasms, T-cell receptor gene rearrangements serve as an important diagnostic indicator of clonality (Figure 8). T-cell receptor gene rearrangements are also supportive evidence of T-cell lineage, since T-cell receptor rearrangements are found in nearly all T cell neoplasms but only infrequently in B-cell neoplasms (Bertness et al., 1985; Flug et al., 1985; Rabbitts et al., 1985; Waldmann et al., 1985) and very rarely in acute myeloblastic leukemia (Cheng et al., 1986). However, crossovers of T-cell receptor gene rearrangements in B-cell neoplasms and immunoglobulin gene rearrangements in T-cell neoplasms do occasionally occur (Pelicci et al., 1985; Tawa et al., 1985), presumably due to utilization of the same recombination signals and enzymatic mechanism; therefore, one must exercise caution when assessing lineage by gene rearrangement analysis alone. In this context, phenotypic markers must be evaluated to assure a correct diagnosis of cellular lineage in lymphoblastic neoplasms.

A major feature of intrathymic T-cell differentiation is the development of the antigen receptor complex in preparation for specific antigen recognition by the mature T cell. By using human precursor T-cell neoplasms as models of stages of intrathymic T-cell differentiation, we have found a program of events which, in sequence, lead to the expression of the T-cell receptor/T3 complex (Pittaluga et al., 1986). Since each step in development represents a sequential point in a cascade, the stages of development of the antigen receptor complex can be considered markers of differentiation among precursor T-cell neoplasms. The earliest recognizable step is immunoreactivity with antibody 3A1 (CD7), followed shortly thereafter by expression of the T1 and T11 markers. At approximately this time,

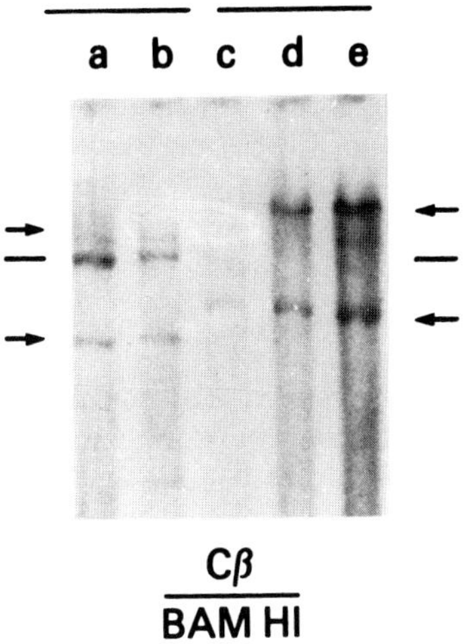

Figure 8 Southern blot analysis of two cases of lymphoblastic lymphoma. Sequential biopsies of two patients (patient 1, A and B; patient 2, C-E) were analyzed for rearrangements of the β subunit of the T-cell receptor. DNA was extracted, digested with the restriction enzyme BamHI and size separated in an agarose gel. Southern filters were hybridized with a constant region segment of β subunit DNA (C_β). Autoradiographs revealed two β gene rearrangements in both lymphomas (arrows). Germline or unrearranged DNA is present (dashed lines), presumably as a result of contaminating normal cells in these lymph nodes. In this example, the identical clone of lymphoma as the original tumor has recurred in both patients, since the relapse specimens (B in patient 1 and D, E in patient 2) are identical to their respective pretreatment gene rearrangement patterns (A in patient 1 and C in patient 2). Thus, gene rearrangement analysis not only diagnoses the clonality of disease but is useful in documenting recurrence of the same neoplastic clone.

the genes for the β subunit of the T-cell receptor and the Tγ gene undergo rearrangement. Concordantly, mRNA encoding the T3 δ chain is transcribed and subsequently message for the β chain appears. Coincident with the appearance of β chain mRNA is the expression of surface membrane T6 (CD1) and intracellular T3 (CD3) molecules (Figure 9). As later events, mRNA of the Tα gene is transcribed and surface T3 protein appears only at the latest stages. It is evident from analyses of T lymphoblastic neoplasms that stages of precursor T-cell development are compartmentalized into a highly regulated and orchestrated pathway of gene expression. By understanding the sequence of events surrounding the acquisition of specific antigen recognition by T cells, we can begin to see how the cell surface markers of early T cells relate to this critical developmental process.

Cell surface markers detected by antibodies 3A1, T1, and T11 may represent cell surface molecules integrally related to the differentiation process. Understanding the coordination of expression between cell surface markers and functional developments not only provides a means for subclassifying T-cell neoplasms but also serves as the framework for dissecting the developmental regulation of T-cell function.

V. DIFFERENTIAL DIAGNOSIS AND CLINICAL IMPLICATIONS

By a combined use of phenotypic analysis with monoclonal antibodies and molecular genetics with probes for the rearranging genes of lymphocytes, one can accurately and reproducibly distinguish lymphoblastic neoplasms from mature lymphocytic neoplasms or from nonlymphoid leukemias and lymphomas (Table 1). For example, as shown in Table 1, the presence of TdT is a useful diagnostic marker to distinguish the lymphoblastic neoplasms from mature lymphoid neoplasms (Braziel et al., 1983). The lymphoid nature of lymphoblastic neoplasms is evidenced by their reactivity with either anti-B-cell antibodies, such as B4 or B1, or anti-T-cell antibodies, such as 3A1 (Leu9), T1, T11, T3, T4, T8, and T6. Although acute leukemias with mixed phenotypes or some myeloid leukemias might express some of these markers in rare instances (Chan et al., 1985; Mirro et al., 1985), careful use of the entire battery of monoclonal antibodies described here should resolve the lymphoid derivation in the vast majority of cases.

The distinction between T-cell or B-cell origin of lymphoblastic neoplasms is very clearly made by the use of two antibodies, 3A1 (Leu9) and B4. As mentioned previously, 3A1 detects all cases of T-cell lymphoblastic neoplasms but does not usually react with precursor B-cell neoplasms, including common ALL. Conversely, B4 antibody reacts with nearly all cases of precursor B-cell neoplasms whether or not their immunoglobulin genes are rearranged, but B4 antibody does not react with precursor T-cell neoplasms. Thus, these two antibodies can readily distinguish the cell of origin in acute lymphoblastic leukemia and lymphoma.

As lineage markers, rearrangements of immunoglobulin genes and T-cell receptor genes are somewhat less specific because β chain genes occasionally may be rearranged in precursor B-cell neoplasms (Pelicci et al., 1985; Tawa et al., 1985); immunoglobulin heavy chain genes may be rearranged in some precursor T-cell neoplasms (Korsmeyer et al., 1983; Ha et al., 1984; Kitchingman et al., 1985); and rare cases of acute myeloblastic leukemia are reported to have rearranged their T-cell receptor β chain or immunoglobulin heavy chain genes (Cheng et al., 1986; Palumbo et al., 1984). However, immunoglobulin light chain genes are generally not rearranged in any cell other than B cells and, thus, rearrangement of both the heavy and light chain genes is indicative of a B-cell lineage (Korsmeyer et al., 1983; Cossman et al., 1986). Expression of the immunoglobu-

Table 1 Cellular Markers in the Differential Diagnosis of Lymphoblastic Neoplasms (Percent of Cases Positive)

	Phenotype								Genotype	
Neoplasm	TdT	CD7 (3A1, Leu9)	CD20 (B1) CD19 (B4)	CD4/CD8 (T4/T8)	CD1 (T6)	CD10 (CALLA)	CD5/CD3/CD2 (T1/T3/T11)	Ig	TCR gene	Ig gene
Mature (peripheral) T	0	50-90%	0	50-90%/0	0	0	50-90%	0	>90%	<15%
Lymphoblastic (pre-) T	>90%	>90%	0	50-90%/50-90%	50-90%	(25%)	50-90%	0	50-90%	<15%
Lymphoblastic (pre-) B	>90%	0	>90%	0/0	0	>90%	0	cIg (20%)	<15%	>90%

Key: TCR gene = T-cell antigen receptor gene rearrangements; Ig gene = immunoglobulin gene rearrangements; cIg = cytoplasmic immunoglobulin.

lin gene appears to be generally restricted to cells of B-cell lineage since immunoglobulin is usually not found in precursor T-cell neoplasms (Greaves et al., 1977; Reinherz et al., 1980; Bernard et al., 1981; Cossman et al., 1983a; Chan et al., 1985). In this context, the T-cell receptor/T3 complex does not appear to be expressed in precursor B-cell neoplasms since the T3 molecule is not identified in precursor B-cell leukemias and lymphomas.

By employing a select battery of monoclonal antibodies in combination with appropriate gene rearrangement analyses, the clonality and lineage of lymphoblastic neoplasms can be identified in nearly every case. These markers serve not only to help diagnose and classify neoplasms at presentation but are useful adjuncts in the diagnosis of recurrence since rare cells can be identified using appropriate marker profiles and flow cytometry or by genetic analysis of patient samples (Table 1). Cell lineage analysis also carries prognostic information since T-cell

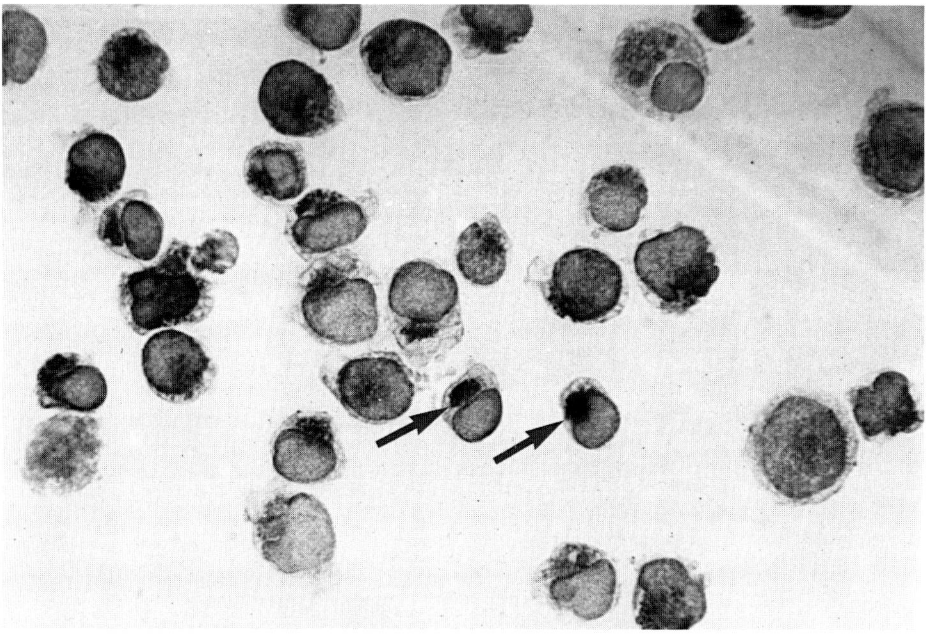

Figure 9 Intracellular T3. Immunostaining of cytocentrifuge preparations of pre T-cell neoplasms with anti-T3 antibodies (such as Leu4 shown here) indicates intracellular T3 molecules. Intracellular T3 appears prior to the expression of surface T3 in pre-T neoplasms and is further evidence of the T-cell lineage of the lymphoblastic neoplasm. The reaction product is often perinuclear (examples are indicated by arrows) and some staining of nuclear membrane appears as well.

forms of lymphoblastic neoplasms often pursue a more aggressive course than their non-T counterparts (Greaves et al., 1977; von Fliedner, 1985). Clearly, few areas of clinical medicine have been more profoundly impacted by the new tools of monoclonal antibodies and recombinant DNA than the laboratory diagnosis of human lymphoblastic neoplasia.

REFERENCES

Alt, F., and Baltimore, D. (1982). Joining of immunoglobulin heavy chain gene segments: Implications from a chromosome with evidence of three D-J_H fusions. *Proc. Nat. Acad. Sci. USA* 79: 4118-4122.

Anderson, K. C., Park, E. K., Bates, M. P., Leonard, R. C. F., Hardy, R., Schlossman, S. F., and Nadler, L. M. (1983). Antigens on human plasma cells identified by monoclonal antibodies. *J. Immunol.* 130: 1132-1138.

Barcos, M. P., and Lukes, R. J. (1975). Malignant lymphoma of convoluted lymphotyces: A new entity of possible T cell type. In *Conflicts in Childhood Cancer: An Evaluation of Current Management Proceedings*, L. F. Sinks and J. O. Godden (eds.). Alan R. Liss, Inc., New York, pp. 147-178.

Bernard, A., Boumsell, L., Reinherz, E. L., Nadler, L. M., Ritz, J., Coppin, H., Richard, Y., Valensi, F., Dausset, J., Flandrin, G., Lamerle, J., and Schlossman, S. F. (1981). Cell surface characterization of malignant T-cells from lymphoblastic lymphoma using monoclonal antibodies. *Blood* 57: 1105-1110.

Bernard, A., Boumsell, L., Dausset, J., Milstein, C., and Schlossman, S. F. (1984). *Leucocyte Typing*, Springer-Verlag, Berlin, Heidelberg, New York, Tokyo.

Bertness, V., Kirsch, I., Hollis, G., Johnson, B., and Bunn, P. A. (1985). T-cell receptor gene rearrangements as clinical markers of human T-cell lymphomas. *N. Engl. J. Med.* 313: 534-538.

Bollum, F. J. (1979). Terminal deoxynucleotidyl transferase as a hematopoietic cell marker. *Blood* 54: 1203-1215.

Borst, J., Alexander, S., Elder, J., and Terhorst, C. (1983). The T3 complex on human T lymphocytes involves four structurally distinct glycoproteins. *J. Biol. Chem.* 258: 5135-5141.

Borst, J., Coligan, J. E., Oettgen, H., Pessano, S., Malin, R., and Terhorst, C. (1985). The delta- and epsilon-chains of the human T3/T-cell receptor complex are distinct polypeptides. *Nature* 312: 455-458.

Braun, M., Martin, P., Ledbetter, J., and Hansen, J. (1983). Granulocytes and cultures of human fibroblasts express common acute lymphoblastic leukemia-associated antigens. *Blood* 61: 718-725.

Braziel, R. M., Keneklis, T., Donlan, J. A., Hsu, S. M., Cossman, J., Bollum, F. J., and Jaffe, E. S. (1983). Terminal deoxynucleotidyl transferase in non-Hodgkin's lymphomas. *Am. J. Clin. Pathol.* 80: 655-659.

Brenner, M. B., Trowbridge, I. S., and Strominger, J. L. (1985). Cross-linking of human T cell receptor proteins: Association between the T cell idiotype beta subunit and the T3 glycoprotein heavy subunit. *Cell* 40: 183-190.

Chan, L. C., Pegran, S. M., and Greaves, M. F. (1985). Contribution of immunophenotype to the classification and differential diagnosis of acute leukemia. *Lancet* 1: 475-479.

Cheng, G. Y., Minden, M. D., Toyonaga, B., Mak, T. W., and McCulloch, E. A. (1986). T cell receptor and immunoglobulin gene rearrangements in acute myeloblastic leukemia. *J. Exp. Med.* 163: 414-424.

Collins, M. K. L., Tanigawa, G., Kissonerghis, A.-M., Ritter, M., Price, K. M., Tonegawa, S., and Owen, M. J. (1985). Regulation of T-cell receptor gene expression in human T-cell development. *Proc. Nat. Acad. Sci. USA* 82: 4503-4507.

Cossman, J., Neckers, L. M., Arnold, A., and Korsmeyer, S. J. (1982). Induction of differentiation in a case of common acute lymphoblastic leukemia. *N. Engl. J. Med.* 307: 1251-1254.

Cossman, J., Chused, T. M., Fisher, R. I., Magrath, I., Bollum, F., and Jaffe, E. S. (1983a). Diversity of immunological phenotypes of lymphoblastic lymphoma. *Cancer Res.* 43: 4486-4490.

Cossman, J., Neckers, L. M., Leonard, W. J., and Greene, W. C. (1983b). Polymorphonuclear neutrophils express the common acute lymphoblastic leukemia antigen. *J. Exp. Med.* 157: 1064-1069.

Cossman, J., Bakhshi, A., and Korsmeyer, S. (1986). Gene rearrangements applied to diagnostic immunopathology. In *Manual of Clinical Laboratory Immunology*, N. R. Rose, H. Friedman, and J. L. Fahey (eds.). American Society for Microbiology, Washington, D.C., pp. 168-173.

Flug, F., Pelicci, P. G., Bonetti, F., Knowles, D. M., II, and Dalla-Favera, R. (1985). T-cell receptor gene rearrangements as markers of lineage and clonality in T-cell neoplasms. *Proc. Nat. Acad. Sci. USA* 82:3460-3464.

Gathings, W. E., Lawton, A. R., and Cooper, M. D. (1977). Immunofluorescent studies of the development of pre-B cells, B lymphocytes and immunoglobulin isotype diversity in humans. *Eur. J. Immunol.* 7: 804-810.

Greaves, M. F., Brown, G., Rapson, N. T., and Lasiter, T. A. (1975). Antisera to acute lymphoblastic leukemia cells. *Clin. Immunol. Immunopathol.* 4: 67-84.

Greaves, M. F., Janossy, G., Roberts, M., Rapson, N. T., Ellis, R. B., Chessels, J., Lister, T. A., and Catovsky, D. (1977). Membrane phenotyping: Diagnosis, monitoring and classification of acute "lymphoid" leukemias. In *Immunological Diagnosis of Leukemias and Lymphomas*, International Symposium of the Institute fur Hamatologie, S. Thierfelder, H. Rodt, and E. Thiel (eds.). Springer-Verlag, Berlin, pp. 61-75.

Greaves, M. F., Hariri, G., Newman, R. A., Sutherland, D. R., Ritter, M. A., and Ritz, J. (1983). Selective expression of the common acute lymphoblast leukemia (gp100) antigens on immature lymphoid cells and their malignant counterparts. *Blood* 61: 628-639.

Ha, K., Minden, M., Hozumi, N., and Gelfand, E. (1984). Immunoglobulin μ-chain gene rearrangement in a patient with T cell acute lymphoblastic leukemia. *J. Clin. Invest.* 74: 1232-1236.

Hannum, C. H., Kappler, J. W., Trowbridge, I. S., Marrack, P., and Freed, J. H. (1984). Immunoglobulin-like nature of the α-chain of a human T-cell antigen/MHC receptor. *Nature* 312: 65-67.

Hayday, A. C., Diamond, D. J., Tanigawa, G., Helig, J. S., Folsom, V., Saito, H., and Tonegawa, S. (1985a). Unusual organization and diversity of T-cell receptor α-chain genes. *Nature* 316: 828-832.

Hayday, A. C., Saito, H., Gillies, S. D., Kranz, D. M., Tanigawa, G., Eisen, H. N., and Tonegawa, S. (1985b). Structure, organization, and somatic rearrangements of T cell gamma genes. *Cell* 40: 259-269.

Haynes, B. F., Mann, D. L., Hemler, M. E., Schroer, J. A., Shelhamer, J. H., Eisenbarth, G. S., Strominger, J. L., Thomas, C. A., Mostowski, H. S., and Fauci, A. S. (1980). Characterization of a monoclonal antibody that defines an immunoregulatory T cell subset for immunoglobulin synthesis in humans. *Proc. Nat. Acad. Sci. USA* 77: 2914-2918.

Hieter, P. A., Korsmeyer, S. J., Waldmann, T. A., and Leder, P. (1981). Human immunoglobulin κ light-chain genes are deleted or rearranged in λ-producing B cells. *Nature* 290: 369-372.

Hokland, P., Rosenthal, P., Griffin, J. D., Nadler, L. M., Daley, J., Hokland, M., Schlossman, S. F., and Ritz, J. (1983). Purification and characterization of fetal hematopoietic cells that express the common acute lymphoblastic leukemia antigen (CALLA). *J. Exp. Med.* 157: 114-129.

Imboden, J. B., and Stobo, J. D. (1985). Transmembrane signalling by the T cell antigen receptor: Perturbation of the T3-antigen receptor complex generates inositol phosphates and releases calcium ions from intracellular stores. *J. Exp. Med.* 161: 446-456.

Kitchingman, G. R., Rovigatti, U., Mauer, A. M., Melvin, S., Murphy, S. B., and Stass, S. (1985). Rearrangement of immunoglobulin heavy chain genes in T cell acute lymphoblastic leukemia. *Blood* 65: 725-729.

Korsmeyer, S. J., Hieter, P. A., Ravetch, J. V., Poplack, D. G., Waldmann, T. A., and Leder, P. (1981). Developmental hierarchy of immunoglobulin gene rearrangements in human leukemic pre-B cells. *Proc. Nat. Acad. Sci. USA* 78: 7096-7100.

Korsmeyer, S. J., Arnold, A., Bakhshi, A., Ravetch, J. V., Siebenlist, V., Hieter, P. A., Sharrow, S. O., LeBien, T. W., Kersey, J. H., Poplack, D. G., Leder, P., and Waldmann, T. A. (1983). Immunoglobulin gene rearrangement and cell surface antigen expression in acute lymphocytic leukemias of T cell and B cell precursor origins. *J. Clin. Invest.* 71: 301-313.

Kranz, D. M., Saito, H., Heller, M., Takagaki, Y., Haas, W., Heisen, H. N., and Tonegawa, S. (1985). Limited diversity of the rearranged T-cell gamma gene. *Nature* 313: 752-755.

Link, M., Warnke, R., Finlay, J., Amylon, M., Miller, R., Dilley, J., and Levy, R. (1983). A single monoclonal antibody identifies T-cell lineage of childhood lymphoid malignancies. *Blood* 62: 722-728.

Lipford, E. H., and Cossman, J. (1986). Biological diagnosis of B-cell neoplasia. *Cancer Invest.* 4: 69-80.

Lobach, D. F., Hensley, L. L., Ho, W., and Haynes, B. F. (1985). Human T cell antigen expression during the early stages of fetal thymic maturation. *J. Immunol.* 135: 1752-1759.

Lopez, M., DeRossi, G., Ronosno, G., Napolitano, M., Pasqualetti, D., Gugliemi, C., Annino, L., and Pandolfi, F. (1985). Relevance of 3A1 monoclonal antibody in the diagnosis of T-cell acute lymphoblastic leukemia. *Diagn. Immunol.* 3: 11-14.

Metzgar, R. S., Borowitz, M. J., Jones, N. H., and Dowell, B. L. (1981). Distribution of common acute lymphoblastic leukemia antigen in non-hematopoietic tissues. *J. Exp. Med.* 154: 1249-1254.

Meuer, S. C., Acuto, O., Hussey, R. E., Hodgon, J. C., Fitzgerald, K. A., Schlossman, S. F., and Reinherz, E. L. (1983). Evidence for the T3-associated 90K heterodimer as the T-cell antigen receptor. *Nature* 303: 808-810.

Mirro, J., Zipf, T. F., Pui, C.-H., Kitchingman, G., Williams, D., Melvin, S., Murphy, S. B., and Stass, S. (1985). Acute mixed lineage leukemia: Clinicopathologic correlations and prognostic significance. *Blood* 66: 1115-1123.

Nadler, L. M., Stashenko, P., Hardy, R., van Agthoven, A., Terhorst, C., and Schlossman, S. F. (1981). Characterization of a human B cell-specific antigen (B2) distinct from B1. *J. Immunol.* 126: 1941-1947.

Nadler, L. M., Ritz, J., Bates, M. P., Park, E. K., Anderson, K. C., Sallan, S. E., and Schlossman, S. F. (1982). Induction of human B cell antigens in non-T cell acute lymphoblastic leukemia. *J. Clin. Invest.* 70: 433-442.

Nadler, L. M., Anderson, K. C., Marti, G., Bates, M. P., Park, E., Saley, J. F., and Schlossman, S. F. (1983). B4, a human B lymphocyte antigen expressed on normal, mitogen activated and malignant B lymphocytes. *J. Immunol.* 131: 244-250.

Nadler, L. M., Korsmeyer, S. J., Anderson, K. C., Boyd, A. W., Slaughenhaupt, B., Park, E., Jensen, J., Coral, F., Mayer, R. J., Sallan, S. E., Ritz, J., and Schlossman, S. F. (1984). B cell origin of non-T cell acute lymphoblastic leukemia. A model for discrete stages of neoplastic and normal pre-B cell differentiation. *J. Clin. Invest.* 74: 332-340.

Ohashi, P. S., Mak, T. W., van den Elsen, P., Yanagi, Y., Yoshikai, Y., Calman, A. F., Terhorst, C., Stobo, J. D., and Weiss, A. (1985). Reconstitution of an active surface T3/T-cell antigen receptor by DNA transfer. *Nature* 316: 606-609.

Palumbo, A., Minowada, J., Erikson, J., Croce, C. M., and Rovera, G. (1984). Lineage infidelity of a human myelogenous leukemia cell line. *Blood* 64: 1059-1063.

Pelicci, P.-G., Knowles, D. M., and Dalla-Favera, R. (1985). Lymphoid tumors displaying rearrangements of both immunoglobulin and T cell receptor genes. *J. Exp. Med.* 162: 1015-1024.

Pittaluga, S., Raffeld, M., Lipford, E. H., and Cossman, J. (1986). 3A1 (CD7) expression precedes T_β gene rearrangements in precursor T (lymphoblastic) neoplasms. *Blood*, in press.

Rabbitts, T. H., Stinson, A., Forster, A., Foroni, I., Luzzatto, L., Catovsky, D., Hammarstrom, L., Smith, C. I. E., Jones, D., Karpas, A., Minowada, J., and Taylor, A. M. R. (1985). Heterogeneity of T-cell β-chain gene rearrangements in human leukaemias and lymphomas. *EMBO J.* 4: 2217-2224.

Raulet, D. H., Garman, R. D., Saito, H., and Tonegawa, S. (1985). Developmental regulation of T-cell receptor gene expression. *Nature* 314: 403-407.

Reinherz, E. L., Kung, P. C., Goldstein, G., Levey, R. H., and Schlossman, S. F. (1980). Discrete stages of human intrathymic differentiation: Analysis of normal thymocytes and leukemic lymphoblasts of T lineage. *Proc. Nat. Acad. Sci. USA* 77: 1588-1592.

Reinherz, E. L., Haynes, B. F., Nadler, L. M., and Bernstein, I. D. (1986). *Leukocyte Typing II*, Vol. 2, *Human T Lymphocytes.* Springer-Verlag, New York, Berlin, Heidelberg, Tokyo.

Ritchie, K. A., Brinster, R. L., and Storb, U. (1984). Allelic exclusion and control of endogenous immunoglobulin gene rearrangement in κ transgenic mice. *Nature* 312: 517-520.

Ritz, J., Pesando, J. M., Notis-McConarty, J., Lazarus, H., and Schlossman, S. F. (1980). A monoclonal antibody to human acute lymphoblastic leukemia antigen. *Nature* 283: 583-585.

Ritz, J., Nadler, L. M., Bhan, A. K., Notis-McConarty, J., Pesando, J. M., and Schlossman, S. F. (1981). Expression of common acute lymphoblastic leukemia antigen (CALLA) by lymphomas of B cell and T cell lineage. *Blood* 58: 648-652.

Royer, H. D., Acuto, O., Fabbi, M., Tizard, R., Ramachandran, K., Smart, J. E., and Reinherz, E. L. (1984). Genes encoding the Ti beta subunit of the antigen/MHC receptor undergo rearrangement during intrathymic ontogeny prior to surface T3-Ti expression. *Cell* 39: 261-266.

Royer, H. D., Ramarli, D., Acuto, O., Campen, T. J., and Reinherz, E. L. (1985). Genes encoding the T-cell receptor α and β subunits are transcribed in an ordered manner during intrathymic ontogeny. *Proc. Nat. Acad. Sci. USA* 82: 5510-5514.

Saito, H., Kranz, D. M., Takagaki, Y., Hayday, A. C., Eisen, H. N., and Tonegawa, S. (1984). A third rearranged and expressed gene in a clone of cytotoxic T lymphocytes. *Nature* 312: 36-40.

Sim, G. K., Yague, J., Nelson, J., Marrack, P., Palmer, E., Augustin, A., and Kappler, J. (1984). Primary structure of human T-cell receptor α-chain. *Nature* 312: 771-775.

Siminovitch, K. A., Bakhshi, A., Goldman, P., and Korsmeyer, S. J. (1985). A uniform deleting element mediates the loss of κ genes in human B cells. *Nature* 316: 260-262.

Siu, G., Clark, S. P., Yoshikai, Y., Malissen, M., Yanagi, Y., Strauss, E., Mak, T. W., and Hood, L. (1984). The human T cell antigen receptor is encoded by variable, diversity, and joining gene segments that rearrange to generate a complete V gene. *Cell* 37: 393-401.

Snodgrass, H. R., Dembic, Z., Steinmetz, M., and von Boehmer, H. (1985). Expression of T-cell antigen receptor during fetal development in the thymus. *Nature* 315: 232-233.

Spits, H., Borst, J., Tax, W., Capel, P. J. A., Terhorst, C., and Devries, J. E. (1985). Characterisation of a monoclonal antibody (WT31) that recognizes a common epitope of the human T-cell receptor for antigen. *J. Immunol.* 135: 1922-1928.

Stashenko, P., Nadler, L. M., Hardy, R., and Schlossman, S. F. (1980). Characterization of a human B lymphocyte specific antigen. *J. Immunol.* 125: 1506-1514.

Tawa, A., Hozumi, N., Minden, M., Mak, T. W., and Gelfand, E. W. (1985). Rearrangement of the T-cell receptor β-chain gene in non-T-cell, non-B-cell acute lymphoblastic leukemia of childhood. *N. Engl. J. Med.* 313: 1033-1037.

Tonegawa, S. (1983). Somatic generation of antibody diversity. *Nature* 302: 575-581.

van den Elsen, P., Shepley, B., Borst, J., Coligan, J. E., Markham, A. F., Orkin, S., and Terhorst, C. (1984). Isolation of cDNA clones encoding the 20k T3 glycoprotein of human T-cell receptor complex. *Nature* 312: 413-418.

Vogler, L. B., Crist, W. M., Bockman, D. E., Pearl, E. R., Lawton, A. R., and Cooper, M. D. (1978). Pre-B-cell leukemia: A new phenotype of childhood lymphoblastic leukemia. *N. Engl. J. Med.* 298: 872-878.

von Fliedner, V. (1985). Contribution of immunological markers to the diagnosis and prognosis of human leukemia. *Eur. J. Cancer Clin. Oncol.* 21: 347-353.

Waldmann, T. A., Davis, M. M., Bongiovanni, K. F., and Korsmeyer, S. J. (1985). Rearrangements of genes for the antigen receptor on T cells as markers of lineage and clonality in human lymphoid neoplasms. *N. Engl. J. Med.* 313: 776-783.

Weiss, A., and Stobo, J. D. (1984). Requirement for the coexpression of T3 and the T cell antigen receptor on a malignant human T cell line. *J. Exp. Med.* 160: 1284-1299.

Yanagi, Y., Yoshikai, Y., Leggett, K., Clark, S., Aleksander, I., and Mak, T. (1984). A human T cell specific cDNA clone encodes a protein having extensive homology to immunoglobulin chains. *Nature* 308: 145-148.

Yanagi, Y., Chan, A., Chin, B., Minden, M., and Mak, T. (1985). Analysis of cDNA clones specific for human T cells and the α and β chains of the T-cell receptor heterodimer from a human T-cell line. *Proc. Nat. Acad. Sci. USA* 82: 3430-3434.

Yoshikai, Y., Clark, S. P., Taylor, S., Sohn, U., Wilson, B. I., Minden, M. D., and Mak, T. W. (1985). Organization and sequences of the variable, joining and constant region genes of the human T-cell receptor α-chain. *Nature* 316: 837-839.

8

Immunophenotype in the Characterization and Diagnosis of Acute Leukemia
Myeloid Markers

JOSEPH MIRRO, JR. *St. Jude Children's Research Hospital and University of Tennessee College of Medicine, Memphis, Tennessee*

FREDERICK G. BEHM *St. Jude Children's Research Hospital, Memphis, Tennessee*

I. INTRODUCTION

In general, human leukemic cells are phenotypically similar to their normal hematopoietic counterparts, suggesting that malignant transformation results in a maturation arrest but permits continued proliferation. The development of monoclonal antibodies (MoAbs) reactive with lineage- and differentiation-associated cell surface antigens has provided highly specific reagents for the identification of these antigens on leukemic cells. In lymphoid leukemia the use of MoAbs that identify T- or B-cell associated antigens has in most cases provided clarification of the cell lineage, which appears to be an important predictor of clinical outcome (Brouet et al., 1976; Flandrin et al., 1975; Chessels et al., 1977). Such findings in childhood acute lymphoblastic leukemia (ALL) have led to treatment modifications with the goal of improving outcome in the poor-risk group and decreasing toxicity in the good-risk group. MoAbs studies of ALL have also provided insights into the probable leukemogenic target cell. Some cell types (e.g., Ia+, CALLA+) appear to become leukemic more often than would be expected based on their apparent normal frequency alone, suggesting that leukemogenesis is not an entirely random event (Greaves et al., 1986).

Myeloid differentiation is more easily studied using morphologic criteria than is lymphoid differentiation. Since acute nonlymphoid leukemia (ANLL) is a morphologically heterogeneous disease composed of atypical cells with characteristics somewhat similar to normal myeloid cells, a standard classification system was developed (Bennett et al., 1976). This French-American-British (FAB) system is based on the morphologic and cytochemical staining characteristics of nonlymphoid cells (Bennett et al., 1985b). It has become a widely used and accepted classification. Although some clinical correlations are clear, such as promyelocytic morphology (FAB-M3) correlated with disseminated intravascular coagulation and monocytic leukemia (FAB-M5) correlated with an overall poorer survival (Bennett and Begg, 1981; Foon et al., 1979), the prognostic significance of the FAB classification has varied between institutions (Head et al., 1985). Furthermore, the value of the FAB classification system continues to be debated (see Chapter 1). This classification system also has not been particularly useful in suggesting directions for future basic research into the biologic characteristics of ANLL. Thus, investigators are attempting to develop new and more useful classification systems for ANLL (Bloomfield et al., 1984; Dinndorf et al., 1986; Griffin et al., 1986; Ball and Fanger, 1983; Drexler et al., 1985; Vaughn et al., 1983). MoAbs reactive with nonlymphoid-associated antigens appear useful in confirming the diagnosis of ANLL in selected cases including undifferentiated leukemia, and in defining prognostically significant subgroups. This immunologic approach has also proven to be important to basic research in hematopoiesis and is beginning to provide new insights into early myelopoiesis. Therefore, an immunological classification system may provide information that is supplemental to the FAB classification.

The major objective of this chapter is to briefly summarize the large volume of published material concerning the MoAbs that identify myeloid-associated cell surface antigens and to discuss their usefulness in studying ANLL. Specific areas of discussion are as follows: (a) clinically relevant data on MoAbs useful in phenotyping myeloid leukemic cells; (b) knowledge of the surface molecules identified by these MoAbs and their role in normal cell function; (c) analysis of normal myelopoiesis using MoAbs; and (d) the use of MoAbs in diagnosing ANLL, the correlation of surface antigen expression with prognosis, and the potential use of myeloid markers to follow residual disease. Finally, the available information about the potential therapeutic use of MoAbs in ANLL will be presented.

II. MONOCLONAL ANTIBODIES REACTIVE WITH MYELOID-ASSOCIATED CELL SURFACE ANTIGENS

Our understanding of myeloid-associated antigens has advanced at a slower pace than that of lymphoid-associated antigens for several reasons. First, there are multiple distinct nonlymphoid cell populations (e.g., granulocytes, monocytes, platelets, and red cells) that must be analyzed for antigen expression. Second, nonlymphoid-associated antigens are biochemically complex; many are composed of carbohydrate or lipid. This area of immunologic investigations has also become increasingly complicated due to the rapidly expanding numbers of available MoAbs, the complex and inconsistent nomenclature used by separate investigators, and the lack of direct comparisons between antibodies. There is also evidence to indicate that the phenotype of clonogenic myeloid leukemia cells is different from the phenotype expressed by the majority of leukemic cells present in the bone marrow at the time of diagnosis.

The First, Second and Third International Workshops on Human Leukocyte Differentiation Antigens were conducted to assess the interrelationships between MoAbs and to determine their reactivities within the hematological system. As a result of these workshops, groups of MoAbs that recognize the same or similar antigens have been identified and these groups have been designated Cluster Groups of Differentiation (CD). Biochemical analysis of the antigens identified by a number of MoAbs within these cluster groups has confirmed that these antibodies often identify the same surface molecule. Some groups of antibodies appear to identify the same or similar molecules by immunofluorescence; however when

Table 1 References for Commonly Used Monoclonal Antibodies (MoAbs)

MoAb	First Author/Reference
Mo1 and OKM1	Griffin, J. (1984) In *Leukocyte Typing,* A. Bernard et al. (eds). Springer-Verlag, Berlin, p. 404
Mo5	Todd, R. F. (1985) *Blood* 95:964
20.2	Kamoun, M. (1983) *Clin. Immunol. Immunopathol.* 29: 181
MY4	Griffin, J. (1981) *J. Clin. Invest.* 69:932
MOP9	Dimitriu-Bona, A. (1983) *J. Immunol.* 130:145
FMC17	Seymour, G. J. (1983) *J. Reticuloendothel. Soc.* 34:463
MA5	Takacs, L. (1983) *Lancet* 2:1500
Ki-M1 and Ki-M5	Parweresch, M. R. (1983) *Blood* 62:585
MY9	Griffin, J. (1984) *Leuk. Res.* 8:521
L4F3, T5A7, L1B3 1G10	Andrews, R. G. (1983) *Blood* 62:124
MY10	Civin, C. I. (1984) *J. Immunol.* 133:157
BI-3C5	Tindle, R. W. Third International Workshop p 74 (abstract)
60.1 and 60.3	Beatty, P. G. (1983) *J. Immunol.* 131:2913
MY8	Griffin (1981) *J. Clin. Invest.* 69:932
80H-3	Mannoni, P. (1982) *Human Immunol.* 5:309
82H5	Janowska-Wieczorek, A. (1984) *Br. J. Haematol.* 58:159
R1B12 and S4-7	Pessano, S. (1984) *Blood* 64:275
MCS.1	Tatsumi, S. (1981) *Proc. Am. Assoc. Cancer Res.* 22: 181

Table 1 continues

Table 1 (*continued*)

MoAb	First Author/Reference
MCS.2	Gregg, S. L. (1984) *Cancer Res.* 44:2724
SJ-D1	Mirro, J. (1984) In *Leukocyte Typing*, A. Bernard et al. (Eds). Springer-Verlag, Berlin, p. 442
M5	Schwarting, R. (1985) *Blood* 65:974
5F1	Bernstein, I. D. (1982) *J. Immunol.* 128:876
My1	Civin, C. I. (1981) *Blood* 57:842
FMC10 and FMC13	Zola, H. (1981) *Br. J. Haematol.* 48:481
DUHL60.1	McKolanis, J. R. (1984) In *Leukocyte Typing*, A. Bernard et al. (eds.) Springer-Verlag, Berlin, p. 387
VEP13	Rumpold, H. (1982) *J. Immunol.* 129:1458
GO22b	Thompson, J. (1984) *J. Am. Ger. Soc.* 32:274
GO35	Thompson, J. (1984) In *Advances in Immunobiology*. J. S. Thompson, et al. (eds.). Alan Liss, Inc., New York, p. 169
MY7	Griffin, J. (1983) *Int. J. Cell Cloning* 1:33
VIE-64	Knapp, W. (1981) In *Leukemia Markers*. W. Knapp (ed.). Academic Press, London, p. 207
SFL23.6	Das Gupta, A. (1985) *Blood* 66:522
LeuM1	Hanjan, S. N. (1982) *Clin. Immunol. Immunopathol.* 23:172
AML2.23	Ball, E. D. (1983) *Blood* 61:456
PMN 6/29	Ball, E. D. (1982) *Proc. Natl. Acad. Sci. USA* 79:5374
CAMAL 1	Malcolm, A. (1984) *Exp. Hematol.* 12:539
MoU48	Winchester, R. (1984) *Med. Oncol. Tumor Pharmacother.* 1:263
MoS1	Winchester, R. (1983) *J. Clin. Invest.* 71:1633
VIMD5	Majdic, O. (1981) *Blood* 58:1127
CLB-FcRgran1 and CLB-LFA-1/1	Miedma, F. (1984) *Eur. J. Immunol.* 14:518
MHM23	Hildreth, J. E. K. (1983) *Eur. J. Immunol.* 13:202
TS1/18.11	Krensky, A. M. (1984) *Am. J. Immunol.* 132:2180
JOAN 1	Peschel, C. (1986) In *Leukocyte Typing II*. E. L. Reinberz, et al. (eds). Springer-Verlag, New York, p. 181

this information has not been confirmed, the cluster group is designated as a provisional working group (CDw). Additionally, when a group of MoAbs cluster by immunofluorescence reactivity but appear to recognize different molecules, this group is also designated as a provisional working group (CDw). The reader is referred to the joint report of these Workshops for an excellent and more comprehensive summary (Bernard, Boumsell and Hill, 1984; Bernstein and Self, 1986). Recently, using molecular biology, the reactivity of certain antibodies with specific antigens has been confirmed by DNA-mediated gene transfer (Look et al., 1985; Look et al., 1986; Peiper, Ashmun and Look, 1986).

It should be emphasized that there are important differences between MoAbs even in the same cluster group. These differences include their stability, isotype, ability to fix complement, and specific binding site (epitope). Investigators interested in specific uses of the MoAbs reacting with myeloid antigens will need to consult the original articles describing these antibodies (see Table 1). The objective

Table 2 Monoclonal Antibodies Reactive with Nonlymphoid Cell Surface Antigens

Group[a]	Antibodies	Antigen
CD11	Mo1, VIM12, 60.1, Ki-M5, OKM1	C3bi (α chain) ppt = 170/95 Kd
CDw12	20.2	
CDw13	My7, SJ-D1, MCS.2 MoU48, MoU28	gp150 kd
CDw14 (55)	MY4, MoP9, FMC17 MoS1, MA5, Mo2	gp55
CDw14 (150,95)	VIM13, Ki-M1, SCHL3, M5	p150, 95
CDw14 (85)	5F1	gp85 kd
CD15	My-1, 1G10, FMC10, FMC13 VIMD5, DUHL60.1	x-hapten
CD16	BW243/41, CLB FcR gran 1 GO22b, VEP13	Fc receptor
CDw17	T5A7, GO35	Lactosylceramide
CDw18	MHM23, CLB-LFA-1/1 60.3, TS1/18.11, 1B4	LFA-1 (α or β chain) ppt = 180/170/150/95 kd
---[b]	MY9, L4F3, L1B3	p67 kd
---[b]	MY10, BI-3C5	gp115 kd

[a]Based on International Workshop nomenclature (see text).
[b]Not yet assigned cluster group designations (see text).
p = protein; gp = glycoprotein; ppt = precipitate. For other abbreviations see text.

Table 3 Monoclonal Antibody Reactivity with Blood Cells[a]

	Myeloblast	Promyelocyte	Myelocyte	Metamyelocyte	Neutrophil	Monoblast/ Promonocyte	Monocyte	Erythroblast	Erythrocyte	Megakaryocyte	Platelet
CD11 (Mo1, OKM1)	–	–	+	+	+	+	+	–	–	–	–
CDw12 (20.2)	–	–	–	–	–		+				
CDw13 (MY7, MCS.2, SJ-D1)	+	+	+	+	+	+	+	–	–		–
CDw14 (MY4, Mo2)	–	–	–	–	–	+	+	–	–	–	–
CDw14 (5F1)	–	–	–	–	–	+	+	+	–		+
CD15 (VIM-D5, DUHL60.1, 1G10)	+	+	+	+	+	–	+	–	–	–	–
CD16 (VEP13, GO22b)					+		+				
CDw17 (T5A7, GO35)	–	–	–	+	+	+	+	–	–	–	–
CDw18 (MHM23, 60.3)					+		+				
MY9, L4F3, L1B3	+	+	+	+	–	+	+	–	–		–
MY10, BI-3C5	+	–	–	–	–	+	–	–	–		–

[a]Results may differ slightly with individual antibodies.

of our present summary is to emphasize similarities among antibodies. The information provided below is a composite of findings from immunologic, biochemical, and molecular studies. The groups of MoAbs discussed are based on the International Workshops cluster group designations (Table 2). The reactivity of the MoAbs on peripheral blood cells is included in the description below and summarized in Table 3.

Cluster group CD11. Antibodies in this group will react with most granulocytes and monocytes and with subsets of lymphoid cells (large granular lymphocytes). This group includes a number of well-known MoAbs (including Mo1, OKM1, VIM12, Ki-M5, and 60.1) and has been shown to react with the C3bi receptor, a 155, 94 kilodalton (kd) heterodimer. The glycoprotein heterodimer identified by this group of MoAbs is a receptor for the binding of particles opsonized with the C3 cleavage product C3bi.

Cluster group CDw12 (provisional). This group appears distinct immunologically and includes antibody 20.2, which reacts with neutrophils and monocytes.

Cluster group CDw13 (provisional). MoAbs in this group will react with peripheral blood neutrophils (40% to 70%) and monocytes (50%). DNA-mediated gene transfer experiments and biochemical analysis have proven these antibodies all react with the same 150 kd glycoprotein, which is the product of a single gene (Look et al., 1985; Look et al., 1986). Immunologic studies indicate that the epitopes for a number of MoAbs in this cluster group are different (Mirro et al., unpublished observations).

Cluster group CDw14 (provisional). By immunological analysis this cluster group includes a heterogenous group of MoAbs. Immunoprecipitation and DNA transfection experiments have identified at least three separate subgroups within CDw14. The first (CDw14, 55) includes MoAbs (e.g., MY4, MoP9, FMC17 and MA5) which react with a 55-kd surface glycoprotein (gp55) expressed primarily on monocytes. The second subgroup (CDw14, 150,95) includes antibodies Ki-M1, SCHL3, VIM13 and M5 which appear to react with a heterodimer of 150,95 kd which appears to be part of the leukocyte functional antigen family (see CDw18). Antibodies in CDw14 (150,95) are reactive with neutrophils, monocytes, and large granular lymphocytes. The third subgroup (CDw14, 85) consists of antibody 5F1, which reacts with an 85-kd surface molecule expressed on monocytes and platelets.

Cluster group CD15. Some MoAbs in CD15 react almost exclusively with neutrophils (FMC10, FMC13) while others also react with peripheral blood monocytes (My-1, 1G10, DUHL60.1). These reactive differences are presumed to be due to antibody affinity or epitope specificity. This group of antibodies reacts with the x-hapten carbohydrate (lacto-N fucopentaosyl III) (Huang, L. C. et al., 1983) which is not restricted to hematopoietic cells but is widely expressed on human malignant cells (neuroblastoma, adenocarcinoma, teratocarcinoma); normal cells (epithelia); and in secretions (urine, milk). The large number of murine MoAbs reacting with the x-hapten suggests that this carbohydrate structure is prominent on the surface of nonlymphoid cells and is highly antigenic in mice.

Cluster group CD16. This group includes antibodies VEP13, CLBFcRgran1 GO22b, and BW243/41, which recognize the Fc receptor on granulocytes. Antibodies in this cluster group react with neutrophils and large granular lymphocytes. There is some heterogeneity in the molecular weights in the molecules precipitated by these antibodies which appears to be a result of glycosylation.

Cluster group CDw17 (provisional). Both antibodies in this group (T5A7 and GO35) are known to react with a glycolipid moiety, lactosylceramide, found on granulocytic and monocytic cells as well as platelets (Symington et al., 1985).

Cluster group CDw18 (provisional). MoAbs in this cluster group identify a group of heterodimers designated as LFA-1 (leukocyte functional antigen), found on monocytes, granulocytes, and large granular lymphocytes. Antibodies in CDw18 precipitate a family of molecules of 180, 170, 150, and 95 kd. The LFA-1 family appears to be composed of heterodimers with a common β chain but different α chains. MoAbs in CDw18 appear to react with the β chain, which explains the common 95-kd molecular weight antigen in this cluster group. This 95-kd β-chain molecule appears to be common to the C3bi molecule (CD11), the granulocyte Fc receptor (CD16), and the heterodimers identified by some antibodies in the CDw14.

Other MoAbs not assigned cluster groups. Testing MoAbs on NIH/3T3 mouse fibroblasts after DNA-mediated gene transfer of human cellular DNA encoding for myeloid-associated antigens has made it possible to determine that specific antibodies react with the same gene product. This molecular approach has identified the following additional MoAb groups:

1. Anti-p67: MoAbs MY9, L4F3 and L1B3 react with a single gene product (Peiper, Ashmun and Look, 1986), a 67-kd cell surface antigen present on approximately half of myelocytic and monocytic cells;
2. Anti-gp115: MoAbs MY10 and BI-3C5 react with a 115-kd surface antigen (Civin et al., 1984; Look et al., 1986). This antigen appears to be present only on early precursors (Civin et al., 1984; Tindle et al., 1986) and therefore may prove extremely useful in studies of hematopoiesis (see below).

III. FUNCTIONS OF CELL SURFACE ANTIGENS IDENTIFIED BY MONOCLONAL ANTIBODIES

The first membrane antigen that was identified as functionally significant was the glycoprotein heterodimer defined by monoclonal antibodies in the CD11 group (e.g., Mo1 and OKM1). This heterodimer is a receptor for the binding of particles opsonized with the C3 cleavage product C3bi (Arnaout et al., 1982; Wright et al., 1983). Antibodies in CD16 (Table 2) identify the Fc receptor on granulocytes and large granular lymphocytes (Linch et al., 1984; Breard et al., 1980). Additional MoAbs have also been reported that identify structures involved in phagocytosis, antigen presentation and migration (Skubitz et al., 1983; Skubitz, Zhen and August, 1983).

The first clinical documentation of a surface antigen deficiency was in a group of patients with recurrent infections (Arnaout et al., 1982; Todd and Arnaout, 1986). These patients did not express antigens identified by MoAbs in CDw18, which implied the importance of these antigens (LFA-1) in normal immunologic function. Several groups of investigators have clarified the structural and functional characteristics of these heterodimers (Wallis et al., 1986; Todd et al., 1984). Briefly, the antigens identified by MoAbs of CD11, CDw14 (150, 95) and CDw18 share a common 95-kd β chain but have different α chains. Functional assays have demonstrated that this family of antigens is important in multiple cell functions. Antibodies of CD11, e.g., Mo1, identify a molecule that has complement receptor type 3 (CR3) activity and may play a role in myeloid cell adhesion phenomena. The LFA-1 antigen, identified by antibodies in CDw18, promotes lymphoid cell adhesion interactions that include lymphocyte proliferation and cytotoxic effector activity. Neutrophil adherence, spreading, aggregation and phagocytosis of zymosan particles can be inhibited in a dose-dependent fashion by MoAb 60.3 (CDw18) and 60.1 (CD11) but not by OKM1 (CD11). Thus the functionally active site on these surface molecules may be near the epitope identified by 60.1 (α chain) or the 60.3 β chain (Wallis et al., 1986). The 150, 95 cell surface antigen (CDw14) has possible phagocyte C3d receptor activity and also appears to be a member of this antigen family. The exact relationship between CDw14 (150,95) CD11 and CDw18 has not yet been completely clarified.

IV. ANALYSIS OF NORMAL MYELOPOIESIS USING MONOCLONAL ANTIBODIES

An important benefit of MoAbs is the increased understanding of hematopoiesis resulting from their use to isolate specific myeloid precursors. The expression of several MoAb-defined myeloid antigens corresponds to pathways of differentiation within the myeloid lineage. These antibodies are therefore useful tools for identifying hematopoietic cells at various stages of maturation and proliferative potential (Andrews, Torok-Storb and Bernstein, 1983; Strauss et al., 1984; Strauss, Stuart and Civin, 1983; Winchester et al., 1977). Using either complement-dependent MoAb-mediated lysis (negative selection) or techniques such as fluorescence-activated cell sorting or immune rosetting (positive selection), it has been possible to determine patterns of antigen expression by multipotent stem cells (CFU-

Table 4 Monoclonal Antibody Reactivity with Hematopoietic Progenitor Cells

Antibodies[a]	CFU-GEMM	CFU-GM (d 14)	CFU-GM (d 7)	BFU-E	CFU-E	CFU-meg
anti-gp115 MY10, BI-3C5	+	+		+		+
anti-p67 MY9	+	+	+	+		
anti-gp150 MY7		+	+			
JOAN 1		+	+	+	+	+
anti-p67 L4F3		+	+	+	+	+
1G10 (CD15)		+	+			
VIM2			+			+
T5A7 (CDw17)			+			
5F1 (CDw14)						

[a]Results from different laboratories using different antibodies have given variable results. See text for abbreviations and details.

GEMM) and by stem cells committed to the myeloid (CFU-GM), erythroid (BFU-E, CFU-E), or megakaryocyte/platelet (CFU-meg) pathways of differentiation. Table 4 briefly summarizes some of the published results and may serve as a general guide. In several reports, myeloid progenitor cells have been purified 50- to 100-fold from bone marrow mononuclear cells, permitting studies of morphologic and functional characteristics of these progenitor-enriched populations (Leary et al., 1985).

The expression of p67 identified by MoAbs MY9, L4F3 and L1B3 has been extensively studied and occurs on CFU-GEMM, CFU-GM (day 14 and day 7), BFU-E and possibly CFU-E (Andrews, Torok-Storb, and Bernstein, 1983 and Griffin et al., 1983b). This antigen is useful in identifying early myeloid precursors and its expression is shown in Figure 1. Likewise the expression of gp150 has been well studied. This antigen is expressed later in myeloid differentiation (Fig. 2) and is useful in studies of myelopoiesis. Certain antigens, such as gp115, appear to be uniquely expressed by progenitor cells; other antigens are detectable on myeloid, erythroid, or platelet precursors corresponding to morphologically and histochemically distinct stages of maturation. In the case of neutrophil differentiation, some antigens are either lost (Ia, MY-10) or acquired (Mo1, MY8, 80H.3, or B34.3) as cells progress from myeloblasts to mature neutrophils (Table 3). Expression of other determinants (82H5, R1B19, S4-7) is maintained on all recognizable myeloid cells (Foon and Todd, 1986). Thus, morphologic differentiation is accompanied by surface antigen changes which can be followed by MoAb reactivity.

V. MONOCLONAL ANTIBODIES IN THE DIAGNOSIS AND PROGNOSIS OF ACUTE NONLYMPHOCYTIC LEUKEMIA AND CHRONIC MYELOGENOUS LEUKEMIA IN BLAST CRISIS

ANLL is a clonal malignancy of nonlymphoid progenitor cells resulting in excessive proliferation and accumulation of immature hematopoietic elements (Fialkow et al., 1981). The diagnosis is made primarily on morphologic and cytochemical evaluation and is usually straightforward. Variants of this disease are generally classified according to the morphologic similarity of the leukemic cell population

Figure 1 Schematic representation of human hematopoietic differentiation indicating the expression of p67 (identified by MoAbs MY9, L4F3, L1B3). Cells expressing p67 are indicated by *. The expression on CFU-GEMM, CFU-GM (day 14 or 7) BFU-E, CFU-E and CFU-meg is based on results of positive and/or negative selection experiments and subsequent colony growth. Expression is down-regulated on nondividing cells of the granulocytic series, bands and segmented forms. Figure used with the kind permission of Dr. Stephen C. Peiper and Anne Williford.

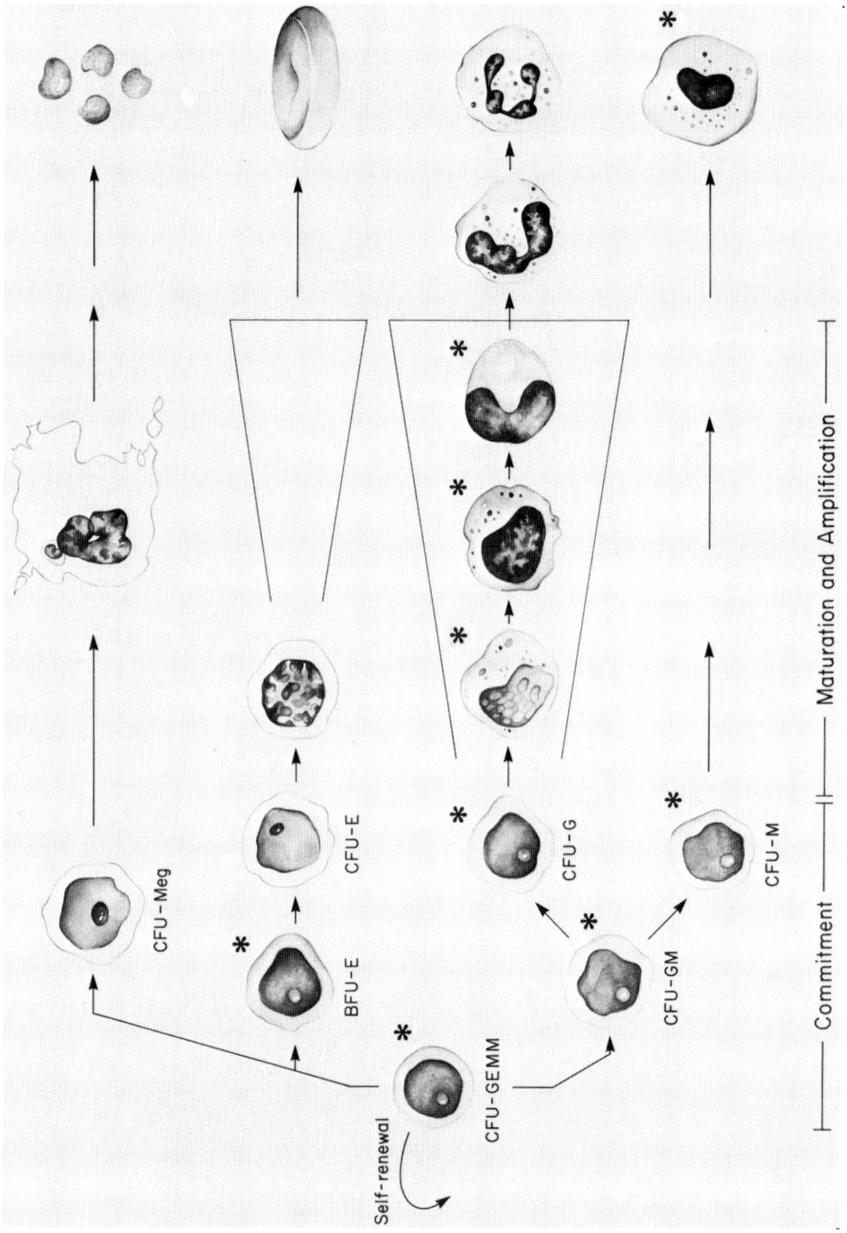
Self-renewal
CFU-GEMM
CFU-Meg
BFU-E
CFU-E
CFU-GM
CFU-G
CFU-M
Commitment
Maturation and Amplification

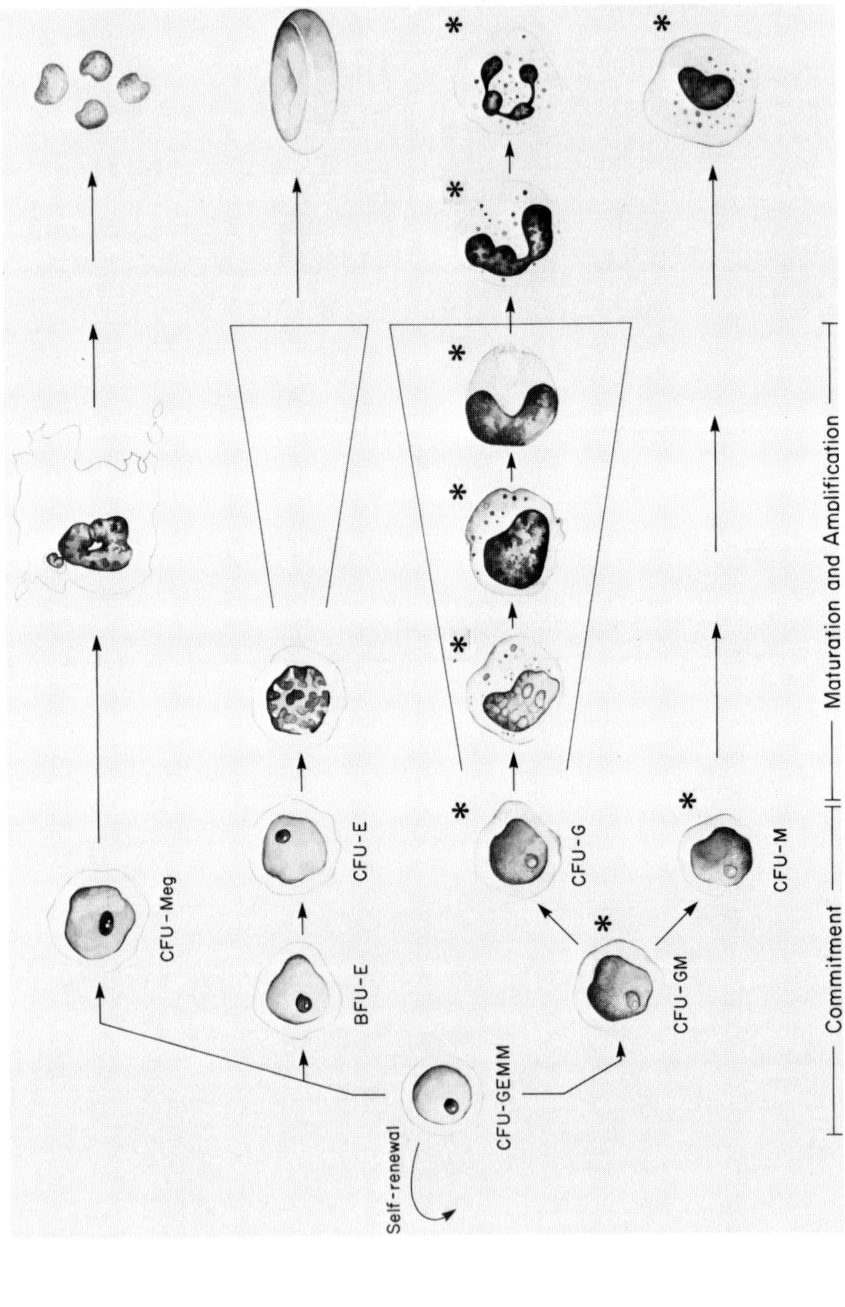
Self-renewal
CFU-GEMM
CFU-Meg
BFU-E
CFU-E
CFU-GM
CFU-G
CFU-M
Commitment
Maturation and Amplification

to normal myeloid precursors (FAB criteria) and identification is usually easy in cases of FAB-M2 through M6, i.e., acute myeloblastic leukemia, acute promyelocytic leukemia, acute monoblastic leukemia and acute erythroleukemia. However, in a small percentage of FAB-M1 cases with very undifferentiated blasts and with megakaryocytic leukemia, FAB-M7, the diagnosis may be a difficult to make (Huang, M.J., et al., 1984). The major difficulty is distinguishing M1 from L2 cases when the cytochemical staining is negative at the light microscopic level (Browman, Neame, Soamboonsrup, 1986).

Numerous MoAbs reactive with myeloid-associated antigens were quickly evaluated to determine their reactivity for human ANLL cells (Linkler-Israeli et al., 1981; Van der Reijden, 1983; Civin, Mirro and Banquerigo, 1981). In all cases, these antibodies identify determinants expressed by either normal circulating myeloid cells or bone marrow progenitors. Although none of these reagents recognizes a leukemia-specific determinant, they can be helpful in the diagnosis. The marked difference in therapy and prognosis between ANLL and ALL make this distinction of primary importance. MoAbs that identify antigens expressed by myeloid but not lymphoid leukemias (or vice versa) have potential diagnostic value in cases of undifferentiated leukemia. Leukemic cells expressing multiple myeloid-associated surface antigens without expressing lymphoid-associated antigens suggests the diagnosis of nonlymphocytic leukemia. However the expression of myeloid-associated cell surface antigens alone cannot be accepted as definitive diagnostic proof of nonlymphoid lineage, since these antigens are not restricted to a single lineage (Dinndorf et al., 1985; Mirro et al., 1985a, 1985b; Greaves et al., 1986; Smith et al., 1983) (see Chapter 12 on Acute Mixed Lineage Leukemia).

Several MoAbs that have been extensively tested are useful reagents to detect myeloid cells since they are reactive with most ANLL cells but are generally nonreactive with lymphoid leukemia. Majdic et al. (1981), studied 208 leukemias and found that 91% of ANLL samples reacted positively with MoAb VIM2 while all nonmyeloid leukemias were negative. Chan, Pegram and Greaves (1985), tested the MY9 antibody against leukemic cells from 100 consecutive cases and found that 86% of the AML cases but none of the 50 ALL cases were reactive with MY9. In a large study with multiple MoAbs, Griffin et al. (1983a) demonstrated that

---

Figure 2 Schematic representation of human hematopoietic differentiation indicating the expression of gp150 (identified by MoAbs in CDw13). The gp150 surface antigen is not expressed on CFU-GEMM, BFU-E, CFU-E or CFU-meg, based on results of positive and/or negative selection experiments and subsequent colony growth. It is expressed on committed granulocytic and monocytic precursors and on all subsequent cells in these lineages. Cells expressing gp150 are indicated by *. Figure used with kind permission of Dr. Stephen C. Peiper and Anne Williford.

Table 5 Monoclonal Antibody Reactivity with Myeloid Leukemia (Percent of Patients Considered Positive)

		FAB Category			
Group	Antibody	M1 + M2	M3	M4 + M5	Overall
anti-p67	MY9	77%	76%	75%	76%
anti-gp150	MY7	71%	73%	63%	67%
	MY8	33%	32%	70%	52%
CD-15	My-1	32%	33%	54%	46%
CD-11	Mo1	38%	40%	84%	46%
anti-gp55	MY4/Mo2	17%	2%	54%	35%

Data compiled from Griffin et al., 1983c, Griffin et al., 1986, Foon and Todd, 1986, Drexler et al., 1985, and Mirro et al. (unpublished).

62 of 70 myeloid leukemias expressed a phenotype corresponding to immature myeloid cells. Drexler et al. (1985) found that cells from most cases of nonlymphocytic leukemia studied expressed the gp150 molecule identified by antibody MCS.2. Table 5 is a compilation of several major reported series in adults (Drexler et al., 1985; Griffin et al., 1986; Foon and Todd, 1986), and our results in childhood ANLL, which are not significantly different from the adult series (Mirro et al., unpublished observation). The data indicate that antibodies recognizing gp150 (MSC.2, MY7, SJ-D1) in CDw13 react with approximately 67% of cases of ANLL and those recognizing p67 (MY9, L4F3) react with 76% of cases. MoAbs against p67 and gp150 would appear to be useful agents for determining the lineage of leukemic blasts.

In some cases the diagnosis may be made rapidly by the use of MoAbs. For example, in a prospective study of over 100 cases of childhood ANLL using MoAbs, we identified two patients whose leukemic blasts demonstrated myeloid-associated surface antigens (gp150) but were morphologically and cytochemically undifferentiated. Leukemic blasts from both patients subsequently demonstrated myeloperoxidase at the electron microscopic level, confirming the diagnosis of AML.

The addition of immunophenotyping information may also improve the intraobserver and interobserver reproducibility in classifying cases. In a study of over 100 cases Browman, Neame and Soamboonsrup (1986) demonstrated improved classification reproducibility when immunophenotype information was provided in addition to Wright-stained and cytochemical preparations.

A. Correlation of MoAb and FAB

There are several subtypes of ANLL that differ in morphology, histochemistry, and surface marker expression. The FAB classification, relating the morphologic appearance of leukemic cells to presumed normal hematopoietic counterparts identifies seven subtypes: M1 and M2 represent undifferentiated and differentiated myeloblastic leukemia; M3, promyelocytic leukemia; M4 and M5, myelomonocytic and monocytic variants; M6, erythroleukemia; and M7, megakaryocytic leukemia (Bennett et al., 1976, 1985a and 1985b; Breton-Gorius et al., 1978). Various investigators have reported briefer remissions or lower response and survival rates in patients with the M5 variant, fewer remissions in erythroleukemia (M6), and longer remissions in promyelocytic leukemia (M3), indicating that this classification has some prognostic importance (Head et al., 1985). The reactivities of a number of MoAbs (MY9, MY7, Mo5, V1M2) have shown no correlation with FAB-classified AML variants M1-M5 in extensive testing; too few patients with M6 and M7 variants were examined to permit conclusions (Griffin et al., 1983a). However, several other antibodies (including MY8, Mo1, MY4 and Mo2) appear to react with antigens expressed on leukemia cells displaying monocytic differentiation (M4 and M5, Table 5) (Griffin et al., 1983a, 1986). Likewise antibody MCS.2 has shown a correlation with FAB-M1 leukemia (Drexler et al., 1985). A myeloid immunophenotypic subclassification has been developed by Neame and coworkers that correlates well with the FAB classification using the pattern of reactivity with MoAbs; MY7, MY9, LeuM1, MY4, AML 2.23 and PMN 6/29 (Neame et al., 1986). If confirmed by other investigators, this immunophenotyping classification could be used to supplement the FAB system.

Antibody VIE-64, which binds to glycoprotein A (Knapp et al., 1981), and MoAb SFL 23.6, which has a well-defined reactivity restricted to the erythroid lineage (Das Gupta et al., 1985) should be useful reagents for distinguishing M6 variant cells. Monoclonal antibodies against platelet glycoproteins Ib, IIb, IIIa, aIIIaa (against factor VIII-related antigen) may be useful in identifying megakaryoblastic leukemia (Tetteroo et al., 1982). However, in our experience, antibodies to glycoprotein IIb may cross-react with myeloid leukemic cells M1-M5 (Mirro and Behm, unpublished observation). Thus, with the exception of FAB M4 through M7, the evidence for a correlation between surface marker expression and FAB classification is not convincing (van der Reijden et al., 1983; Griffin et al., 1986).

B. Cell Markers in CML

MoAbs are important in analyzing the acute phase (blast crisis) of chronic myelogenous leukemia. Chronic myelogenous leukemia (CML) is a myeloproliferative disorder characterized by a specific chromosomal abnormality, the Philadelphia (Ph^1) chromosome, occurring in a hematopoietic stem cell (Janossy,

Roberts and Greaves, 1976; Douer et al., 1981; Fialkow, Jacobson and Papagannopoulou, 1977). The Ph^1 chromosome results from a reciprocal translocation between chromosomes 9 and 22, designated t(9;22), with translocation of the c-abl oncogene from chromosome 9 to the Ph^1 chromosome. In the chronic phase of the disease, CML is characterized by an overproduction of relatively mature granulocytes. After a variable period of time (median of 3 years), most patients enter an acute phase (blast crisis) in which maturation no longer occurs (Griffin, Beveridge and Schlossman, 1982). This phase resembles acute leukemia. Determination of the lineage present in the blast crisis is of major importance to clinicians since the lineage dictates therapy and prognosis. Patients in lymphoid crisis may respond to vincristine and prednisone while those in myeloid blast crisis do not (Janossy et al., 1979). Approximately one-third of acute phase CML patients have cells with lymphoid features that include the expression of TdT, CALLA, Ia, B1, and rarely, rearrangements in immunoglobulin heavy and light chain genes (Janossy et al., 1977; Janossy et al., 1979; Bettelheim et al., 1985; Griffin et al., 1983c; Korsmeyer et al., 1981). Rare cases of lymphoid blast phase with T-cell markers have also been reported (Chan et al., 1986). In blast crisis involving myeloid cells, the cells typically resemble myeloblasts, but erythroblasts, megakaryoblasts, and monoblasts are also observed. Expression of several myeloid markers (MY7, MY9, VIM2, Mo1, and OKM1) on myeloid blast crisis cells and their lack of expression by lymphoid blast crisis cells provides important information for the detection of the lineage expressed during blast crisis.

Bettleheim and coworkers (1985) studied 45 patients with chronic myelogenous leukemia in blast crisis (CML-BC) and, using a large panel of monoclonal antibodies, demonstrated myeloid phenotype in over half; approximately one-third had a lymphoid phenotype, and the remainder were mixed or unclassifiable. In contrast with ANLL, MoAb studies in CML-BC have demonstrated frequent coexpression of megakaryocytic (61%) or erythropoietic (16%) along with myeloid differentiation (Bettleheim et al., 1985). Another large series of CML patients undergoing blast crisis likewise found that most blasts demonstrate a myeloid immunophenotype and confirmed that some patients exhibit surface antigens characteristics of more than one lineage (Griffin, 1983c). The capacity of the leukemic cells in CML to differentiate along several pathways supports the assumption that CML is a disease of the pluripotential hematopoietic stem cell (Parkin, McKenna and Brunning, 1982). As therapy improves, MoAbs may play a larger role in following CML patients.

C. Classifications of ANLL Using MoAbs

As a result of research using immunophenotyping, alternative classifications of ANLL have been proposed (Griffin et al., 1983a; Griffin and Schlossman, 1984; Linch et al., 1984). Drexler and colleagues (1985) have defined three types of nonlymphocytic leukemia based on antigen reactivity with MCS.2, MCS.1, and Ia. These researchers found a significant correlation between their immunologic type 1 (undifferentiated, MCS.2+, Ia+) and the FAB classification M1. Leukemias of FAB-M1 reacted significantly more often with MCS.2, which identifies the gp150 molecule. In this series, immunologic group II (MCS.2+, MCS.1+ and Ia+) or group III (MCS.2+, MCS.1+, Fc receptor positive) did not correlate with FAB classification.

In a series analyzing surface markers in ANLL, Griffin and co-workers (1983a) subdivided 70 patients into four phenotypic groups based on their blast cell pattern of surface antigen expression. Group I AML cases (21% of patients) expressed the antigenic phenotype of the CFU-C-committed myeloid progenitor cell (Ia and MY7 positive); group II cases (26%) displayed phenotypic characteristics of normal myeloblasts (MY7, Ia, Mo1/OKM1 and MY8 positive); group III cells (8%) showed the phenotype of normal promyelocytes (MY7 and Mo1/MY8 positive; Ia negative); and group IV cells (45%) expressed the phenotype characteristic of promonocytes and monocytes (MY4, MY7, MY8/Mo1, and Ia positive). Within these four groups, a large amount of morphologic heterogeneity existed: the myeloid leukemia (M1 and M2) and myelomonocytic leukemia (M4) patients were dispersed among all four groups.

A number of investigators have proposed myeloid differentiation schema to account for these findings. Ball and Fanger (1983) suggested that the normal M4 counterpart is an intermediate bipotential precursor cell capable of differentiating along either the monocytic or granulocytic pathway. In this differentiation schema the myeloblast (M1 and M2), which is the progenitor of the M4 cell, is also bipotential. Although the differentiation schema proposed by these investigators is consistent with some experimental findings, considerable additional data are required before they can be accepted. Furthermore, given the heterogeneity of surface antigen expression in AML, such hypotheses require further immunophenotyping studies of the clonogenic leukemic progenitors.

D. Heterogeneity in ANLL Immunophenotype

In most immunophenotyping studies of ANLL, patients are classified as "positive" for the expression of a marker if greater than 20% of their leukemic cells bear the determinant. Although certain antigens tend to be expressed by most of the leukemic cells (or normal cells), there is considerable variability (Ball et al., 1982b; Clement, Lehmeyer and Gartland, 1983; Sabbath et al., 1985). Marker expression appears to correlate with the level of myeloid differentiation, leading to the conclusion that the leukemic population is heterogeneous in its stage of differentiation; therefore, the block in differentiation which occurs in ANLL appears to be incomplete (Sachs, 1980). Evidence to support this assumption comes from in vitro clonogenic data. Leukemic myeloid progenitor cells from some patients can be grown in vitro in semisolid medium. The clonogenic leukemia cells (L-CFC) are, by definition, capable of limited proliferation (with a subset capable of self-renewal), a feature that distinguishes them from the majority of leukemic cells, which are terminally differentiated. Several groups have investigated the surface marker characteristics of L-CFC and found that the phenotype of the total leukemic cell population may not predict the L-CFC phenotype (Ball et al., 1982a; Ferrero et al., 1983a). In general, the L-CFC has a pattern of antigenic expression that is more "immature" than the predominant phenotype of the total population (Ferrero et al., 1983b).

E. Prognostic Value of MoAbs Studies in ANLL

A major objective in many immunophenotyping studies is to develop a classification system with independent prognostic significance. Recently, a large cooperative group study by Griffin and his colleagues (1986) demonstrated that immunophenotype has independent prognostic significance in adult myeloid leukemia. In this study, expression of several antigens (Ia, MY4, Mo1, Mo2) correlated with FAB M4 or M5. These results are consistent with earlier studies by other investigators (Table 5). The presence of monocytic-associated surface antigens (MY4 and Mo2) correlated with extramedullary disease and elevated white count. Expression of MY7 or MY4 antigen identified patients with a low rate of complete remission (CR). In this study, expression of antigen combinations was even more useful than expression of single antigens. For example, patients whose blasts did not express MY4 or MY7 had a very high CR rate, and the lack of both antigens was more predictive than either considered alone.

Surface antigen expression was also useful in studying patients achieving a complete remission: those whose blasts expressed Ia at diagnosis had a lower one-year continuous CR than those whose blasts did not. Likewise, blast expression of MY8 and Mo1 was associated with decreased continuous CR (median follow-up time of 19 months). This study demonstrated that myeloid marker analysis provides prognostic information independent of FAB classification.

F. MoAbs to Diagnose Residual Disease

Innovative uses of monoclonal antibodies include attempts to diagnose minimal residual disease. A recently developed monoclonal antibody, "CAMAL 1", appears to have strong selective reactivity with myeloid leukemia cells and is only slightly reactive with normal marrow myeloid cells (Levy et al., 1985; Logan, Malcolm and Levy, 1984). This antibody may provide an extremely valuable tool in diagnosing leukemia and evaluating minimal residual disease (Malcolm et al., 1984; Logan, Whitney, Naiman and Levy, unpublished observation). Expression of the CAMAL-1 antigen appears to be useful for predicting relapse after bone marrow transplant. This MoAb may be extremely important in determining the advisability of bone marrow transplant for patients in first complete remission of ANLL. Because of cross-reactivity with normal myeloid cells, no other monoclonal antibody appears to be useful for predicting residual disease in ANLL.

VI. POTENTIAL THERAPEUTIC USES OF MONOCLONAL ANTIBODIES

Cross-reactivity between normal hematopoietic progenitors and leukemic cells limits the therapeutic usefulness of MoAbs to myeloid-associated surface antigens. In some patients the administration of MoAbs led to transient reduction in circulating leukemia cells; there was no sustained effect on the bone marrow, involved lymph nodes or other organs (Ball et al., 1983). Side effects of monoclonal antibody therapy are usually minor. Respiratory distress following the rapid infusion of monoclonal antibody has been described, and some patients have demonstrated transient elevation of creatinine and hepatic enzymes. However, by using MoAbs that react with mature antigens present on leukemic cells but not on early normal hematopoietic progenitors, immunotherapy in ANLL appears promising. MoAbs PM-81 (CD15) and AML 2.23 (CDw14,55) with complement have been used for ex vivo treatment of bone marrow before autologous transplantation in AML patients with excellent early results (Ball et al., 1986). Likewise, monoclonal antibodies conjugated to toxins could serve to eliminate the more "mature" leukemic cells.

With the development of MoAbs to the gp115 surface antigen (MY10, BI-3C5); the potential exists to purify normal hematopoietic progenitors from bone marrow that may be involved with minimal residual leukemia (Civin et al., 1984). Patients could then undergo autologous bone marrow transplant using a marrow enriched for normal hematopoietic progenitors and depleted (possibly by MoAbs) of leukemia.

One major problem with these approaches has been the marked variability in surface phenotype within the ANLL population. The immunofluorescence reactivity of the total leukemic population does not necessarily predict the phenotype of the clonogenic cells. In some patients the clonogenic leukemic cells express a phenotype similar to the relatively mature normal colony forming cells (late CFU-GM), while in others the clonogenic leukemic cell may be similar to the less mature colony forming cells (early CFU-GM or CFU-GEMM); finally, a composite phenotype may exist. Thus, separating leukemic clonogenic cells from normal clonogenic cells using monoclonal antibodies may be difficult and require analysis of the clonogenic leukemic cell in each patient.

VII. SUMMARY

A large number of monoclonal antibodies reactive with myeloid surface antigens have been developed and described. Fortunately, as a result of the First, Second and Third International Workshops, a common nomenclature has been developed. With a common nomenclature, previous publications can be compared and some meaningful conclusions drawn. With the more recent biochemical studies and DNA-mediated gene transfer studies, this complex field is becoming clearer. It is now obvious that a number of monoclonal antibodies react with the same cell surface molecule but often with different epitopes.

Some MoAbs appear useful in identifying cell surface antigens common to most cases of acute nonlymphocytic leukemia, including the antibodies that recognize the gp150 (CDw13) and p67 (MY9, L4F3 and L1B3). Likewise, antibodies that recognize the gp115 (MY10 and BI-1C5) may prove to be useful in identifying even more undifferentiated myeloid cells, although this has not yet been clearly shown.

From the elegant work of Griffin and others, it would appear that reactivity with several monoclonal antibodies, specifically MY7, MY4, Ia, Mo1 and MY8, correlate with prognosis. These MoAbs appear to add prognostic information independent of the FAB classification and, therefore, may prove beneficial in prospective studies of therapy. The recent demonstration that ex vivo bone marrow purging with MoAbs is feasible may lead to additional therapeutic trials using MoAbs. While further information is being generated from prospective studies, it appears warranted to test ANLL blasts with MoAbs from each cluster group identified by the International Workshops. In an effort to correlate immunophenotype with biologic characteristics and clinical outcome, immunophenotyping studies should be done in conjunction with large clinical trials and other biological studies.

ACKNOWLEDGMENTS

We wish to thank the following investigators for kindly supplying unpublished information: Drs. J. D. Griffin, K. A. Foon, R. F. Todd, S. Peiper, A. T. Look, J. Levy, H. G., Drexler, P. B. Neame and W. Knapp. We wish to thank Ms. Christy Wright for editorial assistance and P. Vandiveer, and V. Gray for typing.

REFERENCES

Andrews, R. G., Torok-Storb, B., and Bernstein, I. D. (1983). Myeloid-associated differentiation antigens on stem cells and their progeny identified by monoclonal antibodies. *Blood* 62:124-132.

Arnaout, M. A., Pitt, J., Cohen, J. J., Melamed, J., Rosen, F. S., and Colten, H. R. (1982). Deficiency of a granulocyte-membrane glycoprotein (gp150) in a boy with recurrent bacterial infections. *New Engl. J. Med.* 306:693-699.

Arnaout, M. A., Todd, R. F. III, Dana, N., Melamed, J., Schlossman, S. F., and Colten, H. R. (1983). Inhibition of phagocytosis of complement C3- or immunoglobulin G-coated particles and of C3bi binding by monoclonal antibodies to the monocyte-granulocyte glycoprotein (Mo1). *J. Clin. Invest.* 72:171-179.

Ball, E. D., and Fanger, M. W. (1983). The expression of myeloid-specific antigens on myeloid leukemia cells: correlations with leukemia subclasses and implications for myeloid differentiation. *Blood* 61:456-463.

Ball, E. D., Kadushin, J. M., Schacter, B., and Fanger, M. W. (1982a). Studies on the ability of monoclonal antibodies to selectively mediate complement-dependent cytotoxicity of human myelogenous leukemia blast cells. *J. Immunol.* 128:1476-1481.

Ball, E. D., Graziano, R. F., Shen, L., and Fanger, M. W. (1982b). Monoclonal antibodies to novel myeloid antigens reveal human neutrophil heterogeneity. *Proc. Natl. Acad. Sci. USA* 79:5374-5378.

Ball, E. D., Bernier, G. M., Cornwell, G. G. III, McIntyre, O. R., O'Donnell, J. F., and Fanger, M. W. (1983). Monoclonal antibodies to myeloid differentiation antigens: *In-vivo* studies of three patients with acute myelogenous leukemia. *Blood* 62:1203-1210.

Ball, E. D., Mills, L. E., Coughlin, C. T., Beck, J. R., and Cornwell, G. G. (1986b). Autologous bone marrow transplantation in acute myelogenous leukemia: In vitro treatment with myeloid cell-specific monoclonal antibodies. *Blood* 68: 1311-1315.

Beatty, P. G., Ledbetter, J. A., Martin, P. J., Price, T. H., Hansen, J. A. (1983). Definition of a common leukocyte cell-surface antigen (gp95-150) associated with diverse cell-mediated immune functions. *J. Immunol.* 131:2913-2919.

Bennett, J. M., Begg, C. B. (1981). Eastern Cooperative Oncology Group Study of the cytochemistry of adult acute myeloid leukemia by correlation of subtypes with response and survival. *Cancer Res.* 41:4833-4837.

Bennett, J. M., Catovski, D., Daniel, M. T., Flandrin, G., Galton, D. A. G., Gralnick, H. R., and Sultan, C. (1976). Proposals for the classification of the acute leukemias. *Br. J. Haematol.* 33:451-458.

Bennett, J. M., Catovsky, D., Daniel, M. T., Flandrin, G., Galton, D. A. G., Gralnick, H. R., and Sultan, C. (1985a). Criteria for the diagnosis of acute leukemia of megakaryocytic lineage (M7). A report of the French-American-British co-operative group. *Ann. Int. Med.* 103:460-462.

Bennett, J. M., Catovsky, D., Daniel, M. T., Flandrin, G., Galton, D. A. G., Gralnick, H. R., and Sultan, C. (1985b). Proposed revised criteria for the classification of acute myeloid leukemia: A report of the French-American-British Cooperative Group. *Ann. Int. Med.* 103:620-625.

Bernard, A., Boumsell, L., and Hill, C. (1984). Joint report of the First International Workshop on Human Leucocyte Differentiation Antigens by the investigators of the participating laboratories. In *Leukocyte Typing*, A. Bernard, L. Boumsell, J. Dausset, C. Milstein, S. F. Schlossman (eds.). Springer-Verlag, Berlin, pp. 9-135.

Bernstein, I. D., and Self, S. (1986). Joint report of the myeloid section of the Second International Workshop on Human Leucocyte Differentiation Antigens. In *Leukocyte Typing II*, Vol. 3, E. Reinherz, B. Haynes, L. Nadler, I. D. Bernstein (eds.). Springer-Verlag, New York, pp. 1-25.

Bernstein, I. D., Andrews, R. G., Cohen, S. F., McMaster, B. E. (1982). Normal and malignant human myelocytic and monocytic cells identified by monoclonal antibodies. *J. Immunol.* 128:876-881.

Bettelheim, P., Lutz, D., Majdic, O., Paietta, E., Haas, O., Linkesch, W., Neumann, E., Lechner, K., and Knapp, W. (1985). Cell lineage heterogeneity in blast crisis of chronic myeloid leukaemia. *Br. J. Haematol.* 59:395-400.

Bloomfield, C. D., Goldman, A., Hassfeld, D., and de la Chapelle, A. (1984). Fourth International Workshop of Chromosomes in Leukemia 1982: The clinical significance of chromosomal abnormalities in acute nonlymphoblastic leukemia. *Cancer Genet. Cytogenet.* 11:332-350.

Breard, J., Reinherz, E. L., Kung, P. C., Goldstein, G., and Schlossman, S. F. (1980). A monoclonal antibody reactive with human peripheral blood monocytes. *J. Immunol.* 124:1943-1948.

Breton-Gorius, J., Reyes, F., Vernant, J. P., Tulliez, M., and Dreyfus, B. (1978). The blast crisis of chronic granulocytic leukaemia: megakaryoblastic nature of cells as revealed by the presence of platelet-peroxidase a cytochemical ultrastructural study. *Br. J. Haematol.* 39:295-303.

Brouet, J. C., Valensi, F., Daniel, M. T., Flandrin, G., Preud'homme, J. L., and Seligmann, M. (1976). Immunological classification of acute lymphoblastic leukemia: Evaluation of its clinical significance in a hundred patients. *Br. J. Haematol.* 33:319-328.

Browman, G. P., Neame, P. B., and Soamboonsrup, P. (1986). The contribution of cytochemistry and immunophenotyping to the reproducibility of the FAB classification in acute leukemia. *Blood* 68:900-905.

Burmester, G. R., Winchester, R. J., Dimitriu-Bona, A., Klein, M., Steiner, G., Sissons, H. A. (1983). Delineation of four cell types comprising the giant cell tumor of bones. Expression of Ia and monocyte-macrophage lineage antigens. *J. Clin. Invest.* 71:1633-1648.

Chan, L. C., Furley, A. J., Ford, A. M., Yardumian, D. A., and Greaves, M. F. (1986). Clonal rearrangement and expression of the T cell receptor β gene and involvement of the breakpoint cluster region in blast crisis of CGL. *Blood* 67:533-536.

Chan, L. C., Pegram, S. M., and Greaves, M. F. (1985). Contribution of immunophenotype to the classification and differential diagnosis of acute leukemia. *Lancet* 1:475-479.

Chessels, J. M., Hardisty, R. M., Rapoon, N. T., and Greaves, M. F. (1977). Acute lymphoblastic leukaemia in children: Classification and prognosis. *Lancet* 2: 1307-1309.

Civin, C. I., Mirro, J., and Banquerigo, M. L. (1981). My-1 a new myeloid specific antigen identified by a mouse monoclonal antibody. *Blood* 57:842-845.

Civin, C. I., Strauss, L. C., Brovall, C., Fackler, M. J., Schwartz, J. F., and Shaper, J. H. (1984). Antigenic analysis of hematopoiesis III. A hematopoietic progenitor cell surface antigen defined by a monoclonal antibody raised against KG-1a cells. *J. Immunol.* 133:157-165.

Clement, L. T., Lehmeyer, J. E., and Gartland, G. L. (1983). Identification of neutrophil subpopulations with monoclonal antibodies. *Blood* 61:326-332.

Das Gupta, A., Samoszuk, M. K., Papayannopoulou, T., and Stamatoxannopoulos, G. (1985). SFL 23.6: a monoclonal antibody reactive and CFU-E, erythroblasts and erythrocytes. *Blood* 66:522-526.

Dimitriu-Bona, A., Burmester, G. R., Waters, S. J., Winchester, R. J. (1983). Human mononuclear phagocyte differentiation antigens. I. Patterns of antigenic expression on the surface of human monocytes and macrophages defined by monoclonal antibodies. *J. Immunol.* 130:145-152.

Dinndorf, P. A., Benjamin, D., Ridgway, D., and Bernstein, I. D. (1985). Immunodiagnosis of childhood ALL with monoclonal antibodies to myeloid and lymphoid associated antigens. *Leuk. Res.* 9:449-461.

Dinndorf, P. A., Andrews, R. G., Benjamin, D., Ridgway, D., Wolff, L., and Bernstein, I. D. (1986). Expression of normal myeloid-associated antigens by acute leukemia cells. *Blood* 67:1048-1053.

Douer, D., Levin, A. M., Sparkes, R. S., Fabian, I., Sparkes, M., Cline, M. J., and Koeffler, H. P. (1981). Chronic myelocytic leukaemia: a pluri-potent haemopoietic cell is involved in the malignant clone. *Br. J. Haematol.* 49:615-619.

Drexler, H. G., Sagawa, K., Menon, M., and Minowada, J. (1985). "Pan-myeloid" reagent: the monoclonal antibody MCS-2 in the routine immunodiagnostic service of leukemia phenotyping. *Gann* 76:235-239.

Ferrero, D., Broxmeyer, H. E., Pagliardi, G. L., Venuta, S., Lange, B., Pessano, S., and Rovera, G. (1983a). Antigenically distinct subpopulations of myeloid progenitor cells (CFU-GM) in human peripheral blood and marrow. *Proc. Natl. Acad. Sci. USA* 80:4114-4118.

Ferrero, D., Pessano, S., Pagliardi, G. L., and Rovera, G. (1983b). Induction of differentiation of human myeloid leukemias: surface changes probed with monoclonal antibodies. *Blood* 61:171-179.

Fialkow, P. J., Jacobson, R. J., and Papayannopoulou, T. (1977). Chronic myelocytic leukemia: clonal origin in a stem cell common to the granulocyte, erythrocyte, platelet and monocyte/macrophage. *Am. J. Med.* 63:125-130.

Fialkow, P. J., Singer, J. W., Adamson, J. W., Vaidya, K., Dow, L. W., Ochs, J., and Moohr, J. W. (1981). Acute nonlymphocytic leukemia: Heterogeneity of stem cell origin. *Blood* 57:1068-1073.

Flandrin, G., Brouet, J. C., Daniel, M. T., and Preud'homme, J. L. (1975). Acute leukemia with Burkitt's tumor cells: A study of six cases with special reference to lymphocyte surface markers. *Blood* 45:183-188.

Foon, K. A., Naiem, F., Yale, C., and Gale, R. P. (1979). Acute myelogenous leukemia: morphologic classification and response to therapy. *Leuk. Res.* 3:171-173.

Foon, K. A., and Todd, R. F. (1986). Immunologic classification of leukemia and lymphoma. *Blood* 68:1-31.

Greaves, M. F., Chan, L. C., Furley, A. J. W., Watt, S. M., and Molgaard, H. V. (1986). Lineage promiscuity in hemopoietic differentiation and leukemia. *Blood* 67:1-11.

Gregg, S. L., Gajl-Peczalska, K. J., LeBien, T. W., Bloomfield, C. D., Brunning, R., Sagawa, K. (1984). Monoclonal antibody MCS-2 as the marker of phorbol diester-induced myeloid differentiation in acute undifferentiated leukemia. *Cancer Res.* 44:2724-2730.

Griffin, J. D., and Schlossman, S. F. (1984). Expression of myeloid differentiation antigens in acute myeloblastic leukemia. In *Leukocyte Typing*, A. Bernard, L. Boumsell, J. Dausset, C. Milstein, S. F. Schlossman (eds.). Springer-Verlag, Berlin, pp. 404-410.

Griffin, J. D., Beveridge, R. P., and Schlossman, S. F. (1982). Isolation of myeloid progenitor cells from peripheral blood of chronic myelogenous leukemia patients. *Blood* 60:30-37.

Griffin, J. D., Ritz, J., Nadler, L. M., and Schlossman, S. F. (1981). Expression of myeloid differentiation antigens in normal and malignant myeloid cells. *J. Clin. Invest.* 68:932-941.

Griffin, J. D., Linch, D., Sabbath, K., Larcom, P., Schlossman, S. F. (1984). A monoclonal antibody reactive with normal and leukemic human myeloid progenitor cells. *Leuk. Res.* 8:5221-5234.

Griffin, J. D., Mayer, R. J., Weinstein, H. J., Rosenthal, D. S., Coral, F. S., Beveridge, R. P., and Schlossman, S. F. (1983a). Surface marker analysis of acute myeloblastic leukemia: identification of differentiation-associated phenotypes. *Blood* 62:557-563.

Griffin, J. D., Ritz, J., Beveridge, R. P., Lipton, J. M., Daley, J. F., and Schlossman, S. F. (1983b). Expression of MY7 antigen on myeloid precursor cells. *Int. J. Cell Cloning* 1:33-48.

Griffin, J. D., Todd, F. J. III, Ritz, J., Nadler, L. M., Canellos, G. P., Rosenthal, D., Gallivan, M., Beveridge, R. P., Weinstein, H., Karp, D., and Schlossman, S. F. (1983c). Differentiation patterns in the blastic phase of chronic myeloid leukemia. *Blood* 61:85-91.

Griffin, J. D., Davis, R., Nelson, D. A., Davey, F. R., Mayer, R. J., Schiffer, C., McIntyre, O. R., and Bloomfield, C. D. (1986). Use of surface marker analysis to predict outcome of adult acute myeloblastic leukemia. *Blood* 68:1232-1241.

Hanjan, S. N., Kearney, J. F., Cooper, M. D. (1982). A monoclonal antibody (MMA) that identifies a differentiation antigen on human myelomonocytic cells. *Clin. Immunol. Immunopathol.* 23:172-188.

Head, D. R., Savage, R. A., Cerezo, L., Craven, C. M., Bickers, J. N., Hartsock, R., Hosty, T. A., Saiki, J. H., Wilson, H. E., Morrison, F. S., Coltman, C. A., and Hutton, J. J. (1985). Reproducibility of the French-American-British classification of acute leukemia. The Southwest Oncology Group experience. *Am. J. Hematol.* 18:47-57.

Hildreth, J. E., Gotch, F. M., Hildreth, P. D., McMichael, A. J. (1983). A human lymphocyte-associated antigen involved in cell-mediated lympholysis. *Eur. J. Immunol.* 13:202-208.

Huang, L. C., Civin, C. I., Magnani, J. H., Shaper, J. J., and Ginsberg, V. (1983). My-1, the human myeloid-specific antigen detected by mouse monoclonal antibodies, is a sugar sequence found in lacto-N-fucopentaose III. *Blood* 61: 1020-1023.

Huang, M. J., Li, C. Y., Nichols, W. L., Young, J. H., and Katzmann, J. A. (1984). Acute leukemia with megakaryocytic differentiation: a study of 12 cases identified immunocytochemically. *Blood* 64:427-439.

Janossy, G., Roberts, M., and Greaves, M. F. (1976). Target cell in chronic myeloid leukaemia and its relationship to acute lymphoid leukaemia. *Lancet* 1: 1058-1060.

Janossy, G., Greaves, M. F., Sutherland, R., Durrant, J., and Lewis, C. (1977). Comparative analysis of membrane phenotypes in acute lymphoid leukemia and in lymphoid blast crisis of chronic myeloid leukemia. *Leuk. Res.* 1:289-300.

Janossy, G., Woodruff, R. K., Pippard, M. J., Prentice, G., Hoffbrand, A. V., Paxton, A., Lister, T. A., Bunch, C., and Greaves, M. F. (1979). Relation of "lymphoid" phenotype and response to chemotherapy incorporating vincristine-prednisone in the acute phase of Ph^1 positive leukemia. *Cancer* 43: 426-434.

Janowska-Wieczorek, A., Mannoni, P., Turner, A. F., McGann, L. E., Shaw, A. R. E., and Turc, J.-M. (1984). Monoclonal antibody specific for granulocytic lineage cells and reactive with human pluripotent and committed haematopoietic progenitor cells. *Br. J. Haematol.* 58:159-168.

Kamoun, M., Martin, P. J., Kadin, M. E., Lum, L. G., Hansen, J. A. (1983). Human monocyte-histiocyte differentiation antigens identified by monoclonal antibodies. *Clin. Immunol. Immunopathol.* 29:181-195.

Knapp, W., Majdic, O., Rumpold, H., Bettelheim, P., Kraft, D., Liszka, K., Forster, O., and Lutz, D. (1981). Myeloid differentiation antigens as defined by monoclonal antibodies. In *Leukemia Markers*, W. Knapp (ed.). Academic Press, London, p. 207.

Korsmeyer, S. J., Hieter, P. A., Ravetch, J. V., Poplack, D. G., Waldmann, T. A., and Leder, P. (1981). Developmental hierarchy of immunoglobulin gene rearrangements in human leukemic pre-B-cells. *Proc. Natl. Acad. Sci. USA* 78: 7096-7196.

Krensky, A. M., Robbins, E., Springer, T. A., Burakoff, S. J. (1984). LFA-1, LFA-2, and LFA-3 antigens are involved in CTL-target conjugation. *J. Immunol.* 132:2180-2182.

Leary, A. G., Strauss, L. C., Civin, C. I., and Ogawa, M. (1985). Disparate differentiation in hemopoietic colonies derived from human paired progenitors. *Blood* 66:327-332.

Levy, J. G., Logan, P. M., Whitney, S., Malcolm, A. J., Naiman, S., Powles, R., and Crawford, D. (1985). Demonstration of a leukemia-associated antigen (CAMAL) in peripheral blood leucocytes of bone marrow transplant patients prior to relapse. *Transplantation* 40:167-173.

Linch, D. C., Allen, C., Beverley, P. C. L., Bynoe, A. G., Scott, C. S., and Hogg, N. (1984). Monoclonal antibodies differentiating between monocytic and nonmonocytic variants of AML. *Blood* 63:566-573.

Linkler-Israeli, M., Billing, R. J., Foon, K. A., and Terasaki, P. I. (1981). Monoclonal antibodies reactive with acute myelogeneous leukemia cells. *J. Immunol.* 127:2473-2477.

Logan, P. M., Malcolm, A. J., and Levy, J. G. (1984). Detection of a common leukemia-associated antigen in human myelogenous leukemia using immunoperoxidase. *Diagn. Immunolo.* 2:86-97.

Look, A. T., Peiper, S. C., Rebentisch, M. B., Ashmun, R. A., Roussel, M. F., Rettenmier, C. W., and Sherr, C. J. (1985). Transfer and expression of the gene encoding a human myeloid membrane antigen (gp150). *J. Clin. Invest.* 75:569-579.

Look, A. T., Peiper, S. C., Rebentisch, M. B., Ashmun, R. A., Roussel, M. F., Lemons, R. S., LeBeau, M. M., Rubin, C. M., and Sherr, C. J. (1986). Molecular cloning, expression, and chromosomal localization of the gene encoding a human myeloid membrane antigen (gp150). *J. Clin. Invest.* 78:914-921.

McKolanis, J. R., Borowitz, M. J., Tuck, F. L., Metzgar, R. S. (1984). Membrane antigens of human myeloid cells defined by monoclonal antibodies. In *Leukocyte Typing*, A. Bernard, L. Boumsell, J. Dausset, C. Milstein, and S. F. Schlossman (eds.). Springer-Verlag, Berlin, p. 387.

Majdic, O., Liszka, K., Lutz, D., and Knapp, W. (1981). Myeloid differentiation antigen defined by a monoclonal antibody. *Blood* 58:1127-1133.

Malcolm, A. J., Shipman, R. C., Logan, P. M., and Levy, J. G. (1984). A monoclonal antibody to myelogenous leukemia: isolation and characterization. *Exp. Hematol.* 12:539-547.

Mannoni, P., Janowska-Wieczorek, A., Turner, A. R., McGann, L., Turc, J. M. (1982). Monoclonal antibodies against human granulocytes and myeloid differentiation antigens. *Hum. Immunol.* 5:309-323.

Miedma, F., Tetteroo, P. A. T., Hesselink, W. G., Werner, G., Spits, H., Melief, C. J. M. (1984). Both F_c receptors and lymphocyte-function-associated antigen 1 on human Ty lymphocytes are required for antibody-dependent cellular cytotoxicity (killer cell activity). *Eur. J. Immunol.* 14:518-523.

Mirro, J., Antoun, G. R., Zipf, T. F., Melvin, S., and Stass, S. (1985a). The E-rosette-associated antigen of T-cells can be identified on blasts from patients with acute myeloblastic leukemia. *Blood* 75:363-367.

Mirro, J., Zipf, T. F., Pui, C.-H., Kitchingman, G., Williams, D., Melvin, S., Murphy, S. B., and Stass, S. (1985b). Acute mixed lineage leukemia: clinicopathologic correlations and prognostic significance. *Blood* 66:1115-1123.

Mirro, J., Melvin, S., Metzger, D., Look, A. T., Murphy, S. (1984). Changes in cell surface antigen expression during myelocytic and monocytic cell differentiation. In *Leukocyte Typing*, A. Bernard, L. Boumsell, J. Daussel, C. Milstein, and S. F. Schlossman (eds.). Springer-Verlag, Berlin, p. 442-445.

Neame, P. B., Soamboonsrup, P., Browman, G. P., Meyer, R. M., Benger, A., Wilson, W. E. C., Walker, I. R., Saeed, N., and McBride, J. A. (1986). Classifying acute leukemia by immunophenotyping: A combined FAB-Immunologic classification of AML. *Blood* 68:1355-1362.

Parkin, J. L., McKenna, R. W., and Brunning, R. D. (1982). Philadelphia chromosome-positive blastic leukaemia: ultrastructural and ultracytochemical evidence of basophil and mast cell differentiation. *Br. J. Haematol.* 52:663-677.

Paweresch, M. R., Radzun, H. J., Hansmann, M.-L., Peters, K.-P. (1983). Monoclonal antibody Ki-M4 specificially recognizes human dendritic reticulum cells (follicular dendritic cells) and their possible precursor in blood. *Blood* 62: 585-590.

Peiper, S. C., Ashmun, R. A., and Look, A. T. (1986). DNA-mediated transfer of the gene encoding the p67 myeloid differentiation antigen recognized by MY9, L1B2, and L4F3. (Abstract). Third International Workshop on Human Leukocyte Differentiation Antigens, p. 71.

Perussia, B., Trinchieri, G., Lebman, D., Jankiewicz, J., Lange, B., and Rovera, G. (1982). Monoclonal antibodies that detect differentiation antigens on human myelomonocytic cells. *Blood* 59:382-392.

Peschel, C., Konwalinka, G., Geissler, D., Grunewald, K., Liszka, K., Stockinger, H., Majdic, D., Braunsteiner, H., Knapp, W. (1986). Reactivity of anti-myeloid monoclonal antibodies with committed hematopoietic precursor cells. In *Leukocyte Typing II*, Vol. 3, E. L. Reinherz, B. F. Haynes, L. M. Nadler, and I. D. Bernstein (eds.). Springer-Verlag, New York, pp. 181-192.

Pessano, S., Palumbo, A., Ferrero, D., Pagliardi, G. L., Bottero, L., Lai, S. K., Meo, P., Carter, C., Hubbell, H., Lange, B., and Rovera, G. (1984). Subpopulation heterogeneity in human acute myeloid leukemia determined by monoclonal antibodies. *Blood* 64:275-281.

Rumpold, H., Kraft, D., Obexer, G., Bock, G., Gebhart, W. (1982). A monoclonal antibody against a surface antigen shared by human large granular lymphocytes and granulocytes. *J. Immunol.* 129:1458-1464.

Sabbath, K. D., Ball, E. D., Larcom, P., Davis, R. B., and Griffin, J. D. (1985). Heterogenity of clonogenic cells in acute myeloblastic leukemia. *J. Clin. Invest.* 75:746-753.

Sachs, L. (1980). Constitutive uncoupling of pathways of gene expression that control growth and differentiation in myeloid leukemia. A model for the origin and progression of malignancy. *Proc. Natl. Acad. Sci. USA* 77:6152-6156.

Schwarting, R., Stein, H., Wang, C. Y. (1985). The monoclonal antibodies *α* S-HCL 1 (*α* Leu-14) and *α* S-HCL 3 (*α* Leu-M5) allow the diagnosis of hairy cell leukemia. *Blood* 65:974-983.

Seremetis, S., Cuttner, J., Winchester, R. (1984). Definition of AML susceptibility and classification using monoclonal antibodies. *Med. Oncol. Tumor Pharmacother.* 1:263-267.

Seymour, G. J., Poulter, L. W., Bofill, M., Hobbs, S., Janossy, G., Brooks, D., Zola, H., Bradley, J. (1983). The reactivity of a monoclonal antibody against cells of the monocyte-macrophage series in sections of normal and inflamed human tissues. *J. Reticuloendothel. Soc.* 34:463-473.

Skubitz, K. M., Zhen, Y. S., and August, J. T. (1983). A human granulocyte-specific antigen characterized by use of monoclonal antibodies. *Blood* 61: 19-26.

Skubitz, K., Pessano, S., Bottero, L., Ferrero, D., Rovera, G., and August, T. A. (1983). Human granulocyte surface molecules identified by murine monoclonal antibodies. *J. Immunol.* 131:1882-1888.

Smith, L. J., Curtis, J. E., Messner, H. A., Senn, J. S., Furthmayr, H., and McCulloch, E. A. (1983). Lineage infidelity in acute leukemia. *Blood* 61:1138-1145.

Strauss, L. C., Stuart, R. K., and Civin, C. I. (1983). Antigen analysis of hematopoiesis. I. Expression of the My-1 granulocyte surface antigen on human marrow cells and leukemic cell lines. *Blood* 61:1222-1231.

Strauss, L. C., Skubitz, K. M., August, J. T., and Civin, C. I. (1984). Antigenic analysis of hematopoiesis: II. Expression of human neutrophil antigens on normal and leukemic marrow cells. *Blood* 63:574-578.

Symington, F. W., McMaster, B. E., Hakomori, S., and Bernstein, I. D. (1985). Glycolipid specificites of anti-hematopoietic cell antibodies. In *Leukocyte Typing II*, Vol. 3, E. Reinherz, B. Haynes, L. Nadler, and I. D. Bernstein (eds.). Springer-Verlag, New York, pp. 47-54.

Takacs, L., Szende, B., Monostori, E., Rot, A., Lapis, K., Szecseny, A., Ando, I. (1983). Expression of HLA-DR antigen on bileduct cells of rejected liver transplant. *Lancet* 2:1500. (letter).

Tatsumi, E., Sagawa, K., Mirro, J., Civin, C. I., Preisler, H. D., Henderson, E. S., Minowada, J. (1981). Immunologic membrane phenotypes in human myeloid leukemia by monoclonal antibodies. *Proc. Am. Assoc. Cancer Res.* 22:181. (abstract).

Tetteroo, P. A. T., Lansdorp, P. M., Leeksma, O. C., and Von Dem Borne, A. E. G. K. (1982). Monoclonal antibodies against human platelet glycoprotein IIIa. *Br. J. Haematol.* 55:509-522.

Thompson, J. (1984). In *Advances in Immunobiology*. J. S. Thompson et al. (eds.). Alan Liss, Inc., New York, p. 169.

Thompson, J. S., Wekstein, D. R., Rhoades, J. L., Kirkpatrick, C., Brown, S. A., Roxzman, T., Straus, R., Tietz, N. (1984). The immune status of healthy centenarians. *J. Am. Geriatr. Soc.* 32:274-281.

Tindle, R. W., Katz, F., Martin, H., Watt, S., Catovsky, D., Janossy, G., Greaves, M. (1986). BI-3C5 defines multipotential and lineage restricted haemopoietic progenitor cells and their leukaemic counterparts (abstract). Third International Workshop on Human Leukocyte Differentiation Antigens, p. 74.

Todd, R. F., Roach, J. A., Arnaout, M. A. (1985). The modulated expression of Mo5, a human myelomonocytic plasma membrane antigen. *Blood* 65:946-973.

Todd, R. F. III, and Arnaout, M. A. (1986). Monoclonal antibodies that identify Mo1 and LFA-1, two human leukocyte membrane glycoproteins: A review. In *Leukocyte Typing II*, Vol. 3, E. Reinherz, B. Haynes, L. Nadler, and I. D. Bernstein (eds.). Springer-Verlag, New York, pp. 95-108.

Todd, R. F. III, Arnaout, M. A., Rosen, R. E., Crowley, C. A., Peters, W. A., and Babior, B. M. (1984). Subcellular localization of the large subunit of Mo1 (Mo1*a*: formerly gp110), a surface glycoprotein associated with neutrophil adhesion. *J. Clin. Invest.* 74:1280-1290.

Van der Reijden, H. J., van Rhenen, D. J., Lansdorp, P. M., van't Veer, M., Langehuijsen, M. M. A. C., Engelfrezt, C. P., and von dem Borne, A. E. G. K. (1983). A comparison of surface marker analysis and FAB classification in acute myeloid leukemia. *Blood* 61:443-448.

Vaughn, W. P., Strauss, L. C., Burke, P. J., Skubitz, K. M., Schwartz, J. F., Karp, J. E., and Civin, C. I. (1983). Surface marker phenotype (SMP) predicts response to therapy in acute non-lymphocytic leukemia (ANLL). *Proc. Am. Soc. Clin. Oncol.* 23:183 (abstr).

Wallis, W. J., Kickstein, D. D., Schwartz, B. R., June, C. H., Ochs, H. D., Beatty, P. G., Klebanoff, S. J., and Harlan, J. M. (1986). Monoclonal antibody-defined functional epitopes on adhesion-promoting glycoprotein complex (CDw18) of human neutrophils. *Blood* 67:1007-1013.

Winchester, R. J., Ross, G. D., Jarowski, C. J., Wang, C. Y., Halper, J., and Broxmeyer, H. E. (1977). Expression of Ia-like antigens on human granulocytes during early phases of differentiation. *Proc. Natl. Acad. Sci. USA* 74: 4012-4016.

Wright, S. D., Rao, P. E., Van Voorhis, W. C., Craigmyle, L. S. Iida, K., Talle, M. A., Westberg, E. F., Goldstein, G., and Silverstein, S. C. (1983). Identification of the C3bi receptor of human monocytes and macrophages by using monoclonal antibodies. *Proc. Natl. Acad. Sci. USA* 80:5699-5703.

Zola, H., McNamara, P., Thomas, M., Smart, I. J., Bradley, J. (1981). The preparation and properties of monoclonal antibodies against human granulocyte membrane antigens. *Br. J. Haematol.* 48:481-490.

9

Characterization of Acute Leukemia Using Lineage-Associated Molecular Probes

WINFRIED B. GRANINGER* *Howard Hughes Medical Institute, Washington University School of Medicine, St. Louis, Missouri*

JOHN J. WRIGHT and CAROLYN A. FELIX *National Cancer Institute, National Institutes of Health, Bethesda, Maryland*

STANLEY J. KORSMEYER *Howard Hughes Medical Institute, Washington University School of Medicine, St. Louis, Missouri*

The characterization of leukemic cell populations has recently been improved by the application of molecular biology techniques. These methods provided the tools for a more detailed understanding of the molecular mechanisms involved in the development and maturation of normal bone marrow cells. In return, this body of knowledge provided insights into the clonality, lineage commitment, stage of differentiation, and mechanisms of transformation of lymphocytic leukemias. Prior to recombinant DNA technology, the most dramatic progress in characterizing neoplastic populations was achieved by the immunologic analysis of cell surface antigens associated with cellular lineages and maturational stages (Aisenberg, 1978; Jaffe et al., 1977). This determination of cell surface phenotype helped refine conventional classifications based on morphology and histochemistry.

However, the detection of a given surface antigen relies upon the availability of a specific antibody directed against the molecule of interest. Thus they are of no value in immature cell populations, which do not yet express this antigen. Furthermore, virtually none of these antigens are solely restricted to malignant cells; they are present on normal cellular counterparts as well. Thus, they frequently lack the ability to discriminate between neoplastic and admixed normal cells within a tumor sample. Moreover, before the molecular biology era, the determination that a lymphoid neoplasm was clonal was for all practical purposes limited to B-cell malignancies, which exclusively expressed but one cell surface immunoglobulin light-chain class, kappa (κ) or lambda (λ). Due to these limita-

**Current affiliation*: Second Department of Medicine, University of Vienna, Vienna, Austria

tions of classic immunologic characterization, we have pursued a molecular approach.

In neoplasms of lymphoid lineage, a tumor-specific molecular marker is created by the rearrangement of gene subsegments coding for the antigen receptor molecules. The understanding of the mechanisms involved in the generation of these molecules and the cloning of the immunoglobulin (Ig) and T-cell antigen receptor (TCR) genes has been accomplished using the clonal expansions provided by neoplastic cells. Thus, the leukemias in particular made a big contribution to our understanding of normal development and these observations paid an enormous dividend in resolving uncertain issues within neoplasia. Specifically, the discovery of an ordered sequence of immunoglobulin (Ig) and T-cell receptor (TCR) gene rearrangements during lymphocyte development has defined the state of maturation and the B- versus T-cell lineage commitment of leukemias that were of uncertain classification. In addition, a direct contribution to malignant transformation was identified. Further, recombinations between immunoglobulin or T-cell receptor loci with nonhomologous chromosomes occur in histopathologically distinct neoplasms. A translocation of cellular oncogenes or newly discovered transforming genes into the proximity of Ig gene or TCR loci alters the quality or regulation of these genes' products and provides a growth advantage.

I. ANTIBODY DIVERSITY IS ACHIEVED BY REARRANGEMENT OF GENE SUBSEGMENTS

The genes for immunoglobulin heavy and light chains are organized as discontinuous, separated DNA segments in their embryonic or germline form (Hozumi and Tonegawa, 1976; Brack et al., 1978; Seidman and Leder, 1978). In order to synthesize a functional immunoglobulin molecule, a B cell has to assemble these segments from their germline position, thus generating a different configuration of DNA. This process is called *DNA rearrangement* and occurs early during B-cell development.

A. Light-Chain Genes

Immunoglobulin molecules consist of two identical heavy and two identical light chains. Human B cells can express either the kappa (κ) light-chain class (60% of the time) or the lambda (λ) light-chain class (40%).

The human κ gene locus is located on the short arm of chromosome 2 at band 2p11 (Malcolm et al., 1982). The first 95 amino acids of a κ light-chain molecule are encoded by one of multiple, different V_κ genes. The remaining 13 amino acids that complete the variable portion of the κ light chain are contributed by one of five alternative joining segments (J_κ) (Hieter, Maizel, and Leder, 1982). There is only one constant (C_κ) gene region on each allele and it is separated from the string of J_κ segments by a long intervening sequence (Hieter et al., 1980). The activation of a κ gene is initiated by a DNA rearrangement, which brings a single V_κ gene into continguity with one J_κ segment (Figure 1). This

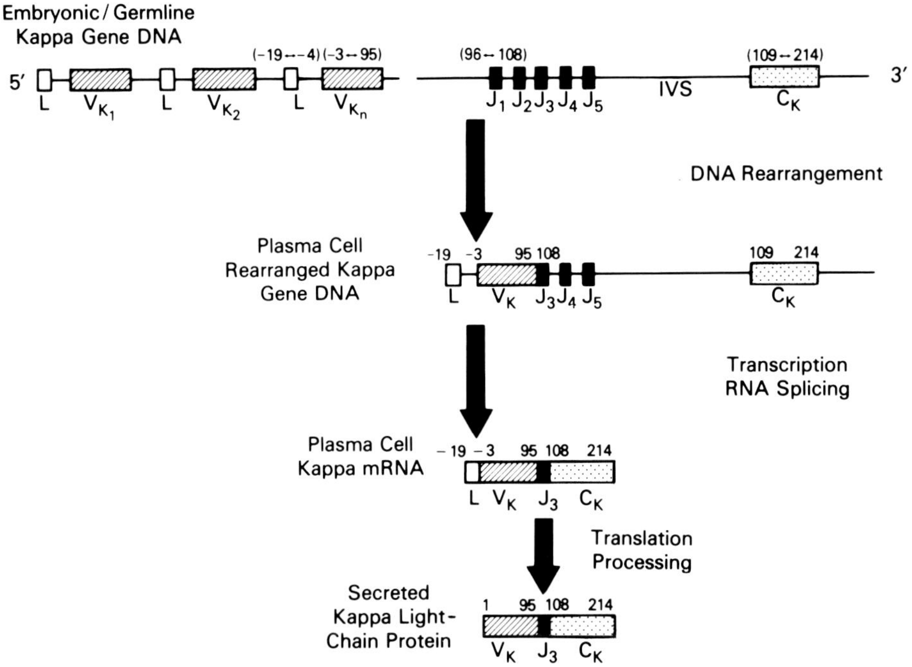

Figure 1 Organization of the germline (unrearranged) κ-gene locus and principle of immunoglobulin gene activation.

rearranged κ gene is then transcribed and the intervening sequence between J_K and C_K is removed by RNA splicing in order to produce a functional messenger RNA. A random recombination process, which juxtaposes one of a large number of germline V_K genes with an alternate J_K segment, generates a large diversity of variable portions of the final immunoglobulin molecule. Moreover, the exact point of recombination between V_K and J_K is flexible, thus generating changes in nucleotide sequence, which alter the amino acid composition of the immunoglobulin (this is called *junctional diversity*) (Max, Seidman, and Leder, 1979). To these mechanisms are added somatic mutation (Pech et al., 1981) and the independent assortment of different heavy and light chains to create the seemingly unlimited number of antibody specificities (Leder, 1982; Tonegawa, 1983).

A slightly different organization of gene subsegments is found at the locus of lambda (λ) light-chain genes, which is on the long arm of chromosome 22 at band 22q11 (McBride et al., 1982). In the germline position, multiple duplicated $J_\lambda C_\lambda$ units are placed in a tandem fashion (Hieter, 1981b). At least six different C_λ genes are present in the human haploid genome; unlike κ genes, they display a germline polymorphism between different individuals, which reflects a varied

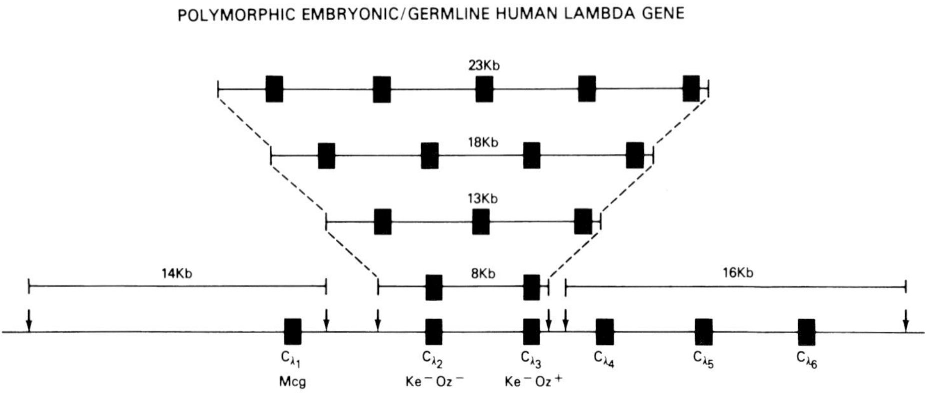

Figure 2 Different human individuals may have different numbers of C_λ genes and therefore display different numbers of restriction fragments hybridizing to a C_λ probe in the germline configuration.

number of C_λ gene segments (Figure 2). Thus different restriction fragment lengths can be observed for the germline configuration of C_λ genes from different individuals (Taub et al., 1983). As with κ genes, a functional DNA rearrangement brings together variable regions (V_λ) and junctional elements (J_λ) before the λ polypeptide can be produced. Only one of the two available light-chain isotypes (κ or λ) is produced by an individual mature B cell; this is called *isotypic exclusion*. Furthermore, only the maternal or paternal allele of the selected class is expressed, termed *allelic exclusion*. Remarkably, the genetic mechanisms that accomplish these phenomena are markedly different in κ- versus λ-producing cells (Hieter et al., 1981a). A monoclonal expansion of κ-producing B cells always possesses one κ gene recombination responsible for the production of the protein. The other κ allele may assume one of three configurations: it may be deleted, ineffectively rearranged, or may remain in the germline form. κ producers retain their λ genes in the germline form, so that they cannot be used for light-chain production. In contrast, λ-producing B cells were found to have either rearranged or deleted their κ genes (Figure 3). This was shown in malignant clonal B-cell populations and then in peripheral-blood polyclonal B cells of a normal individual (Korsmeyer et al., 1982). This finding revealed an ordered developmental sequence of light-chain gene utilization in which κ rearrangement and deletion preceded λ gene recombination (Korsmeyer et al., 1981). The loss of C_κ genes in λ producers is mediated by a uniform genetic element called the *kappa deleting element* (Kde), which was identified and cloned by our laboratory (Siminovitch et al., 1985). The Kde is located on chromosome 2 at band 2p11 and rearranges either to a V_κ region or into a conserved recombinatorial signal within the J_κ-C_κ

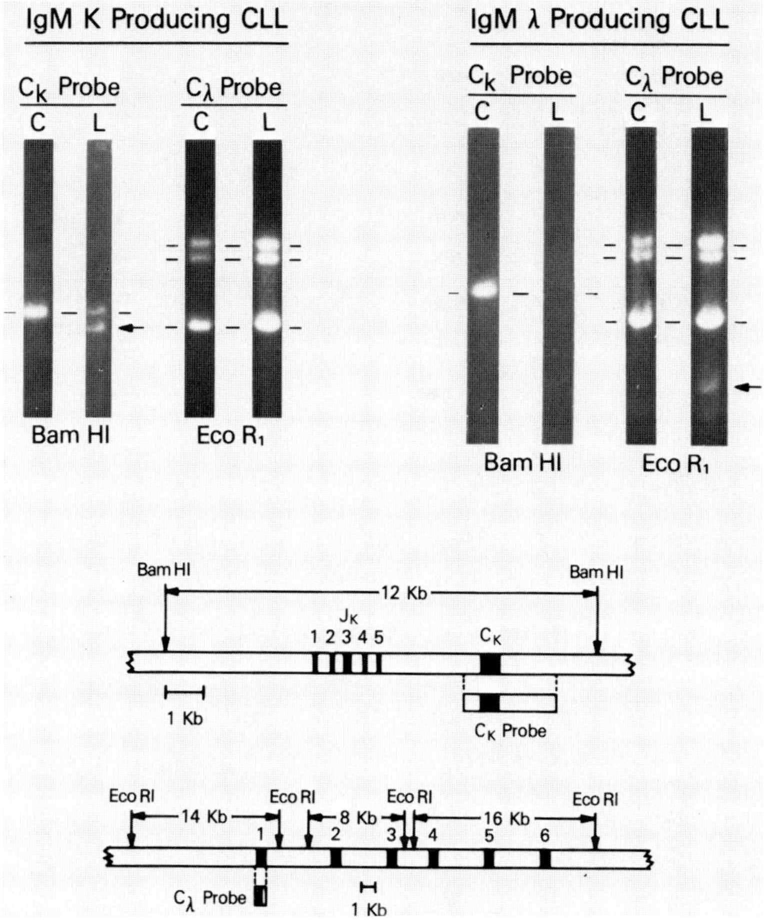

Figure 3 Autoradiography of Southern Blots hybridized to a C_κ or a C_λ probe. The configuration of the germline segments and the location of the probes used is shown in the diagram. C indicates control or germline configuration; L indicates the DNA from the leukemias. Horizontal bars mark the position of the unrearranged (germline) bands; arrows show the different size of the rearranged fragments. The κ producing leukemia shows one germline and one rearranged κ allele, whereas the λ genes are all germline. In contrast, the λ-producing leukemia has deleted both κ alleles.

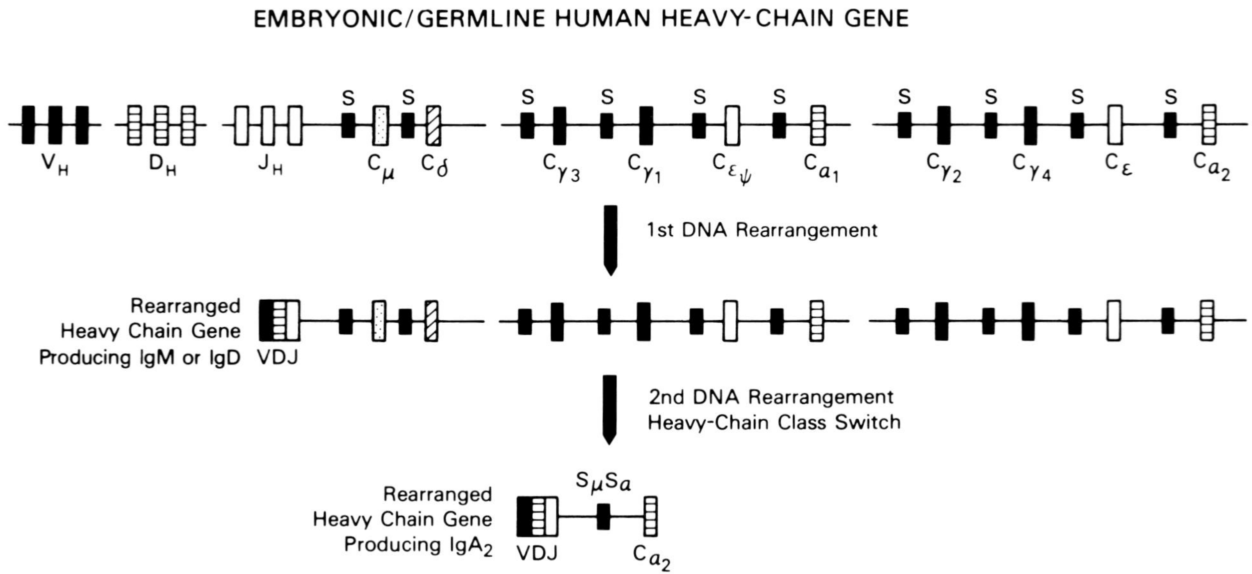

Figure 4 Germline organization of the heavy chain genes. Note, that production of IgM or IgD protein is possible after the first DNA rearrangement and alternative RNA splicing. The heavy chain class switch is a second DNA rearrangement enabling the expression of the distal constant regions.

intervening sequence. This destroys any chance for the locus to make a κ chain and plays a major role in insuring that a B cell makes but a single light-chain molecule.

B. Heavy-Chain Genes

The assembly of gene subsegments for the immunoglobulin heavy chain follows a similar principle to that of the light chains (Figure 4). Additional variation in specificity is achieved by the use of small diversity regions (D_H), which are juxtaposed between V_H and one of six J_H segments on either side (Siebenlist et al., 1981; Ravetch et al., 1981). From the study of neoplastic cell populations at different maturational stages, it appears that a D_H/J_H recombination usually precedes the juxtaposition of a V_H region. This complex recombinatorial sequence does not always yield functional rearrangements, as indicated by the finding that 85% of mature human B cells have rearranged both of their heavy-chain alleles in order to generate a valid V/D/J rearrangement. The heavy-chain gene possesses a variety of constant regions ($C\mu$, $C\delta$, $C\gamma$, $C\alpha$, $C\epsilon$). The capacity of this locus to utilize the same antigenic specificity contributed by the $V_H/D_H/J_H$ rearrangement with different constant regions results in molecules with different effector functions. The alternative use of different constant regions is achieved by two genetic mechanisms. An alternative RNA splicing scheme allows the same V/D/J to be juxtaposed with $C\mu$ or $C\delta$ at the RNA level (Knap et al., 1982; Moore et al., 1981). Use of the more distally located C_H regions is accomplished by a second DNA rearrangement termed *heavy-chain class switch* (Figure 4), which is a deletional rearrangement that moves the selected constant region closer to the assembled V/D/J (Davis, Kim, and Hood, 1980; Marcu et al., 1982).

C. Technical Detection of Gene Rearrangement

The juxtaposition of V and J segments during immunoglobulin gene rearrangement leads to a change in the location of the short nucleotide sequences that are recognized and cleaved by bacterial enzymes known as restriction endonucleases. The relocation of these restriction sites results in altered length restriction fragments in a rearranged gene as compared to a germline form of the gene (Figure 5). These restriction fragments can be size-separated on agarose gels and then transferred to nitrocellulose paper, where they are identified by hybridization to a radiolabeled DNA probe.

Most leukemias appear to be clonal expansions representing the progeny of a single cell. If a gene rearrangement has occurred in the progenitor cell, every cell in the population will bear the same immunoglobulin gene recombination, utilizing the identical V and J segment. The presence of multiple copies of the same Ig rearrangement in a clonal population enables its detection by Southern blot analysis. In contrast, in a polyclonal population of normal cells with numerous different Ig gene rearrangements, none of the rearranged genes in this collective popu-

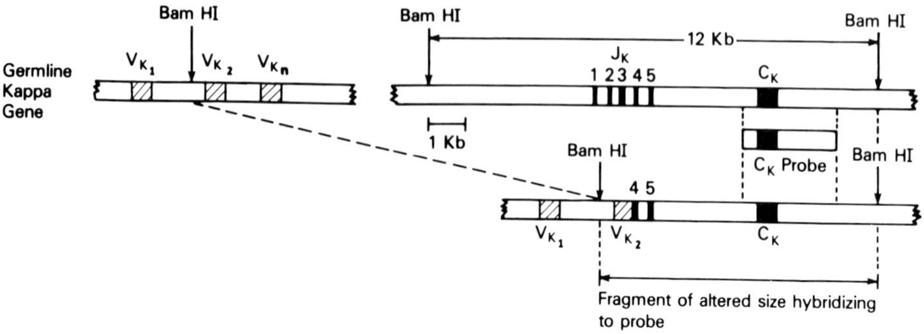

Figure 5 DNA rearrangement of a kappa gene alters the size of the restriction fragment containing the constant region C_K and hybridizing to the C_K probe. [Reprinted, by permission of the *New England Journal of Medicine*, (309: 826-831).]

lation will be discernible by Southern blot analysis, because they fall below the threshold of detection. A DNA rearrangement can be detected within a mixed population of cells if the clonal population comprises as little as 1-5% of all cells. Moreover, individual B cells will rearrange different Ig heavy- and light-chain gene subsegments, creating an Ig gene rearrangement pattern that is unique to each cell. Thus lineage-associated DNA rearrangements serve as sensitive as well as specific clonal markers.

II. PRE-B-CELL COMMITMENT OF NON-T NON-B ALL

Phenotypic analysis of acute lymphoblastic leukemias based on conventional immunologic markers (surface and cytoplasmic immunoglobulins, sheep red blood cell rosetting, and a variety of monoclonal antibodies directed against cell surface determinants) led to a classification scheme with five major subtypes, including B-ALL, T-ALL, common ALL and unclassified or null ALL (Chessels et al., 1977; Foon, Scroff, and Gale, 1982; Brouet et al., 1976). The exact cellular lineage and stage of differentiation of leukemias in the common ALL and null-ALL subgroups had been controversial. Using immunoglobulin gene rearrangement analysis for further characterization (Korsmeyer et al., 1983), we showed that all cases of non-T non-B ALL, that lacked both definitive T-cell markers and surface immunoglobulin had rearranged their Ig genes. All had rearranged heavy-chain segments except for several extremely immature cells which were genetically indeterminant with totally germline genes. Approximately 40% of these leukemias had proceeded further to light-chain gene rearrangement. In contrast, the majority of T-ALLs (90%) have a germline configuration of heavy-chain genes; no light-chain gene rearrangement occurs in T-ALLs. The finding of rearranged Ig genes in the previously uncertain subgroup of "non-T non-B ALLs" indicated that these cells were already commited to the B-cell lineage. Nadler et al. (1984) analyzed the surface expression of B-cell-associated and -restricted antigens in 138 patients with non-T non-B cell ALL. A developmental order of phenotypic expression was found, proceeding from the production of the major histocompatibility antigen HLA-DR antigen alone to a 40, 80 Kd heterodimer, B4 (Nadler et al., 1983), then to the common acute lymphoblastic leukemia antigen (CALLA), and finally the 35-Kd phosphoprotein termed B1 (Nadler et al., 1981) (Figure 6).

Coordinate with the hierarchy of Ig gene rearrangements, ALL patients with surface phenotypic stage II (DR^+ $B4^+$) had rearranged heavy-chain genes but germline light-chain genes and represented the most immature form of pre B cells. Later stages (DR^+ $B4^+$ $CALLA^+$) also displayed some kappa- and lambda-chain gene rearrangements.

The pattern of light-chain gene rearrangement in ALLs further supported a κ-before-λ order. Cells that possessed rearranged κ genes and retained germline λ genes were noted. Moreover, an intermediate set of pre-B cells existed in which the Kde had eliminated the κ genes, yet λ genes were still germline. Those cells that had progressed to λ rearrangement consistently had no remaining germline κ genes, the Kde having removed them. Thus the Ig gene rearrangement patterns within these pre B cells revealed a cascade of events, in which heavy chains preceded light and κ gene rearrangements preceded λ gene recombination.

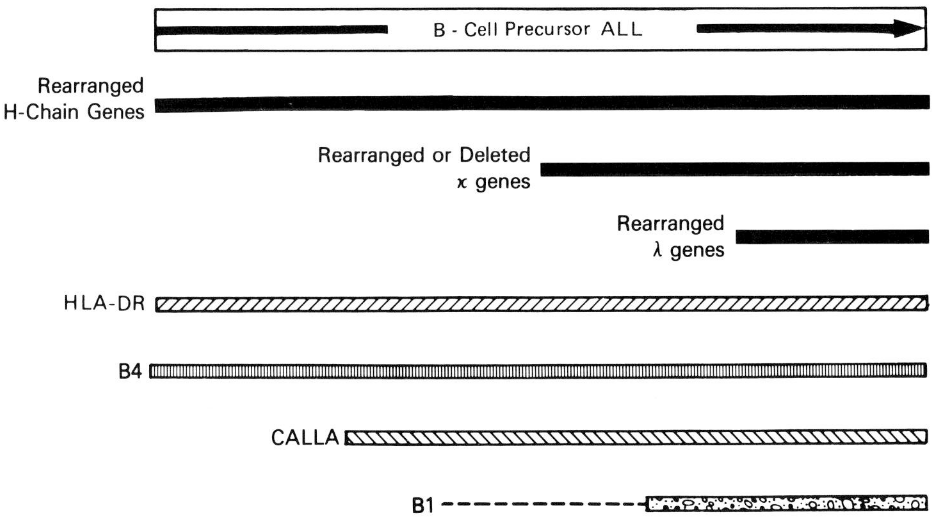

Figure 6 Hierarchial order of Ig gene rearrangement during different maturational stages of B-cell precursor ALL. The time of surface expression of differentiation antigens is shown below.

When examined for the presence of cytoplasmic immunoglobulin, only 25% of these B cells precursor ALLs revealed the production of small amounts of immunoglobulin. These Ig molecules were usually of the μ class, but in one case γ was produced. Some leukemias appear to possess an effective rearrangement with correctly assembled $V_H/D_H/J_H$ regions yet produce no cytoplasmic μ chain. A portion of these leukemias can be induced to differentiate with such agents as phorbol esters. Once they have matured, they at times produce cytoplasmic, and upon one occasion, even surface immunoglobulin (Cossman et al., 1982; Nadler et al., 1982). Some element of the maturational arrest that kept this leukemia at an immature stage appears to have prevented the production of Ig. However, most of these B cell precursor leukemias still fail to make immunoglobulin after exposure to such differentiating agents. The fact that many pre B-cell ALLs do not produce Ig protein reflects a high rate of D/J intermediate or aberrant, ineffective gene recombinations. If a cell fails to properly juxtapose D_H/J_H or V_H/D_H segments, a minor change in the coding sequence may lead to an abnormal transcription product and subsequently make the translation into a mature immunoglobulin impossible. Although the concept of ordered pre B-cell developmental stages primarily evolved from the study of ALLs, normal cellular counterparts to these B-cell differentiation stages were also demonstrated in adult and fetal bone marrow (Nadler et al., 1984).

III. CLONAL EVOLUTION OF ALL

Since pre B-cell ALLs lack surface Ig, they possess no cell surface clonal markers that allow them to be discriminated from non-neoplastic pre B cells. None of the pre-B-associated surface antigens are restricted to malignant cells. Therefore no clonal markers existed to follow the natural history of leukemias at diagnosis and relapse or to permit the search for minimal residual disease during remission. Therefore, we used the DNA rearrangement of Ig gene subsegments as markers specific for individual neoplastic cells in order to follow serial samples from patients (Wright, 1986a). A comparison of Ig heavy and light chain gene configuration revealed that most patients had an identical pattern at diagnosis and relapse. This finding firmly establishes that both leukemic populations represent the expansions of the same clone of malignant cells. In 2 out of 11 patients, a variation in Ig gene rearrangement pattern between diagnosis and relapse was found. However, one identical, rearranged Ig gene allele was present in both leukemic episodes, indicating that these leukemic subclones arose from a common clonal progenitor cell. Thus, none of these leukemias were truly biclonal in that they did not arise from separately transformed cells. Instead, one or more of the Ig alleles may undergo progressive rearrangements over time, leading to the varied patterns. If the maturational arrest of a neoplastic pre B cell occurs at a stage when Ig gene recombinases are still active, further rearrangement might well be expected.

Physiological progressions from intermediate D/J recombinations to completed V/D/J heavy chains and from heavy-chain rearrangement alone to adding a light-chain rearrangement may occur between diagnosis and relapse phases. Furthermore, events such as deletions of gene segments were also seen during clonal evolution of leukemic cell populations in the same patient.

Another example for progressive Ig gene rearrangements in the clonal evolution of ALLs was given by Kitchingman (1985), who found more than two rearranged bands when hybridizing ALL DNA to a Cμ probe. Although the presence of a third chromosome 14 was found in some of these cases, the authors concluded that additional rearrangements of the heavy-chain genes occurred in a subpopulation of leukemic cells after the expansion of the primary malignant clone.

IV. LYMPHOID BLAST CRISIS IN CML: BLASTS ARE B-CELL PRECURSORS

Chronic myelogeneous leukemia (CML) is a clonal proliferation of cells that arise from a remarkably pluripotent stem cell (Barr and Fialkow, 1973). The lymphoid blast crises of this disease demonstrated rearranged heavy and often light chains in almost all cases, indicating that these blasts were genetically committed B cell precursors. Although a T-cell blast crisis in CML has also been described (Chan, 1986) the vast majority of lymphoid blasts are committed to the B-cell lineage (Bakshi et al., 1983).

Clonal evolution of CML lymphoblasts over time has also been documented. In one patient with two separate lymphoid blast crises, we demonstrated that both populations had the same heavy-chain gene rearrangement as well as the same cytogenetic abnormality (a loss of chromosome 7 in addition to the Ph^1 chromosome). Light-chain analysis, however, showed rearranged λ genes in the first blast crisis but a germline configuration of λ genes in the second crisis (Figure 7). This indicates that both populations were the progeny of a common lymphoid progenitor cell with identically rearranged heavy-chain genes and an identical unique cytogenetic aberration. However, the immediate precursor cell which gave rise to each blast crisis varied in its extent of genetic maturation with respect to light-chain gene rearrangements. Thus it was shown that a transformed clone of B-cell precursors in CML can undergo the sequential differentiative steps of heavy- and light-chain rearrangement (Bakshi et al., 1983).

V. MINIMAL RESIDUAL DISEASE

The identification of residual malignant cells or early relapse prior to histopathological evidence of relapse has been previously attempted using immunologic, enzymatic, and cytogenetic markers. These methods are limited, however, because of a lack of tumor specificity or sensitivity.

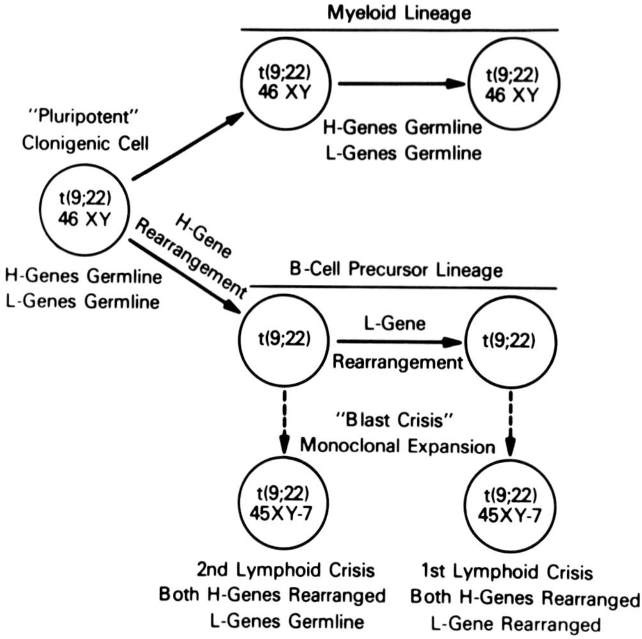

Figure 7 Clonal evolution of a hematopoietic precursor cell carrying the t(9;22) translocation. Cells from two lymphoid blast crises in the same CML patient represent the divergent progeny of a single B-cell clone.

Since the joining of gene subsegments that code for the antigen receptors on B and on T lymphocytes creates a distinct pattern unique to an individual cell, the analysis of gene rearrangements has a high specificity for a given monoclonal population. A distinct DNA rearrangement will only be detectable if an individual cell has clonally expanded. A clonal population must comprise at least 1-5% of all cells present to have its rearrangement seen on a Southern blot analysis (Arnold et al., 1983).

During the early induction phases of chemotherapy in patients with pre-B ALL, the molecular detection of clonal cells paralleled the presence of lymphoblasts in the bone marrow. Disappearance of blasts was marked by the return of a germline pattern of Ig genes. This indicates that the malignant cell population was actually eradicated rather than simply being altered in morphology. Similarly, patients presumed to be cured and who were now off chemotherapy also revealed no clonal cells. In addition, patients with CNS or testicular extramedullary relapse had no molecular evidence for bone marrow reseeding.

Relapses often occur in patients still receiving maintenance chemotherapy. The vast majority of patients in such shorter term periods of remission are also free of clonal disease by gene rearrangement. However, an exception has been noted in which clonal cells were demonstrated by gene rearrangement while bone marrow morphology indicated (clinical) remission. This patient subsequently relapsed 6 months later (Wright, 1986b). Although the detection of a clonal Ig gene rearrangement is not necessarily equivalent to a diagnosis of malignancy, the presence of a clonal pattern identical to that seen during the acute phase of the leukemia indicates that remission is not always an absence of clonal cells. Similar results were reported by Zehnbauer et al. (1986), who found a clonal rearrangement of Ig genes in 3 out of 7 patients with ALL in complete clinical remission. Prospective studies will be needed to determine if the detection of clonality during remission will be an effective clinical test to predict patients who will relapse. Utilizing probes for the immunoglobulin genes, the T-cell receptor genes, and defined breakpoints of chromosomal translocation (see below) should refine our concepts of minimal residual disease.

VI. T-CELL RECEPTOR GENES

Just as the molecular biology of B-cell malignancies allows conclusive determination of the clonality, stages of differentiation, and chromosomal translocations of tumors via specific Ig gene rearrangements, analogous tools are available to study T-cell malignancies. Although a variety of monoclonal antibodies against T-cell-associated antigens can be used to determine the differentiation stage of single thymocytes, they cannot be used to determine the clonality of a population since they are not clone specific.

Since no alternative receptor isotypes equivalent to κ or λ chains had been described for T cells, the determination of T-cell clonality had been limited to cases with cytogenetic abnormalities or distinguishable allelic markers such as G6PD isoenzymes.

The cloning of the T-cell antigen receptor (TCR) genes provided the first clonal markers that could be universally applied to T-cell populations. The antigen-specific T-cell receptor is a cell surface protein complex composed of at least five distinct polypeptide chains. Two of these, termed α and β chains, represent the antigen recognition part and form a disulfide-linked heterodimer. It is associated with the so-called T3 complex (consisting of at least the T3δ, T3ϵ, T3γ and T3 zeta chain). The genes encoding the β subunit of the TCR were the first to be characterized (Yanagi et al., 1984; Hedrick et al., 1984; Hedrick et al., 1985). Very similar to the Ig genes, the β-chain gene consists of a stretch of discontinuous gene subsegments, which have to be juxtaposed before the surface expression of the polypeptide (Sim et al., 1984). The β-chain gene complex is located on chromosome 7 at band 7q35 (Caccia et al., 1984). It consists of two different constant region genes ($C_{\beta}1$ and $C_{\beta}2$) and each of these has associated diversity regions (D_{β}) and junctional regions (J_{β}). The rearrangement of the TCR_{β} genes

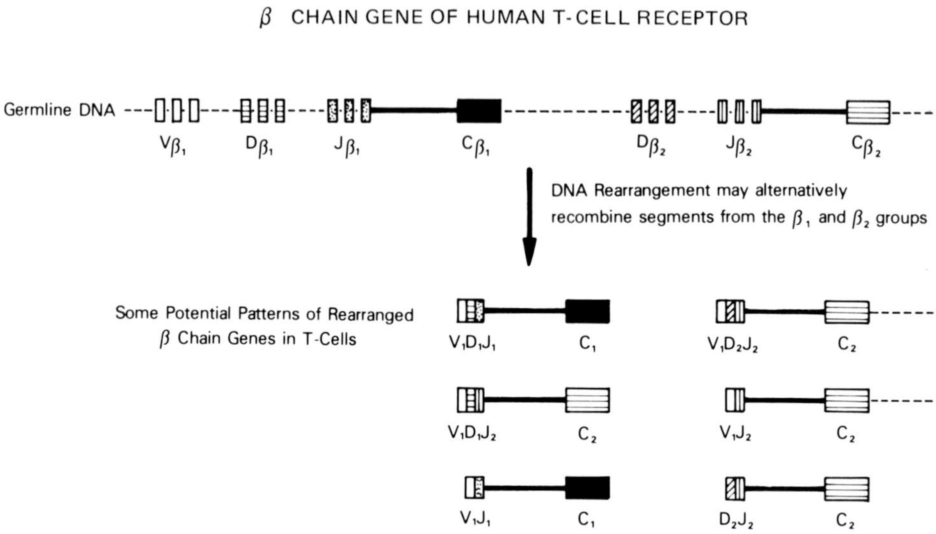

Figure 8 Organization of the T-cell receptor β-chain gene.

may alternatively recombine segments from the TCR_{β_1} and TCR_{β_2} groups (Figure 8). Unlike the Ig genes, the location of at least one V_β gene has been demonstrated to be downstream (3') to the constant regions, indicating that the mechanisms of TCR_β gene rearrangement can involve more complex events like inversion in order to produce a productive VDJ joining (Malissen, 1986). Rearrangement of the TCR_β region can be assessed using the restriction enzyme BamHI (for detection of rearrangement of the entire C_β complex), EcoRI (for rearrangement of $C_\beta1$) or HindIII (for rearrangement of $C_\beta2$).

The organization of the genes for the TCR α chain is somewhat unusual in that a large number of J genes are spread over a very long distance on chromosome segment 14q11 (Sim et al., 1984; Yoshikai et al., 1985) (Figure 9). Analogous to other members of the immunoglobulin gene superfamily, the TCR_α chain genes have to be rearranged before expression. Due to the large number

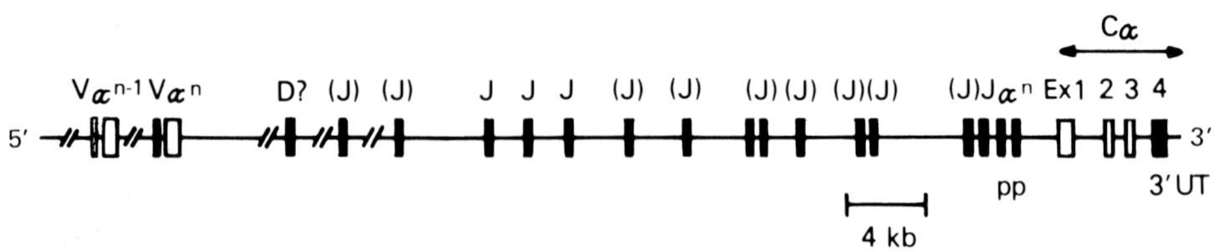

Figure 9 More than 50 J_α gene segments extend over a long chromosomal distance at the T-cell receptor α-chain gene locus.

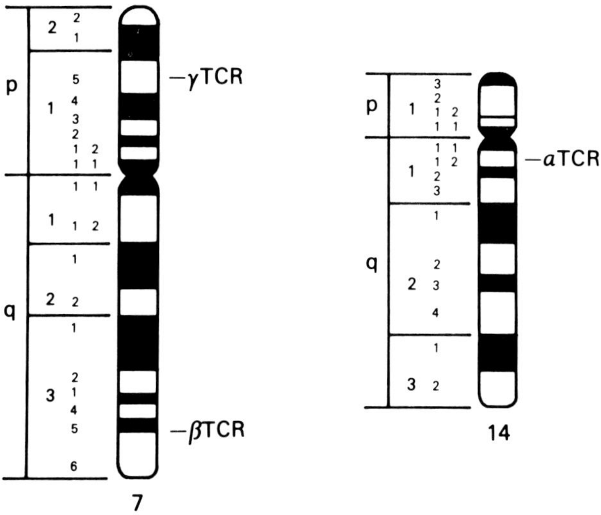

Figure 10 Chromosomal location of human TCR genes.

and the distance covered by J_α segments, the analysis of all TCR_α chain rearrangements is technically difficult. However, activation of this locus can be readily assessed by examining its RNA transcription.

A third rearranging gene complex isolated from T cells is termed the TCR γ chain (not to be confused with the T3γ chain) and is localized to chromosome 7 at band 7p15 (Figure 10). This gene also consists of two constant regions (C_γ), associated J segments (Figure 11), and a limited number of variable regions (Hayday et al., 1985; Quertermous et al., 1986). The structure will predict a membrane receptor protein, but at this writing, the actual protein or its function have not been characterized. This gene complex has been shown to rearrange in thymocytes (Snodgrass et al., 1985), T cells of both helper and suppressor phenotype, and in T cell leukemias (Murre et al., 1985).

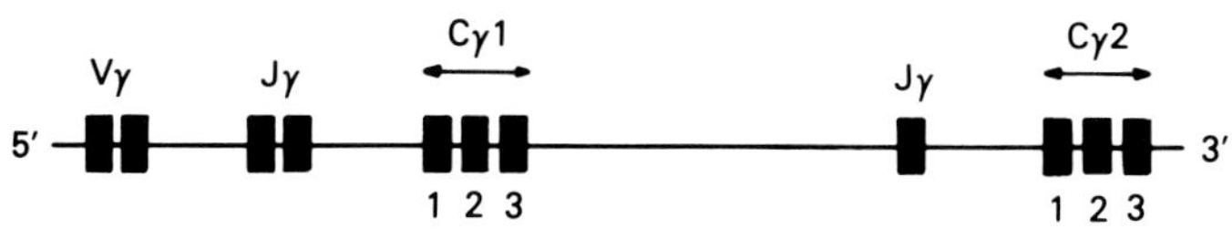

Figure 11 Two constant region genes are present on each allele of the human T-cell receptor γ-chain gene.

Using the rearrangement pattern of the TCR genes as a fingerprint for monoclonal cell populations, the clonal origin of many T-cell malignancies was demonstrated, such as T-cell chronic lymphocytic leukemia (Aisenberg, 1985), T-cell lymphomas (Flug et al., 1985; O'Connor et al., 1985) and Sezary syndrome (Weiss et al., 1985).

In T-cell ALL, Southern blot analysis of restriction-endonuclease-digested genomic DNA showed rearrangements of the TCR β genes in over 90% of the patients; in most cases both alleles were involved (Minden et al., 1985; Tawa et al., 1985; Felix et al., 1986). As in the case of Ig genes, this methodology can be used to assess the presence of residual clonal cells following antileukemic therapy (Waldmann, 1985). Moreover, the existence of monoclonal T-cell populations in diseases like T8 lymphocytosis with hematocytopenia (Berliner, 1986) and angioimmunoblastic lymphadenopathy (Lipford, Smith, and Pittaluga, 1986; Weiss et al., 1986) substantially changes our understanding of these syndromes and in addition might facilitate the early detection of lymphoproliferative disease.

VII. MATURATIONAL STAGE OF T-CELL ALLs

The development of monoclonal antibodies against unique T-cell-specific surface glycoproteins has led to a model of thymocyte differentiation, where the expression of the sheep erythrocyte binding protein (T11) (stage I: $T_{11}^{+} T_3^{-} T_6^{-}$) precedes the production of the T6 antigen (stage II: $T_{11}^{+} T_3^{-} T_6^{+}$) and the coexpression of the T4 and T8 molecules. Subsequently in intrathymic differentiation, the T3 glycoprotein which complexes with the antigen recognizing T_i heterodimer appears on the cell surface (Reinherz et al., 1980). The complex of T3 and T_i is called the T-cell receptor (TCR). Studies of normal thymocyte fractions showed that rearrangement of the TCR β-chain genes occurred prior to the surface expression of the T3 molecule, whereas in stage I thymocytes, the TCR β-chain genes remained in their germline form (Royer et al., 1984, 1985). When we investigated the rearrangement pattern of TCR genes in T-cell precursor ALLs, we found that rearrangement of the TCR β genes occurred prior to the activation of the TCR α-chain locus (Felix et al., 1986). This was consistent with the report of Collins et al. (1985), who also found TCR α-chain RNA only in the phenotypically most mature T-cell ALLs.

90% of T-cell ALLs rearrange and usually express the TCR β genes, whereas only 50% express significant amounts of TCR α RNA; in general only this latter subset possesses an intact cell surface antigen receptor molecule and is $T3^+$. Studies of early thymic development in mice suggested that activation of the TCR γ chain genes might take place before TCR β gene activation (Raulet et al., 1985). In human T-cell ALLs, we found that most of the cases had already rearranged the TCR β and the TCR γ genes (Figure 12). However, we demonstrated examples

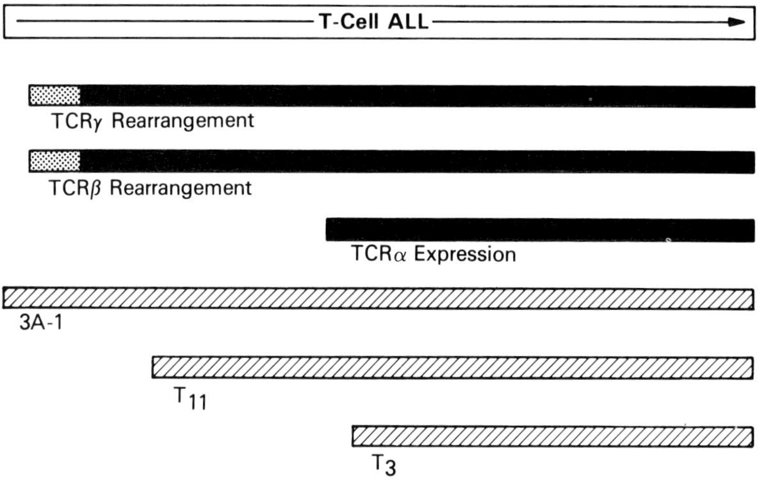

Figure 12 Activation of the T-cell receptor genes follows a sequential order within different maturational stages of T-cell ALL. TCR_α gene transcription occurs only in relatively mature forms of T-ALL, while β and γ TCR occurs early but in a varied order.

of pre T-cell ALL in which TCR γ genes were rearranged and the TCR β locus was still in the germline position. In contrast, we have also noted one example with rearranged TCR β genes and germline TCR γ. Thus, while the earliest steps may often be the TCR γ before TCR β gene rearrangement, this sequence is not invariant (Felix et al., 1986).

While the rearrangement of DNA segments produces a lifelong marker in a clonal population of cells, the transcription of genes reflects regulatory mechanisms operating during cell maturation. Any attempt to determine the maturational stage of cells by the detection of specific mRNAs must consider the potential reversibility of gene transcription during differentiation. It is very likely, for instance, that transcription of the TCR_γ gene occurs only during a certain maturational stage in normal T-cell development. On the other hand, we could demonstrate rare cases of malignant T-cell populations that express TCR_γ and TCR_α genes but not TCR β, suggesting alternative forms of the T cell receptor molecule. The genes for the subunits of the T3 complex ($T3_\gamma$, $T3_\delta$, $T3_\epsilon$) have recently been isolated and characterized (Gold et al., 1986). The availability of cDNA probes for these genes will make it possible to study the developmental order of activation of all subunits of the T3 complex. Since the transcription of these genes might precede the actual appearance of the whole surface molecule, additional information about the maturational stage of normal and malignant T-cell populations may result.

VIII. LINEAGE SPILLOVER

Although mature immunoglobulin-producing B cells must always possess rearranged genes for the Ig heavy and light chains, we and others have noted that Ig heavy-chain genes may be rearranged within T lymphocytes and occasionally even in myeloid cells (Korsmeyer et al., 1983; Arnold et al., 1983; Rivogatti et al., 1984; Ha, 1984; Kitchingman et al., 1985; Greaves et al., 1986).

Likewise, an activation of the TCR genes can be found not only in lymphoid cells clearly committed to T lineage, but occasionally within B cells. Such lineage spillover phenomena are not only observed in malignant cell populations, but also in growth-factor-maintained, nontransformed cells. Approximately 10% of all T-cell neoplasms display rearranged heavy-chain genes, but retain their κ and λ light-chain genes in the germline form. A significantly higher incidence of lineage nonspecific rearrangements of the TCR γ chain (40%) and perhaps the β chain genes (20%) was observed in pre B-cell forms of ALL (Felix et al., 1986). This is a considerably higher incidence of rearrangement than is present in mature B-cell neoplasms or Ebstein-Barr virus cell lines (γ TCR, 0%; β TCR 10%). While the expression of TCR α-chain genes represents a relatively late event in T-cell maturation, it is possible to detect TCR α RNA production in some clear B-lineage-committed cells.

Several explanations exist for this finding of lineage spillover of antigen receptor genes. It is likely that the same recombinase enzymes participate in rearrangement of Ig genes as well as TCR genes (Yoncopoulos et al., 1986). Recognition signals (heptamer, spacer, nonamer) flanking the individual gene subsegments are highly homologous in TCR and Ig genes. A putative transactivating factor, which opens the chromosome structure at the site of rearrangeable genes, might lack complete lineage specificity and occasionally activate the loci for both gene families simultaneously. It is conceivable that the onset of recombinatorial mechanisms occurs in a very early maturation state when a final decision for lineage commitment is not yet made. The higher percentage of TCR rearrangement in very immature pre-B ALLs may indicate a maturational arrest of these malignant cells at a time when recombination of both sets of receptor genes can occur. In contrast, the activation of κ and λ genes seems to be restricted to a later step in B-lymphocyte development, since in all T cells a germline position of these genes was found.

When interpreting gene rearrangement patterns for lineage characterization of a cell, a lineage spillover of at least 10% for Ig H chains and TCR genes must therefore be considered. The apparently more frequent lineage crossover of γ TCR gene rearrangements in pre B leukemias suggests that such events might confer a growth advantage, predispose some cell subsets to malignant transformation, represent unanticipated subpopulations of progenitor cells fortuitously transformed, or alternatively be a secondary change following transformation.

IX. CHROMOSOMAL TRANSLOCATIONS

Specific chromosomal translocations are uniquely or highly associated with histologically distinct neoplasms (Rowley and Testa, 1982; Yunis, 1983; Leder, 1982). It is of particular interest that the sites of typical chromosomal translocations in lymphoid neoplasms involve the very bands that contain the genes for the immunoglobulins or the T cell receptor. This cytogenetic finding can be confirmed at the molecular level in that the use of Ig gene specific probes shows a rearrangement of the respective Ig gene loci in translocation bearing cells. The molecular cloning of the breakpoints of these translocations then allows the precise characterization of the sites and reciprocal partners of these translocations. The classical example of a chromosomal translocation that involves an Ig locus is that of Burkitt's lymphoma (Kirsch et al., 1982; Taub et al., 1982; Dalla Favera et al., 1982).

The most common chromosomal aberration in Burkitt's lymphomas is a reciprocal translocation between chromosome segment 14q32 (the IgH locus) and chromosome segment 8q24. Further variants were described involving the locus of the κ genes (2p11) and the λ genes (22q11) (Lenoit et al., 1982; Hollis et al., 1984; Erikson et al., 1983). The site at chromosome 8q24 was uniformly involved and interestingly proved to be the locus of the cellular oncogene c-myc. These translocations were juxtaposing an active immunoglobulin gene locus with a cellular oncogene, resulting in the deregulation of the translocated proliferation-related gene (Adams, Gerondakis, and Webb, 1985). Other B cell malignancies like multiple myeloma, some lymphomas, and cases of CLL also have a high percentage of translocations involving Ig gene loci. Active research in this field is revealing more information about the genes at the reciprocal sites of the translocations and their potential role in malignant transformation.

Analogous to the involvement of the Ig gene loci in B-cell malignancies, chromosomal translocations into the TCR gene loci have been demonstrated within certain T-cell leukemias and lymphomas. A t(11;14)(p13;q11) breakpoint occurs in perhaps 50% of T-ALLs and breaks within the TCR α-chain locus (Erikson et al., 1985). Two cases of T-ALL with complex chromosomal aberrations including a t(8;14)(q24;q11) translocation possibly involving the TCR α locus and the c-myc locus were reported (Hayashi, Yamamoto, and Kojima, 1986). Thus, there is a remarkable association of T-cell receptor translocations in T cells and Ig gene loci in B cells. However, an inversion of chromosome 14 segments after breaking at the TCR α locus (14q11) and the Ig_H locus (14q32) has been molecularly characterized in T-cell lymphomas (Denny et al., 1986; Baer et al., 1985; Hecht et al., 1984; Baltimore, 1986) but recently also in a case with pre-B ALL (Clare et al., 1986). The translocations which juxtapose Ig and TCR genes suggest that these translocations occur at a developmental stage when both the TCR and Ig gene loci were accessible and normally available for recombinatorial enzymes.

Since distinct chromosomal translocations are found in malignant cells and not in their normal counterparts, a hypothesis that these translocations are contributing to a neoplastic growth advantage has developed. In the case of two known oncogenes, c-myc and c-abl, this hypothesis has already been verified. The antigen receptor genes by analogy can be used as a handle to identify other, unknown genes at the breakpoint sites of translocations that may participate in transformation. Moreover, the cloning of these chromosomal breakpoints generates probes that can be used to molecularly mark transformation events within these malignancies.

X. PERSPECTIVE/OUTLOOK

In this chapter we have shown the usefulness and applicability of molecular biology techniques for the characterization of leukemias. The exploitation of recent insights into the molecular biology of human lymphoid neoplasms and the availability of cloned probes for the immunoglobulin and T-cell receptor genes provide us with sensitive and specific markers for clonality, lineage and stage of differentiation of lymphoid leukemias. Detailed and prospective studies applying this methodology will determine the extent to which this improvement in identification and classification proves to have prognostic or therapeutic impact. For example, improvements in the detection of minimal residual disease may allow earlier and more precise chemotherapeutic strategies for patients. The characterization of specific chromosomal translocations that involve antigen receptor genes and/or growth-regulating genes will also facilitate accurate diagnosis and enable a more precise and sensitive followup of patients with leukemias and lymphomas. Moreover, a more detailed understanding of the function of the genes involved in such translocations may provide us with direct insights into the pathophysiology of transformation and malignant growth. In these revelations also lies the hope for more tailor-made therapies for lymphoid neoplasms.

REFERENCES

Adams, J. M., Gerondakis, S., and Webb, E. (1983). Cellular myc oncogene is altered by chromosome translocation to an immunoglobulin locus in murine plasmacytomas and is rearranged similarly in human Burkitt lymphomas. *Proc. Natl. Acad. Sci. USA* 80:1982.

Aisenberg, A. C. (1978). Cell surface markers in lymphoproliferative disease. *N. Eng. J. Med.* 304:331.

Aisenberg, A. C., Krontiris, T. G., Mak, T. K., and Wilkes, B. M. (1985). Rearrangement of the gene for the beta chain of the T-cell receptor in T-cell chronic lymphocytic leukemia and related disorders. *N. Engl. J. Med.* 313:529.

Arnold, A., Cossman, J., Bakhshi, A., Jaffe, E. S., and Waldmann, T. A. (1983). Immunoglobulin gene rearrangements as unique clonal markers in human lymphoid neoplasms. *N. Engl. J. Med.* 309:1593.

Baer, R., Chen, K. C., Smith, S. D., and Rabbitts, T. H. (1985). Fusion of an immunoglobulin variable gene and a T cell receptor constant gene in the chromosome 14 inversion associated with T cell tumors. *Cell* 143:705.

Bakhshi, A., Minowada, J., Arnold, A., Cossman, J., Jensen, J. P., Whang-Peng, J., Waldmann, T. A., and Korsmeyer, S. J. (1983). Lymphoid blast crises of chronic myelogenous leukemia represent stages in the development of B-cell precursors. *N. Engl. J. Med.* 309:826.

Baltimore, D. (1986). Inversion for gene construction. *Nature* 319:12-13.

Barr, R. D., and Fialkow, P. J. (1973). Clonal origin of chronic myelocytic leukemia. *N. Engl. J. Med.* 289:307.

Berliner, N., Duby, A., Linch, D., Murre, C., Quertermous, T., Knott, L., Azin, T., Newland, A., Lewis, D., Galvin, M., and Seidman, J. (1986). T cell receptor gene rearrangements define a monoclonal T cell proliferation in patients with T cell lymphocytosis and cytopenia. *Blood* 67(4):914-918.

Brack, C., Hirama, M., Lenhard-Schuller, R., and Tonegawa, S. (1978). A complete immunoglobulin gene is created by somatic recombination. *Cell* 15:1.

Brouet, J. C., Valensi, F., Daniet, M. T., Flandrin, G., Preud'Homme, J. L., and Seligmann, M. (1976). Immunological classification of acute lymphoblastic leukemias: Evaluation of its clinical significance in a hundred patients. *Br. J. Haematol.* 33:319.

Chessells, J. M., Hardisty, R. M., Rapson, N. T., and Greaves, M. F. (1977). Acute lymphoblastic leukemia in children: Classification and prognosis. *Lancet* 2: 1307.

Caccia, N., Kronenberg, M., Saxe, D., Haars, R., Bruns, G. A. P., et al. (1984). The T cell receptor β chain genes are located on chromosome 6 in mice and chromosome 7 in humans. *Cell* 37:1091.

Chan, L. C., Furley, A. J., Ford, A. M., Yardumian, D. A., and Greaves, M. F. (1986). Clonal rearrangement and expression of the T cell receptor β gene and involvement of the break point cluster region in blast crisis of CGL. *Blood* 67:533-536.

Clare, N., Bolt, D., Messerschmidt, G., Zeltger, P., Hansen, K., and Manhoff, L. (1986). Lymphocyte malignancy and chromosome 14: structural aberrations involving band q11. *Blood* 67(3):704-709.

Collins, M. K. L., Tanigawa, G., Kissonerghis, A. M., Ritter, M., Price, K. M., Tonegawa, S., and Owen, M. J. (1985). Regulation of T cell receptor gene expression in human T-cell development. *Proc. Natl. Acad. Sci. USA* 82: 4503-4507.

Cossman, J., Neckers, L. M., Arnold, A., and Korsmeyer, S. J. (1982). Induction of differentiation a case of common, acute lymphoblastic leukemia. *N. Engl. J. Med.* 307:1251.

Dalla-Favera, R., Bregni, M., Erikson, J., Patterson, D., Gallo, R. C., and Croce, C. M. (1982). Human c-myc oncogene is located on the region of chromosome 8 that is translocated in Burkitt lymphoma cells. *Proc. Natl. Acad. Sci. USA* 79:7824.

Davis, M. M., Kim, S. K., and Hood, L. E. (1980). DNA sequences mediating class switching α-immunoglobulins. *Science* 209:1360.

de Klein, A., Geurts van Kessel, A., Grosveld, G., Bartram, C. R., Hagemeijer, A., Bottsma, D., Spurr, N. K., Heisterkamp, N., Groffen, J., and Stephenson, J. R. (1982). A cellular oncogene (c-abl) is translocated to the Philadelphia chromosome in chronic myelocytic leukemia. *Nature* 294:765-767.

Denny, C., Yoshikai, Y., Mak, T., Smith, S., Hollis, G., and Kirsch, I. R. (1986). A chromosome 14 inversion in a T cell lymphoma is caused by site specific recombination between Ig and TCR loci. *Nature* 320:549-551.

Erikson, J., Nishikura, K., ar-Rushdi, A., Finan, J., Emanuel, B., Lenoir, G., Nowell, P. C., Croce, C. M. (1983). Translocation of an immunoglobulin kappa locus to a region 3' of an unrearranged c-myc oncogene enhances c-myc transcription. *Proc. Natl. Acad. Sci. USA* 80:7581-7585.

Erikson, J., Williams, D. L., Finan, J., Nowell, P. C., and Croce, C. M. (1985). Locus of the α chain of the T cell receptor is split by chromosome translocation in T cell leukemias. *Science* 229:784.

Felix, C. A., Wright, J. J., Poplack, D. G., Reaman, G., Cole, D., Goldman, P., and Korsmeyer, S. J. (1981). T cell receptor α, β, and γ genes in T cell and pre B cell acute lymphoblastic leukemia. *J. Clin. Invest.* In press.

Flug, F., Pelicci, P.-G., Bonetti, F., Knowles, D. M., and Dalla-Favera, R. (1985). T-cell receptor gene rearrangements as markers of lineage and clonality in T-cell neoplasms. *Proc. Natl. Acad. Sci. USA* 82:3460.

Foon, K. A., Schroff, R. W., and Gale, R. P. (1982). Surface markers on leukemia and lymphoma cells: recent advances. *Blood* 60(1):1-19.

Gold, D., Puck, J., Pettey, C., Cho, M., Coligan, J., Woody, J., and Terhorst, C. (1986). Isolation of cDNA clones encoding the 20 K non-glycosylated polypeptide chain of the human TCR/T3 complex. *Nature* 321:431-434.

Greaves, M. F., Chan, L. C., Furley, A. J. W., Watt, S. M., and Molgaard, H. V. (1986). Lineage promiscuity in hematopoietic differentiation and leukemia. *Blood* 67:1.

Ha, K., Minden, M., Hozumi, N., and Gelfand, E. W. (1984). Immunoglobulin gene rearrangement in acute myelogenous leukemia. *Cancer Res.* 44(10): 4658-4660.

Hayashi, Y., Yamamoto, K., and Kojima, S. (1986). T cell ALL with a t(8;14) possibly involving a c-myc locus and TCR α chain genes. *N. Engl. J. Med.* 314(10):650-651.

Hayday, A. C., Saito, H., Gillies, S. D., Kranz, D. M., Tanigawa, G., Eison, H. N., and Tonegawa, S. (1985). Structure, organization and somatic rearrangement of T-cell gama genes. *Cell* 40:259.

Hecht, F., Morgan, R., and Hecht, B. K. M. (1984). Common region on chromosome 14 in T cell leukemia and lymphoma. *Science* 226:1445-1446.

Hedrick, S. M., Cohen, D. I., Nielson, E. A., and Davis, M. M. (1984). Isolation of cDNA clones encoding T-cell specific membrane-associated proteins. *Nature* 308:149.

Hedrick, S. M., Germain, R. N., Bevan, M. J., Dorf, M., Engel, I., Fink, P., Gascoigne, N., Heber-Katz, E., Kapp, J., Kaufmann, Y., Kaye, J., Melchers, F., Pierce, C., Schwartz, R. H., Sorensen, C., Tanigushi, M., and Davis, M. M.

(1985). Rearrangement and transcription of a T-cell receptor β-chain gene in different T-cell subsets. *Proc. Natl. Acad. Sci. USA* 82:531-535.

Hieter, P. A., Maizel, J. R. Jr., and Leder, P. (1982). Evolution of human immunoglobulin k J region genes. *J. Biol. Chem.* 257:1516.

Hieter, P. A., Max, E. E., Seidman, J. G., Maizel, J. V., Poplack, D. G., Waldmann, T. A., and Leder, P. (1980). Cloned human and mouse kappa immunoglobulin constant and J region genes conserve homology in functional segments. *Cell* 22:197.

Hieter, P. A., Korsmeyer, S. J., Waldmann, T. A., and Leder, P. (1981a). Human immunoglobulin κ light chain genes are deleted or rearranged in λ-producing B cells. *Nature* 290:368.

Hieter, P. A., Hollis, G. F., Korsmeyer, S. J., Waldmann, T. A., and Leder, P. (1981b). Clustered arrangement of immunoglobulin λ constant region genes in man. *Nature* 294:536.

Hollis, G. F., Mitchell, K. F., Battey, J., Potter, J., Taub, R., Lenoir, G. M., and Leder, P. (1984). A variant translocation places the lambda immunoglobulin genes 3' to the c-myc oncogene in Burkitt's lymphoma. *Nature* 307: 752-755.

Hozumi, N., and Tonegawa, S. (1976). Evidence for somatic rearrangement of immunoglobulin genes coding for variable and constant regions. *Proc. Natl. Acad. Sci. USA* 73:3628.

Jaffe, E. S., Braylan, R. C., Nanba, K., Frank, M. M., and Berard, C. W. (1977). Functional markers: A new prespective on malignant lymphomas. *Cancer Treat. Rep.* 61:953.

Kirsch, I. R., Morton, C. C., Nakahara, K., and Leder, P. (1982). Human immunoglobulin heavy chain genes map to a region of translocation in malignant B lymphocytes. *Science* 216:301.

Kitchingman, G., Rovigatti, U., Mauer, A., Melvin, S., Murphy, S., and Stass, S. (1985). Rearrangement of Immunoglobulin Heavy Chain Genes in T cell ALL. *Blood* 65(3):725-729.

Knap, M. R., Liu, C.-P., Newell, N., Ward, R. B., Tucker, P. W., Strober, S., and Blattner, F. (1982). Simultaneous expression of immunoglobulin μ and heavy chains by a cloned B cell lymphoma: A single copy of the V_H gene is shared by two adjacent C_H genes. *Proc. Natl. Acad. Sci. USA* 79:2996.

Korsmeyer, S. J., Nieter, P. A., Ravetch, J. V., Poplack, D. G., Waldmann, T. A., and Leder, P. (1981). Developmental hierarchy of immunoglobulin gene rearrangements in human leukemic pre-B cells. *Proc. Natl. Acad. Sci. USA* 78: 7096.

Korsmeyer, S. J., Hieter, P. A., Sharrow, S. O., Goldman, C. K., Leder, P., and Waldmann, T. A. (1982). Normal human B cells display ordered light chain gene rearrangements and deletions. *J. Exp. Med.* 156:975.

Korsmeyer, S. J., Arnold, A., Bakhshi, A., Ravetch, J. V., Siebenlist, U., Hieter, P. A., Sharrow, S. O., LeBein, T. W., Kersey, J. H., Poplack, D. G., Leder, P., and Waldmann, T. A. (1983). Immunoglobulin gene rearrangements and cell surface antigen expression in acute lymphocytic leukemias of T cell and B cell precursor origins. *J. Clin. Invest.* 71:301.

Leder, P. (1982). The genetics of antibody diversity. *Sci. Amer.* 246:102.

Leder, P., Battey, J., Lenoir, G., Moulding, C., Murphy, W., Potter, H., Stewart, T., and Taub, R. (1983). Translocations among antibody genes in human cancer. *Science* 222:765-771.

Lenoir, G. M., Preud'homme, J. L., Bernheim, A., and Berger, R. (1982). Correlations between immunoglobulin light chain expression and variant translocation in Burkitt's lymphoma. *Nature* 298:474.

Lipford, E. H., Smith, H. R., and Pittaluga, S. (1987). Clonality of angioimmunoblastic lymphadenopathy and implications for its evolution to malignant lymphoma. *J. Clin. Invest.* In press.

McBride, O. W., Hieter, P. A., Hollis, G. F., Swan, D., Otey, M. C., and Leder, P. (1982). Chromosomal location of human κ and λ immunoglobulin light chain constant region genes. *J. Exp. Med.* 155:1480.

Malcolm, S., Barton, P., Murphy, C., Ferguson Smith, M. A., Bentley, D. L., and Rabbitts, T. H. (1982). Localization of human immunoglobulin κ light chain variable region genes to the short arm of chromosome 2 by in situ hybridization. *Proc. Natl. Acad. Sci. USA* 79:4957.

Malissen, M., McCoy, C., Blanc, D., Trucy, J., Devaux, C., Schmitt-Verhulst, A. M., Fitch, F., Hood, L., and Malissen, B. (1986). Direct evidence for chromosomal inversion during T-cell receptor beta-gene rearrangements. *Nature* 319: 28-33.

Marcu, K. B., Lang, R. B., Stanton, L. W., and Harris, L. J. (1982). A model for the molecular requirements of immunoglobulin heavy chain class switching. *Nature* 298:87.

Max, E. E., Seidman, J. G., and Leder, P. (1979). Sequences of five potential recombination sites close to an immunoglobulin κ constant region gene. *Proc. Natl. Acad. Sci. USA* 76:3450.

Minden, M. D., Toyonaga, B., Ha, K., Yanagi, Y., Chin, B., Gelfand, E., and Mak, T. (1985). Somatic rearrangement of T-cell antigen receptor gene in human T-cell malignancies. *Proc. Natl. Acad. Sci. USA* 82:1224.

Moore, K. W., Rogers, J., Hunkapiller, T., Early, P., Nottenburg, C., Weissman, I., Bazin, H., Wall, R., and Hood, L. E. (1981). Expression of IgD may use both DNA rearrangement and RNA splicing mechanisms. *Proc. Natl. Acad. Sci. USA* 78:1800.

Murre, C., Waldmann, R. A., Morton, C. C., Bongiovanni, K. F., Waldmann, T. A., Shows, T. B., and Seidmann, J. G. (1985). Human γ-chain genes are rearranged in leukemic T cells and map to the short arm of chromosome 7. *Nature* 316:549.

Nadler, L. M., Ritz, J., Hardy, R., Pesando, J. M., Schlossman, S. F., and Stashenko, P. (1981). A unique cell surface antigen identifying lymphoid malignancies of B-cell origin. *J. Clin. Invest.* 67:134.

Nadler, L. M., Ritz, J., Bates, M. P., Park, E. K., Anderson, K. C., Sallan, S. E., and Schlossman, S. F. (1982). Induction of human B-cell antigens in non-T cell acute lymphoblastic leukemia. *J. Clin. Invest.* 70:433.

Nadler, L. M., Anderson, K. C., Mouti, G., Bates, M., Park, E., Daley, J. F., and Schlossman, S. F. (1983). B_4, a human B-lymphocyte associated antigen expressed on normal, mitogen-activated, and malignant B lymphocytes. *J. Immunol.* 131:244.

Nadler, L. M., Korsmeyer, S. J., Anderson, K. C., Boyd, A. W., Slaughenhoupt, B., Park, E., Jensen, J., Coral, F., Mayer, R. J., and Sallan, S. E. (1984). The B cell origin of non-T acute lymphoblastic leukemia: A model for discrete stages of neoplastic and normal pre-B cell differentiation. *J. Clin. Invest.* 74: 332.

O'Connor, N. T. J., Wainscoat, J. S., Weatherall, D. J., Gatter, K. C., Issacson, P., Jones, D., Lennert, K., Feller, A. C., Patterson, E., and Ramsey A. (1985). Rearrangement of the T-cell receptor beta chain gene in the diagnosis of lymphoproliferative disorders. *Lancet* 1:1295.

Pech, M., Hochtl, J., Schnell, H., and Zachau, H. G. (1981). Differences between germline and rearranged immunoglobulin V_K coding sequences suggest a localized mutation mechanism. *Nature* 291:668.

Quertermous, T., Murre, C., Dialynas, D., Duby, A. D., Strominger, J. L., Waldmann, T. A., and Seigman, J. G. (1986). Human T-cell gamma genes: Organization, diversity and rearrangement. *Science* 231:252.

Raulet, D. H., Garman, R. D., Saito, H., and Tonegawa, S. (1985). Developmental regulation of T-cell receptor gene expression. *Nature* 314:103.

Ravetch, J. V., Siebenlist, U., Korsmeyer, S. J., Waldmann, T., and Leder, P. (1981). The structure of the human immunoglobulin μ locus: Characterization of embryonic and rearranged J and D genes. *Cell* 27:583.

Reinherz, E. L., Kung, P. C., Goldstein, G., Levey, R. M., and Schlossmann, S. F. (1980). Discrete stages of human intrathymic differentiation: Analysis of normal thymocytes and leukemic lymphoblasts of T-cell lineage. *PNAS* 77: 1588-92.

Rovigatti, U., Mirro, J., Kitchingman, G., Dahl, G., Ochs, J., Murphy, S., and Stass, S. (1984). Heavy chain immunoglobulin gene rearrangement in acute nonlymphocytic leukemia. *Blood* 63:1023.

Rowley, J. D., and Testa, J. R. (1982). Chromosome abnormalities in malignant hematologic diseases. *Adv. Cancer Res.* 36:103.

Royer, H. D., Acuto, O., Fabbi, M., Tizard, R., Ramachandran, K., Smart, J. E., and Reinherz, E. L. (1984). Genes encoding the Ti β subunit of the antigen/MHC receptor undergo rearrangement during intrathymic ontogeny prior to surface T3-Ti expression. *Cell* 39:261.

Royer, H. D., Ramarli, D., Acuto, O., Campen, T. J., and Reinherz, E. L. (1985). Genes encoding the T-cell α and β subunits are transcribed in an ordered manner during intrathymic ontogeny. *Proc. Natl. Acad. Sci. USA* 82:5510.

Saito, H., Kranz, D. M., Takagaki, Y., Hayday, A. C., Eisen, H. N., and Tonegawa, S. (1984). A third rearranged and expressed gene in a clone of cytotoxic T lymphocytes. *Nature* 321:36.

Seidman, J. G., and Leder, P. (1978). The arrangement and rearrangement of antibody genes. *Nature* 276:790.

Siebenlist, U., Ravetch, J. V., Korsmeyer, S. J., Waldmann, T., and Leder, P. (1981). Human immunoglobulin D segments encoded in tandem multigenic families. *Nature* 294:631.

Sim, G. K., Yague, J., Nelson, J., Marrack, P., Palmer, E. Augustin, A., and Kappler, J. (1984). Primary structure of human T-cell receptor α chain. *Nature* 312:771.

Siminovitch, K. A., Bakhski, A., Goldman, P., and Korsmeyer, S. J. (1985). A uniform deleting element mediates the loss of κ genes in human B cells. *Nature* 316:260.

Snodgrass, H. R., Dembic, Z., Steinmetz, M., and von-Boehmer, H. (1985). Expression of T-cell antigen receptor genes during fetal development in the thymus. *Nature* 315:232.

Taub, R., Kirsch, I., Morton, C., Lenoir, G., Swan, D., Tronick, S., Aaronson, S., and Leder, P. (1982). Translocation of the c-myc gene into the immunoglobulin heavy chain locus in human Burkitt lymphoma and murine plasmacy toma cells. *Proc. Natl. Acad. Sci. USA* 79:7837.

Taub, R. A., Hollis, G. F., Hieter, P. A., Korsmeyer, S. J., Waldmann, T. A., and Leder, P. (1983). The variable amplification of immunoglobulin lambda light chain genes in human populations. *Nature* 304:172.

Tawa, A., Hozumi, N., Minden, M., Mak, T. W., and Gelfand, E. W. (1985). Rearrangement of the T cell receptor β chain gene in non-T cell, non-B cell acute lymphoblastic leukemia of childhood. *N. Engl. J. Med.* 313:1033.

Tonegawa, S. (1983). Somatic generation of antibody diversity. *Nature* 302:575.

Tsujimoto, Y., Yunis, J. J., and Onorato-Showe, L. (1984). Molecular cloning of the chromosomal breakpoints of B cell leukemias and lymphoas with the t(11;14) chromosomal translocation. *Science* 224:2403.

Waldmann, T. A., Davis, M. M., Bongiovanni, K. F., and Korsmeyer, S. J. (1985). Rearrangements of genes for the antigen receptor on T cells as markers of lineage and clonality in human lymphoid neoplasms. *N. Engl. J. Med.* 313: 776.

Weiss, L. M., Hu, E., Woods, G. S., Moulds, C., Cleary, M. L., Warnke, R., and Sklar, J. (1985). Clonal rearrangements of T-cell receptor genes in mycosis fungoides and dermatopathic lymphadenopathy. *N. Engl. J. Med.* 313:539.

Weiss, L. M., Strickler, J. G., Dorfman, R. F., Horning, S. S., Warnke, R. A., and Sklar, J. (1986). Clonal T cell populations in angioimmunoblastic lymphadenopathy and anioimmunoblastic lymphadenopathy-like lymphoma. *Am. J. Pathol.* 122:392.

Wright, J. J., Poplack, D. G., Bakhski, A., and Korsmeyer, S. J. (1986a). DNA rearrangements as unique markers of clonal evolution, recurrence, and translocation. In *Minimal Residual Disease in Acute Leukemia*, A. Hagenbeek and B. Lowenberg (Eds.). Dordrecht, The Netherlands: Martinus Nijhoff Publishers.

Wright, J. J., Felix, C., Korsmeyer, S., Reaman, G., Cole, D., Jensen, J., and Poplack, D. (1986b). Immunoglobulin and T cell receptor gene rearrangement as clonal markers in acute lymphoblastic leukemia (ALL). *Proc. Amer. Soc. Clinc. Oncol.* 5:18.

Yanagi, Y., Yoshikai, Y., Leggett, K., Clark, S. P., Aleksander, I., and Mak, T. W. (1984). A human T-cell specific cDNA clone encodes a protein having extensive homology to immunoglobulin chains. *Nature* 308:145.

Yancopoulos, G. D., Blackwell, T. K., Suh, H., Hood, L., and Alt, F. W. (1986). Introduced T cell receptor variable region gene segments recombine in pre-B cells: Evidence that B and T cells use a common recombinase. *Cell* 44:251.

Yoshikai, Y., Clark, S. P., Taylor, S. Sohn, U., Wilson, B. I., Minden, M. D., and Mak, T. W. (1985). Organization and sequences of the variable, joining and constant region genes of the human T-cell receptor α-chain. *Nature* 316:837.

Yunis, J. J. (1983). Chromosomal basis of human neoplasia. *Science* 221:227.

Zehnbauer, B., Pardoll, D., Graham, M., and Vogelstein, B. (1986). Immunoglobulin Gene Rearrangements in Remission Bone Marrow Specimens from patients with ALL. *Blood* 67(3):835-838.

10

Oncogenes and Acute Leukemia

MURRAY B. GARDNER *School of Medicine, University of California–Davis, Davis, California*

I. INTRODUCTION

Cellular oncogenes, otherwise called proto-oncogenes or c-oncs, constitute a limited number of evolutionarily conserved cellular genes that are apparently involved in normal cell growth and differentiation. When activated by mutation or loss of regulatory gene function, the oncogenes are quantitatively or qualitatively altered and they then help to turn normal cells into malignant or immortal cells by molecular genetic mechanisms that are just now becoming visible (1,1a). Most human proto-oncogenes represent the cellular homolog of the oncogenes present in highly tumorigenic retroviruses of animal origin, such as those inducing acute leukemia or sarcoma in chickens, mice, and cats (2). Now that almost all human proto-oncogenes have been mapped to specific chromosomal loci, it has become apparent that c-onc activation often follows chromosomal rearrangements or more subtle genetic alteration by mechanisms completely independent of retrovirus involvement. In addition to such chromosomal aberrations, evidence of proto-oncogene involvement in human neoplasia is provided by in vitro DNA-mediated transfection analysis and by analysis of gene expression in tumor and normal tissues. Transfection experiments have identified one family (ras) of human oncogenes that is related to animal retroviral oncogenes and other oncogenes that are unrelated to retroviruses (3).

In this chapter I will first briefly review the major ways in which cellular oncogenes are activated in nature, and current knowledge of the effector function of cellular oncogenes in normal and malignant cell growth. I will then summarize, in more detail, evidence indicating the involvement of specific cellular oncogenes in human acute leukemia. Although still largely descriptive and speculative, enough evidence has accumulated to link certain proto-oncogenes to acute leukemia in humans. This research should, therefore, soon lead to a deeper understanding of oncogene function in normal and abnormal growth processes and to better practical methods for diagnosis and, possibly, treatment of human cancer.

A. Activation of Cellular Oncogenes by Retrovirus Translocation or Insertion Promotion

Most proto-oncogenes, about 30 in number, represent the normal cellular homolog of genes that were "rescued," mutated, and activated by natural "helper" retrovirus infections of chickens, mice and cats, with single examples from turkey and woolly monkey (4,5). The prototype oncogene of this type is the src gene transduced by avian leukosis virus from chicken DNA many years ago to form the Rous sarcoma virus (6). In several instances, homologous oncogenes have been transduced by different helper viruses from different animal species, indicating perhaps a limited repertoire of proto-oncogenes in nature. An example is the fes oncogene, present in both feline and avian sarcoma viruses (7). Several animal retroviruses even include two separately transduced oncogenes or an oncogene and another cellular gene in the same genome. Examples include the myb and ets oncogenes in an avian acute leukemia virus (8) and the fgr oncogene and actin gene in the GR strain of feline sarcoma virus (9).

By virtue of encoding the enzyme reverse transcriptase, retroviruses insert full-length double-stranded copies (provirus) of their RNA genome into the chromosomal DNA of the infected host cells. Insertion of proviral DNA in the vicinity of a c-onc gene sets the stage for transduction of the cellular proto-oncogene in these animal models. For transduction to occur, a rare event, proviral and c-onc hybrid transcripts undergo recombination during reverse transcription; in this process, the c-onc introns are largely eliminated and the rescued c-onc exons undergo several nucleotide substitutions, deletions, or point mutations (10,10a). Replication of the helper retrovirus in susceptible cells then greatly increases the amount of the transduced oncogene. Activation in situ of c-onc genes in animal cells may follow insertion of exogenous retrovirus whose proviral DNA stimulates c-onc expression by strong promoter or enhancer elements within the proviral long terminal repeat (LTR). Insertional mutation of the c-myc locus by exogenous retrovirus infection in avian B cell (11,12,12a) and rodent (13,14) or feline T-cell lymphomas (15-17) and insertional activation of the int-1 and int-2 loci by the mammary tumor virus in mice (18,19) are prime examples of this phenomenon.

As far as we know, cellular oncogenes have not as yet been transduced from human DNA by the T-cell lymphotropic retroviruses (HTLV-I, II, HTLV-III/LAV) that infect humans (20,21). Nor is there any evidence for direct activation of cellular oncogenes by the LTR sequences or randomly integrated HTLV proviral genomes (22). Instead, HTLV transactivating gene products, similar to those in some DNA tumor viruses, may be a critical determinant of the development of adult T-cell leukemia in infected humans (23,24). It should also be emphasized that humans appear totally resistant to infection with retroviruses from other species, even under conditions of close exposure (25). Thus, activation of human cellular oncogenes in leukemogenesis, or tumorigenesis in general, apparently does not result from transduction or insertional mutagenesis from infection with exogenous retroviruses, unless, of course, such an event has escaped detection. In so much as retroviruses are apparently not involved, what mechanism does account for the activation of human c-onc homologs that has been detected in some human leukemias and other tumors? C-onc activation by insertional mutagenesis of endogenous transposon-like retroviral elements, as occurs in mice (26), remains a theoretical possibility, since endogenous retrovirus-like sequences and their expression have been identified in the human genome (27,28). However, other means of oncogene activation, unrelated to retroviruses, and apparently more directly applicable to human leukemogenesis, include chromosomal gross rearrangements, gene amplification, and subtle point mutations.

B. Activation of Cellular Oncogenes by Chromosomal Rearrangements

Chromosomal abnormalities, as seen at the level of the light microscope, have long been associated with certain human tumors, including many hematological malignancies (29,30). Increased resolution provided by chromosomal banding techniques led to the realization that many of these changes were nonrandom, contrary to previous thought (31). Indeed, a multitude of chromosomal changes, especially translocations, were specifically linked to human malignancies. Soon after the discovery of retroviral oncogenes, they were molecularly cloned and mapped to specific regions of human and animal chromosomes by a combination of somatic cell genetics, Southern blots and in situ hybridization (32). It then became apparent that cellular oncogenes were often positioned close to specific breakpoints at the site of translocation and that expression of these genes was altered as a result of this event. Thus far, two human cellular oncogenes, myc and abl, are strongly implicated in human leukemia as a result of this mechanism. A number of Burkitt's and other B-lymphoma cell lines have translocations that join the c-myc gene on chromosome 8 to one of three immunoglobulin loci on chromosomes 14, 2, or 22 (31a,33-36). The Philadelphia (Ph^1) chromosome, a specific marker for chronic myelogenous leukemia (CML), links c-abl from one end of chromosome 9 to a distal region of chromosome 22 (37-40). Gene amplification, sometimes visible in the form of homogeneously staining regions or double minute chromosomes, has also been shown to occasionally include cellular oncogenes (41). For example, the c-myc and c-myb oncogenes have been found amplified in certain acute myelocytic leukemias (AML) of man (42-45).

C. Activation of Cellular Oncogenes by Point Mutation

Activated oncogenes in animal and human genomes have also been detected by the DNA transfection technique, in which DNA from a variety of human and animal tumors induces neoplastic transformation after introduction into established lines (e.g., NIH 3T3) of rodent fibroblasts (3,46). Transformation of the recipient cells depends upon acquisition of a dominant mutant allele present in the donor DNA. The majority of oncogenes identified in this manner belong to the ras gene family (47). Two members of this family, c-Ha-ras-1 and c-Ha-ras-2, were also identified as retroviral oncogenes. The third member, N-ras, has only been detected by transfection (48-50). Compared to the normal cellular ras proto-oncogene, the activated ras genes detected by the transfection assay have a single nucleotide mutation either at position 12 or 13 or at position 59, 61 or 63, a change which renders the ras protein (p21) oncogenic (51-53). Activated N-ras genes with point mutations at codon 12 or 13 have been described in some cases of human AML (56,57). Activated Ki-ras-2 and activated N-ras have been found in different T-cell acute lymphocytic leukemia (T-ALL) lines (58). Although the point mutations around codons 12, 13, or 59 are assumed to be somatic mutations, direct proof is usually lacking because the homologous sequences from the DNA of normal tissue are not compared. Transfection studies have implicated several other genes as oncogenes distinct from the ras family (3). Based on restriction mapping, these putative oncogenes appear specific for T or B lymphocytes at certain stages of maturation (60-62). However, a sequence comparison of these activated oncogenes with their normal cellular counterparts has also not yet been reported.

D. Effector Functions of Cellular Oncogenes

Various components of the signal pathways controlling cell growth and differentiation are now known to be encoded by cellular oncogenes (63). Not surprisingly, several proto-oncogenes (e.g., c-myc, c-fos, c-myb, c-Ha-ras, c-Ki-ras and c-N-ras) are expressed in a cell-cycle-dependent manner (63a). Other cell-cycle-dependent genes have also been identified which might contribute to the phenotype of human leukemias (63b,c,d). However, we must recognize that finding a high level of cell-cycle-specific RNA in a tumor may simply reflect an increased fraction of cycling cells rather than overexpression of that gene. Clearly, the mechanism of action of growth factors overlaps that of oncogenes and, possibly, other cell-cycle-dependent genes (63e).

Cellular oncogenes can be classified on the basis of the nuclear or cytoplasmic localization of their protein products which correlates with certain functional properties (64). Nuclear oncogenes include c-myc, N-myc, myb, p53, ski and fos. Although not yet well defined, their normal function probably affects transcription of specific cellular genes whose products are critical to growth and differentiation. In normal cells other genes (anti-oncogenes) may control the oncogene expression by encoding binding proteins, which attach to the oncogenic sequences or their upstream promoters (65). Enhanced expression of the nuclear oncogenes may result from their deregulation, for example, by chromosome translocation, and the increased levels of oncogene protein may then lead to an increased transcription of the other cell-cycle-dependent genes involved in continued cell growth or immortalization. Cytoplasmic oncogenes, which include src, ras, erb B, neu, fms, fgr, fes/fps, yes, mil/raf, mos and abl, are usually activated by mutations that alter the structure of the encoded proteins and also sometimes cause increased levels of the oncogene protein. These mutations can be spontaneously arising or chemically induced single nucleotide substitutions, as seen with the ras family; or they can be the result of chromosomal translocation, as seen with abl and myc genes.

Many of the cytoplasmic oncogene proteins are related to growth factors. For example, the sis oncogene controls the synthesis of platelet-derived growth factor (PDGF) (66); the erb B oncogene encodes a protein almost identical with the epidermal growth factor (EGF) receptor (67); the erb A oncogene is related to the human glucocorticoid receptor (68); and the fms oncogene is related to the receptor for the mononuclear phagocyte growth factor, CSF 1 (69). Many of these cytoplasmic oncogene proteins are related to the src protein (pp60) and encode tyrosine protein kinase and lipid kinase activity (70,70a). Although a number of cellular proteins are modified by this phosphokinase activity, none appear directly linked to malignant transformation (70,71). By contrast, phosphorylation of the membrane lipid inositol, by this kinase activity, converts inositol polyphosphate into diacylglycerol and inositol triphosphate which function as second messengers to activate protein kinase C, increase cytoplasmic pH, and mobilize intracellular calcium (72). This second messenger pathway involving inositol lipids is an important signal transduction mechanism for controlling such fundamental cellular processes as secretion, metabolism, phototransduction, and cell proliferation. Protein kinase C may also be the prime target for the action of phorbol esters and other tumor promoters (72a).

The normal cellular ras gene protein (p21) binds to both plasma membrane and guanosine triphosphate (GTP) (73), a property in common with the G proteins, which are known to transduce signals from various cell surface receptors to adenyl cyclase, which also functions as a major second messenger pathway (74). Whereas the normal ras p21 can both bind to and hydrolyze GTP, the oncogenic ras p21, altered by point mutation, can still bind to GTP but fails to hydrolyze this nucleotide (75,76). The loss of GTPase activity allows the continued production of the second messengers (inositol triphosphate and diacylglycerol) in an uncontrolled way, thus stimulating cell proliferation. It therefore appears that cellular oncogenes constitute a "biologic road map" (2) to the various constituents responsible for conveying growth stimuli from the cell surface to the nucleus.

We see that activated oncogenes can function autonomously as growth stimuli by at least four mechanisms: (a) autocrine stimulation by the secretion of growth factors, e.g., sis encoded PDGF' which interacts with receptors on the same cells; (b) constitutive expression of growth factor receptors, e.g., erb B encoded EGF;

Table 1 Candidate Oncogenes Associated with Acute Leukemia in Humans

Gene	Type of leukemia	Primary tumor or cell line	Mechanism of oncogene activation or detection	Ref.
c-myc	Burkitt's lymphoma and other B-cell lymphomas	Cell lines	Translocation	33-36, 100-103
c-myc	APML and AML	Primary tumor and cell line (HL60)	Amplification	42,43
c-myc	AML	Primary tumor	Amplification	42,44
c-myc	T-cell leukemia	Primary tumor and cell lines	Translocation	133,134, 134a
c-abl	CML and its blastic crisis	Cell lines	Translocation	37-40, 120a,120b
c-abl	ALL	Primary tumor	Translocation	122
c-abl	AML	Primary tumor	Translocation	124,125
c-abl	AML	Cell line (K562)	Amplification	120
bcl-1,2	B-cell lymphomas	Primary tumors	Translocation	114,114a
c-mos	AML	Primary tumor	Translocation	32,127
c-ets-1	AMMOL	Primary tumor	Translocation	129,130, 131,132a
c-ets-2	AML	Primary tumor	Translocation	129
c-pim	AML and ?T-cell leukemia	Cell lines	Translocation	136,136a
NGF receptor	APML	Primary tumor	Translocation	138
c-fes or e-erb A	APML	Cell lines	Translocation	139,140
c-myb	AML	Cell lines	Amplification	45
c-fms	AML	Cell lines	Deletion	148,96
C-Ki-ras-2	AML	Cell lines (CEM)	Transfection	58
N-ras	Burkitt's lymphomas	Cell lines	Transfection	160
N-ras	APML	Cell lines (HL60)	Transfection	49

Table 1 continues

Table 1 (continued)

Gene	Type of leukemia	Primary tumor or cell line	Mechanism of oncogene activation or detection	Ref.
N-ras	T-cell leukemia	Cell lines	Transfection	160
N-ras	AML & CML	Primary tumor cell lines	Transfection	58
Blym-1	Burkitt's lymphoma	Cell lines	Transfection	60-62, 170,167a, 169
Tx-2	pre B-cell leukemia	Cell lines	Transfection	60
Tx-3	Mature B-cell leukemia	Cell lines	Transfection	60
Tlym-1	T-cell lymphoma	Cell lines	Transfection	60,61
dbl	Diffuse B-cell lymphoma	Primary tumor	Transfection	169a

AML = Acute myeloblastic leukemia; APML = Acute promyelocytic leukemia; AMMOL = Acute myelomonocytic leukemia; CML = Chronic myelogenous leukemia; NGF = Nerve growth factor.

(c) transduction of growth signals, e.g., src and ras stimulated second messenger activity; and (d) transcriptional deregulation, e.g., myc and fos stimulation of genes involved in cell division. Obviously, oncogenes may function in a variety of ways to convert normal cells into tumor cells.

Using functional assays based on cotransfection of rodent cell lines, oncogenes have been placed in one of two complementation groups: (a) those oncogenes (e.g., myc, polyoma large T, adenovirus Ela) that are primarily responsible for immortalization, and (b) those oncogenes (e.g., ras, polyoma middle T) that are primarily responsible for transformation (64). It appears as if, at least to some extent, most oncogenes will fall within a few functional groups representative of different steps in the pathway of cell growth regulation. Cooperation between members of these groups may promote the stepwise progression of precancerous growths to fully autonomous tumors (77).

We will now examine the involvement of candidate oncogenes in acute human leukemia according to the 3 lines of evidence: (a) expression in normal and tumor tissue, (b) activation by chromosomal rearrangements and (c) DNA-mediated gene transfer. Candidate oncogenes are listed in Table 1 and were also recently reviewed in (78) and (78a).

II. EXPRESSION OF CELLULAR ONCOGENES IN HUMAN LEUKEMIA

A. Commonly Expressed Oncogenes

As one measure of the possible pathogenic role of cellular oncogenes in human leukemogenesis, the expression of these genes has been determined at the RNA level using Northern and dot blots. Five proto-oncogenes, c-myc, c-fos, c-rel, c-Ha-ras and c-K-ras, were expressed in nearly all primary hematologic malignancies and cell lines (79,80,81). However, comparable levels of expression of these oncogenes were generally found in actively growing normal peripheral blood leukocytes and in some nonhematopoietic cell types. Expression of ras specific protein (p21) was observed in AML, in the blastoid crises of CML, and in some B-cell malignancies. However, proteins (p21) related to c-ras were found by Western blot analysis in almost all tested tumors, regardless of tumor type (81a). Quantitative variations or abnormal electrophoretic mobility of ras p21 were not correlated with any specific hematologic tumor; such correlations were observed in human carcinomas (81b,c,d).

The expression of c-myc 2.4-2.7 kilobase (kb) transcripts varied 25-fold in leukemias of myeloid and lymphoid origin with no apparent pattern of specificity (59,80,82). The expression of c-myc and c-fos appeared related to normal cell growth and differentiation as evidenced by increased levels of c-myc and c-fos RNA following mitogenic stimulation of resting cells (83-87) and the decreased levels following growth arrest of lymphoid cells (88,89) or DMSO-induced differentiation of the HL60 promyelocytic cell line (90). Sustained suppression of c-myc expression appeared to be required for terminal macrophage differentiation of HL60 cells (90). C-myc expression in normal human B lymphocytes also appeared cell-cycle-dependent, but in fact was elevated in all phases of the cell cycle (90).

Other oncogenes modulated in their expression during the differentiation of hematopoietic precursor cells included c-myb (91) and c-fms (95,96). The level of c-myb RNA decreased, whereas the levels of c-fos and c-fms expression increased following differentiation of the HL60 cells to macrophages (93). Although normal macrophages expressed high levels of both c-fms and c-fos RNA (92,93), c-fos expression was probably not required for myeloid differentiation to macrophages (94). Expression of c-fms 3.6 kb RNA was detected infrequently in various leukemias (80). Since levels of c-myc, c-fos, c-fms, c-rel, c-Ha-ras, and c-K-ras RNA expression are not clearly elevated in leukemias, as compared to normal dividing leukocytes or macrophages, these genes, if involved in leukemogenesis, probably exhibit more subtle alterations or operate in conjunction with other oncogenes. The activation of c-ras by point mutation and the cooperation of c-ras and c-myc in rodent cell transformation illustrate these points.

B. Uniquely Expressed Oncogenes

By contrast, c-abl, c-myb, c-fes/fps and c-src RNA were sometimes detected in leukemia cells but rarely in normal cells (79,80,81). In CML, translocation of c-abl from chromosome 9 to chromosome 22 accounts for the activation of this c-onc and expression of an altered RNA transcript and protein product (37-40). The high level of c-abl RNA in the K-562 erythroleukemia cell line is due to amplification of the gene (97,97a). Elevated expression of c-abl is not commonly seen in other hematopoietic neoplasms. Increased expression of c-myb 4.5 kb RNA transcripts compared to normal leukocytes was found primarily associated with myeloid leukemias (80,82). As seen with c-myc, the levels of c-myb RNA also decreased when the HL60 line was induced to differentiate (82). The c-myb gene apparently has a general function in cellular proliferation and a specific function in thymic differentiation (97b). Expression of c-fes/fps 2.6 kg RNA transcripts was detected at higher levels in some hematopoietic tumors than in normal cells, with highest levels in AML cells (80). Expression of c-fes/fps tyrosine protein kinase is mainly restricted to hematopoietic cells of myeloid lineage and the c-fes/fps oncogene is closely linked upstream to a gene encoding a receptor-like protein (80a). The differential expression of c-fes/fps RNA and protein suggested an involvement of these oncogenes in leukemogenesis, perhaps based on cell lineage or stage of maturation. C-fgr RNA was recently found at high levels in EBV-positive Burkitt's lymphoma cell lines and Epstein-Barr virus (EBV) transformed normal lymphocytes indicating, for the first time, the induction of a proto-oncogene by infection with a DNA tumor virus (98).

Only an infrequent hematopoietic malignancy had detectable expression of c-src or c-erb RNA transcripts (79-80). Compared to normal peripheral blood leukocytes, several AML samples showed markedly elevated levels of c-erb RNA. C-src RNA expression was increased in only an occasional T-cell ALL, AML or CML. A strong correlation found between levels of c-src kinase activity (pp60) and degree of monocyte differentiation of cells from patients with AML suggests that activation of c-src is a normal physiologic step in myeloid differentiation (79a). Blood platelets also express high levels of c-src pp60 protein, indicating that expression of this tyrosine kinase activity is not exclusively associated with proliferating cells (79b).

Transcripts of c-mos, c-sis and c-yes genes were not detected in any hematopoietic tumor (80). C-sis activation appeared rather specific to human tumors of connective tissue or glial origin (80,81,82). However, activated human monocytes were recently shown to express the c-sis oncogene and release PDFG activity (99). The pathogenic role of these uniquely expressed oncogenes in initiation or promotion of human leukemia or other tumors will remain uncertain until more comparisons are done with normal immature cells and until the expression of oncogene proteins is more critically evaluated.

In summary, findings based mainly on detection of c-onc RNA suggest that several c-onc genes are expressed in virtually all human leukemias; some are expressed infrequently but with consistent patterns; and others are not detectable. The data are consistent with but by no means conclusive for cooperation between oncogenes, e.g., c-myc or c-myb and c-ras in some AML or B-cell malignancies. However, the relative lack of specificity and the variation between c-onc expression and type of leukemia indicate that, in general, transformation of human hematopoietic cells must also involve oncogenes other than those related to animal retroviruses.

III. ACTIVATION OF ONCOGENES BY CHROMOSOMAL REARRANGEMENT IN HUMAN LYMPHOMA AND LEUKEMIA

Many cellular proto-oncogenes are located in the chromosomal bands that are consistently the site of translocations associated with specific hematologic and other malignancies. Of the many specific chromosomal defects found in leukemias and non-Hodgkin's lymphomas, an associated oncogene activation has been well established in several instances. Best understood are the c-myc and c-abl translocations specific to Burkitt's lymphoma and CML, respectively.

A. Translocation of c-myc and Immunoglobulin Genes in B-Cell Lymphomas

In Burkitt's lymphoma a reciprocal translocation is responsible for moving c-myc from its normal location on chromosome 8 band q24 to chromosome 14, band q32 (100), where it becomes activated by joining with the immunoglobulin heavy-chain genes (IgH) within their switch region (35,36,101,102). The same t(8;14) translocation involving c-myc and IgH occurs in some small noncleaved and large cell immunoblastic lymphomas. As a result of the translocation, the c-myc locus is altered and usually becomes rearranged with the immunoglobulin genes in such a way as to result in an increased level of transcription that fails to respond to normal transcriptional control (103-106). The chromosome 8 translocation breakpoint usually occurs in the first intron or exon of c-myc, a region that may be the binding site of a trans-acting repressor which regulates c-myc expression (107). In addition, other mutations resulting from this t8;14 rearrangement may lead to an altered c-myc product (108). Because recombination of c-myc with the heavy chain cluster occurs at the switch region in the allelically excluded locus, the cells are still able to make immunoglobulin from the other allele (109,110). The c-myc oncogene on the normal chromosome 8 is transcriptionally silent (110, 111). In about 10% of Burkitt's lymphomas, c-myc stays on chromosome 8 but rearranges with the kappa or lambda immunoglobulin light-chain genes translocated to chromosome 8 from chromosomes 2p13 or 22q11, respectively. In these variant translocations, the type of light chain produced correlates with the type of light chain encoded by the translocated locus. Interestingly, the site of chromosomal breakpoint and the type of structural alteration of the myc gene differ in endemic and sporadic forms of Burkitt's lymphoma, probably as a function of different stages of B-cell differentiation (110a). A similar rearrangement between c-myc and the immunoglobulin heavy-chain genes within their switch regions occurs in murine plasmacytomas (112,113), suggesting a common genetic mechanism in nature for induction of B-cell neoplasms.

The 8;14 translocation characterizing most Burkitt's lymphomas is also found in about 25% of diffuse large-cell lymphomas, but in the apparent absence of c-myc rearrangements (31a). C-myc rearrangement, apparently not involving the Ig loci, was found in only one diffuse large-cell lymphoma among 16 tumors of this type and 22 lymphomas of other types examined. In these tumors, activation of c-myc may occur by other mechanisms, including translocation more distal to the gene. Trisomy for chromosome 8 occurs rather frequently in AML (31), but it is as yet unknown if c-myc is altered. In addition to c-myc, some Burkitt's lymphomas contain other activated transforming genes (N-ras, Blym-1, and c-fgr) detected by DNA transfer and molecular hybridization, respectively.

B. bcl-1, bcl-2, and Other Putative Oncogenes

Translocations involving the IgH band q32 of chromosome 14 often occur with one of several chromosomes other than chromosome 8 and may point the way to other, as yet unknown oncogenes (30,32). In this manner, a putative oncogene, termed bcl-1, located on chromosome 11 band q13, rearranges with the IgH locus at chromosome 14q32 in some patients with small lymphocytic cell lymphoma and diffuse large-cell lymphoma (114). A reciprocal translocation between chromosome 14q32 and chromosome 18q21 also occurs in many follicular B-cell lymphomas. The putative bcl-2 oncogene is located at the q21 breakpoint on chromosome 18 and is interrupted or split by the t14;18 translocation (114a) in a manner similar to the splitting of the c-myc gene in some Burkitt's lymphomas carrying the t(8;14) translocation. About 30% of pre B-cell acute lymphoblastic leukemias have a t(1;19) (q23, p13) translocation and 25% of T-cell acute lymphoblastic leukemias contain a t(11;14) (p13; q13) translocation. Oncogenes remain to be identified at these chromosomal breakpoints.

C. c-abl, the Philadelphia Chromosome, and Chronic Myelogenous Leukemia

In CML, the c-abl proto-oncogene moves from the distal end of the long arm of chromosome 9 band q34 to chromosome 22 band q11, thereby generating the Ph^1 chromosome and an abnormal c-abl transcript (115,116,40,118). The breakpoints on chromosome 9q34 are variable and located far upstream ($\geqslant$ 40 kb) from c-abl, whereas the breakpoints on chromosome 22q11 are concentrated in a more restricted region ($\sim$ 5 kb) referred to as the "breakpoint cluster region" (bcr) (40,120b). Juxtaposition of c-abl and the 5' portion of bcr results in a novel 8 kb fused abl/bcr transcript and an altered c-abl protein (p210), which acquires activated tyrosine kinase activity (97,120). This altered c-abl protein (p210) is expressed in Ph^1 positive cell lines and bone marrow cells of Ph^1 positive CML patients, and is strongly implicated in the pathogenesis of CML (117,119). In addition, the c-abl gene becomes amplified and may undergo other mutations in the

Ph^1 chromosome. When Ph^1-positive CML patients enter the blastic or terminal phase of the disease, they usually express greater levels of the 8 kb RNA and acquire an extra Ph^1 chromosome (32). The Ig lambda light-chain gene retained on chromosome 22 and the sis oncogene translocated to chromosome 9 during formation of the Ph^1 chromosome are not considered critical to the pathogenesis of CML because both loci are located far distant from bcr (118). Nor has expression of c-sis been detected in Ph^1-positive cells (97). The same genomic change as occurs in Ph^1 positive CML has been observed in some CML patients with apparently normal karyotype or "masked" Ph^1 chromosomes (120a). In this situation, a separate mechanism, other than chromosomal translocation, must juxtapose c-abl and bcr DNA within the leukemic cells. A few Ph^1-negative CML patients show no genomic rearrangement of c-abl and bcr and thus may suffer from a different hematologic disease.

D. c-abl and Acute Lymphocytic Leukemia

About 10% of human ALL cases carry a t(9;22) chromosomal translocation, cytogenetically indistinguishable from the Ph^1 chromosome (121). In adult ALL of this type, the same genetic rearrangement of c-abl and bcr loci may occur as is seen in CML. However, in childhood ALL, the chromosome 22 breakpoint occurs proximal (5') to the bcr locus, which is thus not involved in this translocation (122). Moreover, normal-sized bcr and c-abl transcripts were observed in one childhood ALL cell line carrying the t(9;22) translocation. Therefore, if c-abl expression is found altered in Ph^1 ALL cells of childhood, the genetic mechanism of activation must be different from that of CML. It has now been shown that Ph^1 ALL cells express unique abl-derived tyrosine kinoses of 185 and 180 kilodaltons that are distinct from the bcr-abl-derived p210 protein of CML (122a).

In view of the critical role of c-abl in the pathogenesis of CML, other malignancies involving changes of chromosome 9 at band q34 might also be expected to involve this oncogene. Furthermore, somatic cell hybrids between Ph^1-positive CML cells and mouse fibroblasts have shown that expression of the altered c-abl gene is not myeloid-cell specific, but the effect of the altered c-abl protein may, of course, differ for different cell types (123). A candidate is the t(6;9) of AML with increased basophils, in which a reciprocal translocation occurs between chromosome 6p23 and chromosome 9q34 (124). However, in two such cases the breakpoint on chromosome 9 was distal (3') to c-abl, which was therefore not translocated (125). Furthermore, an abnormal c-abl protein was not detected. Thus, if the t(6;9) translocation of AML activates c-abl, it does so by a mechanism different from its activation in CML. In one AML patient the c-abl gene was duplicated and translocated to the junction of a reciprocal translocation between chromosomes 4 and 10 on the 4q+ chromosome. It remains possible that c-abl is an innocent bystander of this t(4;10) variant translocation and is not involved in the pathogenesis of this type of AML. In this disease other sequences distal to c-abl on chromosome 9 may become oncogenic by movement to chromosone 6.

E. c-myb and Acute Lymphocytic Leukemia

The c-myb gene is located on chromosome 6 at band q 22-24 (126), a region often deleted in one chromosome in ALL. Mentioned above was the finding that immature T-cell ALL sometimes shows expression of c-myb RNA (82). A deletion of band 6q24 has also been seen in AML cell lines, in association with amplification of the c-myb gene (45). However, the significance of c-myb activation by these chromosomal aberrations remains uncertain.

F. c-mos and Acute Myeloblastic Leukemia

Oncogene c-mos is located on chromosome 8 band q 22 (127), the site of the breakpoint on chromosome 8 in the t(8;21) translocation which occurs in about 8% of AMLs (32). However, rearrangements or altered expression of c-mos have not as yet been reported in AML with the t(8;21) translocation, so the relationship of c-mos to this type of leukemia is currently unknown.

G. c-ets-1 and c-ets-2 and Acute Myelomonocytic Leukemia

The human ets oncogene has two separate loci: ets-1 is on chromosome 11, band q23; ets-2 is on chromosome 21, band 22 (128). The ets-1 gene was translocated from chromosome 11 to chromosome 4 in certain stem cell leukemias of infants (129) and from chromosome 11 to chromosome 9 in about 10% of adults with AMMOL (130). The c-ets-1 gene was translocated adjacent to interferon B1 genes on the short arm of chromosome 9 (131). The break on chromosome 9 split the interferon genes and the interferon B1 gene was translocated to chromosome 11. The juxtaposition of c-ets-1 just 3' to the B1 interferon gene suggests that factors that regulate expression of interferon genes may also activate c-ets-1 expression. Other alterations involving both rearrangement and amplification of the c-ets-1 locus have been detected by Southern blotting in AML and lymphoma patients with chromosomal abnormalities involving chromosome band 11q22 (132a). The ets-2 gene was found translocated from chromosome 21 to 8 in the M2 subtype of AML (129). Both c-ets-1 and c-ets-2 translocations are associated with alteration and overexpression of the ets-1 and ets-2 RNS. It seems likely that the c-ets-2 locus is involved in the abnormalities of chromosome 21, in particular trisomy 21, which occurs in Down's syndrome (132) in association with an increased incidence of AML. Further molecular analysis of the c-ets-1 and c-ets-2 genes and their products and the breakpoints underlying their translocations will help determine the function of these genes in acute leukemogenesis.

H. Translocation of the T-Cell Receptor, Activation of c-myc, and T-Cell Leukemia

In a manner similar to myc and bcl deregulation in Burkitt's lymphoma and other B-cell malignancies, it appears that c-myc may be activated in some T-cell leukemias by translocation of the α locus of the T-cell receptor downstream to c-myc on chromosome 8 (133,134). The gene encoding the α chain of the T-cell receptor is located at chromosome 14, band q11. A common chromosome alteration in ALL of T-cell type is a t(8;14) translocation in which the chromosome 14 breakpoint lies between the V α and C α genes. In two patients with T-cell leukemias, the C α locus on chromosome 14 was translocated to a region some distance (~38kb) 3' to c-myc, resulting in its transcriptional deregulation. In other patients with T-cell leukemia, a similar break on chromosome 14 translocated the C α locus to chromosome 11 at band p13, which may therefore be the site of an as yet unidentified proto-oncogene (134a). Apparently the α chain of the T-cell receptor contains genetic elements capable of activating transcription of c-myc and possibly other genes over considerable chromosomal distances.

I. c-pim and Acute Leukemia

Another putative oncogene, possibly activated by proximity to the α-chain locus of the T-cell receptor, is the c-pim locus on chromosome 6, band p21. Translocations between chromosomes 6p21 and 14q11 have been described in human leukemias (135). C-pim is the human homolog of the murine pim-1 gene, which is activated in murine T-cell lymphomas by insertion promotion of exogenous provirus (13). Translocation of chromosome 6p21 to chromosome 9q33-34 occurs in some cases of AML (136). It has not yet been determined whether the c-pim gene is directly involved in this translocation. C-pim 3.2 kb RNA is actively transcribed at various levels in many cell lines of hematopoietic lineage, including lines of lymphoblastoid, CML, and Burkitt's lymphoma origin. However, the level of c-pim RNA was low or undetected in human cell lines of T-cell origin (136a). The possible involvement of c-pim in different translocations, t(6;9) and t(6;14), suggests that this gene may be activated by different mechanisms and have an important role in human leukemia.

J. Nerve Growth Factor Receptor Gene and Acute Promyelocytic Leukemia

Yet another putative oncogene is the nerve growth factor (NGF) receptor gene located close to the chromosome 17 breakpoint seen in the t(15;17) (q22;q21) translocation associated with acute promyelocytic leukemia (137,138). However, the growth factor receptor gene is apparently distal to the breakpoint on chromosome 17 and appears to be in a germline configuration, suggesting that its structure is not grossly altered.

K. c-fes or c-erb A and Acute Promyelocytic Leukemia

Oncogene c-fes is located on chromosome 15 on the long arm (band q25-q26) (139,126), which is frequently translocated to the long arm (band q21-q22) of chromosome 17 in patients with acute promyelocytic leukemia (31). Although c-fes could be involved in the pathogenesis, the critical recombinant locus appears to be located elsewhere on chromosome 15. Another c-onc which might be involved in this translocation is c-erb A, located near the breakpoint on chromosome 17 (140).

L. Amplification or Deletion of c-onc Genes

In addition to chromosomal translocation and point mutation, somatic gene amplification or deletion represent other ways in which oncogene expression can be altered in human tumors. Regions of amplified DNA are sometimes detected by cytogenetic analysis in the form of double minute chromosomes or homogeneously staining regions (41). Examples include c-myc amplification in a few cases of human AML and in an acute promyelocytic leukemia cell line (HL60) and primary tumor (42,43). High levels of c-myc RNA were detected in proliferating HL60 cells but decreased when the cells stopped growing (82). C-myc amplification has also been observed in CML, Burkitt's lymphoma, glioblastoma, neuroendocrine tumors and in colon, breast and lung carcinoma cell lines (141,142, 143,144). A 3' c-myc rearrangement and enhanced RNA transcription were found in the human leukemic T-cell line, HUT 78, associated with a trisomy of chromosome 8 (143a). N-myc amplification was also relatively common in carcinomas and sarcomas and was associated with aggressive biologic behavior (144,144a, 145,146). A striking degree of amplification and expression of the N-myc gene is associated with neuroblastomas, retinoblastomas, and small cell lung cancers (144b). Antisera against the N-myc protein could detect this protein in the nuclei of neuroblastoma cells (147). However, no evidence of c-myc or N-myc amplification was found in most primary leukemias and lymphomas.

The c-myb oncogene was also found amplified in several primary cell lines cultured from a patient with AML (45). C-myb transcription was increased 5- to 10-fold and chromosomal instability was noted in the chromosomal 6 region q22-24 where the c-myb locus is located. Whether amplification was present in nonleukemic cells from the same individual was not determined. Such an amplification may prevent the normal physiologic suppression of c-myb which appears to correlate with a switch from cell proliferation to differentiation. However, an amplification of c-myb has not been observed in most AML or other hematopoietic tumor DNA. C-ets-1 has been found amplified in one case of AMML. C-ki-ras-2 is amplified in some primary carcinomas of lung, colon, bladder and rectum and in neuroendocrine tumors but, as yet, has not been found amplified in human leukemia cell DNA. C-abl is amplified 4- to 8-fold and over expressed in the K562 Ph^1-positive erythroleukemic cell line derived from a patient with CML in blast crisis (97,97a). However, amplification of c-abl is not common in CML.

Apparent allelic deletions of c-Ha-ras and c-myb were also relatively common in human carcinomas and sarcomas, although not seen in leukemias and lymphomas (144). These changes may be random or may be related to the disease. A deletion of the gene for the granulocyte/macrophage colony stimulating factor

(GM-CSF) receptor which corresponds to the c-fms oncogene on chromosome 5, bands q23 to q32, frequently occurs in patients with AML or refractory anemia (148,96). This loss of part or all of chromosome 5 has been observed in AML either de novo or following cytotoxic therapy for a previous different malignancy, suggesting that it may be a marker for mutagen-induced leukemias (29). It seems likely that loss of the GM-CSF receptor gene is involved in the pathogenesis of these hematologic disorders. Such a deletion of a wild-type gene might allow the expression of a recessive mutant allele on the homologous chromosome, a mechanism proposed for the pathogenesis of retinoblastoma and Wilms tumor (54,55,149,150).

IV. DETECTION OF ACTIVATED ONCOGENES BY TRANSFECTION OF DNA FROM HEMATOPOIETIC NEOPLASMS

A. c-ras

Cellular oncogenes capable of transforming NIH 3T3 mouse cells have been found in many primary human tumors and cell lines, including leukemias (3,46,58,151). The majority of these activated oncogenes are members of the ras gene family which are detected in about 10-15% of tumors tested, albeit with rather little tissue specificity. The ras gene family consists of 5 separate cellular genes, c-Ha-ras 1 and 2, c-Ki-ras 1 and 2, and N-ras. The first 4 members are closely related to the viral oncogenes in the Harvey (Ha) and Kirsten (Ki) strains of murine sarcoma viruses (47). The fifth member, N-ras, is more distantly related and has been detected only by transfection (152). Activated c-Ha-ras-1 oncogenes in bladder tumor cell lines were the first activated oncogenes to be detected by transfection (155,156). However this oncogene has been detected only in a few carconomas and melanomas and not, as yet, in any leukemias or other hematopoietic tumors. By contrast, activated c-Ki-ras-2 and c-N-ras have been found in many human tumors, including leukemias (49,50,58,153,154,159-161,163). C-Ha-ras-2 and c-Ki-ras-1 are nonfunctioning pseudogenes (157,158). Activated c-Ki-ras-2 was found in an intermediate T-cell ALL line (CEM) (58) and activated N-ras was found in cell lines or fresh bone marrow cells from CML and AML (58,159) and in cell lines from acute promyelocytic leukemia (HL60) (90), Burkitt's lymphoma (Ramos), immature T-leukemia (RPMI 8402) and intermediate T leukemia (Molt 3, Molt 4, T-ALL-1, p12) (160). Activated N-ras was found particularly often ($\geqslant$50%) in AML, making this the human tumor type from which activated ras oncogenes could most predictably be detected. Levels of N-ras 2.0-2.2 kb RNA were similar in normal and tumor cells. Instead of an increased level of expression, activation of N-ras, like c-Ha-ras-1 and c-Ki-ras-2, depends on point mutation around amino acids 12, 13 and 61 (57). The mutant N-ras proteins migrate with an altered mobility on SDS gel electrophoresis (50). The failure to detect mutant ras genes in normal tissues by transfection or restriction enzyme digestion strongly suggests that activation of ras oncogenes occurs only in somatic cells (161-163). The bias toward activation of N-ras in leukemias suggests that this gene, rather than other ras genes, may be involved in regulating hematopoietic cell proliferation and differentiation. The reproducible pattern of Ha-ras-1 gene activation by single point mutation in animal tumors induced by the same chemical carcinogen (164,164a) suggests that a specific carcinogenic agent may similarly be responsible for N-ras activation in AML.

B. Cellular Oncogenes Unrelated to Viral Oncogenes

In contrast to activated ras genes, which show little tissue specificity, other 3T3 cell transforming genes, unrelated to ras or other viral oncogenes, do appear to have tissue specificity (3,60-62). A transforming gene of this type was first detected in DNA from chicken B cell lymphomas induced by avian leukosis virus (165). This gene, named Blym, was cloned, sequenced (166) and found to be different than the c-myc gene which is activated by LTR insertion in these tumors (11). At least five different transforming genes of this type have been detected in DNA from B- and T-lymphocytic neoplasms and, based on restriction endonuclease digestion, these oncogenes appear specific to particular stages of differentiation and lymphoid cell lineage. Such genes may, therefore, be involved in normal cell differentiation. Moreover, these oncogenes appear to be the same in mouse and human tumors of the same type. Thus, oncogenes apparently specific to tumors of pre-B cells (Tx-2), Burkitt's lymphoma (Blym-1), mature B cells (Tx-3), intermediate T cells (Tlym-1) and mature T cells (Tx-4) have been identified by the transfection technique.

The Blym-1 oncogene is a small gene of about 550 base pairs encoding a protein of 65 amino acids (mol wt 7800) which is distantly related to a growth factor, transferrin (167a). Activation of Blym-1 in some Burkitt's lymphomas is detected by transfection (62) and this oncogene represents the human homolog of the Blym-1 oncogene activated in avian leukosis virus-induced bursal lymphomas in the chicken. Blym-1 is also related to a family of conserved repeated DNA sequences called LINES present in mouse and human DNA (167). In fact, the "chicken" Blym-1 oncogene apparently is a portion of a mouse LINES element whose transforming potential was activated during molecular cloning. The human Blym-1 gene is 50-60% homologous to the mouse LINES sequences but does not show significant homology to the human LINES element (168). The human Blym-1 gene, although distantly related to repetitive DNA sequences, represents a unique sequence mapped to a unique chromosomal locus (62,169). The chicken and human Blym-1 genes have been molecularly cloned and sequenced, but it is not yet known how the transforming gene differs from the normal allele. The activated Blym-1 gene has identical nucleotide sequences with its normal allele and no significant increase is noted in the level of Blym-1 RNA in Burkitt's lymphoma tissue compared to EBV immortalized lymphoid cell lines (170). These results suggest that Blym-1 activation may result by a more subtle deregulation, perhaps involving flanking control sequences (171).

The Tlym-1 oncogene is also small (1-2 kb) and appears to have homology to class -1 histocompatibility antigens (60,61). The mechanism of activation of Tlym-1 is, as yet, also unknown. Much more remains to be learned about these putative oncogenes and their transcriptional and translational products in relation to human leukemogenesis.

A new transforming gene, called dbl, encoding a 2.9 kb RNA and a 66 kb protein, was recently isolated from a human B-cell lymphoma (169a), but the significance of this gene remains to be determined. The NIH 3T3 transfection assay may yet reveal other transforming genes, distinct from the ras gene family, in human leukemias.

V. CONCLUSION

Numerous cellular oncogenes have been identified as candidates for involvement in the genesis of human hematopoietic malignancies. However, the evidence for their etiologic role in the pathogenesis of human leukemia remains largely indirect and circumstancial. The most direct evidence exists for c-myc and c-abl because of their reproduceable activation by specific chromosomal translocations in different tumors of the same type, namely, Burkitt's lymphoma and CML. Other oncogenes that show promise of a pathogenic role in human leukemia include c-myb, c-fes/fps, c-ets-1 and c-ets-2, c-pim, N-ras and the α T-cell receptor. Putative differentiation or lineage-specific oncogenes identified by transfection analysis are also promising leads, awaiting further confirmation. The evidence for c-onc involvement based on altered RNA expression is quite inconclusive. Most human leukemias appear to express multiple oncogenes without tissue specificity. However, the lack of adequate normal tissue controls makes interpretation of these findings quite uncertain. Many of the c-oncs (e.g., c-myc, c-fos) may be expressed because they are related more to normal cell division than to malignancy per se. Obviously, other genes—e.g., cell-cycle-dependent or differentiation-stage-specific genes—in addition to the currently defined oncogenes may be instrumental in the neoplastic process and multiple routes of oncogenesis in the same tissue undoubtably exist.

More direct evidence for the involvement of cellular oncogenes in human cancer will come from transfection experiments or construction of transgenic animals in which the activated or normal counterpart genes are introduced into normal cells from the same tissue and compared for phenotypic effect. In this way, microinjection of activated c-myc into 3T3 cells was shown to stimulate DNA synthesis (172) and c-myc transgenic mice developed increased numbers of lymphoid malignancies (173). Microinjection of cells with purified proto-oncogene proteins, e.g., c-ras p21, or with monoclonal antibody to such proteins will help determine the function of these proteins (174,175). Future studies will also entail transfection of oncogenes after site-specific mutagenesis and linkage of oncogenes to different expression vectors. Further study of c-onc protein expression in normal and malignant tissue and use of immunocytochemistry and in situ hybridization to detect RNA and protein expression in individual cells is a current frontier.

Screening of human tissues or secretions with oncogene probes and specific antisera to oncogene proteins or their synthetic peptides (176) should lead to more precise diagnosis of tumor cell lineage, earlier diagnosis of malignant or premalignant lesions, and should provide useful prognostic information. Genetic susceptibility to cancer may be linked to detection of unusual alleles of cellular oncogenes as determined by restriction fragment heterogeneity (177). Oncogenes as targets for tumor therapy remain further in the future. The close link between oncogenes, chromosomal break points and growth factors presages the identification of yet more oncogenes and a clearer picture of their function in normal cell growth. Included here will be an understanding of the proto-oncogene promoters upstream of the transcriptional start sites and their regulation by DNA binding factors. One such transcription factor, Spl, has been shown to bind to the c-Ha-ras-1 promoter region and thereby to regulate the expression of this proto-oncogene (178). Identification of anti-oncogenes and other nucleic acid sequences regulating oncogene expression depends on development of novel assay systems and promises to become another area of vigorous research.

ACKNOWLEDGMENTS

I wish to thank Ms. Faith Betti for typing the manuscript, Ms. Betsy Bencken for editorial help, and my wife Alice for her patience.

REFERENCES

1. Varmus, H. E. (1984). The molecular genetics of cellular oncogenes. *Ann. Rev. Genet.* 18:553-612.
1a. Duesberg, P. H. (1983). Retroviral transforming genes in normal cells? *Nature* 304:219-225.
2. Bishop, J. M. (1985). Viral oncogenes. *Cell* 42:23-38.
3. Cooper, G. M. (1982). Cellular transforming genes. *Science* 217:801-806.
4. Gardner, M. (1980). Historical background. In *Molecular Biology of RNA Tumor Viruses*, J. R. Stephenson (ed.). Academic Press, NY, pp. 1-46.
5. Bishop, J. M. (1983). Cellular oncogenes and retroviruses. *Ann. Rev. Biochem.* 52:301-354.
6. Swanstrom, R., Parker, R. C., Varmus, H. E., and Bishop, J. M. (1981). Transduction of a cellular oncogene: The genesis of Rous sarcoma virus. *Proc. Natl. Acad. Sci. USA* 80:2519-2523.
7. Shibuya, M., Hanafusa, T., Hanafusa, H., and Stephenson, R. (1980). Homology exists among the transforming sequences of avian and feline sarcoma viruses. *Proc. Natl. Acad. Sci. USA* 77:6536-6540.

8. Duesberg, P. H., Bister, K., and Moscovici, C. (1980). Genetic structure of avian myeloblastosis virus released from transformed myeloblasts as a defective virus particle. *Proc. Natl. Acad. Sci. USA* 77:5120-5124.
9. Naharro, G., Robbins, K. C., and Reddy, E. P. (1984). Gene product of v-fgr onc: hybrid protein containing a portion of actin and a tyrosine-specific protein kinase. *Science* 223:63-66.
10. Varmus, H. E. (1982). Form and function of retroviral proviruses. *Science* 216:812-820.
10a. Levy, J. B., Iba, H., and Hanafusa, H. (1986). Activation of the transforming potential of $p60^{c\text{-}src}$ by a single amino acid change. *Proc. Natl. Acad. Sci. USA* 83:4228-4232.
11. Hayward, W. S., Neel, B. G., and Astrin, S. M. (1981). Activation of a cellular onc gene by promoter insertion in ALV-induced lymphoid leukosis. *Nature* 209:475-449.
12. Fung, Y. K. T., Fadly, A. M., Crittenden, L. B., and Kung, H. J. (1981). On the mechanism of retrovirus-induced avian lymphoid leukosis: deletion and integration of the proviruses. *Proc. Natl. Acad. Sci. USA* 78:3418-3422.
12a. Payne, G. S., Bishop, J. M., and Varmus, H. E. (1982). Multiple arrangements of viral DNA and an activated host oncogene in bursal lymphomas. *Cell* 31:99-109.
13. Cuypers, H. T., Selten, G., Quint, W., Zijlstra, M., Maandag, E. R. Boelns, W., van Wezenbeck, P., Melief, C., and Berns, A. (1984). Murine leukemia virus-induced T-cell lymphomagenesis: integration of proviruses in a distinct chromosomal region. *Cell* 37:141-150.
14. Steffen, D. (1984). Proviruses are adjacent to c-myc in some murine leukemia virus-induced lymphomas. *Proc. Natl. Acad. Sci. USA* 81:2097-3001.
15. Neil, J. C., Hughes, D., McFarlane, R., Wilkie, N. M., Onions, D. E., et al. (1984). Transduction and rearrangement of the myc gene by feline leukemia virus in naturally occurring T-cell lymphomas. *Nature* 308:814-820.
16. Mullins, J. J., Brody, D. S., Binart, K. C., Jr., and Cotter, S. M. (1984). Viral transduction of c-myc gene in naturally occuring feline leukemia. *Nature* 308:856-858.
17. Levy, L. S., Gardner, M. B., and Casey, J. W. (1984). Isolation of a feline leukemia provirus containing the oncogene myc from a feline lymphosarcoma. *Nature* 308:853-856.
18. Nusse, R., and Varmus, H. E. (1982). Many tumors induced by the mouse mammary tumor virus contain a provirus integrated in the same region of the host genome. *Cell* 31:99-109.
19. Dickson, C., Smith, R., Brookes, S., and Peters, G. (1984). Tumorigenesis by mouse mammary tumor virus: proviral activation of a cellular gene in the common integration region int-2. *Cell* 37:529-536.
20. Poiesz, B. J., Ruscetti, F. W., Gazdar, A. F., Bunn, P. A., Minna, J. D., and Gallo, R. C. (1980). Detection and isolation of type C retrovirus particles from fresh and cultured lymphocytes of a patient with cutaneous T-cell lymphoma. *Proc. Natl. Acad. Sci. USA* 77:7415-7419.

21. Yoshida, Miyoshi, I., and Hinuma, Y. (1982). Isolation and characterization of a retrovirus from cell lines of human adult T-cell leukemia and its implications in the disease. *Proc. Natl. Acad. Sci. USA* 79:2031-2035.
22. Seiki, M., Eddy, R., Snows, I. B., and Yoshida, M. (1984). Nonspecific integration of the HTLV provirus genome into adult T-cell leukemia cells. *Nature* 309:640-642.
23. Sodroski, J. G., Rosen, C., and Haseltine, W. A. (1984). Transfecting transcriptional activation in the long terminal repeat of human T lymphotropic viruses in infected cells. *Science* 225:381-385.
24. Cann, A. J., Rosenblatt, J. D., Wachsman, W., Shah, N. P., and Chen, I. S. Y. (1985). Identification of the gene responsible for human T-cell leukemia virus transcriptional regulation. *Nature* 318:571-574.
25. Gardner, M. B., Rasheed, S., Shimizu, S., Rongey, R. L., Henderson, B. E., McAllister, R. M., Klement, V., Charman, H. D., Gilden, R. V., Heberling, R. L., and Huebner, R. J. (1977). Search for RNA tumor virus in humans. In *Origins of Human Cancer*, H. H. Hiatt, J. D. Watson, J. A. Winsten (eds.). Cold Spring Harbor Lab, Cold Spring Harbor, New York, pp. 1235-1251.
26. Rechavi, G., Givol, D., and Canaani, E. (1982). Activation of a cellular oncogene by DNA rearrangement: possible involvement of an IS-like element. *Nature* 300:607-610.
27. Martin, M. A., Bryant, T., Rasheed, S., and Kahn, A. S. (1981). Identification and cloning of endogenous retroviral sequences present in human DNA. *Proc. Natl. Acad. Sci. USA* 78:4892-4896.
28. Bonner, T. I., O'Connell, C., and Cohen, M. (1982). Cloned endogenous retroviral sequences from human DNA. *Proc. Natl. Acad. Sci. USA* 79: 4709-4713.
29. Rowley, J. D., and Testa, J. R. (1982). Chromosome abnormalities in malignant hematologic disease. *Adv. in Cancer Research.* 36:103-148.
30. Yunis, J. J. (1983). The chromosomal basis of human neoplasia. *Science* 221:227-235.
31. Rowley, J. D. (1982). Identification of the constant chromosome regions involved in human hematologic malignant disease. *Science* 216:749-751.
31a. Trench-Cherevix, G., Brown, J. A., and Western, E. H. (1986). Somatic rearrangement of the c-myc oncogene in primary diffuse large cell lymphoma. In *RNA Tumor Viruses*. Cold Spring Harbor Laboratory, p. 175 (abstract).
32. Rowley, J. D. (1983). Human oncogene location and chromosome aberrations. *Nature* 301:290-291.
33. Klein, G. (1983). Specific chromosomal translocations and the genesis of B cell derived tumors in mice and men. *Cell* 32:311-315.
34. Perry, R. P. (1983). Consequences of myc invasion of immunoglobulin loci: facts and speculations. *Cell* 33:647-649.
35. Erikson, J., Finan, J., Nowell, P. C., and Croce, C. M. (1982). Translocation of immunoglobulin V_H genes in Burkitt's lymphoma. *Proc. Natl. Acad. Sci. USA* 79:5611-5615.

36. Dalla-Favera, R., Martinotti, S., Gallo, R. C., Erikson, J., and Croce, C. M. (1983). Translocation and rearrangements of the c-myc oncogene locus in human undifferentiated B-cell lymphomas. *Science* 219:963-967.
37. Heisterkamp, J., Stephenson, J. R., Groffen, J., Hansen, P. F., de Klein, A., et al. (1983). Localization of the c-abl oncogene adjacent to a translocation breakpoint in chronic myelocytic leukaemia. *Nature* 306:239-242.
38. de Klein, A., Guerts van Kessel, A., Grosveld, G., Bartram, C. R., Hagemeijer, A., et al. (1982). A cellular oncogene is translocated to the Philadelphia chromosome in chronic myeloid leukaemia. *Nature* 300:765-767.
39. Rabbits, T. H., Forster, S., and Matthews, J. G. (1983). The breakpoint of the Philadelphia chromosome 22 in chronic myeloid leukaemia is distal to the immunoglobulin lambda light chain constant region genes. *Mol. Biol. Med.* 1:119-129.
40. Groffen, J., Stephenson, J. R., Heisterkamp, N., de Klein, A., Bartram, C. R., et al. (1984). Philadelphia chromosomal breakpoints are clustered within a limited region, bcr, on chromosome 22. *Cell* 36:93-99.
41. Cowell, J. K. (1982). Double minutes and homogeneously staining regions: gene amplification in mammalian cells. *Ann. Rev. Genet.* 16:21-59.
42. Collins, S. J., and Groudine, M. (1982). Amplification of endogenous myc-related DNA sequences in a human myeloid leukaemia cell line. *Nature* 298: 679-681.
43. Dalla-Favera, R., Wong-Staal, F., and Gallo, R. C. (1982). Onc gene amplification in promyelocytic leukaemia cell line HL-60 and primary leukaemic cells of the same patient. *Nature* 299:61-63.
44. Nowell, P. C., Finan, J., Dalla-Favera, R., Gallo, R. C., ar-Rushdi, A., et al. (1983). Association of amplified oncogene c-myc with an abnormally banded chromosome 8 in a human leukaemia cell line. *Nature* 306:494-497.
45. Pelicci, P. G., Lanfrancone, L., Brantwaite, M. D., Wolman, S. R., and Dalla-Favera, R. (1984). Amplification of the c-myb oncogene in a case of human acute myelogeneous leukemia. *Science* 224:1117-1120.
46. Weinberg, R. A. (1981). Use of transfection to analyze genetic information and malignant transformation. *Biochem. Biophy. Acta* 651:25-35.
47. Chang, E. H., Gonda, M. A., Ellis, R. W., Scolnick, E. M., and Lowy, D. R. (1982). Human genome contains four genes homologous to transforming genes of Harvey and Kirsten murine sarcoma viruses. *Proc. Natl. Acad. Sci. USA* 79:4848-4852.
48. Hall, A., Marshall, C. J., Spurr, N. K., and Weiss, R. A. (1983). Identification of transforming gene in two human sarcoma cell lines as a new member of the ras gene family located on chromosome one. *Nature* 303:396-400.
49. Murray, M. J., Cunningham, J. M., Parada, L. F., Dautry, F., Lebowitz, P., and Weinberg, R. A. (1983). The HL-60 transforming sequences: a ras oncogene coexisting with altered myc genes in hematopoietic tumors. *Cell* 33: 749-757.
50. Shimizu, K., Goldfarb, M., Suard, Y., Perucho, M., Li, Y., Kamata, T., Feramisco, J., Stavnezer, E., Fogh, J., and Wigler, M. H. (1983). Three human

transforming genes are related to the viral ras oncogenes. *Proc. Natl. Acad. Sci. USA* 80:2112-2116.
51. Reddy, E. P., Reynolds, R. K., Santos, E., and Barbacid, M. (1982). A point mutation is responsible for the acquisition of transforming properties by the T24 human bladder carcinoma oncogene. *Nature* 300:149-152.
52. Tabin, C. J., Bardley, S. M., Bargmann, C. I., Weinberg, R. A., Papageorge, A. G., Scolnick, E. M., Dhar, R., Lowy, D. R., and Chang, E. H. (1982). Mechanism of activation of a human oncogene. *Nature* 300:143-149.
53. Taparowsky, E., Suard, Y., Fasano, O., Shimizu, K., Goldfarb, M., and Wigler, M. (1982). Activation of the T24 bladder carcinoma transforming gene is linked to a single amino acid change. *Nature* 30:762-765.
54. Murphree, A. L., and Benedict, W. F. (1984). Retinoblastoma: clues to human oncogenesis. *Science* 223:1028-1033.
55. Benedict, W. F., Murphree, A. L., Benerjee, A., Spina, C. A., and Sparkes, R. S. (1983). Patient with 13 chromosome deletion: evidence that the retinoblastoma gene is a recessive cancer gene. *Science* 219:974-974.
56. Gambke, C., Hall, A., and Moroni, C. (1985). Activation of an N-ras gene in acute myeloblastic leukemia through somatic mutation in the first exon. *Proc. Natl. Acad. Sci. USA* 82:879-882.
57. Bos, J. L., Toksoz, D., Marshall, C. J., Verlaan-de Vries, M., Veeneman, G. H., Vander Eb, A. J., van Boom, J. H., Janssen, J. W. G., and Steenvoorden, A. C. M. (1985). Amino-acid substitutions at codon 13 of the N-ras oncogene in human acute myeloid leukaemia. *Nature* 315:726-730.
58. Eva, A., Tronick, S. R., Gol, R. A., Pierce, J. H., and Aaronson, S. A. (1983). Transforming genes of human hematopoietic tumors: frequent detection of ras-related oncogenes whose activation appears to be independent of tumor phenotype. *Proc. Natl. Acad. Sci. USA* 80:4926-4930.
59. Eva, R., Robbins, K. C., Andersen, P. R., Srinivasan, A., Tronick, S. R., et al. (1982). Cellular genes analogous to retroviral onc genes are transcribed in human tumor cells. *Nature* 295:116-119.
60. Lane, M. A., Sainten, A., and Cooper, G. M. (1982). Stage-specific transforming genes of human and mouse B- and T-lymphocyte neoplasms. *Cell* 28:873-880.
61. Lane, M. A., Sainten, A., Doherty, K. M., and Cooper, G. M. (1984). Isolation and characterization of a stage-specific transforming gene, Tlym-I, from T cell lymphomas. *Proc. Natl. Acad. Sci. USA* 81:2227-2231.
62. Diamond, A., Cooper, G. M., Ritz, J., and Lane, M. A. (1983). Identification and molecular cloning of the human Blym transforming gene activated in Burkitt's lymphomas. *Nature* 305:112-116.
63. Heldin, C.-H., and Westermark, B. (1984). Growth factors: mechanism of action and relation to oncogenes. *Cell* 37:9-20.
63a. Kaczmarek, L. (1986). Biology of disease: protooncogene expression during the cell cycle. *Lab. Invest.* 54:365-376.
63b. Calabretta, B., Kaczmarek, L., Mars, W., Ochoa, D., Gibson, C. W., Hirschhorn, R. R., and Baserga, R. (1985). Cell-cycle-specific genes differentially expressed in human leukemias. *Proc. Natl. Acad. Sci. USA* 82:4463-4467.

63c. Kaczmarek, L., Calabretta, B., and Baserga, R. (1985). Expression of cell-cycle-dependent genes in phytohemagglutinin-stimulated human lymphocytes. *Proc. Natl. Acad. Sci. USA* 82:5375-5379.

63d. Calabretta, B., Venturelli, D., Kaczmarek, L., Narni, F., Talpaz, M., Anderson, B., Beran, M., and Baserga, R. (1986). Altered expression of G_1-specific genes in human malignant myeloid cells. *Proc. Natl. Acad. Sci. USA* 83:1495-1498.

63e. Goustin, A. S., Leof, E. B., Shipley, G. D., and Moses, H. L. (1986). Growth factors and cancer. *Cancer Res.* 46:1015-1029.

64. Weinberg, R. A. (1985). The action of oncogenes in the cytoplasm and nucleus. *Science* 230:770-776.

65. Sager, R. (1986). Genetic suppression of tumor formation: A new frontier in cancer research. *Cancer Research.* 46:1573-1580.

66. Doolittle, R. F., Hunkapiller, M. W., Hood, L. E., DeVare, S. G., Robbins, K. C., Aaronson, S. A., and Antoniades, H. N. (1983). Simian sarcoma virus onc gene, v-sis, is derived from the gene (or genes) encoding a platelet-derived growth factor. *Science* 221:275-276.

67. Downward, J., Yarden, Y., Mayes, E., Scrace, G., Totty, N., et al. (1984). Close similarity of epidermal growth factor receptor and v-erb-B oncogene protein sequences. *Nature* 307:521-527.

68. Weinberger, C., Hallenberg, S. M., Rosenfeld, M. G., and Evans, R. M. (1985). Domain structure of human glucocorticoid receptor and its relationship to the v-erb-A oncogene product. *Nature* 318:670-672.

69. Sherr, C. J., Rettenmier, C. W., Sacca, R., Roussel, M. F., Look, A. T., and Stanley, E. R. (1985). The c-fms proto-oncogene product is related to the receptor for the mononuclear phagocyte growth factor, CSF-1. *Cell* 41: 665-676.

70. Hunter, T. (1984). Oncogenes and protooncogenes: how do they differ? *J. Natl. Cancer Inst.* 73:773-786.

70a. Erikson, R. L., Collett, M. S., Erikson, E., and Purchio, A. F. (1979). Evidence that the avian sarcoma virus transforming gene product is a cycle AMP-independent protein kinase. *Proc. Natl. Acad. Sci. USA* 76:6260-6264.

71. Radke, K., and Martin, G. S. (1979). Transformation by Rous sarcoma virus—effects of src gene expression on the synthesis and phosphorylation of cellular polypeptides. *Proc. Natl. Acad. Sci. USA* 76:5212-5216.

72. Berridge, M. J., and Irvine, R. F. (1984). Inositol triphosphate, a novel second mesenger in cellular signal transduction. *Nature* 312:315-321.

72a. Nishizuka, Y. (1984). The role of protein kinase C in cell surface signal transduction and tumour promotion. *Nature* 308:693-698.

73. Shih, T. Y., Papageorge, A. G., Stokes, P. E., Weeks, M. O., and Scolnick, E. M. (1980). Guanine nucleotide-binding and autophosphorylating activities associated with $p21^{src}$ protein of Harvey murine sarcoma virus. *Nature* 287:686-691.

74. Gilman, A. G. (1984). G proteins and dual control of adenylate cyclase. *Cell* 36:577-579.

75. Gibbs, J. B., Sigal, I. S., Poe, M., and Scolnick, E. M. (1984). Intrinsic GTPase activity distinguishes normal and oncogenic ras p21 molecules. *Proc. Natl. Acad. Sci. USA* 81:5704-5708.
76. McGrath, J. P., Capon, D. J., Goeddel, D. V., and Levinson, A. D. (1984). Comparative biochemical properties of normal and activated human ras p21 protein. *Nature* 310:644-649.
77. Land, H., Parada, L. J., and Weinberg, R. A. (1983). Cellular oncogenes and multistep carcinogenesis. *Science* 227:771-778.
78. Marshall, C. (1985). Human oncogenes. In *RNA Tumor Viruses: Molecular Biology of Tumor Viruses*, 2nd ed. R. Weiss, Teich, N., Varmus, H., and Coffin, J. (eds.). Cold Spring Harbor Laboratory, Cold Spring Harbor, New York, pp. 478-558.
78a. Willeche, K., and Schafer, R. (1984). Human oncogenes. *Human Genetics* 66:132-142.
79. Rosson, D., and Tereba, A. (1983). Transcription of hematopoietic-associated oncogenes in childhood leukemia. *Cancer Research* 43:3912-3918.
79a. Gee, C. E., Griffen, J., Sastre, L., Miller, L. J., Springer, T. A., Prunica-Wormus, H., and Roberts, T. M. (1986). Differentiation of myeloid cells is accompanied by increased levels of pp60 c-src protein kinase activity. *RNA Tumor Viruses. Cold Spring Harbor Laboratory*, p. 208 (abstract).
79b. Golden, A., Nemeth, S. P., and Brugge, J. S. (1986). Blood platelets express high level of the $pp60^{c\text{-}src}$-specific tyrosine kinase activity. *Proc. Natl. Acad. Sci. USA* 83:852-856.
80. Slamon, D. J., deKernion, J. B., Verma, I. M., and Cline, M. J. (1984). Expression of cellular oncogenes in human malignancies. *Science* 224:256-262.
80a. Schalkren, J. A., Roebroek, A. J. M., Leunissen, J. A. M., Dubryune, F. M. J., Bloemers, H. P. J., and Vande Ven, W. J. M. (1986). The c-fes/fps proto-oncogene is closely linked to a gene encoding a receptor-like protein. *RNA Tumor Viruses. Cold Spring Harbor Laboratory*, p. 198 (abstract).
81. McClain, K. L. (1984). Expression of oncogenes in human leukemias. *Cancer Res.* 44:5382-5389.
81a. Tanaka, T., Slamon, D. J., Battifora, H., and Cline, M. J. (1986). Expression of p21 ras oncoproteins in human cancers. *Cancer Res.* 46:1465-1470.
81b. Kurzrock, R., Gallick, G. E., and Gutterman, J. U. (1986). Differential expression of $p21^{ras}$ gene products among histological subtypes of fresh primary human lung tumors. *Cancer Res.* 46:1530-1534.
81c. Viola, M. V., Fromowitz, F., Oravex, S., Deb, S., Finkel, G., Lundy, J., Hand, P., Thor, A., and Schlom, J. (1986). Expression of ras oncogene p21 in prostate cancer. *New Eng. J. of Med.* 314:134-137.
81d. Gallick, G. E., Kurzrock, R., Kloetzer, W. S., Arlinghaus, R. B., and Gutterman, J. U. (1985). Expression of $p21^{ras}$ in fresh primary and metastatic human colorectal tumors. *Proc. Natl. Acad. Sci. USA* 82:1795-1799.
82. Westin, E. H., Wong-Staal, F., Gelmann, E. P. Favera, R. D., Papas, T. S., et al. (1982). Expression of cellular homologues of retroviral onc genes in human hematopoietic cells. *Proc. Natl. Acad. Sci. USA* 79:2490-2494.

83. Kelly, K., Cochran, B. H., Stiles, C. D., and Peder, P. (1983). Cell-specific regulation of the c-myc gene by lymphocyte mitogens and platelet-derived growth factor. *Cell* 35:603-610.
84. Campisi, J., Gray, H. E., Pardee, A. B., Dean, M., and Sonenshein, G. E. (1984). Cell-cycle control of c-myc but not c-ras expression is lost following chemical transformation. *Cell* 36:241-247.
85. Greenberg, M. E., and Ziff, E. B. (1984). Stimulation of 3T3 cells induces transcription of the c-fos protooncogene. *Nature* 311:433-438.
86. Kruijer, W., Cooper, J. A., Hunter, T., and Verma, I. M. (1984). Platelet derived growth factor induces rapid but transient expression of the c-fos gene and protein. *Nature* 312:711-716.
87. Muller, R., Bravo, R., Burckhardt, J., and Curran, T. (1984). Induction of c-fos gene and protein by growth factors precedes activation of c-myc. *Nature* 312:716-720.
88. Jonak, G. J., and Night, E. (1984). Selective reduction of c-myc mRNA in Daudi cells by human interferon. *Proc. Natl. Acad. Sci. USA* 81:1747-1750.
89. McCormack, J. E., Pepe, V. H., Kent, R. B., Dean, M., Marshak-Rothstein, A., and Sonenshein, G. E. (1984). Specific regulation of c-myc oncogene expression in a murine B-cell lymphoma. *Proc. Natl. Acad. Sci. USA* 81:5546-5550.
90. Ely, C., Lefturich, J., Hall, R., and Westin, E. (1986). Sustained suppression of c-myc gene expression is required for terminal macrophage-like differentiation of HL60 cells. *RNA Tumor Viruses. Cold Spring Harbor Laboratory*. p. 176. (abstract).
91. Gonda, T. J., and Metcalf, D. (1984). Expression of myb, myc, and fos proto-oncogenes during differentiation of a murine myeloid leukemia. *Nature* 310:249-251.
92. Muller, R., Muller, D., and Guilbert, L. (1984). Differential expression of c-fos in hematopoietic cells: correlation with differentiation of monomyelocytic cells in vitro. *EMBO J.* 3:1887-1890.
93. Mitchell, R. L., Zokas, L., Scheiber, R. D., and Verma, I. M. (1985). Rapid induction of the expression of protooncogene fos during human monocyte differentiation. *Cell* 40:209-217.
94. Mitchell, R. L., Chubb-Henning, C., Huberman, E., and Verma, I. M. (1986). C-fos expression is neither sufficient nor obligatory for differentiation of monomyelocytes to macrophages. *Cell* 45:497-504.
95. Seriban, E., Mitchell, T., and Kufe, D. (1985). Expression of the c-fms protooncogene during human monocyte differentiation. *Nature* 316:64-66.
96. Nienruis, A. W., Bunn, H. F., Turner, P. H., Gopai, T. V., Nash, W. B., O'Brien, S. J., and Sheri, C. J. (1985). Expression of the human c-fms protooncogene in hematopoietic cells and its deletion in the $5q^-$ syndrome. *Cell* 42:421-428.
97. Collins, S. J., Kubonishi, I., Miyoshi, I., and Groudine, M. (1984). Altered transcription of the c-abl oncogene in K-562 and other chronic myelogeneous leukemia cells. *Science* 225:72-74.

97a. Collins, S. J., and Groudine, M. (1983). Rearrangement and amplification of c-abl sequences in the human chronic myelogenous leukemia cell line K562. *Proc. Natl. Acad. Sci. USA* 80:4813-4817.
97b. Thompson, C. B., Challoner, P. B., Neiman, P. E., and Groudine, M. (1986). Expression of the c-myb proto-oncogene during cellular proliferation. *Nature* 319:374-380.
98. Cheah, M. S. C., Ley, T. J., Tronick, S. R., and Robbins, K. C. (1986). Fgr proto-oncogene mRNA induced in B lymphocytes by Epstein-Barr virus infection. *Nature* 319:238-240.
99. Martinet, Y., Bitterman, P. B., Mornex, J.-F., Grotendorst, G. R., Martin, G. R., and Crystal, R. G. (1986). Activated human monocytes express the c-sis proto-oncogene and release a mediator showing PDGF-like activity. *Nature* 319:158-160.
100. Manolova, Y., Manolov, G., Kieler, J., Levan, A., and Klein, G. (1979). Genesis of the 14q+ marker in Burkitt's lymphoma. *Hereditas* 90:5-10.
101. Dalla-Favera, R., Bregni, M., Erikson, J., Patterson, D., Gallo, R. C., and Croce, C. M. (1982). Human c-myc oncogene is located on the region of chromosome 8 that is translocated in Burkitt lymphoma cells. *Proc. Natl. Acad. Sci. USA* 79:7824-7827.
102. Hayday, A. C., Gillies, S. D., Saito, H., Wood, C., Wiman, K., Hayward, W. S., and Tonegawa, S. (1984). Activation of a translocated human c-myc gene by an enhancer in the immunoglobulin heavy-chain locus. *Nature* 307:334-340.
103. Erikson, J., ar-Rushdi, A., Drowinga, H. I., Nowell, P. C., and Croce, C. M. (1983). Transcriptional activation of the translocated c-myc oncogene in Burkitt lymphoma. *Proc. Natl. Acad. Sci. USA* 80:820-824.
104. Taub, R., Kirsch, I., Morton, C., Lenoir, G., Swan, S., Trownick, S., Aaronson, S., and Leder, P. (1982). Translocation of the c-myc gene into the heavy chain locus in human Burkitt lymphoma and murine plasmacytoma cells. *Proc. Natl. Acad. Sci. USA* 79:7837-7841.
105. Davis, M., Malcolm, S., and Rabbits, T. H. (1984). Chromosomal translocation can occur on either side of the c-myc oncogene in Burkitt lymphoma cells. *Nature* 308:286-288.
106. Hollis, G. F., Mitchell, K. F., Battey, J., Potter, M., Taub, R., Lenoir, G. M., and Leder, P. (1984). A variant translocation places the immunoglobulin genes 3' to the c-myc oncogene in Burkitt's lymphoma. *Nature* 307:752-755.
107. Leder, P., Battey, J., Lenoir, G., Moudlig, C., Murphy, W., Potter, H., Stewart, T., and Taub, R. (1983). Translocations among antibody genes in human cancer. *Science* 222:765-771.
108. Rabbits, T. H., Hamlyn, P. H., and Baer, R. (1983). Altered nucleotide sequences of a translocated c-myc gene in Burkitt lymphoma. *Nature* 306:760-765.
109. Nishikura, K., ar-Rushdi, A., Erickson, J., Watt, R., Rovera, G., and Croce, C. M. (1983). Differential expression of the normal and of the translocated human c-myc oncogenes in B cells. *Proc. Natl. Acad. Sci. USA* 80: 4822-4826.

110. ar-Rushdi, A., Nishikura, K., Erikson, J., Watt, R., Rovera, G., and Croce, C. M. (1983). Differential expression of the translocated and the untranslocated c-myc oncogene in Burkitt lymphoma. *Science* 222:390-393.

110a. Pelicci, P.-G., Knowles, D. M., Magrath, I., and Dalla-Favera, R. (1986). Chromosomal breakpoints and structural alterations of the c-myc locus differ in endemic and sporadic forms of Burkitt lymphoma. *Proc. Natl. Acad. Sci. USA* 82:2984-2988.

111. Taub, R., Moulding, C., Battey, J., Murphy, W., Vasicek, T., Lenoir, G. M., and Leder, P. (1984). Activation and somatic mutation of the translocated c-myc gene in Burkitt lymphoma cells. *Cell* 36:339-348.

112. Crews, S., Barth, R., Hood, I., Prenn, J., and Calame, K. (1982). Mouse c-myc oncogene is located on chromosome 15 and translocated to chromosome 12 in plasmacytomas. *Science* 218:1319-1321.

113. Adams, J. M., Gerondakis, S., Webb, E., Corcoran, L. M., and Cory, S. (1983). Cellular myc oncogene is altered by chromosome translocation in murine plasmacytomas and is rearranged similarly in human Burkitt lymphomas. *Proc. Natl. Acad. Sci. USA* 80:1982-1986.

114. Tsujimoto, Y., Yunis, J., Onorato-Shoew, L., Erikson, J., Nowell, P. C., et al. (1984). Molecular cloning of the chromosomal breakpoint of B-cell lymphomas and leukemias with the t(11;14) chromosomal translocation. *Science* 224:249-306.

114a. Tsujimoto, Y., Cossman, J., Jaffe, E., and Croce, C. M. (1985). Involvement of the bcl-2 gene in human follicular lymphoma. *Science* 228:1440-1442.

115. Nowell, P. C., and Hungerford, D. A. (1960). A minute chromosome in human chronic granulocytic leukemia. *Science* 132:1197.

116. Caspersson, T., Gahrton, G., Lindstein, J., and Zech, L. (1970). Identification of the Philadelphia chromosome as a number 22 by quinacrine mustard fluorescence analysis. *Exp. Cell Res.* 63:238-240.

117. Canaani, E., Steiner-Saltz, D., Aghai, E., Gale, R. P., Berrebia, A., and Januszewicz, E. (1984). Altered transcription of an oncogene in chronic myeloid leukaemia. *Lancet* 1:593-595.

118. Bartram, C. R., de Klein, A., Hagemeijer, A., Grosveld, G., Heisterkamp, N., and Groffen, J. (1984). Localization of the human c-sis oncogene in Ph^1-positive and Ph^1-negative chronic myelocytic leukemia by in situ hybridization. *Blood* 63:223-225.

119. Konopka, J. B., Watanabe, S. M., Singer, J. W., Collins, S. J., and Witte, O. N. (1985). Cell lines and clinical isolates derived from Ph^1-positive chronic myelogeneous leukemia patients express c-abl proteins with a common structural alteration. *Proc. Natl. Acad. Sci. USA* 82:1810-1814.

120. Konopka, J. B., Watanabe, S. M., and Witte, O. N. (1984). An alteration of the human c-abl protein in K562 leukemia cells unmasks associated tyrosine kinase activity. *Cell* 37:1035-1042.

120a. Morris, C. M., Reene, A. E., Fitzgerald, P. H., Hallings, P. E., Beard, M. E. J., and Keaton, D. C. (1986). Genomic diversity correlates with clinical variation in Ph^1 negative chronic myeloid leukemia. *Nature* 320:281-283.

120b. Heisterkamp, N., Stam, K., and Groffen, J. (1985). Structural organization of the bcr gene and its role in the Ph[1] translocation. *Nature* 315: 758-761.

121. Catovsky, D. (1979). Ph[1] positive acute leukaemia and chronic granulocytic leukaemia: one or two diseases? *Br. J. Hematol.* 42:493-498.

122. Erikson, J., Griffin, C. A., ar-Rushdi, A., Valtieri, M., Hoxie, J., Finan, J., Emanuel, B. S., Rovera, G., Nowell, P. C., and Croce, C. M. (1986). Heterogeneity of chromosome 22 breakpoint in Philadelphia-positive (Ph^+) acute lymphocytic leukemia. *Proc. Natl. Acad. Sci. USA* 83:1807-1811.

122a. Clark, S., McLaughlin, J., Crist, W., Champlin, R., Witte, O. (1987). Unique forms of the abl-tyrosine kinose distinguish Ph[1]-positive CML from Ph[1]-positive ALL. *Science* 235:85-88.

123. Kozbor, D., Giallong, A., Sierzega, M. E., Konopka, J. B., Witte, O. N., Showe, L. C., and Croce, C. M. (1986). Expression of a translocated c-abl gene in hybrids of mouse fibroblasts and chronic myelogeneous leukaemia cells. *Nature* 319:331-333.

124. Rowley, J. D., and Potter, P. (1976). Chromosome banding patterns in acute nonlymphocytic leukemia. *Blood* 47:705-721.

125. Westbrook, C. A., Le Beau, M. M., Diaz, M. O., Groffen, J., and Rowley, J. D. (1985). Chromosomal localization and characterization of c-abl in the t(6;9) of acute nonlymphocytic leukemia. *Proc. Natl. Acad. Sci. USA* 82:8742-8746.

126. Harper, M. E., Franchini, G., Love, J., Simon, M. I., Gallo, R. C., and Wong-Staal, F. (1983). Chromosomal sublocalization of human c-myb and c-fes cellular onc genes. *Nature* 304:169-171.

127. Neil, B. G., Jhanwar, S. C., Chagarti, R. S. K., and Haywood, W. S. (1982). Two human c-onc genes are located on the long arm of chromosome 8. *Proc. Natl. Acad. Sci. USA* 79:7842-7846.

128. Watson, D. K., McWilliams-Smith, M. J., Kozak, C., Reeves, R., Gearhart, Nunn, M. F., Nash, W., Fowle, J. R., Duesberg, P., Papas, T. S., and O'Brien, S. J. (1986). Conserved chromosomal positions of dual domains of the ets protooncogene in cats, mice, and humans. *Proc. Natl. Acad. Sci. USA* 83:1792-1796.

129. Sacchi, N., Watson, D. K., Guerts van Kessel, A. H. M., Hagemeijer, A., Kersey, J., Drabkin, H. D., Patterson, D., and Papas, T. S. (1986). Hu-ets-1 and Hu-ets-2 genes are transposed in acute leukemias with (4;11) and (8;21) translocations. *Science* 231:379-382.

130. Rovigatti, U., Watson, D. K., and Yunis, J. J. (1986). Amplification and rearrangement of Hu-ets-1 in leukemia and lymphoma with involvement of 11q23. *Science* 232:398-400.

131. Diaz, M. O., Le Beau, M. M., Pitha, P., and Rowley, J. D. (1986). Interferon and c-ets-1 genes in the translocation (9;11)(p22;q23) in human acute monocytic leukemia. *Science* 231:265-267.

132. Rosner, F., and Lee, S. L. (1972). Down's syndrome and acute leukemia: myeloblastic or lymphoblastic? *Am. J. Med.* 53:202-218.

132a. Rovigatti, D., Carrall, M. A., Sacher, R. A., Jacobson, R. J., Gallie, B. L., and Yunis, J. J. (1986). Alterations of c-ets oncogene in human neoplasia. *RNA Tumor Viruses. Cold Spring Harbor Laboratory.* p. 211 (abstract).

133. Erikson, J., Finger, L., Sun, L., ar-Rushdi, A., Nishikura, K., Minowada, J., Finan, J., Emanuel, B. S., Nowell, P. C., and Croce, C. M. (1986). Deregulation of c-myc by translocation of the α-locus of the T-cell receptor in T-cell leukemias. *Science* 232:884-886.

134. Shima, E. A., LeBeau, M. M., McKerthan, T. W., Minowada, J., Sharne, L. C., Mak, T. W., Minden, M. D., Rowley, J. D., and Diaz, M. O. (1986). Gene encoding the chain of the T-cell receptor is moved immediately downstream of c-myc in a chromosomal 8;14 translocation in a cell line from a human T-cell leukemia. *Proc. Natl. Acad. Sci. USA* 83:3439-3443.

134a. Lewis, W. H., Michalopoulos, E. E., Williams, D. L., Minden, M. D., and Mak, T. W. (1985). Breakpoints in the human T cell antigen receptor and α chain locus in two T cell leukaemia patients with chromosomal translocations. *Nature* 317:544-546.

135. Philip, P., Jensen, M. K., Killman, S. A., Briushlom, A., and Hansen, N. E. (1978). Chromosomal banding patterns in 88 cases of acute nonlymphocytic leukemia. *Leuk. Res.* 2:201-212.

136. Nagarajan, L., Louie, E., Tsujimoot, Y., ar-Rushdi, A., Huebner, K., and Croce, C. M. (1986). Localization of the human pim oncogene (PIM) to a region of chromosome 6 involved in translocations in acute leukemias. *Proc. Natl. Acad. Sci. USA* 83:2556-2560.

136a. Nagarajan, L., Louie, E., Tsujmoto, Y., ar-Rushdi, A., Huebner, K., and Croce, C. M. (1986). Molecular cloning and chromosomal mapping of h Pim-1 putative oncogene. *RNA Tumor Viruses, Cold Spring Harbor Laboratory*, p. 166 (abstract).

137. Rowley, J. D., Golomb, H. M., Vardimar, J., Fukuhara, S., Dougherty, C., and Potter, D. (1977). Further evidence for a non-random chromosomal abnormality in acute promyelocytic leukemia. *Int. J. Cancer* 20: 869-872.

138. Huebner, K., Isobe, M., Chao, M., Bothwell, M., Ross, A. H., Finan, J., Hoxie, J. A., Sehgal, A., Buck, R., Lanahan, A., Nowell, P. C., Koprowski, H., and Croce, C. M. (1986). The nerve growth factor receptor gene is at human chromosome region 17q22, distal to the chromosome 17 breakpoint in acute leukemias. *Proc. Natl. Acad. Sci. USA* 82:1403-1407.

139. Dalla-Favera, R., Franchini, G., Martinotti, S., Wong-Staal, F., Gallo, R. C., and Croce, C. M. (1982). Chromosomal assignment of the human homologues of feline sarcoma virus and avian myeloblastosis virus onc genes. *Proc. Natl. Acad. Sci. USA* 79:4714-4717.

140. Dayton, A. I., Selden, J. R., Laws, G., Dorney, D. J., Finan, J., Tripputi, P., Emanuel, B. S., Rovera, G., Nowell, P. C., and Croce, C. M. (1984). A human c-erb-A oncogene homologue is closely proximal to the chromosome 17 breakpoint in acute promyelocytic leukemia. *Proc. Natl. Acad. Sci. USA* 81:4495-4499.

141. Alitalo, K., Schwab, M., Lin, Varmus, H. E., and Bishop, J. M. (1983). Homogeneously staining chromosomal regions contain amplified copies of an abundantly expressed cellular oncogene (c-myc) in malignant neuroendocrine cells from a human colon carcinoma. *Proc. Natl. Acad. Sci. USA* 80:1707-1711.

142. Kozbor, D., and Croce, C. M. (1984). Amplification of the c-myc oncogene in one of five human breast carcinoma cell lines. *Cancer Res.* 44: 438-441.
143. Little, C. D., Nau, M. M., Carney, D. N., Gazdar, A. F., and Minna, J. D. (1983). Amplification and expression of the c-myc oncogene in human lung cancer cell lines. *Nature* 306:194-196.
143a. Saglio, G., Emanuel, B. S., Guerrasio, A., Tiubellino, M. C., Serra, A., Lusso, P., Cambrin, G. R., Mazza, U., Malavasi, F., Pegoraro, L., and Foa, R. (1986). 3' c-myc rearrangement in a human leukemic T-cell line. *Cancer Res.* 46:1413-1417.
144. Yokota, J., Tsunetsugu-Yokota, Y., Battifora, H., Le Fevre, C., and Cline, M. J. (1986). Alterations of myc, myb, and ras^{Ha} proto-oncogenes in cancers are frequent and show clinical correlation. *Science* 231:261-265.
144a. Trent, J., Meltzer, P., Rosenblum, M., Harsh, G., Kinzler, K., Mashal, R., Feinberg, A., and Vogelstein, B. (1986). Evidence for rearrangement, amplification, and expression of c-myc in a human glioblastoma. *Proc. Natl. Acad. Sci. USA* 83:470-473.
144b. Nau, M. M., Brooks, B. J., Jr., Carney, D. N., Gazdar, A. F., Battey, J. F., Sausville, E. A., and Minna, J. D. (1986). Human small-cell lung cancers show amplification and expression of the N-myc gene. *Proc. Natl. Acad. Sci. USA* 83:1092-1096.
145. Schwab, M., Ellison, J., Busch, M., Rosenau, W., Varmus, H. E., and Bishop, J. M. (1984). Enhanced expression of the human gene N-myc consequent to amplification of DNA may contribute to malignant progression of neuroblastoma. *Proc. Natl. Acad. Sci.* 81:4940-4944.
146. Lee, W. H., Murphree, A. L., and Benedict, W. F. (1984). Expression and amplification of the N-myc gene in primary retinoblastoma. *Nature* 309: 458-460.
147. Slamon, D. J., Boone, T. C., Seeger, R. C., Keith, D. E., Chazin, V., Lee, H. C., and Souza, L. M. (1986). Identification and characterization of the protein encoded by the human N-myc oncogene. *Science* 232:768-772.
148. Le Beau, M. M., Westbrook, C. A., Diaz, M. O., Larson, R. A., Rowley, J. D., Gasson, J. C., Golde, D. W., and Sherr, C. J. (1986). Evidence for the involvement of GM-CSF and FMS in the deletion (5q) in myeloid disorders. *Science* 231:948-987.
149. Kousfos, Hausen, M. F., Lampkin, B. C., Workman, M. L., Copeland, N., Jeukris, N. A., and Cavenee, W. K. (1984). Loss of alleles at loci on human chromosome 11 during genesis of Wilm's tumor. *Nature* 309:171-172.
150. Orkin, S. H., Goldman, D. S., and Sallan, S. E. (1984). Development of homozygosity for chromosome 11p markers in Wilm's tumor. *Nature* 309:172-174.
151. Pulciani, S., Santos, E., Lauver, A. V., Long, L. K., and Barbacid, M. (1982). Oncogenes in solid human tumors. *Nature* 300:539-542.
152. Davis, M., Malcolm, S., Hall, A., and Marshall, C. J. (1983). Localization of the human N-ras oncogene to chromosome 1 cen p 21 by in situ hybridization. *EMBO J.* 2:2281-2283.

153. Hall, A., Marshall, C. J., Spurr, N. K., and Weiss, R. A. (1983). Identification of transforming gene in two human sarcoma cell lines as a new member of the ras gene family located on chromosome one. *Nature* 303:396-400.
154. Perucho, M., Goldfarb, K., Shimizu, K., Lowa, C., Fogh, J., and Wigler, M. (1981). Human tumor derived cell lines contain common and different transforming genes. *Cell* 27:467-476.
155. Shih, C., and Weinberg, R. A. (1982). Isolation of transforming sequence from a human bladder carcinoma cell line. *Cell* 29:161-169.
156. Der, C. J., Krontiris, T. G., and Cooper, G. M. (1982). Transforming genes of human bladder and lung carcinoma cell lines are homologous to the ras genes of Harvey and Kirsten sarcoma viruses. *Proc. Natl. Acad. Sci. USA* 79:3637-3640.
157. McGrath, J. P., Capon, D. J., Smith, D. H., Chen, E. Y., Seeburg, P. H., Goeddel, D. V., and Levinson, A. D. (1983). Structure and organization of the human Ki-ras protooncogene and a related processed pseudogene. *Nature* 304:501-506.
158. Mijoshi, J., Kogimoto, M., Salda, E., and Sakakir, Y. (1984). The human C-Ha-ras-2 is a processed pseudogene inactivated by numerous base substitutions. *Nucleic Acids Res.* 12:1821-1828.
159. Gambke, C., Signer, E., and Moroni, C. (1984). Activation of N-ras in bone marrow cells from a patient with acute myeloblastic leukemia. *Nature* 307:476-477.
160. Soujri, M., and Flessiner, F. (1983). Identification by transfection of transforming sequences of human T-cell leukemias. *Proc. Natl. Acad. Sci. USA* 80:6676-6679.
161. Feig, L. A., Bast, R. C., Knapp, R. C., and Cooper, G. M. (1984). Somatic activation of ras^k gene in a human ovarian carcinoma. *Science* 223:698-701.
162. Fujita, J., Yoshida, O., Yuasa, Y., Rhim, J. B., Hatanaka, M., and Aaronson, S. A. (1984). Ha-ras oncogenes are activated by somatic alterations in human urinary tract tumors. *Nature* 309:464-466.
163. Santos, E., Martin-Zanca, D., Reddy, E. P., Pierott, M. A., Della Porta, G., and Barbacid, M. (1984). Malignant activation of a K-ras oncogene in lung carcinoma but not in normal tissue of the same patient. *Science* 223:661-664.
164. Sukumar, S., Notario, V., Martin-Zouka, D., and Barbacid, M. (1983). Induction of mammary carcinomas in rats by nitoso-methylurea involves malignant activation of Ha-ras-1 locus by single point mutation. *Nature* 306:658-661.
164a. Balmain, A., and Pragnell, I. B. (1983). Activation of the mouse cellular Harvey ras gene in chemically induced benign skin papillomas. *Nature* 307:658-660.
165. Cooper, G. M., and Nieman, P. E. (1980). Transforming genes of neoplasms induced by avian lymphoid leukosis viruses. *Nature* 287:656-659.

166. Goubin, G., Goldman, D. S., Luce, J., Nieman, P. E., and Cooper, G. M. (1983). Molecular cloning and nucleotide sequence of a transforming gene detected by transfection of chicken B-cell lymphoma DNA. *Nature* 302:114-119.

167. Rogers, J. (1986). Relationship of Blym genes to repeated sequences. *Nature* 320:579.

167a. Neiman, P. (1985). The BLYM oncogenes. *Adv. in Cancer Res.* 45:107-123.

168. Cooper, G. M., Gaubin, G., Diamond, A., and Neiman, P. (1986). Relationship of Blym genes to repeated sequences. *Nature* 320:579-580.

169. Morton, C. C., Taub, R., Diamond, A., Lone, M. R., Cooper, G. M., and Leder, P. (1984). Mapping of the human B-lym-1 transforming gene activated in Burkitt lymphomas to chromosome 1. *Science* 223:173-175.

169a. Eva, A., Pierce, J., and Aaronson, S. A. (1985). Interactions of oncogenes with hematopoietic cells. In *Leukemia Recent Advances in Biology and Treatment*, R. P. Gale and D. W. Golde (eds.). Alan R. Liss, Inc., New York, pp. 3-15.

170. Devine, J. M. (1986). Mechanism of activation of Hu Blym-1 gene unresolved. *Nature* 321:437-438.

171. Cooper, G. M., and Diamond, A. (1986). Mechanism of activation of Hu Blym-1 gene unresolved. *Nature* 321:438-439.

172. Kaczmarek, L., Hyland, J. K., Watt, R., Rosenberg, M., and Baserga, R. (1985). Microinjected c-myc as a competence factor. *Science* 228:1313-1315.

173. Adams, J. M., Harris, A. W., Pinkert, C. A., Corcoran, L. M., Alexander, W. S., Cary, S., Palmiter, R. D., and Brinster, R. L. (1986). The c-myc oncogene driven by immunoglobulin enhancers induces lymphoid malignancy in transgenic mice. *Nature* 318:533-538.

174. Clark, R., Wong, G., Arnheim, N., Nitecki, D., and McCormick, F. (1985). Antibodies specific for amino acid 12 of the ras oncogene product inhibit GTP binding. *Proc. Natl. Acad. Sci. USA* 82:5280-5284.

175. Hagag, N., Nalegoua, S., and Viola, M. (1986). Inhibition of growth factor-induced differentiation of PC12 cells by microinjection of antibody to ras p21. *Nature* 319:680-682.

176. Niman, H. L., Thompson, A. M. H., Yu, A., Markman, M., Willems, J. J., Herwig, K. R., Habib, N. A., Wood, C. B., Houghten, R. A., and Lerner, R. A. (1985). Anti-peptide antibodies detect oncogene-related proteins in urine. *Proc. Natl. Acad. Sci. USA* 82:7924-7928.

177. Krontiris, T. G., DiMartino, N. A., Colb, M., and Parkinson, D. R. (1985). Unique allelic restriction fragments of the human Ha-ras locus in leukocyte and tumour DNAs of cancer patients. *Nature* 313:369-373.

178. Ishii, S., Kadonoga, J. T., Tjian, R., Brady, J. N., Merlino, G. T., and Poston, I. (1986). Binding of the Spl transcription factor by the human Harvey ras-1 protooncogene promoter. *Science* 232:1410-1413.

11

Tissue Culture in Acute Leukemia
Implications for Characterization and Therapy

ARNON NAGLER* *Rambam Medical Center and Technion Israel Institute of Technology, Haifa, Israel*

GARY SPITZER *The University of Texas System Cancer Center, M. D. Anderson Hospital and Tumor Institute, Houston, Texas*

I. INTRODUCTION

Recent advances in in vitro techniques and the development of semisolid and liquid culture techniques have broadened understanding of the hematopoietic process in normal and leukemic states. These techniques have made it possible to detect, quantify, and characterize major subsets of hemopoietic stem and progenitor cells and have led to the discovery of colony-stimulating and synergistic growth factors. The colony-stimulating factors are the proteins necessary for the survival, proliferation, and differentiation of the committed hematopoietic progenitor cells (1,2). Synergistic factors increase the number of both giant macrophage and blast cell colonies (3), the frequency of which bear a close relationship to hematopoietic repopulating ability. Moreover, a number of polypeptide hematopoietic growth factors have recently been purified and cloned. Two of the human colony-stimulating factors have been purified to homogeneity; complementary DNAs encoding them have been cloned (4-7).

The pluripotent hematopoietic stem cells are responsible for the normal production of all hematopoietic cell lines: granulocytic, erythroid, megakaryocytic, and lymphoid cells. The pluripotent hematopoietic stem cell is characterized by both the ability of self-renewal and differentiation to give rise to daughter cells. Present-day cloning techniques from human hematopoietic tissue, however, probably measure progenitor cells already committed in the erythroid, granulocyte macrophage series, and lymphoid series with limited self-renewal ability.

**Current affiliation*: Stanford Medical Center, Stanford, California
This work was supported by a grant from The National Cancer Institute (CA31536).

In leukemia, the proliferation of clones of abnormal hematopoietic stem cells, with variable degrees of abnormalities in cellular differentiation, regulation, and proliferation, is established. In leukemic, myelodysplastic and myeloproliferative syndromes, the normal and leukemic clones may coexist within the bone marrow. The growth advantage for the leukemic over the normal clone appears to be due to abnormal balance of both stimulatory and inhibitory signals and an abnormal response to these regulatory influences, which favors leukemia clone expansion in vivo. Abnormalities frequently occur at the progenitor level, which we can evaluate in vitro. In this chapter, we will try to emphasize the contribution of in vitro marrow myeloid culture techniques to our understanding of the leukemic and preleukemic process and its therapeutic implications.

II. NORMAL HEMATOPOIESIS

A. The Hierarchy of the Hematopoietic System

The hematopoietic system is a cell renewal system responsible for maintaining an enormous number of cells. It contains a full spectrum of variably differentiated cells, from almost immortal primitive stem cells to fully differentiated, nondividing cells with a limited life span. The continued production of differentiated elements with a limited life span requires the existence of stem cells. The hematopoietic system is a pyramid-shaped one with relatively few stem cells and a very large number of mature end cells: red cells, granulocytes, macrophage, platelets and lymphocytes. The hemopoietic population is hierarchically composed of several subpopulations: (1) pluripotent lymphohematopoietic stem cells; (2) the lymphoid and the hematopoietic committed progenitor cells; (3) the bone marrow precursor cells; and (4) the mature peripheral blood end cells. In general, only the most mature cells enter the circulation. The stem cells are located mainly in the bone marrow, with a small population in the spleen and a few in the circulation. As the hematopoietic cells move forward in the hemopoiesis hierarchy, i.e., differentiate, there is loss of self-renewal capacity (8-10). However, in vivo and in vitro data show that the mature B and T lymphocytes can proliferate in response to antigenic presentation.

B. Clonal Assays in Hematopoiesis

Till and McCulloch (11), using the spleen colony-forming technique, documented the existence of the hematopoietic stem cells (CFUs). Johnson and Metcalf (12) and Fauser and Messner (13) developed cloning techniques that supported the growth of colonies with multiple hematopoietic lineages (multipotential colonies). The multipotential hematopoietic colonies (CFU-GEMM) can contain erytrhoid cells, granulocytes, macrophages, eosinophils, megakaryocytes and T-cells and are the immediate precursors of committed cells. The cells that form the multipotential colonies in vitro from murine tissue contain CFUs (14). That the pluripotent

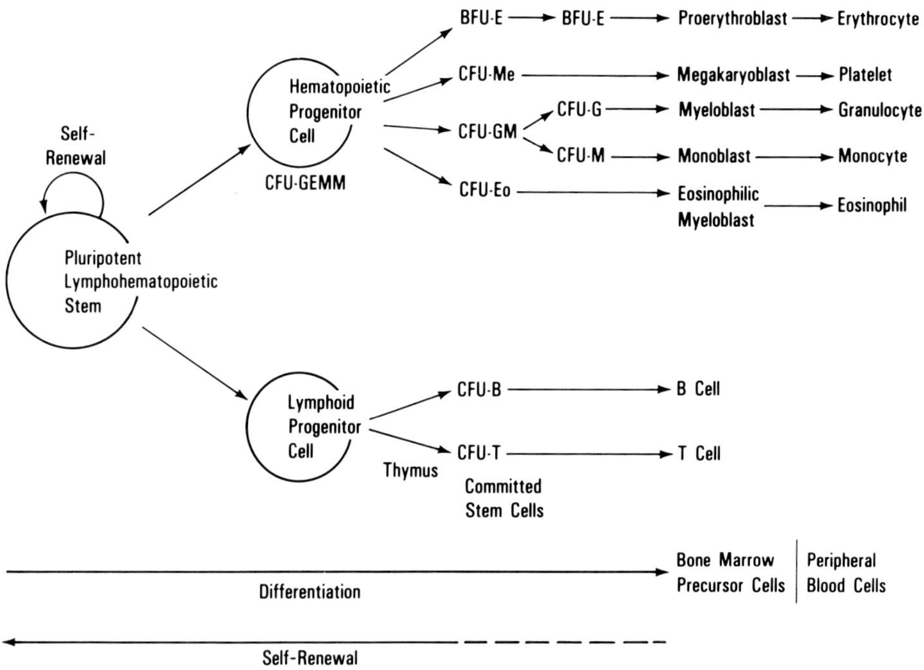

Figure 1 Schematic diagram of hematopoiesis.

stem cell can give rise to lymphoid cell type is suggested by the fact that the multipotent hemopoietic colonies can contain T lymphocytes (15). Random retroviral insertion of genetic material into hematopoietic cells in mice has shown the constant integration site in all cell lineages following radiation and transplantation, providing convincing evidence for a common hematopoietic stem cell (16).

In the semisolid clonal assay technique, the committed progenitor cells generate colonies of a single lineage. The myeloid-committed progenitor cells are the granulocyte-macrophage colony-forming units (CFU-GM) (8,17). The erythroid committed progenitor cells are the burst- and erythroid-colony forming units (BFU-E and CFU-E) (18). The megakaryocytic committed progenitor cells are the megakaryocytic colony-forming units (CFU-Mega) (19). The colonies, when derived from cultures with limited cell numbers, are indeed clones. The committed progenitor cells of the various lineages give rise to the bone marrow precursor cells and the peripheral blood end cells.

C. Hematopoietic Stimulatory Factors

Normal hematopoiesis is under the control of two important mechanisms: the microenvironment and colony-stimulating factor, and other growth factors. The Dexter long-term culture technique provides us with a tool to investigate adherent marrow stromal cells (20). The stromal cells may have a regulatory effect on the self-renewal capacity of the progenitor cells, either by direct cell-cell contact or by secretion of unique, poorly described growth factors (21,22).

The colony-stimulating factors (CSF) are specific growth stimuli that control the proliferation and differentiation of the hemopoietic progenitor cells. In the murine system, four regulatory glycoproteins have been identified: (1) the granulocyte-macrophage colony-stimulating factor (GM-CSF); (2) the macrophage colony-stimulating factor (M-CSF); (3) the multilineage hematopoietic growth factor, or interleukin 3 (IL_3); and (4) granulocyte colony-stimulating factors (G-CSF) (23-25). The IL_3 and GM-CSF genes have been cloned (26-28). The human equivalent of the murine GM-CSF gene has been isolated and the human macrophage colony-stimulating factor (M-CSF) and, recently, granulocyte colony-stimulating factor (G-CSF) genes have been cloned (4-7). The ability of the hematopoietic growth factors to regulate proliferation and differentiation of the hematopoietic progenitor cells appears to be receptor mediated (28-31). One growth factor can down-regulate the receptor of others, effecting the subsequent differentiation (30). In the leukemic and preleukemic states, there is most probably pathology in these regulatory mechanisms and uncoupling between the various progenitor cells, or even more primitive hematopoietic cell proliferation and differentiation (32).

III. LEUKEMIC HEMATOPOIESIS

A. Acute Myelogenous Leukemia

Clonal Nature of Acute Myelogenous Leukemia

Acute myelogenous leukemia (AML) is characterized by a relative or absolute accumulation of immature granulocyte-monocyte blast cells with minimal or no evidence of maturing granulocyte-monocyte cells. Leukemia is a clonal disease. The clonality of the hematopoietic system in leukemia has been documented by using the X-chromosome-linked enzyme glucose 6 phosphate dehydrogenase (G6PD) technique (33,34), by demonstrating nonrandom cytogenetic changes (35), and recently by recombinant DNA techniques which take advantage of X-chromosome-linked DNA polymorphism (36). At the same time, AML is a heterogeneous disease. In some patients, G6PD analysis has demonstrated that the disease involves a stem cell with multiple differentiative expression similar to chronic myelogenous leukemia (CML), whereas in others, the disease involves progenitors with differentiative expression restricted to the granulocyte-macrophage (GM) pathway. A number of clinical circumstances also suggest that leukemia arises from a pluripotent stem cell. The blast crisis in chronic myeloid leukemia can be lymphoid (37-39): Philadelphia-positive lymphoid cells have been identified in CML patients (40), and the same clonality was observed in the lymphoid and myeloid cells of a patient with refractory anemia with ring sideroblasts (41). There are also several reported cases of myelodysplastic syndrome preceding acute lymphoblastic leukemia (42,43). Above all, it was recently shown that immunoglobulin gene rearrangements that are thought to be a characteristic of lymphoid differentiation are present also in patients with AML (36).

Multistep Mechanism of AML

According to the multistep theory of leukemogenesis, three steps are involved in the emergence of AML: an early event that leads to clonal proliferation of pluripotent stem cells that are genetically unstable; leukemic and preleukemic development of distinctive chromosomal abnormalities; and a later event that results in emergence of overt leukemia. It is likely that oncogenes are involved at one or more steps (34).

During the past few years, a number of proto-oncogenes and transforming genes have been mapped to the chromosomal breakpoints involved in specific structural rearrangements. Genes that are located at these breakpoints may have a significant role in leukemogenesis (44,31). A high frequency of ras oncogenes and amplification of the proto-oncogene C-myb have been reported recently in cultures from AML cells lines and AML patients (45,46).

Moreover, chromosomal abnormalities bear a significant relation to prognosis in preleukemic patients. Cytogenetic abnormalities have been demonstrated in 50% to 60% of preleukemic patients, and these patients have a high frequency of leukemic transformation. A study evaluating the cytogenetic markers in 34 preleukemic patients demonstrated that all patients with exclusively abnormal marrow metaphases developed acute leukemia, whereas only one patient with solely normal marrow metaphases subsequently developed leukemia (47). In some preleukemic cases, new cytogenetic lesions occur at the time of acute transformation, suggesting clonal evolution (48,49).

The Coexistence of Normal and Leukemic Clones

In the leukemic states, the normal and transformed clone coexist. In AML, the production of normal hematopoietic cells persists, although often at markedly reduced levels. There is usually anemia, thrombocytopenia and a relative absence of mature granulocytes and monocytes. Thus, the goal of antileukemic therapy is to destroy the transformed blastic clone and await repopulation by the residual normal hematopoietic progenitors. The precise interrelationship between the transformed and normal hematopoietic progenitor are the subject of extensive investigation. The maturation of the transformed clone in AML is arrested.

The degree and location of the maturation arrest within the granulomonocytic lineage varies from patient to patient. At the biologic level, the maturation arrest is the result of uncoupling of the genes which control cellular proliferation and differentiation of the myeloid elements (33).

Response of Myeloid Leukemia to Hematopoietic Growth Factors

The transformed hematopoietic progenitor cell may have an enhanced responsiveness to positive humoral proliferative stimuli like GM-CSF and a decreased responsiveness to a negative proliferation signal like leukemic inhibitor activity or prostaglandin E (50-52).

Human myeloid leukemic cells are dependent on extrinsic colony-stimulating factors (CSF) for growth in vitro and the pathogenesis, at least initially, is likely to be more than just simply an autocrine mechanism. Leukemic cells cannot exhibit sustained proliferation in vitro in culture lacking added CSF in concentrations similar to those required to stimulate normal GM proliferation. No sequence homology was found between the purified and cloned CSFs and the known oncogenes. Finally, CSF receptor numbers on a number of myeloid cell lines have been found to be abnormally high (53). Recently, human meyloid leukemic cell lines have been shown to bind specific growth factors and to express membrane receptors for G-CSF (4-7,54). However, a short-circuiting of the CSF stimulation pathway or dysregulated CSF synthesis may have a role in leukemic transformation. Studies in murine nonleukemic but immortalized hematopoietic cells that are dependent on extrinsic IL_3 or GM-CSF for survival and proliferation have shown that the emergence of subclones capable of autonomous proliferation is associated with the capacity to produce leukemia in vivo (55). Other studies have shown that such cells can become CSF-independent secondary to a spontaneous mutation, and transformation with Abelson virus (56), or transformation with a retroviral vector containing an expressible GM-CSF cDNA clone (57). Only the insertion of GM-CSF material is associated with autocrine stimulation. Transformation of murine bone marrow with retroviral vectors containing *both* V-mil and V-myc induces macrophage leukemic lines secreting murine macrophage colony-stimulating factor (CSF-1) (58). The relevance of these in vitro retroviral insertion of oncogenes or other genetic messages into hematopoietic cells to human AML is uncertain.

Clonality of Remission

In most patients in whom chemotherapy has induced a complete remission, the hematopoietic population is karyotypically normal during remission and appears to be derived from the regeneration of a previously suppressed normal hematopoietic precursor. It was hypothesized that the transformed hematopoietic progenitors cannot initiate or complete the differentiation processes leading to mature cells (59). However, Fearon et al. (36) have recently shown evidence of in vivo differentiation of blast cells from five patients with active AML to mature granulocytes by using restriction fragment length polymorphism and differential methylation patterns of the hypoxanthine phosphoribosyl transferase (HPRT) locus on the X chromosome in female patients. It has been shown that apparently normal colonies from bone marrow at remission remain positive for leukemia-specific antiserum (60,61). An occasional G6PD heterozygote has shown evidence for persistence of an abnormal clone during remission but disappearance of karyotypic abnormalities (34). Thus, it seems that the persistence during remission of a leukemic or preleukemic clone with near normal maturation is quite common.

In Vitro Growth Characteristics of AML in Semisolid Media

AML is subclassified according to the predominant cell type using morphological, cytochemical, and immunological techniques. However, the morphological and cytochemical techniques usually give very little information concerning the normal progenitor cell that gave rise to the leukemic clone and the proliferative and differential potential of this cell. Important insights into myeloid differentiation and the cellular origins of leukemia have been gained through the use of monoclonal antibodies that define cell surface antigens and through molecular probes that identify gene rearrangements (62). Recently, Griffin et al. have subclassified AML into four phenotypes according to differentiation associated surface antigen expression as identified by monoclonal antibodies (63).

However, the clonal culture of hematopoietic cells has provided the most useful technique for assessing the cellular and hematopoietic growth factors involved in regulating leukemic hematopoiesis. The in vitro myeloid culture systems provide us with the tool for better understanding of the biology of AML. The most useful techniques are the semisolid media culture technique (using agar gel or methylcellulose as the support media) (64,65) and the liquid suspension culture technique (66). The semisolid technique permits clonal growth of the myeloid progenitor cells, whereas the liquid suspension culture permits determination of cell proliferative and maturation parameters of the morphologically recognizable myeloid precursors. Moreover, these methods, as discussed previously, can be used to assess the responsiveness of the myeloid leukemic progenitor cells to CSF and the growth requirements of these cells (67,68); the physical characteristics of the leukemic cells (69); the self-renewal and proliferative capacity of the leukemic progenitor cell (70,71); the sensitivity of the leukemic cells to various chemotherapeutic agents (72-75); the sensitivity of leukemic cells to maturation-induced agents (76-78); and the functional capabilities of the cells (79).

Senn et al. (80) reported decreased or absent colony formation in the first publication on human CFU-GM grown from patients with leukemia with human embryo kidney feeder cells. Moore et al. (81) and others (65) cultured bone marrow from patients with leukemia over normal peripheral blood feeder cells immobilized in agar and succeeded in growing blast cell colonies (CFU-L). The growth patterns of the leukemic cells in cultures is highly abnormal. The cloning efficiency of the leukemic cells varies widely from one patient to another. In most studies, clonogenic cells cannot be grown in 30% to 50% of the AML patients. The number of leukemic CFU (CFU-L) and clusters varies from patient to patient, ranging from one colony per 100 blast cells to one colony per 1000 blast cells plated. Usually one of four growth patterns is observed: (1) no growth; (2) formation of small clusters; (3) formation of large clusters; and (4) formation of colonies and clusters but with a high cluster-to-colony ratio (82,83). The small number of colonies is probably due to the fact that only a small proportion of the blast cells are capable of colony formation in vitro (84). Usually no correlation was found between the growth pattern and the morphological subtype of AML. However, the growth pattern of AML cells could be correlated to the clinical outcome of the AML patients in terms of remission induction and the duration of remission (84,85). Moreover, a leukemic growth pattern of bone marrow progenitor cells from preleukemic cells (absent colonies, increased clusters) is associated with a high frequency and rate of leukemic progression. Usually, the growth of the leukemic blast cell colonies requires the presence of a leukocyte-conditioned medium (LCM) that has been prepared in the presence of phytohemagglutinin (PHA) (64,81,86).

Using 10% PHA-LCM, McCulloch et al. observed blast colonies of a relatively uniform phenotype in peripheral blood samples of nearly all patients with AML. Blast colonies usually developed within three to seven days after plating and could reach the size of 20 to 200 cells. The leukemic nature of these colonies is suggested by the primitive blastlike morphologic appearance of their cells (86). The cell from the CFU-L demonstrated the same chromosomal marker as the fresh blasts of the AML patient (87). The CFU-L express cell surface antigens that are usually more immature than that of the fresh leukemic cell population (88).

The frequency of the primary blast colonies showed very little relation to clinical outcome. However, in a series of replating experiments (71,72), the self-renewal capability of the blast cells, i.e., the capacity of the blast cell progenitors to form secondary colonies, was stable during the course of the disease in each patient and was related to remission induction and survival (71). Only a small fraction of the blast cells had the ability to form secondary colonies, possibly representing the true stem cells in the leukemic population. These data suggest again that the CFU-L are a distinct subset of clonogenic cells among the total leukemia population.

The proliferative status of this subpopulation of leukemic blasts was assessed by tritiated thymidine suicide. In this technique, the proliferative status of the progenitor is measured by the capacity of the tritiated thymidine to deactivate the cells during DNA synthesis. All the CFU-L progenitor cells had a high proportion of cells in the S phase of the cell cycle (13), indicating maintenance of the leukemic blast cell populations by the proliferative activity of a small subpopulation of blasts (81). According to these studies, it was postulated the leukemic blast cells are a heterogeneous population; some have proliferative capacity and others have lost this ability.

These heterogeneous blast populations may explain leukemia relapses after long remissions: they may result from leukemic cells that are out of cycle and so escape the cytotoxic effects of the chemotherapeutic agents. Furthermore, indolent leukemia could be the result of leukemic blasts that are not capable of self-renewal, whereas aggressive disease may be the outcome of blasts with high self-renewal potential.

Recently it was reported that conditioned medium from a human bladder carcinoma cell line 5637 can replace PHA-LCM in stimulating the growth of CFU-L from myeloblastic leukemia patients (89). However, the factors in PHA-LCM required for the growth of blast colonies were not identified and, furthermore, there are routinely great variations in potencies of different batches of PHA-LCM. A stable source of leukemic blast growth factor (LBGF) would be valuable. Recent studies have shown that recombinant human GM-CSF (r-GM-CSF) can stimulate in vitro leukemic growth (90,91) but is less effective than the bladder cell line conditioned medium. This may suggest that leukemic growth is dependent on more than one factor, GM-CSF. Griffin et al. (90) have succeeded in growing CFU-L from 12 AML patients with r-GM-CSF. Hoang et al. (91) reported that r-GM-CSF stimulates both the formation of blast colonies from AML patients in methylcellulose and the growth of the blast progenitors in suspension.

Growth of AML Cells in Suspension Culture

One of the problems of the blast assay in methylcellulose is that only a minority of the blast cells form colonies and the plating efficiency from a single colony (secondary plating) declines with repeated passages. Nara et al. (92) have succeeded in growing blast cells of AML patients in suspension cultures. Using E-rosette depleted blast cell populations in the presence of 10% PHA-LCM, they were able to maintain blast colony precursor in exponential growth for a period of 7 to 70 days. When the cells were transferred to methylcellulose cultures, they formed typical blast colonies. Moreover, the degree of proliferation in the liquid suspension culture exceeded that observed in semi-solid medium. The higher degree of proliferation in liquid culture was explained by the assumption that the blast cells in liquid culture stimulate their own growth: membranes from fresh blast cells added to the suspension cultures showed growth-promoting activity (93).

The success in growing leukemic blast cells in liquid culture creates a valuable tool for studying the biologic characteristics of the blast population in AML patients. The proliferative rate in liquid culture may serve as a prognostic indicator for leukemia patients—self-renewal in suspension cultures was found to be related to the survival of the AML patients. Interestingly, in this system there is no selection against malignant cells in favor of their normal counterparts—unlike Dexter type long-term culture system in both AML and CML (94). This method can be used to ascertain the effect of prolonged exposure of the blast cells to colony-stimulating factors, differentiation factors and drugs.

Evaluating Drugs, Biologies, and Radiation

CFU-L grown in culture were used in order to assess the sensitivity of the leukemic blasts to drugs and, more important, to try and correlate the drug sensitivity with the prognosis. Greenberg et al. (74) and others (95,96) have evaluated the cytotoxic effect of various drugs such as cytosine arabinoside (ara-C) and 6-thioguanine, on the granulocytic progenitor cells and have found the optimal dose and time of exposure for maximal cytotoxic effects. However, the results of studies comparing drug sensitivity and patient outcome are conflicting. Marie et al. (73) have found a good in vitro to in vivo correlation for ara-C. Georgoulias et al. (97) and Chan et al. (98) found a good correlation between drug sensitivity of the CFU-L in vitro sensitivity and the remission status of the AML patients. However, others did not find any statistically significant correlation (99,100). Dow et al. (75) recently reported that Adriamycin sensitivity in vitro correlated with remission induction and cytosine arabinoside sensitivity correlated with remission duration.

The in vitro blast assay system can be used to evaluate other modes of therapy in AML. The radiation sensitivity of leukemic progenitor cells may serve to predict the clinical response of AML to chemoradiotherapy before bone marrow transplantation (101). The efficacy of purging residual clonogenic leukemia cells from autologous bone marrow grafts with chemotherapy of monoclonal antibodies can be evaluated (102). Future possible modes of therapy in AML patients can also be evaluated. Leukemic blast cells in suspension culture have been found recently to acquire susceptibility to cytotoxic effects of activated natural killer cells (103). Colony growth in AML patients showed a dose-dependent suppression by cloned interferons (104). Thus, the application of these techniques seems almost unlimited.

Induction of Differentiation

One of the fundamental questions in AML is whether the leukemic cells are capable of maturation under certain environmental circumstances or whether the defect is complete and unchangeable by external conditions (76). Although, as already mentioned, there is most probably uncoupling of the proliferation and differentiation processes in AML, this assumption does not necessarily imply that the maturation block is irreversible. The leukemic blast cells are heterogeneous in their differentiation capacity and it is believed that a cell renewal hierarchy probably continues to function in the leukemic clone (71); some blasts differentiate to form mature cells (36). Initially studies evaluated the effect of maturation-inducing agents such as: 13 cis retinoic acid (13 Cis RA); 1, 25 dihydroxyvitamin D_3 (1,25,$(DH)_2D_3$); and small doses of ara-C on the proliferation and differentiation patterns of normal human bone marrow progenitor cells (105,106). Earlier studies investigated the possibility of inducing differentiation in leukemic cell lines. Abe et al. (107) have shown that 1,25$(DH)_2D_3$ induces mouse leukemia cell lines to differentiate into macrophages. The human promelocytic cell line (HL60) has been shown to differentiate into monocytes by 1,25$(DH)_2D_3$ and into granulocytes by 13 Cis RA (108,109). Ara-C was reported to induce differentiation in murine myeloid leukemia cells (110) and in human HL60 promyelocytic cell lines (111). During the last several years, evidence has accumulated that human myeloid progenitor cells from myelodysplastic (MDS) and leukemic patients can be induced to differentiate (76). We (112) and others (111,113) have shown that 1,25$(DH)_2D_3$ can induce progenitor cells from MDS and acute and chronic myeloid leukemia patients to differentiate along the monocyte-macrophage pathway. Retinoic acid has been shown to inhibit clonal growth and proliferation and to induce differentiation of leukemic cell lines and human leukemic blasts from AML patients (76,114-116). Lately, MDS patients have been treated with 13 Cis RA, 1,25$(DH)_2D_3$, and small doses of ara-C, i.e., maturation-inducing agents, but with equivocal success (117-121).

The mechanisms involved in leukemic cell differentiation have been studied thoroughly. The HL60 cell line has been used as a model to study regulatory sequences that control gene activity during terminal differentiation. Recently, 20 cDNA clones corresponding to mRNAs whose expression is strongly regulated during the differentiation process have been isolated. Furthermore, the levels of these genomic clones have been found to be markedly modulated during cellular differentiation (122).

In recent years, interest has focused on the identification and potential clinical use of physiological hematopoietic growth factors that can interfere with leukemic cell growth by inducing differentiation. Serum from patients following treatment with endotoxin (123,124), human T-lymphocyte leukemia virus-positive (HTLV-positive) cell line conditioned medium (125) PHA-LCM (124), and gamma interferon (126) have all been shown to have differentiation-inducing activities for myeloid leukemic cells. Metcalf et al. (127,128) have shown that the mouse granulocyte colony-stimulating factor (G-CSF) is a human hematopoietic growth factor that has differentiation potential (129) and it has been shown to induce differentiation in WEH1-3B leukemic colonies (26,129). Furthermore, leukemic cells from patients with acute and chronic myelogenous leukemia have been shown to bind G-CSF in the same levels as normal myeloid cells (54).

Recently two other human growth factors, pluripoietin (PPO) and pluripoietin Alpha (PPO A), which have been purified from human bladder carcinoma cell line 5637, have been shown to induce the differentiation of human leukemic cell lines (130). They are probably identical to G-CSF and GM-CSF. Thus human recombinant CSF may be of therapeutic value in inducing differentiation and reducing proliferation of leukemic cells as well as stimulating growth of the normal clone in AML patients. The first in vivo study evaluating the effect of recombinant human GM-CSF in monkeys has shown a dramatic leukocytosis and a substantial reticulocytosis with continuous infusion of the r-GM-CSF (131). However, at this point, the therapeutic role of biologic modifiers of myeloid differentiation remains undefined. Meanwhile, the liquid suspension culture technique and the self-renewal ability of the blast cells is a useful way to evaluate various differentiation-inducing agents (132).

The Interaction Between the Leukemic and Normal Clone

Another aspect that is studied using clonal assays is the interrelationship between the leukemic blasts, the normal clone, the microenvironment, and normal hematopoietic growth factors. Do leukemic cells themselves produce CSF and can leukemic cells suppress the normal clone? Are there differential responses between the normal and the leukemic clone, and finally, can leukemic cells be suppressed by manipulation of the hematopoietic growth factors? Greenberg et al. (133) studied the production of CSF from marrow cells of patients with AML and in half of the patients they found decreased marrow cell CSF production as compared with normal bone marrow. Induction of remission was higher in those with normal CSF production, suggesting that adequate marrow CSF provision may be essential for sustaining normal granulopoiesis in AML. Adherent cells from bone marrow of patients with chronic myelomonocytic leukemia were found to inhibit normal colony formation and on the other hand patients showed elevated colony-stimulating activity (134), suggesting that the leukemic population might be subjected to higher-than-normal proliferative stimulation. In contrast, the frequency of fibroblast colonies and their capacity to produce CSF is reduced in AML patients (135,136). The interpretation of the various studies is difficult, and more information is required before the overall role of CSFs in myeloid leukemia can be characterized and the interrelationship between normal and leukemic cells more carefully characterized.

Leukemic clones have been shown to produce various growth factors. Murine myeloid leukemia lines can produce factors identical to IL_3 (55). Pre-B and B ALL cell lines have been found to produce a growth factor (137). HL60 cell line secretes a glycoprotein factor which stimulates HL60 and myeloid cell growth and colony formation in vitro (138). However, as we have mentioned earlier, the AML blast cells exhibit dependency on exogenous stimulation and have receptors to the normal growth factors (54). Furthermore, antigrowth factors receptor antibodies may inhibit the growth of the malignant clone. Antitransferrin receptor antibody has been recently found to inhibit the growth of myeloid leukemic cell lines (139).

The complete suppression of the pre-existing normal clone by the leukemic clone is one of the striking features in AML. Broxmeyer et al. (51,52) have reported that leukemic cells produce an inhibitory factor (LIA) that inhibits normal but not leukemic CFU. This factor is possibly acidic isoferritin (140). Lactoferrin is another suppressing factor that inhibits CSF production by monocytes (141). Leukemic cells have been shown to be less sensitive to lactoferrin inhibition of CSF release (142). Another possible explanation for the suppression effect of the leukemic cell is via the microenvironment, which was found to produce reduced amounts of CSF in AML patients (135,136).

In Vitro Growth During Remission in AML

Following induction of a complete remission, the growth pattern of the bone marrow progenitor returns to normal and cultured cells form normal numbers of colonies and clusters that exhibit apparently normal differentiation, but frequently in reduced numbers (85,143). Thus, in remission, the hematopoiesis appears to be normal. Chemotherapy-induced remission is usually accompanied by disappearance of the chromosomal markers of the malignant clone and reappearance of functionally normal blood cells of polyclonal origin (144). However, in some cases, although the patient is in complete remission, there is persistent evidence for a clonal origin of the repopulating normal blood cells (145), an observation that was confirmed recently by the restriction fragment length polymorphism technique (36). Thus, one can assume that successful chemotherapy may suppress the blast population and the chromosomal marker, leaving both the clonal leukemic precursors and the normal ones in variable proportions to reemerge as hematologically normal blood cell elements.

B. Acute Lymphoblastic Leukemia

Clonal Nature of Acute Lymphoblastic Leukemia

Acute lymphoblastic leukemia (ALL) is also a clonal disease. The clonal nature of ALL has been demonstrated by the use of the G6PD isoenzyme. Dow et al. (146) used this technique and found only single G6PD isoenzyme in bone marrow and peripheral blood lymphoblasts in 19 patients with ALL. Double enzyme phenotypes were detected in erythrocytes, granulocytes, and platelets. Thus, the progenitors involved by ALL appear to have differentiative expression limited to the lymphoid pathway. These data were confirmed by the finding of an abnormal karyotype in the lymphoblasts. Characteristic fragile chromosomal sites with typical chromosomal breakpoints and translocations such as t(4;11) (q21;q23) have been found in ALL. Proto-oncogenes have been mapped to the chromosomal breakpoints in ALL patients. In the B-cell type ALL, chromosomal translocation between the immunoglobulin regions on chromosomes 2, 14, 22 and the region of c-Myc oncogene on chromosome 8 occurs.

These newer techniques with molecular probes that identified clonal rearrangement of the immunoglobulin genes and the T-cell receptor genes support the clonal origin of ALL (See other chapters in this book). Thus, the blast cells in ALL are the result of the clonal expansion of a single transformed cell. However, it is still not known if all cases of ALL involve a progenitor committed to lymphoid differentiation or a pluripotent stem cell in which myeloid differentiation is blocked. The development of pre B-cell leukemia with a Philadelphia chromosome marker following chemotherapy-induced remission of CML (147) suggests a single stem cell origin and perhaps multiple transformational events. Based on the previous studies (148-152), it is reasonable to believe that the malignant transformation of the lymphoid leukemic stem cell usually occurs at or following immunoglobulin gene rearrangement (153).

In Vitro Growth of Normal Colonies in ALL

Although myeloid progenitor cells are not part of the leukemic clone, most patients with ALL frequently have reduced myelopoiesis as reflected by the presence of anemia, granulocytopenia, and thrombocytopenia. The lymphoid leukemic stem cell and its progeny may inhibit the normal myeloid stem cell, as discussed earlier. However, the complete suppression of normal GM cells and other clonogenic progenitor cells in AML is not generally seen in ALL (65). In ALL the reduced level of normal CFU-GM parallels the mass of the lymphoblast cell infiltrating the bone marrow. In general, attempts at growing progenitor cells such as myeloid, erythroid, and pluripotent colony-forming units from the marrow of patients with ALL are unsuccessful or the number of colonies obtained are very few. The mechanism is probably mechanical crowding of the bone marrow by the malignant cells. This mechanism is supported by the finding that the blood levels of CFU-GM are elevated in ALL patients, whereas in AML patients CFU-GM are absent from the peripheral blood (65).

In Vitro Growth of ALL

In ALL, attempts at growing lymphoblastic leukemic colonies, as in AML, (CFU-L) are frequently not successful. Positive results on the growth of ALL colonies were first reported by Smith et al. (154). They grew malignant lymphoid CFU from the bone marrow and cerebrospinal fluid of children with ALL using agar with a feeder layer and in relative hypoxia. The colony cells grew without lymphoid mitogen, but at a slower rate than the normal cells. The colony cells had the same morphological staining pattern and monoclonal markers as the bone marrow lymphoblasts. Izaguirre et al. (155,156) grew CFU-L from ALL patients using conditioned medium from T cells and irradiated underlayers of T cells. The colonies contained cells that had the same morphological and cell surface antigens as the leukemic blasts. Some of the colonies had the stem cell characteristics of self-renewal. However, the plating efficiency was very low (0.1% to 1%). Recently,

Tomm et al. (157) have reported on the successful culturing of leukemic colonies in ALL patients, including the immunological subtypes pre-B, common, and unclassified ALL. They incorporated PHA or phorbol ester, feeder leukocytes, and IL2. They also showed that the leukemic cells express IL2 receptors after the in vitro exposure to PHA and phorbol ester, receptors that had been lacking from the fresh ALL cells. Immunophenotyping demonstrated the presence of the original leukemia marker on the colony cells. Linearity was observed between colony response and cell numbers plated. Lately a more effective cloning method for ALL was used to evaluate the efficacy of different methods in removing residual clonogenic leukemia cells from autologous marrow grafts in ALL patients (158). Persisting ALL leukemic colonies have been detected during remission and have been used to predict relapse (159), using techniques incorporating PHA, T-cell conditioned media, irradiated adherent cells, and a T-cell depleted target populations immobilized in methylcellulose.

The ability to grow CFU-L from ALL patients will have significant application for studying cell biology as well as the proliferation and differentiation patterns in ALL. The relationship between the lymphoid leukemic stem cell and the normal clone and the response of the leukemic progenitor to normal hematopoietic growth and differentiation factors as well as their sensitivity to cytotoxic chemicals will be studied. The in vitro regulation and growth factor needed for ALL cell growth is poorly understood. The recent development of cloning methods for ALL leukemic cells should facilitate this.

IV. SUMMARY

Recent advances in in vitro culture systems and particularly the ability to grow leukemic progenitor cells in semisolid, liquid, and long-term culture and to evaluate their self-renewal, proliferation, and differentiation capacities have resulted in better understanding of the biology of AML. AML is a clonal disease. The early event in leukemogenesis may be the emergence of a clone of hematopoietic preleukemic progenitors capable of essentially normal differentiation, but with proliferative advantages over the normal progenitors. The overt blastic stage would supervene with a second somatic genetic event. AML is a heterogenous disease. A complete block of maturation is not a consistent feature of AML. Inducing leukemic cells to become mature cells with little or no proliferative potential may represent an effective alternative or adjunct to a cytoreductive modality. Both chemical cytodifferentiation agents and natural growth factors can modify the expression of developmental potential. The purification and cloning of several human hematopoietic growth factors occupies a key position in attempts to understand the nature of AML, and potentially would have an important therapeutic role. These recent advances provide major insights into pathogenic mechanisms underlying leukemia and hopefully will increase survival of our leukemic patients. The recent cloning of ALL cells may help in identifying novel approaches for refractory cases.

REFERENCES

1. Metcalf, D. (1985). *Science* 229:16.
2. Metcalf, D. (1984). *The Haemopoietic Colony Stimulating Factors*. Elsevier, Amsterdam.
3. Stanley, E. R., Bartocci, A., Patinkin, D., Rosendaal, M., and Bradley, T. R. (1986). *Cell* 45:667.
4. Gasson, J., Weisbart, R. H., Kaufman, S. E., Clark, S. C., and Golde, D. W. (1984). *Science* 226:1339.
5. Wong, G. G., Witek, J. S., Temple, P. A., Wilkens, K. M., Leary, A. C., Luxenberg, D. P., Jones, S. S., Brown, E. L., Kay, R. M., Orr, E. C., Shoemaker, C., Golde, D. W., Kaufman, R. J., Hewick, R. M., Wang, E. A., and Clark, S. C. (1985). *Science* 228:810.
6. Souza, L. M., Boone, T. C., Gabrilove, J., Lai, P. H., Esebo, K. M., Murdock, D. C., Chazin, V. R., Bruszewske, J., Lue, H., Chen, K. K., Barendt, J., Platzer, E., Moore, M. A. S., Martelsmann, R., and Welte, K. (1986). *Science* 232:61.
7. Metcalf, D. (1985). *Cell* 43:5.
8. Metcalf, D., and Moore, M. A. S. (1971). In *Haemopoietic cells—Frontiers of Biology*, A. Neuberger and E. Tatum (eds.). North Holland Publ. Co., Amsterdam, London.
9. McCulloch, E. A. (1983). *Blood* 62:1.
10. Lotem, J., and Sachs, L. (1982). *Proc. Natl. Acad. Sci. USA* 79:4347.
11. Till, J. E., and McCulloch, E. A. (1961). *Radiat. Res.* 14:213.
12. Johnson, G. R., and Metcalf, D. (1977). *Proc. Natl. Acad. Sci. USA* 74:3879.
13. Fauser, A. A., and Messner, H. A. (1979). *Blood* 53:1023.
14. Metcalf, D., and Johnson, G. R. (1979). *J. Cell Physiol.* 99:159.
15. Messner, H. A., Izaguirre, C. A., and Jamal, N. (1981). *Blood* 58:402.
16. Lemischka, I. R., Raulet, D. H., and Mulligan, R. C. (1986). *Cell* 45:917.
17. Pluznik, D. H., and Sachs, L. (1965). *J. Cell Comp. Physiol.* 66:319.
18. Strome, J. E., McLeod, D. L., and Shreeve, M. M. (1978). *Exp. Hematol.* 6:461.
19. Mazur, E. M., Hoffman, R., and Bruno, E. (1981). *J. Clin. Invest.* 68:733.
20. Dexter, T. M., Allen, T. D., and Lajtha, L. G. (1977). *J. Cell Physiol.* 91:335.
21. Zipori, D. (1981). *J. Supramol. Struct. Cell Biochem.* 17:347.
22. Zipori, D., Moulds, C., and Lee, F. (1986). *Exp. Hematol.* 14:499.
23. Burgess, A. W., Camakaris, J., and Metcalf, D. (1977). *J. Biol. Chem.* 252:1998.
24. Das, S. K., Stanley, E. R., Guilbert, L. J., and Forman, L. W. (1981). *Blood* 58:630.
25. Ihle, J. N., Keller, J., Henderson, L., Klein, F., and Palaszynski, E. (1982). *J. Immunol.* 129:2431.

26. Nicola, N. A., Metcalf, D., Matsumoto, M., and Johnson, G. R. (1983). *J. Biol. Chem.* 258:9017.
27. Fung, M. C., Hapel, A. J., Ymer, S., Cohen, D. R., Johnson, R. M., Campbell, H. D., and Young, I. G. (1984). *Nature* 307:233.
28. Gough, N. M., Gough, J., Metcalf, D., Kelso, A., Grail, D., Nicola, N. A., Burgess, A. W., and Dunn, A. R. (1984). *Nature* 309:763.
29. Kawasaki, E. S., Lander, M. D., Wang, A. M., Arsdell, J. V., Warren, M. K., Coyne, M. Y., Schwiekart, V. L., Lee, M. T., Wilson, K. J., Bossman, A., Stanley, E. R., Ralph, P., and Mark, D. V. (1985). *Science* 230:295.
30. Walker, F., Nicola, N. A., Metcalf, D., and Burgess, A. W. (1985). *Cell* 43: 269.
31. de Taisne, G., Gegonne, A., Stehelin, D., Bernheim, A., and Berger, R. (1984). *Nature* 310:581.
32. Sachs, L. (1982). *J. Cell Physiol.* 110:151.
33. Till, J. E., and McCulloch, E. A. (1980). *Biochem. Biophys. Acta* 605:431.
34. Fialkow, P. J. (1984). Clonal evolution of human myeloid leukemias. In *Genes and Cancer*, J. M. Bishop, J. D. Rowley, and M. Greaves (eds.). Alan R. Liss, Inc., New York, p. 215.
35. Le Beau, M. M. (1986). *Blood* 67:849.
36. Fearon, E. R., Burke, P. J., Schiffer, C. A., Zehnbauer, B. A., and Vogelstein, B. (1986). *New Eng. J. Med.* 315:15.
37. Bunch, T. A., and Greaves, M. F. (1979). *Cancer* 43:426.
38. Hernandez, P., Carrot, J., and Cruz, C. (1982). *Br. J. Haematol.* 51:175.
39. Beveridge, R. P., Daley, J. F., Lane, H., and Schlossman, S. F. (1983). *Blood* 61:640.
40. Chan, L. C., Furley, A. J., Ford, A. M., Yardumian, D. A., and Greaves, M. F. (1986). *Blood* 67:533.
41. Prchal, J. T., Throckmorton, D. W., Carroll, A. J., Fuson, E. W., Ganis, R. A., and Prchal, J. F. (1978). *Nature* 274:590.
42. Berneman, Z. N., Van Bockstaele, D., De Meyer, P., Van Der Planken, M., Vertessen, F., De Bodk, R., and Peetermans, M. E. (1985). *Br. J. Haematol.* 60:353.
43. Pereira, A. M., De Castro, J. T., Santos, E. G., Perloiro, M. C., and Catovsky, D. (1985). *Clin. Lab. Haemat.* 7:89.
44. Neel, B. G., Jhanwar, S. C., Chaganti, R. S. K., and Hayward, W. S. (1982). *Proc. Natl. Acad. Sci. USA* 79:7842.
45. Needleman, S. W., Kraus, M. H., Srivastava, S. K., Levine, P. H., and Aaronson, S. A. (1986). *Blood* 67:753.
46. Gamble, C., Singer, E., and Moroni, C. (1984). *Nature* 307:476.
47. Pelicci, P. G., Lanfrancone, L., Brathwalte, M. D., Wolman, S. R., and Dalla Favera, R. (1984). *Science* 224:1117.
48. Gold, E. J., Conjalka, M., Pelus, L. M., Jhanwar, S. C., Broxmeyer, H., Middleton, A. B., Clarkson, B. O., and Moore, M. A. S. (1983). *J. Clin. Oncol.* 1:627.
49. Greenberg, P. L. (1983). *Blood* 61:1035.

50. Metcalf, D., Moore, M., Sheridan, J., and Spitzer, G. (1974). *Blood* 43:847.
51. Broxmeyer, H., Jacobsen, M., Kurland, J., Mendelsohn, N., and Moore, A. S. (1978). *Natl. Canc. Inst.* 60:497.
52. Pelus, L., Broxmeyer, L., Clarkson, B., and Moore, M. (1985). *Can. Res.* 40: 2512.
53. Metcalf, D. (1986). *Blood* 67:257.
54. Nicola, N. A., Begley, C. G., and Metcalf, D. (1985). *Nature* 314:625.
55. Schrader, J. W., and Crapper, R. M. (1983). *Proc. Natl. Acad. Sci. USA* 80: 6892.
56. Cook, W. D., Metcalf, D., Nicola, N. A., Burgess, A. W., and Walker, F. (1985). *Cell* 41:677.
57. Lang, R. A., Metcalf, D., Gough, N. M., Dunn, A. R., and Gonda, T. J. (1985). *Cell* 43:531.
58. Graf, T., Weizsaeker, F. V., Grieser, S., Coll, J., Stehelin, D., Patschinsky, T., Bister, K., Bechade, C., Calothy, G., and Leutz, A. (1986). *Cell* 45:357.
59. Sachs, L. (1980). *Proc. Natl. Acad. Sci. USA* 77:6152.
60. Davis, F. M., Dicke, K. A., Jagannath, S., and Rao, P. N. (1983). *J. Immunol. Methods* 58:349.
61. Malcolm, A. J., Logan, P. M., Shipman, R. C., Kurth, R. C., and Levy, J. G. (1983). *Blood* 61:858.
62. Kenneth, A. F., and Robert, F. T. (1986). *Blood* 68:1.
63. Griffin, J. D., Mayer, R. J., Weinstein, H. J., Rosenthal, D. S., Coral, F. S., Beveridge, R. P., and Schlossman, S. F. (1983). *Blood* 62:557.
64. Dicke, K. A., Spitzer, G., and Ahearn, M. J. (1976). *Nature* 259:129.
65. Spitzer, G., Verma, D. S., Dicke, K. A., and McCredie, K. B. (1978). *Sem. Hematol.* 15:352.
66. Aye, M. T., Niho, Y., Till, J. E., and McCulloch, E. A. (1974). *Blood* 44:205.
67. Buick, R. N., Miden, M. D., and McCulloch, E. A. (1979). *Blood* 54:95.
68. Greenberg, P. L., Mara, B., and Heller, P. (1978). *Blood* 52:362.
69. Chang, L. J.-A., Till, J. E., and McCulloch, E. A. (1980). *J. Cell. Physiol.* 102:217.
70. McCulloch, E. A., Curtis, J. E., Messner, H. A., Senn, J. S., and Gormanson, T. P. (1982). *Blood* 59:601.
71. Minden, M., Major, P., Griffin, J., Wu, A., and Keefe, D. (1983). *Cell. Tiss. Kinet.* 16:577.
72. Nara, N., Curtis, J. E., Senn, J. S., Tritchler, D. L., and McCulloch, E. A. (1986). *Blood* 67:762.
73. Marie, J. P., Zittoun, R., Thevenin, D., Mathieu, M., and Viguie, F. (1983). *Brit. J. Haematol.* 55:427.
74. Greenberg, P. L., Vankersen, I., and Mosny, S. (1976). *Can. Res.* 35:4412.
75. Dow, L. W., Dahl, G. V., Kalwinsky, D. K., Mirro, J., Nash, M. B., and Roberson, P. K. (1986). *Blood* 68:400.
76. Koeffler, H. P. (1983). *Blood* 62:709.
77. Nagler, A., Riklis, I., Tatarsky, I., and Fabian, I. (1984). *Blood* 64:170.
78. Nagler, A., Riklis, I., Tatarsky, I., and Fabian, I. (1985). *Blood* 66:205.
79. Kletter, J., and Nagler, A. (1984). *Acta Hematol.* 72:379.

80. Senn, J. S., McCulloch, E. A., and Till, J. E. (1967). *Lancet* 2:597.
81. Moore, M. A., Spitzer, G., Williams, N., Metcalf, D., and Buckley, J. (1974). *Blood* 44:1.
82. Spitzer, G., Dicke, K. A., Gehan, E. A., Smith, T., and McCredie, K. B. (1976). *Blood Cells* 2:139.
83. Dicke, K. A., Tindle, S., and Jagannath, S. (1983). *J. Cell. Biochem. Suppl.* 78:55.
84. Greenberg, P. L., Williams, C., Nichols, B. A., and Schrier, S. L. (1971). *New Eng. J. Med.* 284:1225.
85. Spitzer, G., Dicke, K. A., McCredie, K. B., and Barlogie, B. (1977). *Brit. J. Haematol.* 35:411.
86. Buick, R. N., Till, J. E., and McCulloch, E. A. (1977). *Lancet* 1:82.
87. Minden, M. D., Till, J. E., and McCulloch, E. A. (1978). *Blood* 52:592.
88. Lange, B., Ferrero, D., Pessano, S., Palumbo, A., Faust, J., Meo, P., and Rovera, G. (1984). *Blood* 64:693.
89. Hoang, T., and McCulloch, E. A. (1985). *Blood* 3:748.
90. Griffin, J. D., Young, D., Herrmann, F., Wiper, D., Wagner, K., and Sabbath, K. D. (1986). *Blood* 67:1448.
91. Hoang, T., Nara, N., Wong, G., Clark, S., Minden, M. D., and McCulloch, E. A. (1986). *Blood* 68:313.
92. Nara, N., and McCulloch, E. A. (1985). *Blood* 65:1484.
93. Nara, N., and McCulloch, E. A. (1986). *Leuk. Res.* 10:273.
94. Coulombel, L., Kalousek, D. K., Eaves, C. J., Gupta, C. M., and Eaves, A. C. (1983). *New Eng. J. Med.* 308:1493.
95. Dresch, C., Kebier, N. E., Mertal, J., and Karsdorf, A. (1983). *Exp. Haematol.* 11:187.
96. Niho, Y., Till, J. E., and McCulloch, E. A. (1976). *Exp. Haematol.* 6:63.
97. Georgoulias, V., Iskandar, Y. L., Amesland, F., Riband, P., Mathe, G., and Jasmin, C. (1984). *J. Clin. Oncol.* 2:1215.
98. Chan, C. H., Wiernik, P. H., Morrison, F. S., Amare, M., Van Sloten, K., and Maloney, T. R. (1983). *Cancer Res.* 43:2346.
99. Curtis, J. E., Messner, H. A., Hasselback, R., Elhakim, T. M., and McCulloch, E. A. (1984). *J. Clin. Oncol.* 2:253.
100. Preisler, H. D., and Azarnia, N. (1984). *Brit. J. Haematol.* 58:633.
101. Ozawa, K., Miura, Y., Suda, T., Motoyoshi, K., and Takaku, F. (1983). *Cancer Res.* 43:2339.
102. Taetle, R., and Honeysett, J. M. (1985). *Cancer* 56:1957.
103. Moingeon, P., Ythier, A., Nowill, A., Delmon, L., Bayle, C., Pico, J. L., Bohmon, C., and Hercend, J. (1986). *Blood* 67:777.
104. Freedman, M. H., Fish, E., Estrov, Z., Grunberger, T., and Williams, B. R. G. (1985). *Exp. Haematol.* 13:932.
105. Nagler, A., Riklis, I., Kletter, J., Tatarsky, I., and Fabian, I. (1986). *Exp. Haematol.* 14:60.
106. Nagler, A., Kletter, J., Riklis, I., Gazit, E., Tatarsky, I., and Fabian, I. (1986). *Exp. Haematol.* 14:241.

107. Abe, E., Miyaura, C., Sakagami, H., Taked, M., Konno, K., Yamarzaki, T., Yoshiki, S., and Suda, T. (1981). *Proc. Natl. Acad. Sci. USA* 78:4990.
108. McCarthy, D. M., San Miguel, J. F., Freaks, H. C., Green, P. M., Zola, H., Catovsky, D., and Goldman, J. M. (1983). *Leu. Res.* 7:51.
109. Hemmi, H., and Breitman, T. R. (1982). *Biochem. Biophys. Res. Commun.* 109:669.
110. Lotem, J., and Sachs, L. (1974). *Proc. Natl. Acad. Sci. USA* 71:3507.
111. Griffin, J. D., Munroe, D., Major, P., and Keefe, D. (1982). *Exp. Haematol.* 10:774.
112. Fabian, I., Riklis, I., Tatarsky, I., and Nagler, A. (1986). *Cancer Res.* 46: 2596.
113. Koeffler, H. P., Armatruda, T., Ikekawa, N., Kobayaski, Y., and Deluca, H. F. (1984). *Cancer Res.* 44:5624.
114. Douer, D., and Koeffler, H. P. (1982). *Exp. Cell Res.* 138:193.
115. Douer, D., and Koeffler, H. P. (1982). *J. Clin. Invest.* 69:1039.
116. Tobler, A., Dawson, M. I., and Koeffler, H. P. (1986). *J. Clin. Invest.* 78: 303.
117. Koeffler, H. P., Hirji, K., and Itri, L. S. (1985). *Can. Chem. Rep.* 69:1399.
118. Winter, J. N., Variakojis, D., Gaynor, E. R., Larson, R. A., and Miller, K. B. (1985). *Cancer* 56:443.
119. Griffin, J. D., Spriggs, D., Wisch, J. S., and Keefe, D. W. (1985). *J. Clin. Oncol.* 3:982.
120. Swanson, G. F., Picozzi, V. J., Morgan, R., Hecht, F., and Greenberg, P. L. (1986). *Blood* 67:1154.
121. Picozzi, V. J., Swanson, G. F., Morgan, R., Hecht, F., and Greenberg, P. L. (1986). *J. Clin. Oncol.* 4:589.
122. Concannon, P., Teraoka, S. N., Nelson, R., and Sales, W. A. (1985). HL-60 cells regulate the expression of transfected genes during *in vitro* cellular differentiation. In *Leukemia: Recent Advances in Biology and Treatment*, R. B. Gale and D. W. Golde (eds.). Alan R. Liss, Inc., New York, p. 71.
123. Moore, M. A. S., Gabrilove, J., and Sheridan, A. P. (1983). *Blood Cells* 9: 125.
124. Ralf, P., Harris, P., Punjabi, C. J., Welte, K., Litkovsky, P. B., Ho, M. K., Robin, B. Y., Moore, M. A. S., and Springer, F. A. (1983). *Blood* 62:1169.
125. Koeffler, H. P., Clen, I. S. Y., and Golde, D. W. (1984). *Blood* 64:482.
126. Elias, L., Wogenvich, F., Wallace, J., and Longmire, J. (1980). *Leuk. Res.* 4:301.
127. Metcalf, D. (1983). *Leuk. Res.* 7:117.
128. Metcalf, D., and Nicola, N. A. (1982). *Int. J. Cancer* 30:773.
129. Nicola, N. A., and Metcalf, D. (1985). *Cancer Surveys* 4:791.
130. Welte, K., Platzer, E., Lu, L., Gabrilove, J. L., Levi, E., Mertelsmann, R., and Moore, M. A. S. (1985). *Proc. Natl. Acad. Sci. USA* 82:1526.
131. Donahue, R. E., Wang, E. A., Stone, D. K., Kamen, R., Wong, G. G., Shegal, P. K., Nathan, D. G., and Clark, S. C. (1986). *Nature* 321:872.
132. Motozi, T., Hoang, T., Tritchler, D., and McCulloch, E. A. (1985). *Blood* 65:894.

133. Greenberg, P. L., Mara, B., and Heller, P. (1978). *Blood* 52:362.
134. Ohyashiki, K., Ohyashiki, J., Oshimura, M., Miyasaka, Y., Sakai, N., Osamura, S., Tonomura, A., and Ito, H. (1984). *Cancer* 54:2468.
135. Kaneko, S., Motomura, S., and Ibayashi, H. (1982). *Brit. J. Haematol.* 51: 217.
136. Greenberg, B. R., Wilson, F. D., and Wao, L. (1981). *Blood* 58:557.
137. Blazer, B. A., Sutton, L. M., and Strome, M. (1983). *Cancer Res.* 43:4562.
138. Perkins, S. L., Andreotti, P. E., Sinha, S. K., Wu, M. C., and Yunis, A. A. (1984). *Cancer Res.* 44:5169.
139. Taetle, R., Rhyner, K., Castagnola, J., To, O., and Mendelsohn, J. (1986). *J. Clin. Invest.* 75:1061.
140. Broxmeyer, H. E., Bognacki, J., Dorner, M. M., and de Sousa, M. (1981). *J. Exp. Med.* 153:1426.
141. Bagby, G. D., McCall, E., and Layman, D. L. (1983). *J. Clin. Invest.* 71: 340.
142. Broxmeyer, H. E., Mendelsohn, N., and Moore, M. A. S. (1977). *Leu. Res.* 1:3.
143. Moore, M. A. S., Williams, N., and Metcalf, D. (1973). *J. Natl. Cancer Inst.* 50:603.
144. Fialkow, P. J., Singer, J. W., Adamson, J. W., Vaidya, K., Dow, L. W., Ochs, J., and Moohr, J. W. (1981). *Blood* 57:1068.
145. Jacobson, R. J., Temple, M. J., Singer, J. W., Raskind, W., Powell, J., and Fialkow, P. J. (1984). *New Eng. J. Med.* 310:1513.
146. Dow, L. W., Martin, P., Moohr, J., MacDougall, L. G., Najfeld, V., Greenberg, M., and Fialkow, P. J. (1985). *Blood* 66:901.
147. Lebien, T. W., Hozier, J., Minowada, J., and Kersey, H. (1979). *New Eng. J. Med.* 301:144.
148. Leder, P. (1982). *Sci. Amer.* 246:102.
149. Tonegawa, S. (1983). *Nature* 302:575.
150. Nadler, L. M., Korsmeyer, S. J., Anderson, K. C., Boyd, A. W., Slaughenhoupt, B., Park, E., Jensen, J., Coral, F., Mayer, R. J., Sallan, S. E., Ritz, J., and Schlossman, S. F. (1984). *J. Clin. Invest.* 74:332.
151. Korsmeyer, S. J., Arnold, A., Bakhshi, A., Ravetch, J. V., Siebemlist, M., Hieter, P. A., Sharrow, S. O., Lebien, T. W., Kersey, J. H., Poplack, D. G., Leder, P., and Waldmann, T. A. (1983). *J. Clin. Invest.* 71:301.
152. Korsmeyer, S. J., Hieter, P. A., Ravetch, J. V., Poplack, D. G., Waldmann, T. A., and Leder, P. (1981). *Proc. Natl. Acad. Sci. USA* 78:7096.
153. Greaves, J. F. (1978). "Target" cells, differentiation and clonal evolution in chronic granulocytic leukemia: A "model" for understanding the biology of malignancy. In *Chronic Granulocytic Leukemia*, M. T. Shaw (ed.). Praeger, New York, p. 15.
154. Smith, S. D., Uyeki, E. M., and Lowman, J. T. (1978). *Blood* 52:712.
155. Izaguirre, C. A., Curtis, J., Messner, H., and McCulloch, E. A. (1981). *Blood* 57:823.
156. Izaguirre, C. A. (1984). *Clin. Haematol.* 13:405.

157. Tomm, I., Delwel, R., Bolhuis, R., Van Zanen, G., and Lowenberg, B. (1985). *Blood* 66:556.
158. Uckun, F. M., Peczalska, K. J. G., Kersey, J. H., Houston, L. L., and Vallera, D. A. (1986). *J. Exp. Med.* 163:317.
159. Estrov, Z., Grunberger, T., Dube, I. D., Wang, Y.-P., and Freedman, M. H. (1986). *New Eng. J. Med.* 315:538.

12

Lineage Heterogeneity in Acute Leukemia
Acute Mixed Lineage Leukemia and Lineage Switch

JOSEPH MIRRO, JR. *St. Jude Children's Research Hospital and University of Tennessee College of Medicine, Memphis, Tennessee*

GEOFFREY R. KITCHINGMAN *St. Jude Children's Research Hospital, Memphis, Tennessee*

SANFORD A. STASS *The University of Texas System Cancer Center, M. D. Anderson Hospital and Tumor Institute, Houston, Texas*

Most contemporary models of hematopoietic differentiation are predicated on the principle of "lineage fidelity," which is based on in vitro and in vivo studies of normal hematopoiesis that suggest that pluripotent hematopoietic precursors commit irreversibly to a single lineage as a discrete differentiation step. Since leukemogenesis uncouples proliferation and differentiation, leukemic cells are thought to represent clonal expansions of target cells "frozen" in one of these discrete differentiation stages. Recently, however, many investigators have identified leukemic blasts that simultaneously express characteristics of more than one lineage, suggesting that lineage fidelity is violated in a significant percentage of acute leukemias (1,2,3). We have termed this *acute mixed lineage leukemia* (3). In the first section of this chapter, we focus on demonstrations of lineage heterogeneity in acute leukemia based on morphologic, cytochemical, and immunologic studies. The second section discusses molecular evidence for acute mixed lineage leukemia. We then consider the specific role of specific chromosomal translocations involving the 11q23 breakpoint in pathogenesis of such cases. In the fourth section we examine lineage switch, the sequential expression of lymphoid and myeloid characteristics, which provides further evidence of lineage heterogeneity. The fifth section focuses on the clinical importance of these observations. Finally, the major implications of these studies for our concepts of hematopoietic differentiation, leukemogenesis, and the control of gene expression are discussed.

I. MIXED LINEAGE LEUKEMIA: MORPHOLOGIC, CYTOCHEMICAL, AND IMMUNOLOGIC STUDIES

The initial immunologic and molecular investigations indicated that acute leukemia is a monoclonal disease with either myeloid or lymphoid characteristics, supporting the notion of lineage fidelity (4-7). Although leukemic phenotypes may not be perfect replicas of normal cells, normal target cells expressing a similar pattern of antigen expression can be identified. Since there is usually minimal deviation of the maturation-linked phenotype in leukemic cells at diagnosis, it appears that leukemogenesis is not an absolute block in differentiation, but rather a variable uncoupling of differentiation and proliferation (8,9).

The first indication that leukemic cells do not uniformly adhere to a lymphoid or myeloid lineage came from morphologic studies showing lymphoid characteristics in chronic myelogenous leukemia (CML) cells undergoing blast crisis (10). Laboratory support for lineage heterogeneity in CML came from the biochemical demonstration of terminal deoxynucleotidyl transferase (TdT) activity in the cells of some patients in blast crisis. These findings led to the conclusion that CML is a disease of stem cell origin (leukemogenesis in a pluripotent progenitor). Other early evidence for lineage heterogeneity was provided by the identification of TdT- and Auer rod-positive cases of leukemia (11,12). These studies, describing leukemic cells that expressed characteristics of multiple lineages, provided the conceptual framework for studies of lineage infidelity.

Table 1 Morphologic and Immunologic Demonstrations of Lineage Heterogeneity in Leukemia

Type of lineage heterogeneity	Ref.
Mixed lineage	
CML	10
Philadelphia chromosome positive ALL	87
AML with TdT	11,12
AML with erythroid characteristics	40
ALL with myeloid surface antigens or AML with lymphoid surface antigens	3,22-23,28-31,88-90
11q23 abnormalities	32,71,75,91,92
Biclonal leukemia (separate populations)	
Lymphoid + monocytoid	24-25
Lymphoid + myeloid	26-28
Sequential expression (lineage switch)	
ALL to AML	28,77-79
AML to ALL	79

CML = chronic myelogenous leukemia.
TdT = terminal deoxynucleotidyl transferase.
ALL = acute lymphocytic leukemia.
AML = acute myelogenous leukemia.

The development of lineage-associated monoclonal antibodies (MoAbs), along with techniques for simultaneous detection of multiple antigens, provided the means to confirm and extend the early studies on mixed lymphoid-myeloid leukemias. Table 1 summarizes the published studies on mixed lineage leukemias, as well as the related topics of biclonal leukemia, 11q23 abnormalities, and lineage switch, which will be discussed in subsequent sections.

The early studies of mixed lineage leukemia using MoAbs have been criticized because of the assumptions made about the specificity of the antibodies and the anticipated phenotypes of normal equivalent cells. The most common problem with any such study is that the MoAbs have not been evaluated extensively enough to ensure that they react with cells of only one lineage. For example, the X-hapten was identified by many MoAbs and at first was reported to be myeloid-specific. However, this antigen, which is a carbohydrate (3-fucosyl-N-acetyllactosamine), was subsequently identified on the surface of cells of several other lineages and is the same as the SSEA-1 antigen of teratocarcinoma. Furthermore, the X-hapten can be exposed on the surface of some acute lymphoblastic leukemia cells by neuraminidase treatment (13,14). This antigen is therefore not lineage-specific and its expression alone cannot be used as proof of multiple lineage characteristics.

Another criticism of studies using MoAbs is the implied assumption that MoAbs are monospecific. As is well known, antigenic specificity is never absolute, as antibodies recognize a small epitope, usually a short stretch of amino acids within a much larger molecule. Therefore, MoAbs can potentially react with other proteins that have the same epitope. Immunoprecipitation of the protein, which eliminates the possibility of cross-reacting epitopes, has been used by some investigators to confirm multiple lineage characteristics with individual leukemic cases.

Finally, reports of mixed lineage characteristics have been criticized because of our limited knowledge of the true progenitor phenotype. Clearly, selective studies of the multipotential progenitor cell must be undertaken before final conclusions can be drawn.

We undertook a prospective study of acute leukemias in an attempt to confirm that cases of acute mixed lineage leukemia do exist, and to determine their clinical significance. If they are frequent, such cases could largely nullify the concept of lineage fidelity and would carry important implications for our understanding of leukemogenesis and normal hematopoietic differentiation. These studies included multiple MoAbs to minimize the risk of individual cross-reactivity or lack of lineage specificity. In most cases, detection of antigens of two separate lineages on individual cells was done simultaneously by use of flow cytometry or microsphere binding. In addition, immunoprecipitation of important antigens was performed to ensure their presence on malignant cells. Finally, and possibly most significantly, these studies included careful molecular analysis of the DNA to extend and expand the concept of lineage heterogeneity to the gene level.

In these studies, we analyzed blast cells from 260 children with acute leukemia and 90 adults with acute or chronic leukemia with monoclonal antibodies for T-cell (4,15-18) and B-cell (5,19) surface antigens, and for myeloid characteristics such as myeloperoxidase positivity or reactivity with myeloid-associated MoAbs (3,6,8,9,20,21). The proportion of patients whose blast cells expressed characteristics of more than one lineage was surprisingly high. Of 207 children diagnosed as having acute lymphocytic leukemia (ALL) by standard criteria, 26 (12.6%) had blast cells showing evidence of myeloid differentiation, as determined by reactivity with MoAbs used to identify myeloid-related cell surface antigens (My-1, MCS.2, Mol, SJ-D1 and 5F1) (3; unpublished results). These early results in childhood ALL have been confirmed by the Pediatric Oncology Group in a larger study of over 800 children (22). In the adult patients we studied, 2 of 28 (7%) with typical ALL expressed myeloid-associated cell surface antigens (MY7 or MY9). A large study of adult patients by Cancer Leukemia Group B likewise demonstrated mixed lineage characteristics in 21% of 129 ALL cases of acute and chronic nonlymphocytic leukemia (Stass et al., unpublished results).

Similarly, blast cells from 10 of the 53 (18.9%) children studied, which otherwise showed typical morphologic and cytochemical features of acute nonlymphocytic leukemia (ANLL), also expressed lymphoid-associated surface antigens (T11, T3, CALLA, and T101) (3; unpublished results). Reactivity with lymphoid-associated MoAbs (T3, T4, T11 and T101) was observed for 22 of 62 (34%) adult cases of acute and chronic nonlymphocytic leukemia (23).

Such patients were originally felt to have biphenotypic leukemia—leukemia in which cells showing myeloid characteristics apparently coexisted with those showing lymphoid features (24-28). One could thus argue that lineage fidelity was maintained because of the existence of separate populations of lymphoid and myeloid blasts. However, when the percentage of cells expressing myeloid characteristics plus the percentage expressing lymphoid characteristics exceeded 100% (29), it implied that at least some cells were expressing antigens of both lineages. The use of dual staining techniques such as microsphere-conjugated MoAbs, immunoperoxidase cytochemistry, and dual laser flow cytometry disclosed simultaneous expression of lymphoid and myeloid characteristics on individual blast cells (3,30-32). Leukemic cells expressing only lymphoid or myeloid features were also identified in these studies. There was no evidence for independent clones; rather, cytogenetic analysis clearly demonstrated that the blast cells represented a single malignant clone in each patient, consistent with glucose-6-phosphate dehydrogenase (G6PD) analysis indicating that acute leukemia is a clonal disease (33).

We estimate from these studies that approximately 25% of cases diagnosed as nonlymphoblastic will possess lymphoid-associated surface antigens, while 13% to 20% of those that appear to be typical ALL will have surface markers common to the myeloid lineage. These observations do not by themselves eliminate the possibility that antigens previously regarded as specific for a single lineage may in fact be expressed on cells of the opposite lineage (34-38). However, the expression of multiple lymphoid-associated and multiple myeloid-associated antigens on individual leukemic cells makes this unlikely. Two other possible explanations for the apparently inappropriate expression of lineage-specific antigens that have strong implications for hematopoietic differentiation are: (a) leukemogenesis occurs in a pluripotent progenitor that normally expresses antigens of several different lineages (2,39), or (b) leukemogenesis results in a derangement of the control of normal gene expression (40,41) and mixed leukemias therefore represent aberrant cell types.

We are not aware of any evidence that normal hematopoietic cells express the degree of interlineage heterogeneity we have noted in acute leukemia, although previously published data indicate that T4 may be expressed on normal or neoplastic monocytes-histiocytes (42). Furthermore, it is difficult to explain the expression of a mature T-cell antigen such as T3 on the surface of an otherwise typical myeloid leukemic cell if the leukemogenic event occurred in a pluripotent progenitor cell. In addition, we have immunoprecipitated the E-rosette receptor from leukemic myeloblasts (31) and found that it has the same molecular weight as the receptor from T lymphocytes. It is clear that further work characterizing the inappropriately expressed antigens will be required before it is possible to draw definitive conclusions regarding lineage fidelity. In addition, more studies on normal hematopoietic progenitor cells in children and during fetal development are needed to clarify the ontogeny of different lineage-specific characteristics and determine whether they are "normally" coexpressed during early development.

Until further information is available, we believe any model of differentiation and leukemogenesis must take into account the possibility of a limited stage of early differentiation where pluripotent cells express characteristics of multiple lineages. Although we hypothesize that aberrant gene expression is also responsible for mixed lineage leukemia, we believe both mechanisms may be occurring and have proposed a model incorporating both possibilities (Figure 1). These possibilities are discussed in detail in section VI.

In the next section we discuss evidence obtained through the use of molecular biological techniques for the existence of mixed lineage leukemias.

II. MOLECULAR STUDIES OF LINEAGE HETEROGENEITY IN ACUTE LEUKEMIA USING IMMUNOGLOBULIN AND T-CELL RECEPTOR GENES

The formation of functional immunoglobulin (Ig) or T-cell receptor (Ti) genes requires the rearrangement and juxtaposition of segments of DNA encoding the variable, diversity (present in the immunoglobulin heavy chain and T-cell receptor β-chain genes), and joining regions through the process of DNA rearrangement (43-49). These rearranged segments are then joined to the appropriate

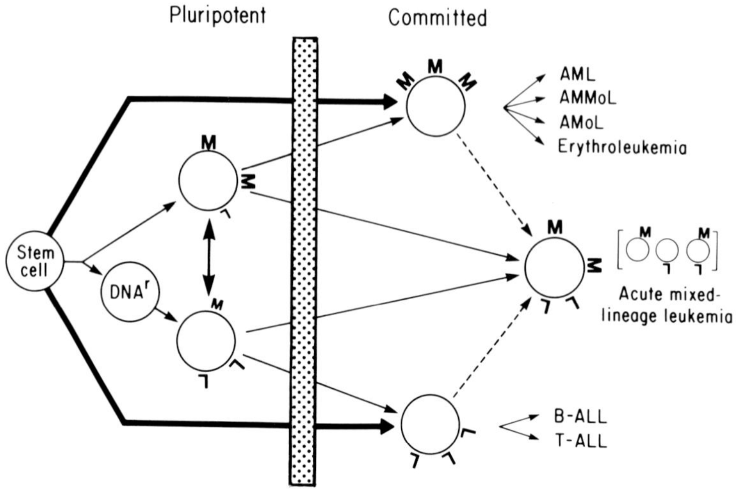

Figure 1 Model of hematopoietic differentiation and leukemogenesis. The leukemogenic event may occur in a stem cell or in a pluripotent progenitor that may express antigens of both lineages. Differentiation in these situations would be normal but could result in mixed lineage leukemia. Alternatively, leukemogenesis may occur in a committed progenitor and result in abnormal control of gene expression leading to mixed-lineage cases. Normal differentiation is demonstrated by ——→, aberrant gene expression by – – –→. Myeloid surface antigen, M, lymphoid surface antigens, L, are represented on pluripotent and committed cells. DNA^r indicates rearrangement in the immunoglobulin heavy chain or T-cell receptor β-chain genes.

Table 2 Molecular Demonstrations of Lineage Heterogeneity in Acute Leukemia

Type of study	Ref.
Immunoglobulin gene rearrangements	
In AML	56, 57, 60
In T-cell ALL	58, 61-63
T-cell receptor gene rearrangements	
In AML	3
In B-precursor cell ALL	63, 66, 67

AML = acute myelogenous leukemia.
ALL = acute lymphocytic leukemia.

constant region by RNA splicing. The expression of functional proteins resulting from the rearrangement process is confined to the appropriate lineage of cells. However, it was discovered several years ago that in mouse tumors the rearrangement process itself did not adhere to lineage fidelity (50-52); that is, rearranged Ig heavy chain genes (in all cases, we are referring to the mu heavy-chain genes only) were found in cell lines derived from T-cell and myeloid tumors. The presence of gene rearrangements in human cell types that do not express functional protein has recently been documented, extending the findings from mouse tumor cell lines to human cell lines (53-58) and to fresh leukemic cells (53-62, see also Chapter 9). A summary of published studies using molecular probes which support the concept of mixed lineage leukemia is given in Table 2.

Initial studies using human-tumor-derived cell lines identified several examples of rearranged Ig heavy-chain genes in T-cell lines, but not in fresh T-ALL cells from patients (53,55), indicating that perhaps the rearrangements were present only after culture of the leukemic cells. The initial molecular evidence for the violation of lineage fidelity in leukemic cell DNA was from a study of Ig heavy-chain gene rearrangements in children with ANLL (56). Blast cells from 2 of 14 patients with ANLL had at least one Ig heavy-chain gene rearranged. We continued these studies and to date 8 of 47 (17%) DNAs from patients with ANLL have shown Ig heavy-chain gene rearrangements. Rearrangement of the heavy-chain gene has also been demonstrated in the myeloid cell line, ML-1, derived from a malignant lymphoma of the T-cell type that underwent lineage switch to ANLL (56,57). Similar results with myeloid cell lines and fresh myeloid leukemia cells have been obtained by several other laboratories (57,60). In all cases examined only the Ig heavy-chain gene is rearranged; the kappa and lambda light-chain genes are in the germline configuration, as was found in the mouse tumor cell lines (50-52). Gene rearrangement studies have also demonstrated that the Ig heavy-chain genes can be rearranged in T-cell ALL (58,61-63). In our own studies, 6 of 22 (27%) T-ALLs were found to have rearranged heavy-chain genes (61; unpublished data).

The utility of genetic studies to demonstrate lineage heterogeneity (or acute mixed lineage leukemia) has been recently extended through the use of probes for the β chain of the T-cell receptor (β-Ti) (64,65), and the unexpected demonstration of its rearrangement in cells of B lymphoid precursor origin (63,66,67), and in nonlymphocytic leukemias (3; unpublished results). To date, we have examined the DNAs of 62 patients with non-T-cell leukemias for the arrangement of the β-Ti, and have found that 13 of 49 (26.5%) with B precursor ALL and 1 of 13 (8%) patients with ANLL have at least one rearranged β-Ti gene. These results are summarized in Figure 2. As all of the B precursor ALLs also have rearranged Ig heavy-chain genes (and all T-ALLs with rearranged Ig heavy-chain genes also have rearranged β-Ti genes), these cells thus have genetic changes

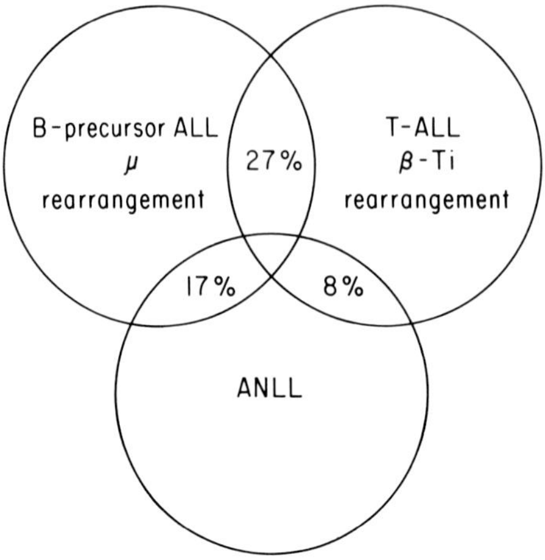

Figure 2 Summary of molecular studies demonstrating lineage heterogeneity. B-precursor ALL is defined by expression of multiple B lineage surface antigens and at least immunoglobulin heavy-chain gene rearrangements. T-cell ALL is defined by the expression of multiple T-cell-associated antigens and rearrangements in the β-Ti gene. ANLL is defined by the standard French-American-British classification and must express myeloid-associated cytochemistries in greater than 3% of leukemic blasts.

found in two distinct lineages. It should be emphasized that the cases with apparently inappropriate gene rearrangements constitute a separate but overlapping group with the mixed lineage patients identified by immunologic and cytochemical methods. Thus, the actual percentage of mixed lineage leukemias may exceed the numbers obtained from either type of analysis alone and greater than 30% of all leukemias may have mixed lineage characteristics.

Analysis of the gene rearrangements does not suffer from the same potential problems alluded to earlier for studies using monoclonal antibodies, such as cross-reactivity of epitopes or the lack of lineage specificity. While the presence of both Ig and Ti gene rearrangements may be explained on the basis of "cross-talk" of the enzymes involved in the recognition of the rearrangement signals present in these two gene families, the rearrangement of either of these genes in myeloid cells cannot be explained on this basis. The correlation of the relative percentage of leukemias demonstrating mixed phenotypes by immunological and cytochemical methods with the gene probing method supports the concept of mixed leukemias representing the transformed counterparts to oligopotential precursor cells.

Analysis of leukemic cells with the molecular probes has identified another type of lineage heterogeneity; the presence of multiple clones with a single leukemic population. Our studies with B precursor ALLs have demonstrated that 24% (36 of 149 cases) have more than two copies of the Ig heavy-chain gene (68; unpublished results). The presence of more than two genes indicates that two separate clones are present, which could arise either by transformation of two separate cells (biclonal leukemia) or by the continuing rearrangement of the heavy-chain genes during outgrowth of a single transformed clone (clonal evolution). In none of the cases studied was there cytogenetic evidence to support the concept of biclonal leukemia (68). In about 30% of the cases, the extra copy or copies of the Ig heavy-chain gene can be explained by a corresponding increase in the number of copies of chromosome 14. For the remaining cases, the simplest explanation is that the leukemic cells continue to differentiate after leukemogenesis, resulting in subclones with different rearrangements in the Ig genes. This is reminiscent of the continued rearrangement of Ig heavy-chain genes in mouse lymphoid cells transformed by the Abelson murine leukemia virus, where up to six sublines have been observed to arise from a single clone over several months in culture (69,70).

The detection by molecular techniques of two clones within a leukemic cell population indicates an intralineage heterogeneity not previously appreciated. The presence at diagnosis of what is probably a major subclone could have important ramifications for the treatment of these leukemias. This will be discussed in more detail in section V.

III. IMPORTANCE OF THE 11q23 BREAKPOINT IN EXPRESSION OF MULTIPLE LINEAGE-ASSOCIATED CHARACTERISTICS

In their review of reported cases of so-called biphenotypic or biclonal leukemia, Ben-Bassat and Gale called attention to the high frequency of the 4;11 chromosomal translocation (71). Our recent review of the t(4;11), with involvement of 11q23 breakpoint, indicates that it occurs in approximately 2.5% of children with acute leukemia and is usually, but not always, associated with lymphoid morphology (32,72-74). The majority of blasts in such cases express lymphoid-associated surface antigens and have undergone Ig heavy-chain gene rearrangement (32,73). However, all cases which we were able to carefully analyze by dual laser flow cytometry had blasts that simultaneously expressed both lymphoid- and myeloid-associated cell surface antigens. Ultrastructural study of the cells from several patients confirmed the dual-lineage characteristics of individual leukemic blasts (32). Adult cases with the t(4;11) were usually classified as lymphoid, although isolated instances of acute myelomonocytic leukemia and acute undifferentiated leukemia were observed. Interestingly, in several cases that were classified as ALL by morphologic, cytochemical, and immunophenotypic criteria, electron microscopy disclosed a small second population of monoblasts with myeloperoxidase-positive granules and/or fibrillary bundles. Thus, there is also good ultrastructural evidence that t(4;11) adult cases are commonly mixed lineage leukemias. These findings confirm previous reports suggesting that the t(4;11) translocation is more likely to occur in cases of mixed lymphoid-myeloid leukemia.

A study of translocations involving the 11q23 breakpoint by other investigators (75) suggested that this is the important abnormality in the pathogenesis of mixed lineage leukemia. Blast cells from a number of patients expressed surface characteristics of both myeloid and lymphoid lineages, and one patient underwent a lineage switch from ALL to AML. The recent localization of the c-*ets* 1 proto-oncogene to this region of chromosome 11 (76) implicates this gene as having a role in the expression of dual lineage characteristics. However, cloning of the breakpoints and analysis of the effects of the translocation on the expression of the c-*ets* 1 gene will be required before a definitive association between this gene and mixed leukemias can be made.

IV. LINEAGE SWITCH: ADDITIONAL EVIDENCE FOR LINEAGE HETEROGENEITY

In addition to acute mixed lineage leukemia, there is a second group of leukemic patients whose blast cells express the characteristics of lymphoid and myeloid cells. In these patients, blast cells undergo a phenotypic conversion from ALL to ANLL, or the reverse, and therefore sequentially express antigens of two separate lineages (28,77-79). Such cases of leukemia have been called *lineage switch* by us. By using a combination of morphologic, cytochemical, and immunologic techniques, we have been able to establish the frequency and spectrum of changes that define such cases. In our initial retrospective study, the frequency of lineage switch was 6.7%. A subsequent retrospective analysis of more than 552 cases of newly diagnosed ALL and ANLL revealed a slightly higher frequency, with 13 of 150 patients (8.5%) who had bone marrow relapses undergoing lineage switch within 1-4 years from diagnosis (79; unpublished results).

Eight of thirteen patients had T-cell-associated characteristics at diagnosis or at the time of lineage switch; otherwise, there were no obvious similarities in clinical or biologic features, except that all patients had been treated with intensive multiagent chemotherapy.

What causes the lineage switch? There is evidence for three different possible mechanisms as a cause of lineage switch. First, within the single leukemic clone there could be subpopulations of cells expressing markers of different lineages. The predominant lineage which is evident at diagnosis is eradicated by chemotherapy directed toward this lineage, allowing the second population to expand and be evident at relapse. The second possibility is that chemotherapy modifies the original leukemic clone by altering gene expression, perhaps through changes in DNA methylation, thereby causing a shift in the expression of phenotypic features. These first two possibilities are supported by the finding of the same karyotypic abnormality at diagnosis and relapse in our studies and those of others (77-79). Further evidence comes from the isolation of a cell line from one of these patients which will express lymphoid or myeloid phentoypes depending on drug exposure. Recent findings suggest that a third possibility exists, that is, that the relapse represents a second, independent malignancy. In this latter case, the original blast cell karyotype is replaced by an entirely different karyotype. Although such findings could result from expansion of a subclone present at diagnosis, they suggest that a second leukemogenic event, rather than mutation or an alteration in gene regulation in an existing malignant clone, is causal.

V. CLINICAL SIGNIFICANCE

The clinical significance of acute mixed lineage leukemia is just beginning to emerge. Patients who meet FAB criteria for ANLL but express the antigen associated with E-rosette formation (T11) appear to have a poor response to induction therapy. In our studies, 5 of 9 patients in this category who received therapy directed to ANLL entered complete remission, but 3 had relatively brief periods of disease-free survival (3; unpublished observation). Of the 4 who failed ANLL therapy, three entered complete remissions when treated with ALL therapy (vincristine, prednisone, and L-asparaginase), while the fourth had a dramatic response but died of sepsis during marrow aplasia. To identify such patients, we suggest that clinical investigators routinely test typical cases of ANLL for reactivity with MoAbs to the E-rosette receptor.

In our original report, we described 18 children with a diagnosis of ALL whose blasts expressed myeloid-associated cell surface antigens. At that time, all patients had been in continuous complete remission for 3 to 14+ months. However, with longer followup, CNS relapses have occurred in 5 patients, 2 of whom subsequently developed bone marrow involvement (unpublished observations). In a larger series of pediatric patients, children with ALL expressing myeloid-associated surface antigens had a lower complete response rate to induction therapy with vincristine, prednisone and asparaginase (22). Similarly, adult patients with ALL having blasts that expressed myeloid-associated antigens had a lower chance of achieving complete remission (23).

The prognostic implications of lineage infidelity based on the presence of inappropriate immunoglobulin and T-cell receptor gene rearrangements will require a larger series of patients and longer followup. Such studies are being performed at our institution and by other groups in both children and adults.

Clinical experience with patients whose blast cells demonstrate lineage switch indicates that a better response is achieved when chemotherapy is directed to the lineage evident at relapse (79). This clinical experience emphasizes the importance of early recognition of lineage switch in the formulation of reinduction therapy.

VI. IMPLICATIONS FOR HEMATOPOIETIC DIFFERENTIATION

Until recently, lineage fidelity was thought to be preserved in leukemic cells, which showed surface marker and enzymatic patterns characteristic of an appropriate normal cell lineage and stage of differentiation. Our data indicate that this theory is too restrictive. If our studies of leukemic cells accurately reflect what occurs in pluripotent progenitors, then the data are best explained by a model of differentiation in which lymphoid and myeloid antigens are expressed simultaneously until the progenitor cell commits to a single lineage. This period of mosaic gene expression is illustrated in Figure 1. Transformation of the progenitors would result in the leukemic phenotypes we have described as *mixed lineage*. Lineage commitment could involve external factors (e.g., growth factors) that cause genes specific for the opposite lineage to be switched off. If further differentiation occurs in such cases under the selective pressure of chemotherapy, such cases may appear to be those we have described as *lineage switch*. Studies of the hypothetical pluripotent progenitor cells that have been invoked to explain these findings in acute leukemias are needed.

Little is known about the chromosomal locations of the genes coding for the various lineage-associated markers or about how their expression is controlled. However, recent studies indicate that most, if not all, leukemic cells contain chromosomal abnormalities, many involving rearrangements of DNA (80,81). Since the control of eukaryotic gene expression is known to involve numerous sequence elements, some, like enhancers, acting at a distance from the site of transcription, genetic perturbations within the cell (e.g., a reciprocal translocation) could be expected to deregulate certain genes, leading to their underexpression or overexpression (82). An example of this would be the activation of the c-*myc* proto-oncogene by the 8;14 translocation in Burkitt's lymphoma (83). Furthermore, translocations may result in abnormal proteins that directly affect cell growth (84-86). Changes in the expression of such genes could result in an almost infinite variety of cell-lineage-related phenotypes, even if the transforming event did not involve a pluripotent progenitor. This explanation of lineage infidelity, brought about by derangement of the control of gene expression, would be an alternative to the mechanism whereby mixed lineage leukemias are derived from the transformation of progenitor cells that express multiple lineage characteristics. Since both possible mechanisms may be responsible for mixed lineage leukemia or lineage switch, we have incorporated both into our proposed model of hematopoietic differentiation (Figure 1).

It is now clear that unusual combinations of myeloid and lymphoid cell lineages are much more common in acute leukemia than has been generally recognized. The traditional division of the acute leukemias into lymphocytic and nonlymphocytic may not be the most accurate way to represent this group of hematologic malignancies. That mixed lineage leukemia may require therapy directed against the secondary phenotype of the blast cells is a clinically important observation and underscores the need for comprehensive testing of blast cells at diagnosis. Similarly, improved treatment responses in patients with lineage switch whose therapy was directed to the lineage evident at relapse warrants careful reclassification of blast cells in patients with recurrent leukemia.

Future studies clarifying the regulation of lineage-associated gene expression and the mechanism of lineage commitment will be essential to understanding mixed lineage leukemia. One clue has been provided by the finding that chromosomal translocations involving 11q23 define a unique subset of patients presenting typically with acute mixed lineage leukemia.

ACKNOWLEDGMENTS

The authors would like to thank Drs. R. Goorha, F. Behm and N. Bunin for molecular and immunophenotyping studies; Drs. D. Williams and S. Raimondi for cytogenetics studies; and L. Woodruff for technical assistance. We also thank Christy Wright for editorial assistance, and Peggy Vandiveer for typing.

REFERENCES

1. Stass, S. A., and Mirro, J. (1986). Lineage heterogeneity in acute leukemia: acute mixed lineage leukemia and lineage switch. *Clin. in Haem.* 15:811-827.
2. Greaves, M. F., Chan, L. C., Furley, A. J. W., Watt, S. M., and Molgaard, H. V. (1986). Lineage promiscuity in hemopoietic differentiation and leukemia. *Blood* 67:1-11.
3. Mirro, J., Zipf, T. F., Pui, C.-H., Kitchingman, G., Williams, D., Melvin, S., Murphy, S. B., and Stass, S. (1985). Acute mixed lineage leukemia: clinicopathologic correlation and prognostic significance. *Blood* 66:1115-1123.
4. Reinherz, E. L., Kung, P. C., Goldstein, G., Levey, R. H., and Schlossman, S. F. (1980). Discrete stages of human intrathymic differentiation: Analysis of normal thymocytes and leukemic lymphoblasts of T cell lineage. *Proc. Natl. Acad. Sci. USA* 77:1588-1592.
5. Nadler, L. M., Anderson, K. C., Marti, G., Bates, M., Park, E., Daley, J. F., and Schlossman, S. F. (1983). B4, a human B lymphocyte-associated antigen expressed on normal, mitogen-activated, and malignant B lymphocytes. *J. Immunol.* 131:244-250.
6. Bernstein, I. D., Andrews, R. G., Cohen, S. F., and McMaster, B. E. (1982). Normal and malignant human myelocytic and monocytic cells identified by monoclonal antibodies. *J. Immunol.* 128:876-881.
7. Griffin, J. D., Linch, D., Sabbath, K., Larcom, P., and Schlossman, S. F. (1984). A monoclonal antibody reactive with normal and leukemic human myeloid progenitor cells. *Leukem. Res.* 8:521-534.
8. Gregg, S. L., Gajl-Peczalska, K. J., LeBien, T. W., Bloomfield, C. D., Brunning, R., and Sagawa, K. (1984). Monoclonal antibody MCS-2 as the marker of phorbol diester-induced myeloid differentiation in acute undifferentiated leukemia. *Canc. Res.* 44:2724-2730.

9. Todd, R. F. III, Griffin, J. D., Ritz, J., Nadler, L. M., Abrams, T., and Schlossman, S. F. (1981). Expression of normal monocyte-macrophage differentiation antigens in HL60 promyelocytes undergoing differentiation induced by leukocyte-conditioned medium or phorbol diester. *Leukem. Res.* 5:491-495.
10. Boggs, D. R. (1974). Hematopoietic stem cell theory in relation to possible lymphoblastic conversion of chronic myeloid leukemia (editorial). *Blood* 44:449-453.
11. Stass, S., Veach, S., Pasquale, S. M., Schumacher, H. R., and Bollum, F. J. (1978). Terminal deoxynucleotidyl transferase positive acute lymphoblastic leukemia with Auer rods. *Lancet i*:1042-1043.
12. Lanham, G. R., Bollum, F. J., Williams, D. L., and Stass, S. A. (1984). Simultaneous occurrence of terminal deoxynucleotidyl transferase and myeloperoxidase in individual leukemic blasts. *Blood* 64:318-320.
13. Stockinger, H., Majdic, O., Liszka, K., Aberer, W., Bettelheim, P., Lutz, D., and Knapp, W. (1984). Exposure by desialylation of myeloid antigens on acute lymphoblastic leukemia cells. *J. Natl. Cancer Inst.* 73:7-11.
14. Tetteroo, P. A. T., van't Veer, M. B., Tromp, J. F., and von dem Borne, A. E. G. Kr. (1984). Detection of the granulocyte-specific antigen 3-fucosyl-N-acetyl-lactosamine on leukemic cells after neuraminidase treatment. *Int. J. Cancer* 33:355-358.
15. Reinherz, E. L., Kung, P. C., Goldstein, G., and Schlossman, S. F. (1979). Separation of functional subsets of human T cells by a monoclonal antibody. *Proc. Natl. Acad. Sci. USA* 76:4061-4065.
16. Kamoun, M., Martin, P. J., Hansen, J. A., Brown, M. A., Siadak, A. W., and Nowinsky, R. C. (1981). Identification of a human T lymphocyte surface protein associated with the E-rosette receptor. *J. Experim. Med.* 153:207-212.
17. Verbi, W., Greaves, M. F., Schneider, C., Koubek, K., Janossy, G., Stein, H., Kung, P., and Goldstein, G. (1982). Monoclonal antibodies OKT-11 and OKT-11A have pan-T reactivity and block sheep erythrocyte "receptors." *Eur. J. Immunol.* 12:81-86.
18. Royston, I., Majda, J. A., Baird, S. M., Meserve, B. L., and Griffin, J. C. (1980). Human T cell antigens defined by monoclonal antibodies: the 65,000-Dalton antigen of T cells (T65) is also found on the chronic lymphocytic leukemia cells bearing surface immunoglobulin. *J. Immunol.* 125:725-731.
19. Ritz, J., Pesando, J. M., Notis-McConarty, J., Lazarus, H., and Schlossman, S. F. (1980). A monoclonal antibody to human acute lymphoblastic leukaemia antigen. *Nature* 283:583-585.
20. Civin, C. I., Mirro, J., and Banquerigo, M. L. (1981). My-1 a new myeloid-specific antigen identified by a mouse monoclonal antibody. *Blood* 57:842-845.
21. Andrews, R. G., Torok-Storb, B., and Bernstein, I. D. (1983). Myeloid-associated differentiation antigens on stem cells and their progeny identified by monoclonal antibodies. *Blood* 62:124-132.

22. Weiner, M., Borowitz, M., Boyett, J., Civin, C., Metzger, R., McKolnis, J., Crist, W., Dowell, B., Pullen, J. (1985). Clinical pathologic aspects of myeloid antigen positivity in pediatric patients with acute lymphoblastic leukemia (ALL). *Proc. Amer. Soc. Clin. Oncol.* 4:C671.
23. Sobel, R. E., Royston, I., Mick, R., Cuttner, J., Ellison, R. R., Davey, F., Nelson, D., and Bloomfield, C. D. (1986). Clinical significance of mixed lymphoid and myeloid characteristics in adult acute lymphoblastic leukemia. *Proc. Amer. Soc. Clin. Oncol.* 5:C623.
24. Mertelsmann, R., Koziner, B., Ralph, P., Filippa, D., McKenzie, S., Arlin, Z. A., Gee, T. S., Moore, M. A. S., and Clarkson, B. D. (1978). Evidence for distinct lymphocytic and monocytic populations in a patient with terminal transferase-positive acute leukemia. *Blood* 51:1051-1056.
25. Ueda, T., Kita, K., Kagawa, D., Tamori, S., Ando, S., Sasada, M., Yoshida, Y., Uchino, H., and Nakamura, T. (1984). Acute leukemia with two cell populations of lymphoblasts and monoblasts. *Leukem. Res.* 8:63-69.
26. Perentesis, J., Ramsay, N., Brunning, R., Kersey, J., and Filipowich, A. (1983). Biphenotypic leukemia: immunologic and morphologic evidence for a common lymphoid-myeloid progenitor in humans. *J. Pediatrics* 102: 63-67.
27. Paietta, E., Bettleheim, P., Schwarzmeier, J. D., Lutz, D., Majdic, O., and Knapp, W. (1983). Distinct lymphoblastic and myeloblastic populations in TdT positive acute myeloblastic leukemia: evidence by double-fluorescence staining. *Leukem. Res.* 7:301-307.
28. Neame, P. B., Soamboonsrup, P., Browman, G., Barr, R. D., Saeed, N., Chan, B., Pai, M., Benger, A., Wilson, W. E. C., Walker, I. R., and McBride, J. A. (1985). Simultaneous or sequential expression of lymphoid and myeloid phenotypes in acute leukemia. *Blood* 65:142-148.
29. Pui, C.-H., Dahl, G. V., Melvin, S., Williams, D. L., Peiper, S., Mirro, J., Murphy, S. B., and Stass, S. (1984). Acute leukemia with mixed lymphoid and myeloid phenotype. *Brit. J. Haematol.* 56:121-130.
30. Bettelheim, P., Paietta, E., Majdic, O., Gadner, H., Schwarzmeier, J., and Knapp, W. (1982). Expression of a myeloid marker on TdT-positive acute lymphocytic leukemia cells: evidence by double-fluorescence staining. *Blood* 60:1392-1396.
31. Mirro, J., Antoun, G. R., Zipf, T. F., Melvin, S., and Stass, S. (1985). The E-rosette-associated antigen of T-cells can be identified on blasts from patients with acute myeloblastic leukemia. *Blood* 65:363-367.
32. Mirro, J., Kitchingman, G., Williams, D., Lauzon, G. J., Lin, C. C., Callihan, T., and Zipf, T. (1986). Clinical and laboratory characteristics of acute leukemia with the 4;11 translocation. *Blood* 67:689-697.
33. Dow, L. W., Martin, P., Moohr, J., Greenberg, M., Macdougall, L. G., Najfeld, V., and Fialkow, P. (1985). Evidence for clonal development of childhood acute lymphoblastic leukemia. *Blood* 66:902-907.
34. Braun, M. P., Martin, P. J., Ledbetter, J. A., and Hansen, J. A. (1983). Granulocytes and cultured human fibroblasts express common acute lymphoblastic leukemia-associated antigens. *Blood* 61:718-725.

35. Metzgar, R. S., Borowitz, M. J., Jones, N. H., and Dowell, B. L. (1981). Distribution of common acute lymphoblastic leukemia in nonhematopoietic tissues. *J. Exper. Med.* 154:1249-1254.
36. Mills, K. H. G., and Cawley, J. C. (1985). Stimulated lymphoid cells of B lineage, but not plasma or myeloid cells, can express E receptor. *Leukem. Res.* 9:375-380.
37. Girardet, C., Ladisch, S., Heumann, D., Mach, J.-P., and Carrel, S. (1983). Identification by a monoclonal antibody of a glycolipid highly expressed by cells from the human myeloid lineage. *Int. J. Cancer* 32:177-183.
38. Huang, L. C., Civin, C. I., Magnani, J. L., Shaper, J. H., and Ginsberg, V. (1983). My-1, the human myeloid-specific antigen detected by mouse monoclonal antibodies, is a sugar sequence found in lacto-N-fucopentaose III. *Blood* 61:1020-1023.
39. Fialkow, P. J., Singer, J. W., Adamson, J. W., Vaidya, K., Dow, L. W., Ochs, J., and Moohr, J. W. (1981). Acute nonlymphocytic leukemia: heterogeneity of stem cell origin. *Blood* 57:1068-1973.
40. Smith, L. J., Curtis, J. E., Messner, H. A., Senn, J. S., Furthmayr, H., and McCulloch, E. A. (1983). Lineage infidelity in acute leukemia. *Blood* 61: 1138-1145.
41. Stass, S., and Mirro, J. (1985). Unexpected heterogeneity in acute leukemia: mixed lineages and lineage switch. *Human Pathol.* 16:864-866.
42. Wood, G. S., Warner, N., and Warnke, R. (1983). Anti-Leu-3/T4 antibodies react with cells of monocyte-macrophage and Langerhans lineage. *J. Immunol.* 131:212-216.
43. Early, P., Huang, H., Davis, M., Calame, K., and Hood, L. (1980). An immunoglobulin heavy chain variable region is generated from three segments of DNA: V_H, D and J_H. *Cell* 19:981-992.
44. Ravetch, J. V., Siebenlist, U., Korsmeyer, S., Waldmann, T., and Leder, P. (1981). Structure of the human immunoglobulin μ locus: characteristics of embryonic and rearranged J and D genes. *Cell* 27:583-591.
45. Kurosawa, Y., Boehner, V. H., Haas, W., and Sakano, A. (1981). Identification of D segments of immunoglobulin heavy chain genes and their rearrangement in T lymphocytes. *Nature (London)* 290:565-570.
46. Cory, S., Adams, J. M., and Kemp, D. J. (1980). Somatic rearrangements forming active immunoglobulin genes in B and T lymphoid cell lines. *Proc. Natl. Acad. Sci. USA* 77:4943-4947.
47. Tonegawa, S. (1983). Somatic generation of antibody diversity. *Nature* 302: 575-581.
48. Toyonaga, B., Yanagi, Y., Suciu-Foca, N., Minden, M., and Mak, T. W. (1984). Rearrangements of T-cell receptor gene YT35 in human DNA from thymic leukaemia, T-cell lines and functional T-cell clones. *Nature* 311:385-387.
49. Yanagi, Y., Yoshikai, Y., Leggett, K., Clark, S. P., Aleksander, I., and Mak, T. W. (1984). A human T cell-specific cDNA clone encodes a protein having extensive homology to immunoglobulin chains. *Nature* 308:145-149.

50. Kemp, D. J., Harris, A. W., Cory, S., and Adams, J. M. (1980). Expression of the immunoglobulin Cμ gene in mouse T and B lymphoid and myeloid cell lines. *Proc. Natl. Acad. Sci. USA* 77:2876-2810.
51. Kurosawa, T., von Boehmer, H., Haas, W., Sakano, H., Travneker, A., and Tonegawa, S. (1981). Identification of D segments of immunoglobulin heavy-chain genes and their rearrangement in T lymphocytes. *Nature* 290: 565-570.
52. Zuniga, M. C., D'Eustachio, P., and Ruddle, N. H. (1982). Immunoglobulin heavy chain gene rearrangement and transcription in murine T cell hybrids and T lymphomas. *Proc. Natl. Acad. Sci. USA* 79:3015-3019.
53. Korsmeyer, S. J., Arnold, A., Bakhshi, A., Ravetch, J. V., Siebenlist, U., Hieter, P. A., Sharrow, S. O., LeBien, T. W., Kersey, J. H., Poplack, D. G., Leder, P., and Waldmann, T. A. (1983). Immunoglobulin gene rearrangement and cell surface antigen expression in acute lymphocytic leukemias of T-cell and B-cell precursor origins. *J. Clin. Invest.* 71:301-313.
54. Korsmeyer, S. J., Hieter, P. A., Ravetch, J. V., Poplack, D. G., Waldmann, T. A., and Leder, P. (1981). Developmental hierarchy of immunoglobulin gene rearrangements in human leukemic pre-B cells. *Proc. Natl. Acad. Sci. USA* 78:7096-7100.
55. Ford, A. M., Molgaard, H. V., Greaves, M. F., and Gould, H. J. (1983). Immunoglobulin gene organisation and expression in haemopoetic stem cell leukaemia. *EMBO J.* 2:997-1001.
56. Rovigatti, U., Mirro, J., Kitchingman, G., Dahl, G., Ochs, J., Murphy, S. B., and Stass, S. (1984). Heavy chain immunoglobulin gene rearrangement in acute nonlymphocytic leukemia. *Blood* 63:1023-1027.
57. Palumbo, A., Minowada, J., Erikson, J., Croce, C. M., and Rovera, G. (1984). Lineage infidelity of a human myelogenous leukemia cell line. *Blood* 64: 1059-1063.
58. Forster, A., Hobart, M., Hengartner, H., and Rabbitts, T. H. (1980). An immunoglobulin heavy-chain gene is altered in two T-cell clones. *Nature* 286: 897-899.
59. Arnold, A., Cossman, J., Bakhshi, A., Jaffe, E. S., Waldmann, T. A., and Korsmeyer, S. J. (1983). Immunoglobulin gene rearrangements as unique clonal markers in human lymphoid neoplasms. *New Eng. J. Med.* 309:1593-1599.
60. Ha, K., Minden, M., Hozumi, N., and Gelfand, E. W. (1984). Immunoglobulin gene rearrangement in acute myelogenous leukemia. *Cancer Res.* 44: 4658-4660.
61. Kitchingman, G. R., Rovigatti, U., Mauer, A. M., Melvin, S., Murphy, S. B., and Stass, S. (1985). Rearrangement of immunoglobulin heavy chain genes in T cell acute lymphoblastic leukemia. *Blood* 65:725-729.
62. Ha, K., Minden, M., Hozumi, N., and Gelfand, E. W. (1984). Immunoglobulin μ-chain gene rearrangement in a patient with T cell acute lymphoblastic leukemia. *J. Clin. Invest.* 73:1232-1236.

63. Pelicci, P.-G., Knowles, D. M., II, and Favera, R. D. F. (1985). Lymphoid tumors displaying rearrangements of both immunoglobulin and T cell receptor genes. *J. Exper. Med.* 162:1015-1024.
64. Minden, M., Toyonaga, B., Ha, K., Yanagi, Y., Chin, B., Gelfand, E., and Mak, T. (1985). Somatic rearrangements of T-cell antigen receptor gene in human T-cell malignancies. *Proc. Natl. Acad. Sci. USA* 82:1224-1227.
65. Acuto, O., Hussey, R. E., Fitzgerald, K. A., Protentis, J. P., Meuer, S. C., Schlossman, S. F., and Reinherz, E. L. (1983). The human T cell receptor: appearance in ontogeny and biochemical relationship of α and β subunits on IL-2 dependent clones and T cell tumors. *Cell* 34:717-726.
66. Tawa, A., Hozumi, N., Minden, M., Mak, T., and Gelfand, E. (1985). Rearrangement of T-cell receptor β-chain gene in non-T-cell, non-B-cell acute lymphoblastic leukemia of childhood. *New Eng. J. Med.* 313:1033-1037.
67. O'Connor, N. T. J., Weatherall, D. J., Feller, A. C., Jones, D., Pallesen, G., Stein, H., Wainscoat, J. S., Gatter, K. C., Isaacson, P., Lennert, K., Ramsey, A., Wright, D. H., and Mason, D. Y. (1985). Rearrangement of the T-cell-receptor β-chain gene in the diagnosis of lymphoproliferative disorders. *Lancet* 1:1295-1297.
68. Kitchingman, G. R., Mirro, J., Stass, S., Rovigatti, U., Melvin, S. L., Williams, D. L., Raimondi, S. C., and Murphy, S. B. (1986). Biologic and prognostic significance of the presence of more than two μ heavy-chain genes in childhood acute lymphoblastic leukemia of B-precursor cell origin. *Blood* 67:698-702.
69. Alt, F., Rosenberg, N., Lewis, S., Thomas, E., and Baltimore, D. (1981). Organization and reorganization of immunoglobulin genes in A-MuLV-transformed cells: rearrangement of heavy but not light-chain genes. *Cell* 27:381-390.
70. Whitlock, C. A., Ziegler, S. F., Treiman, L. J., Stafford, J. I., and Witte, O. N. (1983). Differentiation of cloned populations of immature B cells after transformation with Abelson murine leukemia virus. *Cell* 32:903-911.
71. Ben-Bassat, I., and Gale, R. P. (1984). Hybrid acute leukemia (editorial). *Leukem. Res.* 8:929-936.
72. Arthur, D. C., Bloomfield, C. D., Lindquist, L. L., and Nesbit, M. E. (1982). Translocation 4;11 in acute lymphoblastic leukemia: clinical characteristics and prognostic significance. *Blood* 59:96-99.
73. Crist, W. M., Cleary, M. L., Grossi, C. E., Prasthofer, E. F., Heggie, G. D., Omura, G. A., Carroll, A. J., Link, M. P., and Sklar, J. (1985). Acute leukemias associated with the 4;11 chromosome translocation have rearranged immunoglobulin heavy chain genes. *Blood* 66:33-38.
74. Nagasaka, M., Maeda, S., Maeda, H., Chen, H.-L., Kita, K., Mabuchi, O., Misu, H., Matsuo, T., and Sugiyama, T. (1983). Four cases of t(4;11) acute leukemia and its myelomonocytic nature in infants. *Blood* 61:1174-1181.
75. Kaneko, Y., Maseki, N., Takasaki, N., Sakurai, M., Hayashi, Y., Nakazawa, S., Mori, T., Sakurai, M., Takeda, T., Shikano, T., and Hiyoshi, Y. (1986). Clinical and hematologic characteristics in acute leukemia with 11q23 translocations. *Blood* 67:484-491.

76. de Taisne, C., Gegonne, A., Stehelin, D., Bernheim, A., and Berger, R. (1984). Chromosomal localization of the human proto-oncogene c-*ets*. *Nature* 310: 581-583.
77. Hershfield, M. S., Kurtzberg, J., Harden, E., Moore, J. O., Whang-Peng, J., and Haynes, B. F. (1984). Conversion of a stem cell leukemia from a T-lymphoid to a myeloid phenotype induced by adenosine deaminase inhibitor 2'-deoxycoformycin. *Proc. Natl. Acad. Sci. USA* 81:253-257.
78. Murphy, S. B., Stass, S. A., Kalwinsky, D., and Rivera, G. (1983). Phenotypic conversion of acute leukemia from T-lymphoblastic to myeloblastic induced by therapy with 2'-deoxycoformycin. *Brit. J. Haematol.* 55:285-293.
79. Stass, S., Mirro, J., Melvin, S., Pui, C.-H., Murphy, S. B., and Williams, D. (1984). Lineage switch in acute leukemia. *Blood* 64:701-706.
80. Yunis, J. J., Bloomfield, C. D., and Ensurd, K. (1981). All patients with acute nonlymphocytic leukemia may have a chromosomal defect. *New Eng. J. Med.* 305:135-139.
81. Williams, D. L., Raimondi, S., Rivera, G., George, S., Berard, C. W., and Murphy, S. B. (1985). Presence of clonal chromosome abnormalities in virtually all cases of acute lymphoblastic leukemia. *New Eng. J. Med.* 313:640-641.
82. Dynan, W. S., and Tjian, R. (1985). Control of eukaryotic messenger RNA synthesis by sequence-specific DNA-binding proteins. *Nature* 316:774-778.
83. Dalla-Favera, R., Martinotti, S., Gallo, R. C., Erikson, J., and Croce, C. M. (1983). Translocation and rearrangements of the c-*myc* oncogene locus in human undifferentiated B cell lymphomas. *Science* 219:963-967.
84. Konopka, J. B., Watanabe, S. M. Singer, J. W., Collins, S. J., and Witte, O. N. (1985). Cell lines and clinical isolates derived from Ph-positive chronic myelogenous leukemia patients express c-*abl* proteins with a common structural alteration. *Proc. Natl. Acad. Sci. USA* 82:1810-1814.
85. Stam, K., Heisterkamp, N., Grosveld, G., de Klein, A., Verma, R., Coleman, M., Dosik, H., and Groffen, J. (1985). Evidence of a new chimeric *bcr*/c-*abl* mRNA in patients with chronic myelocytic leukemia and the Philadelphia chromosome. *New Eng. J. Med.* 313:1429-1432.
86. Shitrelman, E., Lifshitz, B., Gale, R. P., and Canaani, E. (1985). Fused transcript of *abl* and *bcr* genes in chronic myelogenous leukemia. *Nature* 315: 550-554.
87. Chessells, J. M., Janossy, G., Lawler, S. D., and Secker-Walker, L. M. (1979). The Ph chromosome in childhood leukaemia. *Brit. J. Haematol.* 41:25-41.
88. Smith, L. J., and McCulloch, E. A. (1984). Lineage infidelity following exposure of T lymphoblasts (MOLT-3 cells) to 5-azacytidine. *Blood* 63:1324-1330.
89. Terrin, B. N., Studer, E. J., Wood, N., Mohanakumar, T., and Russell, E. C. (1985). Childhood leukemia with simultaneously expressed myeloid and lymphoid markers suggesting stem cell origin. *Amer. J. Hematol.* 20:175-181.

90. Paietta, E., Dutcher, J. P., and Wiernik, P. H. (1985). Terminal transferase positive acute promyelocytic leukemia: In vitro differentiation of a T-lymphocytic/promyelocytic hybrid phenotype. *Blood* 65:107-114.
91. Strong, R. C., Korsmeyer, S. J., Parkin, J. L., Arthur, D. C., and Kersey, J. H. (1985). Human acute leukemia cell line with the t(4;11) chromosomal rearrangement exhibits B-lineage and monocytic characteristics. *Blood* 65: 21-31.
92. Parkin, J. L., Arthur, D. C., Abramson, C. S., McKenna, R. W., Kersey, J. H., Heideman, R. L., and Brunning, R. D. (1982). Acute leukemia associated with the t(4;11) chromosome rearrangement: ultrastructural and immunologic characteristics. *Blood* 60:1321-1331.

13

Leukemic Cell Characterization
Clinical and Therapeutic Implications in Childhood Acute Leukemia

GARY V. DAHL* *St. Jude Children's Research Hospital, Memphis, Tennessee*

DAVID K. KALWINSKY *St. Jude Children's Research Hospital and University of Tennessee College of Medicine, Memphis, Tennessee*

I. INTRODUCTION

With improved diagnostic methods, better understanding of hematopoietic cell biology, and advances in supportive care and therapeutics, the childhood acute leukemias are now recognized as biologically heterogeneous diseases that can be cured in a substantial proportion of patients. An increasing number of clinical and biologic features have been shown to have prognostic importance in the acute leukemias (George et al., 1974; Miller, 1975; Greaves et al., 1981; Kalwinsky et al., 1985); however, the efficacy of therapy remains the most important factor influencing outcome, and the significance of a given leukemic cell characterization must a priori be assessed in the context of the therapy given. Current intensive therapy will undoubtedly change the prognostic strength of most clinical and biologic variables.

II. ACUTE LYMPHOCYTIC LEUKEMIA (ALL)

In most current treatment protocols, patients are stratified to receive "standard" or more intensive chemotherapy based on their initial presenting risk features. Although various risk categories have been used to determine the intensity of the treatment used, leukocyte count, age, and race are almost invariably included. With advances in technology, biologic cell characteristics have been related closely to treatment outcome and have been increasingly used to determine treatment assignment. At the present time leukemia cell genetic features are emerging as a

**Current affiliation*: University of California–Davis Medical Center, Sacramento, California key prognostic factor in childhood ALL (Look, 1985; Bloomfield et al., 1986; Williams et al., 1986).

More than 60% of children with average-risk ALL are expected to be long-term survivors after modern therapy (Lampert et al., 1984; Sallan et al., 1981), while only 20% of those with very high-risk leukemia are likely to be cured with most treatment programs (Aur et al., 1978; Camitta et al., 1980). In a recent clinical trial at St. Jude Children's Research Hospital (Memphis, Tennessee), the addition of a teniposide-cytarabine combination to an otherwise standard treatment regimen resulted in over 50% long-term disease-free survival for patients with very high-risk leukemia. As expected, the improved result abolished the prognostic impact of most clinical and biological features. Similar results have been reported by others utilizing intensive chemotherapeutic programs (Lampert et al., 1984; Dahl et al., 1986; Steinberg et al., 1986).

Since 1979, we have prospectively studied leukemia cell characteristics in a large group of newly diagnosed patients. The biological characteristics and their correlation with treatment responses from our study at St. Jude Children's Research Hospital are discussed below.

A. Morphology

Acute lymphoblastic leukemia can be classified morphologically into three subtypes: L1, L2 and L3, as defined by criteria of the French-American-British (FAB) cooperative group (Bennett et al., 1976). In children, the small homogeneous L1 lymphoblast with scant cytoplasm and inconspicuous nucleoli predominates in more than three-fourths of all cases (Wagner and Baehner, 1979; Miller et al., 1983; Hann et al., 1979; van Eys et al., 1986). The L2 blast, larger than the L1 lymphoblast with variable nuclear heterogeneity, prominent nucleoli and abundant cytoplasm, is more frequently reported in adult ALL (Brearley et al., 1979). The L3 or Burkitt's leukemia cell is found in less than 5% of both childhood or adult ALL cases and appears by surface marker typing and cytogenetics to be diagnostic of B-cell leukemias and lymphomas. The L3 cells demonstrate both surface immunoglobulin positivity and 8;14 translocations (Hann et al., 1979; Bennett et al., 1981; Coccia, Miller, and Kersey, 1980; Berger and Bernheim, 1982).

Of 435 children with ALL consecutively admitted to St. Jude Children's Hospital, 366 (84%) had FAB L1 blast cell morphology; 56 (13%) L2; and 13 (3%), L3. Early reports linked L1 morphology with improved duration of complete remission and survival (Wagner and Baehner, 1979; Hann et al., 1979; Keleti, Révéz and Schuler, 1978; Miller et al., 1980). Some centers have established complicated scoring systems based on FAB subgroups, total white blood cell count, and cytochemical periodic acid-Schiff (PAS) reactivity to predict treatment outcome (Palmer et al., 1980). Difficulties in applying the FAB system became apparent, however, because some patients have mixtures of L1 and L2 blasts (Vecchi et al., 1980; Miller et al., 1981). Also, individual hematologists differ by 30% in their assignments of morphologic subtypes (Viana, Maurer, and Ferenc, 1980). A revised semiquantitative scoring system for the FAB has recently been published and should improve reproducibility of this morphologic classification system (Bennett et al., 1981).

L2 morphology appears to represent a poor prognostic feature in ALL (Miller et al., 1983; Hann et al., 1979; Miller et al., 1981; Viana, Maurer, and Ferenc, 1980), and several clinical trials have incorporated this feature into risk assignment (Coccia et al., 1983). At St. Jude Hospital, L2 morphology is associated with poorer outcome when considered as an individual variable (see Table 1) and appears independent of clinical features such as initial white blood cell count, age, and race of patients (see Table 2) (Kalwinsky et al., 1985).

The L3 morphologic type, synonymous with B-cell ALL, denotes a biologically distinctive subtype of ALL noted for its high proliferative growth potential, metabolic complications, and extramedullary involvement. This group of disorders has an extremely poor response to conventional leukemia therapies. More aggressive therapy with high-dose methotrexate, cytosine arabinoside (ara-C) and alkalating agents might improve the current dismal outlook for FAB L3 ALL (Murphy et al., 1985).

B. Cytochemistry

Despite the large number of publications on cytochemical studies, special stains have offered little advantage over Romanowsky-stained smears for morphologic diagnosis of ALL (Flandrin and Daniel, 1973).

The periodic acid-Schiff (PAS) reaction is an insensitive marker for ALL, with up to 43% of cases being essentially negative. At our center, PAS staining was positive in 276 of 402 cases, yet positivity lacked any prognostic impact in predicting induction response on overall treatment outcome (Table 1). While a number of authors report a better prognosis for patients with strongly positive PAS blasts (Laurie, 1968; Feldges et al., 1974; Vowels and Willoughby, 1973), others (Shaw et al., 1977; Humphrey, Nesbit, and Brunning, 1974) failed to demonstrate a relationship of PAS reactivity to outcome. Some authors suggest that the importance of PAS positivity might be secondary to a more significant feature such as T-cell immunophenotype or level of white blood cell count (Catovsky et al., 1974). We have recently reviewed 250 consecutive cases of childhood ALL to determine if a more quantitative scoring system for PAS (score of 0-400) would be useful in predicting patient response, but again found this lacking in independent prognostic significance (Lanham et al., 1985).

The DNA polymerase enzyme terminal deoxynucleotidyl transferase (TdT) is positive in virtually all cases of childhood ALL (Coleman et al., 1976; Janossy et al., 1980a). TdT, however, is also present in the blasts of a small subset of patients with ANLL and acute mixed lineage leukemias (Gordon et al., 1978; Srivastava et

Table 1 Univariate Assessment of Clinical and Biologic Features in Relationship to Time to Failure

	Category (No. of patients)			
Variable[a]	Better	Worse	P value[b]	Estimated ratio of hazard function[c]
WBC ($\times 10^9$/L)	<50 (325)	≥50 (102)	0.0002	1.84
Age (yr)	2-10 (300)	Other (127)	0.0001	2.05
Race	White (380)	Other (47)	0.0014	1.85
CNS leukemia	No (388)	Yes (37)	0.0098	1.87
Sex	Female (120)	Male (257)	0.057	1.34
Morphology	L1 (366)	L2 (56)	0.0008	1.95
Ploidy	Nonpseudo (329)	Pseudo (91)	0.004	1.67
DNA index	≥1.16 (77)	<1.16 (276)	0.0001	3.42
Translocations	No (191)	Yes (52)	0.0003	2.25
PAS reactivity	POS (276)	NEG (126)	0.2817	1.19
Glucocorticoid receptors	≤16 $\times 10^3$/cell (103)	>16 $\times 10^3$/cell (145)	0.9730	1.01
Immunophenotype	Common ALL (294)	T, undiff. (85)	0.008	1.53

[a]Biological variables could not be determined for all patients. Analyses were based on patient subsets for which relevant variables were known.
[b]From likelihood ratio test, which estimates whether or not the proportional hazards model including a given variable provides a better fit to the data than one without the variable.
[c]Ratio of hazard function estimates the proportional increase in risk of failure for a patient having a "worse" value of a given variable compared to a patient with a "better" value.

Table 2 Contribution of Selected Biological Variables to a Clinical Multivariate Model Predictive of Time to Failure

Multivariate model[a]	Category (No. of Patients)		P value[b]	Estimated ratio of hazard function[c]
	Better	Worse		
(A) Morphology	L1 (366)	L2 (56)	0.0194	1.59
Ploidy	Nonpseudo (329)	Pseudo (91)	0.0986	1.35
DNA index (DI)	⩾1.16 (77)	<1.16 (276)	0.0001	3.03
Translocations	No (191)	Yes (52)	0.0037	1.94
Immunophenotype	Common ALL (294)	T, undiff. (85)	0.274	1.23
(B) Ploidy/translocation	Nonpseudo (168)	Pseudo (75)	0.5901	0.8758
Morphology/translocation	L1 (203)	L2 (39)	0.0122	1.84
Translocation/morphology	No (190)	Yes (52)	0.0027	1.99
DI/translocation	⩾1.16 (28)	<1.16 (187)	0.0179	2.87
Translocation/DI	No (165)	Yes (50)	0.0258	1.68
DI/morphology	⩾1.16 (76)	<1.16 (275)	0.0001	3.07
Morphology/DI	L1 (300)	L2 (51)	0.0091	1.72
(C) DI/translocation + morphology	⩾1.16 (28)	>1.16 (186)	0.0087	2.87
Translocation/DI + morphology	No (164)	Yes (50)	0.0188	1.74
Morphology/DI + translocation	L1 (178)	L2 (36)	0.0257	1.76

[a]Multivariate models based on variables of WBC, age and race. (A) tests the addition of a single biological variable to the predictive power of this model. (B) evaluates the information gained by adding ploidy to a model containing these clinical variables as well as translocations (ploidy/translocations), morphology to a clinical model plus translocations (morphology/translocations), etc., testing the addition of a single biological feature to the clinical model containing an added biologic parameter. (C) evaluates the impact of DI, translocations or morphology added to the basic clinical model which contained the other two biologic variables.

[b]From likelihood ratio test, which estimates whether or not the proportional hazards model including a given variable provides a better fit to the data than one without the variable.

[c]Ratio of hazard function estimates the proportional increase in risk of failure for a patient having a "worse" value of a given variable compared to a patient with a "better" value. For example, without adjusting for any other feature, a patient with translocations is 1.94 times as likely to fail at any given point than a nontranslocation patient.

al., 1976; Lanham et al., 1984; Kalwinsky et al., 1981) and cannot be considered specific for lymphoid malignancy. In our studies, this enzyme, when used as a cytochemical stain or measured quantitatively, did not distinguish immunologic subtypes of ALL (Kalwinsky et al., 1981). As a cytochemical stain, TdT is a useful adjuvant for the diagnosis of ALL in extramedullary sites (CSF and testes) (Bradstock et al., 1980), although the presence of small numbers of TdT-positive cells in regenerating marrows as well as in the stem cell compartment limits its utility as a cytochemical stain for minimal residual leukemia (Janossy et al., 1980a). It cannot reliably be utilized to monitor patients for early relapse in ALL (Winick, Steinherz, and Miller, 1985).

Acid phosphatase is an additional cytochemical stain frequently noted for positivity, particularly in T-cell ALL. In our laboratory, the majority of blasts in children with both ALL or ANLL are positive for acid phosphatase. A focal perinuclear Golgi-localized acid phosphatase stain pattern (Catovsky et al., 1974; Catovsky, 1975), which is closely associated with T-cell ALL, has been described, but this finding has also been made in occasional cases of common ALL, thereby lessening its utility as a predictor of immunophenotype (Chessells et al., 1977). By itself, acid phosphatase staining cannot replace accurate surface immunophenotype determinations.

Rare cases with Sudan-black-B-positive ALL have been described in children (Stass et al., 1984) and adults (Tricot et al., 1982). While these cases readily respond to lymphoid directed therapy, the overall prognostic significance of this subset of ALL is yet to be determined.

C. Immunophenotype

B-cell ALL is identified by the presence of surface immunoglobulin and L3 FAB morphology. It is an extremely rare phenotype in ALL, accounting for approximately 2-3% of all childhood cases. This is a disseminated phase of Burkitt's lymphoma in which the marrow is essentially replaced with L3 lymphoblasts that are characterized by unique chromosomal translocations, t(8;14), t(2;8), and t(8;22). One of these three translocations is usually found in the blast cells from patients with B-cell ALL. Important clinical features include massive extramedullary lymphoma in the abdomen or head and neck, CNS involvement manifested by cranial nerve palsies, hyperuricemia, and the highest blast cell proliferative rate among the acute leukemias (Magrath and Ziegler, 1979).

In B-cell ALL, the blood counts at diagnosis are consistent with an extramedullary origin for this disease. In eight children with B-cell ALL seen at our institution over a 4-year period, the median hemoglobin level was 10.0 g/dL, median platelet count was 108×10^9/L, median white blood cell count was 15.6×10^9/L (range, 8.0 to 39.1) and the percentage of circulating blasts was 18% (range, 0-25%). The medium lactate dehydrogenase (LDH) in these children was 1568 IU/L (normal values, 30 to 300 IU/L), consistent with a massive tumor burden.

Lumbar puncture performed at the time of diagnosis revealed that five of the eight children had cells in their spinal fluid at diagnosis.

Therapy for B-cell ALL based on conventional ALL regimens yield uniformly poor results. B-cell ALL is now most often treated with very aggressive chemotherapy including cyclophosphamide, methotrexate, vincristine, doxorubicin, and cytarabine. Treatment is usually of short duration, 5 to 12 months. Although remission is usually readily achieved, most children eventually relapse, especially those with CNS disease present at the time of diagnosis. Only one of seven B-cell ALL patients who achieved complete remission at our institution is a long-term disease-free survivor (Murphy et al., 1986). Recent results from the Germany Berlin-Frankfurt-Munster (BFM) 81/83 trial are particularly encouraging and indicate that a substantial number of children with B-cell ALL will remain disease-free over 2 years from diagnosis (Müller-Weihrich et al., 1985). At the present time the two factors predicting a poor outcome for B-cell ALL patients are the presence of CNS involvement at diagnosis and an initial serum LDH greater than 1000 IU/L, a measure of extensive tumor burden (Murphy et al., 1986).

Common ALL is identified by the presence of the common acute lymphoblastic leukemia (CALLA) and HLA-DR antigens on the surface of lymphoblasts. CALLA is present on the blasts of most children (~80%) with ALL and has been associated with a favorable prognosis. Rearranged immunoglobulin genes are consistently identified in common ALL blasts, demonstrating that these cells are of B-cell lineage. The presence or absence of cytoplasmic immunoglobulin has been used to subclassify non-B, non-T ALL into pre-B (15%) and early pre-B (85%) (Pullen et al., 1984).

Children with common ALL generally do well with standard chemotherapy; however, if the tumor burden is large as indicated by a high initial leukocyte count $>25 \times 10^9$/L or an LDH greater than 1000 IU/L (Pui et al., 1985), their prognosis is worse. When quantitative expression of the CALLA antigen was studied at our institution, it was found that the mean amounts of CALLA for each patient ranged widely from very high to marginally detectable. By statistical analysis, patients with relative amounts of CALLA less than the median for the entire CALLA-positive group had a greater failure rate and shorter remissions (Look et al., 1984).

The presence of cytoplasmic heavy-chain immunoglobulin (CIg) identifies pre-B ALL (Vogler et al., 1978). These cells are either CALLA$^+$ or CALLA$^-$. At our institution, 24% of newly diagnosed cases were found to have the pre-B immunophenotype, with the majority (92%) expressing CALLA. When compared with CALLA$^+$, CIg$^-$ ALL blasts, pre-B cells were more likely to have a DNA index of less than 1.16, pseudodiploid karyotype, and chromosomal translocations. Patients with pre-B ALL were also more likely to have an elevated serum LDH. These features are known to be associated with a poor treatment outcome (Pui et al., 1986b).

Although there is no specific karyotype characteristic of common ALL, approximately one-third of the patients with pre-B ALL have recently been noted to have a nonrandom cytogenetic abnormality, the t(1;19)(q23;p13,3) (Williams et al., 1984; Carroll et al., 1984). In general, children with chromosomal translocations do worse than those without a translocation. As a group, the pre-B patients have shorter remissions than do those with common ALL who lack CIg. The poor outcome for pre-B cases has been substantiated by the Pediatric Oncology Group with large numbers of cases (Crist et al., 1984). The treatment outcome for pre-B cases may be in part explained by the frequent association of known adverse chromosomal abnormalities and high serum LDH levels in these patients (Pui et al., 1986).

T-cell ALL is identified by the presence of blasts reactive with a pan-T antibody and the absence of HLA-DR antigen. Approximately one-half of the cases will demonstrate heat-stable E-rosettes. The overall incidence of this phenotype in children is 15%. Clinically, T-cell ALL is characterized by male sex predominance, older age at diagnosis, high initial leukocyte count and mediastinal mass in about one-half of the patients (Crist et al., 1985; Bowman et al., 1981). The T lymphoblasts can be categorized according to stages of differentiation into early, intermediate, or mature thymocyte subtypes, with about one-third of the T-cell patients falling into each category (Borowitz et al., 1985). The potential clinical relevance of this subset designation has not yet been demonstrated. Investigators have identified the T-cell receptor and are trying to understand the sequence of its development and how T-cell differentiation is regulated (Reinherz et al., 1984). T lymphoblasts that contain cytoplasmic T3 antigen but not surface T3 may represent a "pre-T" stage of thymocyte development. Whether or not this "pre-T" stage is of any prognostic importance awaits correlation with clinical studies.

Standard treatment used for children with common ALL is ineffective for the majority of patients with T-cell ALL, resulting in very poor survival (Sen and Borella, 1975; Pullen et al., 1981). Recent studies suggest that the prognosis of patients with T-ALL may be improving in that over 50% of patients sustained complete remission after aggressive multidrug treatment (Steinberg et al., 1986; Riehm, Fieckert, and Lampert, 1986; Dahl et al., 1986). The more intensive schedules utilizing drugs such as teniposide, ara-C, cyclophosphamide, L-asparaginase, and anthracyclines appear to increase the proportion of successfully treated T-cell patients regardless of other clinical features.

Undifferentiated ALL is identified by the absence of CALLA and the presence of the HLA-DR antigens. Approximately 7% of childhood cases with leukemia of lymphoid morphology demonstrate this phenotype. With the identification of new lineage-associated markers, some cases were found to be of myeloid origin (Kita et al., 1985) and some, to have cytoplasmic immunoglobulins (Pui et al., 1986; Crist et al., 1984), indicative of pre-B ALL. At St. Jude Hospital, most of the cases tested have demonstrated immunoglobulin gene rearrangement and expression of the B4 antigen, indicating that undifferentiated ALL is of B-cell origin.

When compared to $CALLA^+$ ALL, patients having undifferentiated phenotype are more likely: to be children less than 2 years of age; to have higher initial leukocyte counts; and to have blast cells with a DNA index of less than 1.16, a pseudodiploid karyotype, and a chromosomal translocation (Pui et al., 1986). These patients with an undifferentiated phenotype appeared to have lower remission rates and shorter event-free survival than did those with common ALL.

The increased frequency of pseudodiploid karyotypes and chromosomal translocations in undifferentiated ALL may explain the lack of long-term response to chemotherapy for this immunophenotype. Recently, chromosomal derangements involving the distal long arm of chromosome 11 (band q23) were associated with undifferentiated ALL (Nagasaka et al., 1983). Moreover, the c-ets-1 oncogene has been mapped to this chromosomal region (Diaz et al., 1986) and may contribute to the malignant transformation or cell proliferation in these cases.

D. Cytogenetics

Genetic alteration in leukemia cells appears to be associated with the process of malignant transformation. By identifying the karyotypic features most closely related to prognosis in ALL, it has been possible to redefine criteria for assignment of patients to "poor risk" or "favorable risk" therapy groups. These abnormalities are generally defined as changes in either chromosome number (ploidy) or chromosome structure (deletions, translocations, etc.). Banded chromosomes from 330 newly diagnosed patients with ALL were studied at The Third International Workshop on Chromosomes in Leukemia in 1980 (Third International Workshop, 1983). Clonal chromosomal abnormalities were identified in 218 (66%) patients. Based on groupings of specific abnormalities and modal number, relationships were found with various presenting features such as age, leukocyte count, FAB types, and immunologic phenotypes, and with respect to frequency and duration of complete remission and survival. Most interestingly, karyotype pattern was found to be an independent prognostic factor for survival when age, initial leukocyte count and FAB type were considered. Recently, these results were updated, and the analysis shows that karyotype remains an independent prognostic factor for duration of first remissions as well as for survival (Bloomfield et al., 1986).

Leukemia cell ploidy is the enumeration of the modal number of chromosomes in metaphase preparations. The distribution of chromosome numbers is bimodal, with the first peak occurring at 46 chromosomes (representing mainly patients with pseudodiploid karyotype) and the second at 55 chromosomes (Fig. 1). An abnormal clone is indicated if the same cytogenetic abnormalities are present in at least two pseudodiploid, two hyperdiploid, or three hypodiploid cells. Flow cytometry (FCM) has been used as an alternative method to detect hyperdiploid, diploid, near haploid and multiple leukemic stem lines (Look et al., 1985). A DNA index (DI) is used to identify the relationship of leukemic to normal cell DNA content. For normal diploid cells the DI is equal to 1.0. The DI can be used to

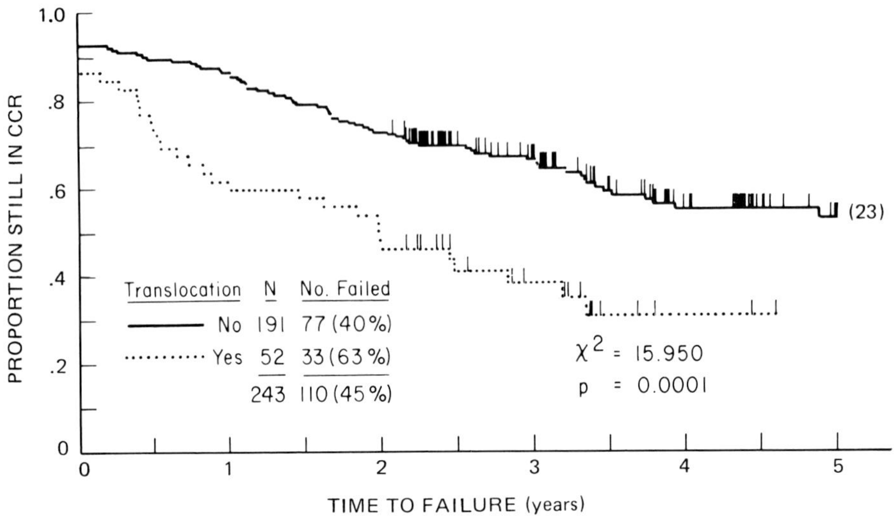

Figure 1 Completely banded karyotypes were obtained in 243 children with non-B ALL. This Kaplan-Meier curve depicts the difference in time to failure for those with and without chromosomal translocations. Remission induction rates differ as indicated by the starting point at time zero. A remission marrow must have no identifiable blasts to achieve M-1 status.

characterize leukemic cell populations at diagnosis from freshly obtained marrow samples. There is excellent correlation between cytogenetic determinations of ploidy and FCM DNA measurements (Look et al., 1982). In large populations of children with ALL, treatment outcome is correlated with DI values. About 30% of children have DNA indexes ≥1.16 (or ≥53 chromosomes) and are likely to be cured (Table 1). This ploidy group appears to be a subset of children with common ALL. A DI ≥1.16 is most frequently seen in early pre-B (common) ALL. With two favorable prognostic features, a hyperdiploid DI ≥1.16 and presenting leukocyte count ≤25,000, one can identify a group of children with ALL who have the lowest probability of relapse when treated with current therapy. Pseudodiploid cases with 46 chromosomes and structural abnormalities confer a poor prognosis. Sixty-five percent of children with ALL have normal and near-diploid ALL (44 to 49 chromosomes) and have an intermediate prognosis. With improved cytogenetic techniques, most cases are found to have chromosomal abnormalities and hence belong to the pseudodiploid category. In early studies, the pseudodiploid karyotype conferred the poorest response to therapy (Kalwinsky et al., 1985). It now appears that chromosomal translocations confer the poorest prognosis, regardless of the ploidy group (Williams et al., 1986). Near haploid (26 to

28 chromosomes) is extremely rare and the few patients with this abnormality have relapsed. Cases with multiple stem lines do poorly and should be classified according to the leukemic line of lowest ploidy.

Chromosomal translocations involving reciprocal DNA exchanges are the most significant biologic abnormality identified in leukemia. Translocations have been identified as the abnormality most frequently associated with treatment failure (Williams et al., 1986). They are linked to immunophenotype in ALL (Williams et al., 1984) and to FAB classification in ANLL (Fourth International Workshop, 1984). Translocations are found in approximately 40% of childhood ALL and are more frequent in the pseudodiploid group (55%). This offers an explanation for the prognostic strength of ploidy groups. The development of refined techniques for direct preparation of karyotypes results in successfully banded karyotypes in greater than 90% of cases of ALL. The relatively small number of translocations in the hyperdiploid group is consistent with their low failure rate and the lack of clinical high-risk features. The hyperdiploid ALL cases have a pattern of whole chromosome addition, forming trisomies, that is not seen in the other ploidy groups. Thus hyperdiploid ALL with 51 or more chromosomes represents

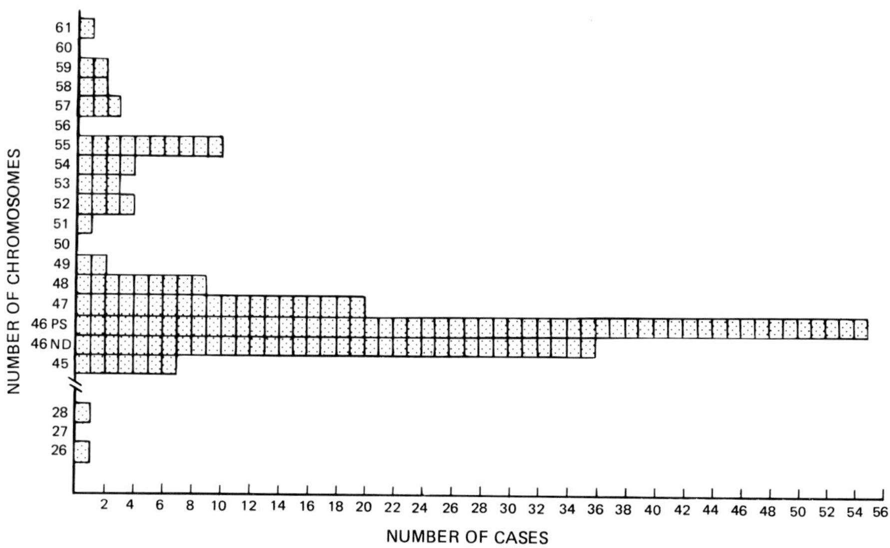

Figure 2 The distribution of chromosome numbers at diagnosis among 161 cases of childhood ALL. The distribution pattern is bimodal with the first peak occurring at 46 chromosomes (pseudodiploid) and the second at 55 chromosomes. ND = normal diploid; PS = pseudodiploid. The percentage of ND cases should decrease as methods of analysis improve.

a distinct unique subset of patients with a better prognosis, except for those whose karyotype contains a translocation.

When times to failure in three recent childhood ALL studies were compared, translocations (specific plus random) were found to confer the worst prognosis (Figure 2). With improved cytogenetic techniques, translocations once considered random may prove to be specific or nonrandom. In ALL, no specific translocation has been found to be associated with a relatively favorable prognosis. Further studies may reveal some heterogeneity of responses among translocations as new specific subgroups are identified or treatment is improved.

Specific Chromosomal Translocations

t(8;14)(q24;q33). This translocation was initially associated with Burkitt's lymphoma. Subsequently, two variant translocations, t(2;8) and t(8;22), were noted in a minority of cases (Bernheim et al., 1981). This abnormality is usually found in B-cell ALL or disseminated Burkitt's lymphoma. In this translocation, the c-myc oncogene is translocated from the long arm of chromosome 8 to the immunoglobulin heavy-chain locus on chromosome 14 or to either light-chain locus on chromosome 2 or 22. The translocation appear to affect B-cell differentiation and may lead to the abnormal proliferation (Klein, 1983).

t(9;22)(q34;q11). The $22q^-$ chromosomal marker, or Philadelphia chromosome (Ph^+), is found at diagnosis in most cases of chronic myelocytic leukemia. In childhood ALL, the Ph^+ is relatively rare (Third International Workshop, 1983). Of 366 children with ALL and complete G-banding studies, 18 (4.9%) were found to have the Ph chromosome (Ribeiro et al., 1986). Their clinical characteristics differ from all other children with ALL only in that they tend to be older, have a higher leukocyte count (47.3×10^9/L) and are more likely to have CNS involvement at diagnosis (7 of 18). The distribution of blast cell immunophenotypes is similar to that of Ph^- cases.

Only 13 of 18 Ph^+ ALL cases achieved complete remission. Cytogenetic studies obtained in remission (n = 5) revealed normal karyotypes in 4 children, while one retained an abnormal Ph negative clone. Three of the five patients have subsequently relapsed with reappearance of the Ph^+ chromosome. In our series two are long-term survivors (51+ and 56+ months), both with variant forms of the Ph chromosome, supporting an improved prognosis for patients with specific chromosomal abnormalities who have karyotypes with breakpoints or rearrangements differing from that found with the classical Ph chromosome.

It is evident that the presence of the Ph chromosome confers a very poor prognosis for children with ALL. For these children, bone marrow transplantation in first remission or intensive experimental treatments should be considered (Bloomfield et al., 1986).

Preliminary data suggest that the breakpoint on chromosome 22 is different from that in CML (Rodenhuis et al., 1985). Molecular probes are available to identify translocations in this region as an alternative to cytogenetic analysis. This may help us identify and understand these differences in this disease phenotype.

t(4;11)(q21;q23). This abnormality is found in approximately 5% of children with ALL. These children tend to be young (often less than 1 year of age), female, and have hyperleucocytosis with CNS involvement at diagnosis (Mirro et al., 1986). Although in most cases the leukemic cells have a lymphoid appearance, recent studies have demonstrated simultaneous expression of lymphoid- and myeloid-associated antigens on individual blasts from some patients tested (Mirro et al., 1985a). This provides evidence for mixed lineage leukemia with the involvement of a multipotential progenitor cell. Of interest is the breakpoint on the number 11 chromosome. Recently, the cellular ets oncogene has been localized to the q23-q24 region of chromosome 11 (Sacchi et al., 1986). Whether it is involved in the pathogenesis of this leukemia is unknown, although it appears involved in the regulation of monocytic differentiation in myelomonocytic and monocytic ANLL, both diseases of younger age and cases with frequent CNS disease (see IIIA and IIIC).

Currently, even with extremely intensive chemotherapy regimens, most of these children relapse. Of the seven patients followed here since 1981, all achieved complete remission. Six of the seven have relapsed, five in the marrow and one in the CNS, from 6 to 48 months of remission. Because the prognosis for children with the t(4;11) is poor, bone marrow transplantation should be considered early in first remission, and children not eligible for transplant should be treated with intensive chemotherapy (Bloomfield et al., 1986).

t(11;14)(p13;q11). This translocation is specific for T-cell ALL (Williams et al., 1984). The locus of the alpha chain of the T-cell antigen receptor has been assigned to chromosome 14, bands q11-q12. This site is often involved in translocations and inversions in T-cell malignancies (Croce et al., 1985). In the t(11;14) (p12;q11), the gene encoding the alpha chain is bisected and may activate an as yet unidentified oncogene. Translocations involving the band q23-q36 region of chromosome 7, the beta-chain encoding regions, have been seen in malignant T-cell lines (Hect et al., 1985) and in the blasts of a number of patients with T-cell ALL (Raimondi et al., 1986). This location may be a preferential site for chromosomal rearrangements in leukemic T lymphocytes. An increasing number of patients with chromosomal rearrangements of the 7q region are being reported, but at present the prognostic importance of this abnormality is unknown (Rainondi et al., 1987).

Children with the t(11;14) have mediastinal masses and high initial leukocyte counts. There is no sex predominance. This translocation was found in one-fourth of the cases of T-cell ALL with completely banded chromosome studies. It is too early to tell whether or not the t(11;14) carries a distinct prognosis, as some patients with the translocation who were treated with intensive chemotherapy regimens continue in remission for at least 3 years.

t(1;19). This chromosomal translocation has been found in approximately 30% of children with pre-B ALL whose fully banded karyotypes have been studied (Williams et al., 1984; Carroll et al., 1984). It has rarely been found in association with the Ph chromosome. Clinically, children with the t(1;19) have high initial leukocyte counts and increased serum LDH (Pui et al., 1986). Since this translocation was discovered relatively recently, its prognostic impact is less certain; however, 10 of 19 patients followed at our institution have already relapsed.

t(10;14)(q24;q11). The t(10;14) involves a reciprocal translocation between chromosome 10 and a locus on the short arm of chromosome 14 which contains the gene that encodes the alpha chain of the T-cell receptor antigen. This translocation was present at diagnosis in 2 of 164 cases of childhood ALL (2 of 22 T-cell ALL). Clinically, these patients had marked leucocytosis and T-cell phenotype but no specific identifying laboratory features. Both are still in remission for over 8 months (Dubé et al., 1986).

The gene for terminal deoxynucleotidyl transferase is on the distal long arm of chromosome 10, and a common fragile site has been observed at 10q25. Since fragile sites are considered to predispose to chromosomal mutation, the translocation could involve the 10q24 because of the general fragility of this area. However, genes important in T-cell differentiation may reside at this location.

12p12. Twenty-three (10%) completely banded cases of ALL seen at St. Jude Hospital over a 3-year period demonstrated 12p abnormalities (Raimondi et al., 1986a). Most of these patients had the common ALL phenotype. One-half of the cases had only 12-12 terminal deletions, while the remainder were involved in translocations (Raimondi et al., 1986a). The specific prognostic significance of this common-ALL-associated abnormality is not known.

With the advent of improved cytogenetic techniques and better characterization of malignant cells, it is apparent that cytogenetic changes are clearly of diagnostic and, more recently, of prognostic importance. Reports indicate that response to therapy can be accurately predicted when classification is based on specific chromosome abnormalities. In addition, even within specific chromosome groups, patients who had karyotypes with different breakpoints than the standard ones may have a better prognosis (Bloomfield et al., 1986). Based on specific translocations, children with ALL who invariably respond poorly to current therapy can be identified. These children, although most frequently achieving complete remissions, inevitably have short remissions. The translocations t(4;11), t(9;22) and t(8;14) consistently predict a poor outcome; other specific and at the present time seemingly random translocations predict a poor prognosis, but none as poor as for these three. Since therapeutic outcome is so poor in patients with translocations, consideration needs to be given to novel chemotherapeutic strategies or ablative therapies with marrow engraftment.

E. Glucocorticoid Receptors

Several investigators had reported that lower levels of glucocorticoid receptors (GR) in ALL are associated with decreased clinical responsiveness to glucocorticoids and a poorer clinical outcome (Costlow, Pui, and Dahl, 1982; Lippman, 1979). The prognostic value of GR levels in childhood ALL had disappeared with more intensive modern therapies (Pui et al., 1984). GR levels are associated with immunophenotype: the GR level in common ALL > pre-B ALL > T-cell ALL > B-cell ALL (Costlow, Pui, and Dahl, 1982).

Insulin receptors are present in most human malignant cells, including ALL, and significant differences in receptor levels have been observed among subtypes of ALL (Esber, Buell, and Leiken, 1976). Lower levels are correlated with T-cell surface markers, presence of a mediastinal mass, lower glucocorticoid receptor levels, higher platelet count, age less than 2 or greater than 10 years, leukocyte count $\geq 100 \times 10^9$/L, and higher labeling index. There is no correlation with CNS disease, FAB type, or sex (Pui et al., 1985a). There is no obvious relationship with insulin receptor level and treatment outcome.

F. Statistical Analysis

The influence of single clinical and biological features in predicting treatment response for 427 children with newly diagnosed ALL treated at St. Jude Children's Research Hospital since 1978 is depicted in Table 1. These variables were analyzed in a proportional hazards model without adjusting for competing effects or covariates. By this analyses, clinical features such as age, initial white blood cell count (WBC), race, CNS leukemia as well as biologic variables of immunophenotype, FAB morphology, and karyotype (ploidy classification, DNA index, and translocations) contributed to outcome. Immunophenotype, PAS reactivity and levels of glucocorticoid receptors showed insignificant effects and were excluded from subsequent analyses.

A clinical model consiting of age, race, and initial WBC was predictive of outcome for these 427 ALL patients. Each of these clinical features made a significant independent contribution to this model after adjusting for the other factors ($p < .01$), while other clinical features such as sex or initial CNS leukemia failed to improve the fit of this model and were therefore excluded from further consideration. Biologic features were then added to this clinical model, to determine if they individually improve the prognostic information available in this multivariate system (Table 2, part A). After accounting for these clinical features immunophenotype no longer added prognostic information independent of age, WBC, and race. Biologic features of morphology and chromosomal features (ploidy group, DNA index and presence or absence of translocations) each added prognostic information to this clinical model. By multivariate analyses, ploidy classification was not an independent feature and failed to add additional information gained by determination of translocation status (Table 2, part B). For these ALL patients, however, FAB morphology, DNA index, as well as chromosomal translocations each appeared to add significant independent biological information to the basic clinical parameters predictive of overall treatment outcome using modern ALL therapy (Table 2, part C).

III. ACUTE NONLYMPHOID LEUKEMIA (ANLL)

A. Morphology and Cytochemistry

The stringent FAB classification system for the myeloid leukemias, while of biologic and clinical importance, is difficult to apply rigorously (Bennett et al., 1985). Approximately one-half of all cases of ANLL in children and adults are myelocytic leukemias and one-half are monocytic variants (Creutzig et al., 1985; Dahl et al., 1982; Bennett, 1982). Progranulocytic leukemia with its numerous bundles of Auer rod structures and distinctive granules is associated with significant early mortality from disseminated coagulopathies (Cordonnier et al., 1985; Bernard et al., 1973; Chan, Steinberg, and Miller, 1981). While patients with this subtype are noted to have long remissions with the advent of more modern therapy (Bernard et al., 1973), its sluggish response to early treatment has only recently been appreciated (Kantarjain et al., 1985; Stone et al., 1985). The monocytic leukemias (FAB M4/M5) are characterized by higher initial leukocyte counts and frequent extramedullary disease including skin, CNS, and gum involvement (Shaw, 1978; Toblem et al., 1980). A syndrome of extreme leukocytosis, respiratory insufficiency, and disseminated intravascular coagulopathy with frequent mortality is a rare complication for patients with monocytic subtypes of ANLL (Lester, Johnson, and Cuttner, 1985). It is unclear if there are significant clinical differences between myelomonocytic leukemia (FAB-M4) and pure monocytic leukemias (M5a, M5b). It has been reported that pure monocytic leukemia in children less than 2 years of age may be a distinct biologic subgroup with impressive treatment responses to monotherapy with the epipodophyllotoxin, VP-16 (Odom and Gordon, 1984). It remains to be established in a larger series whether infants form a prognostically significant subgroup when compared to older children or adolescents with monocytic disease. The micromegakaryocytic form of ANLL (FAB-M7) and the erythroid leukemias (FAB-M6) are rare variants in children and adults for which conventional therapies appear ineffective (Bennett et al., 1980; Huang et al., 1984).

B. Immunophenotype

While batteries of monoclonal antibodies have been developed to identify differentiation-associated antigens of myeloid and monocytic lineage, the relationship of surface antigen expression to response and outcome remains to be determined. A current Cancer and Leukemia Group (CALGB) multiinstitutional study of the relationship of surface marker immunophenotyping in ANLL to a clinical outcome might provide insights into this area (see Chapter 8).

C. Chromosomal Abnormalities in de Novo ANLL

Chromosomal studies have begun to provide meaningful biologic information for the clinician regarding distinctive subtypes of ANLL, information that relates to treatment outcome as well as to possible mechanisms of pathogenesis. By the mid-1970s, approximately 50% of all childhood and adult cases of ANLL had detectable chromosomal abnormalities (Second International Workshop, 1980; Sakuii and Sandberg, 1976; Larson et al., 1983; Brodeur et al., 1983). Initial reports suggested that patients with a normal karyotype responded best; those with a mixture of normal and abnormal cells, intermediately; and those with abnormal metaphases, very poorly (Second International Workshop, 1980; Sakuii and Sandberg, 1976). With improvements in therapies, as well as techniques for karyotype preparation, this distinction is no longer valid (Larson et al., 1983; Brodeur et al., 1983; Rowley, 1985; Woods et al., 1985). Using modern banding and culture techniques, nearly 100% of ANLL cases have been found to have a chromosomal defect, lessening the impact of aneuploidy on prognosis (Yunis, Bloomfield, and Ensrud, 1981). What has emerged, however, are several chromosomal abnormalities of specific biologic and clinical interest in this family of leukemias.

Specific Chromosomal Abnormalities

t(15;17)(q22;q12 or 21). This structural rearrangement involves translocations of the long arm of chromosomes number 15 and 17. Its identity was firmly established in the Second International Workshop (Second International Workshop, 1980), and more recent technical improvements have successfully classified the breakpoints of this translocation and its apparent presence in virtually all cases of acute promyelocytic leukemia (FAB-M3). This chromosomal abnormality is also found in a microgranular variant of acute promyelocytic leukemia (APML) (Golomb, Rowley, and Vadiman, 1980). The biologic significance of this translocation is unknown, since both the c-fes and erb A oncogenes are at some distance, on chromosomes 15 and 17, respectively, from the breakpoints in APML. As noted in Section III.A., APML has a high initial mortality from disseminated coagulopathy and a sluggish induction response. Long-lasting remissions are common in this morphologic and karyotypically identified subgroup.

t(8;21)(q22,q22). This chromosomal translocation is among the most frequent abnormalities noted in most series of childhood (Woods et al., 1985) and adult ANLL (Larson et al., 1983) and is associated primarily with differentiated myelocytic leukemia (FAB-M2). There is frequently a loss of a sex chromosome, a rare event in ANLL (Fourth International Workshop, 1984). The c-mos gene is localized in band 8q22, but whether it plays a role in the development of this leukemia is unknown (Rowley, 1984). In the Fourth International Workshop, cases of t(8;21) had a male predominance (75%) and a younger median age than did the other cases of M2 ANLL. As a group, patients with this abnormality demonstrated superior complete remission rates (75%) by comparison with other

FAB-M2 cases (49%) (Rowley, 1985; Fourth International Workshop, 1984). Despite the higher complete remission rate, however, survival time in cases of t(8;21) is not impressive (Fourth International Workshop, 1984).

t(6;9)(p23,q34). This is a rare chromosomal abnormality in cases of de novo ANLL, with relatively few cases reported (Pearson et al., 1985). Those carefully studied appeared to have an increase in marrow basophilia and a particularly poor response to conventional induction therapy.

11q abnormalities. Rearrangements involving the long arm of chromosome 11, t(9;11) or t(11;17), have been frequently reported in childhood and adult acute monocytic leukemia (AMOL), particularly in cases of undifferentiated FAB-M5a (Brodeur et al., 1983; Fourth International Workshop, 1984; Ferro et al., 1985). The majority of breakpoints are in the 11q23,24 region (Rowley, 1984). Recently, molecular genetic studies have demonstrated that these specific breakpoints on chromosome 9 and 11 result in the juxtaposition of the interferon gene and the cellular proto-oncogene c-ets, thus giving rise to speculation that this rearrangement may specifically deregulate monocytic proliferation (Diaz et al., 1986). In our most recent clinical trials 10 of 23 fully banded cases of acute monocytic leukemia demonstrated t(9;11) or $11q^-$ abnormalities. In a subset of these children less than 1 year of age at diagnosis, 5 of 8 AMOL patients demonstrated a t(9;11) in their diagnostic marrow. Over one-half of the children with a t(9;11) remain in continuous complete remission. The prognostic importance of 11q abnormalities in ANLL is not yet defined.

Inversion 16. Inversion of chromosome 16, inv(16)(p33,q22), or a deletion (16)(q22) has been associated with myelomonocytic leukemia (FAB-M4) and excess eosinophils (>8%). This morphologic subtype includes a proportion of cases with scant numbers of eosinophils, yet morphologically these eosinophils are aberrant with large basophilic granules (Rowley, 1984). From studies of the Fourth International Workshop, it appears that this chromosomal abnormality is subtle and often may be overlooked (Fourth International Workshop, 1984). Preliminary reports suggest that ANLL with inversion 16 syndrome has an improved induction response and relapse-free survival (Hogge et al., 1984; Holmes et al., 1985). Intracerebral myeloblastomas and leptomeningeal CNS leukemias are frequently found in these patients (Holmes et al., 1985).

Monosomy 7. ANLL arising secondary to occupational or mutagenic agents frequently is associated with abnormalities of chromosome 5 or monosomy of chromosome 7 (Fourth International Workshop, 1984). De novo monosomy 7 has been reported in childhood ANLL (Brodeur et al., 1983; Woods et al., 1985) and appears to have a particularly dismal prognosis (Woods et al., 1985), marked by failure to respond to conventional antileukemic therapies. At St. Jude Hospital, 11 of 237 children referred for various hematologic disorders, including

ANLL, pancytopenia, and myeloproliferative syndromes between 1979 and 1984, had monosomy for chromosome 7. Preleukemia was diagnosed in 8 cases (5 evolved to ANLL) and de novo ANLL in 3. There was a striking predominance of males in this series (M:F ratio, 10:1). Although intensive chemotherapy regimens were used, none of the 7 patients who were treated achieved complete remission. The median survival for those who presented with preleukemia was 18 months, while those presenting with de novo ANLL lived for a median of 11 months.

D. Clonogenic Assays in ANLL

The major culture system developed to study myeloid cells in vitro, the Robinson-Pike system, grows marrow cells in a mixture of agar and sera over a feeder layer that serves as a source of colony-stimulating factor, or CSF (Robinson, Kurnick, and Pike, 1971; Moore et al., 1974; Spitzer et al., 1976; Spitzer et al., 1978; Lihou and Smith, 1985). One disadvantage of this method lies in the variation from laboratory to laboratory in assay standardization due to differences in serum, media, sources of CSF, and incubation conditions (Spitzer et al., 1978). The number of cells used to define different stages of leukemic growth, i.e., clusters or colonies, varies by investigator (Moore et al., 1974; Lihou and Smith, 1985; Vincent et al., 1977). An alternative culture system for ANLL cells involves methylcellulose with PHA/leukocyte conditioned feeder layers (Minden, Till, and McCulloch, 1978; Buick, Minden, and McCulloch, 1979). The advantage of this latter system is a more uniform source of CSF and improved adaptation for electron microscopy and karyotypic studies.

Despite the variability in these assays, four independent laboratories have correlated growth patterns of ANLL cells at diagnosis or relapse with response to chemotherapeutic treatments (Moore et al., 1974; Spitzer et al., 1976; Vincent et al., 1977; Buick, Minden, and McCulloch, 1979). In these studies, patients whose cells form abundant clusters or colonies in vitro do poorly; it has been hypothesized that cells capable of luxurious growth under adverse in vitro conditions may naturally be resistant to chemotherapy (Preisler, 1982).

Use of in vitro clonogenic assays to predict drug sensitivity in vivo has been much more difficult. Several laboratories have reported a correlation between in vitro cell kill after daunorubicin or daunorubicin/ara-C and treatment response (Preisler, 1982; Marie et al., 1983; Park et al., 1983; Gustavsson and Olofsson, 1984; Dow et al., 1986), specifically with regards to obtaining of a complete remission. Using this assay methodology, Dow et al. (1986) were able to correlate increased in vitro sensitivity of childhood ANLL cells to ara-C, daunorubicin or a combination of these agents to increased duration of complete remission. The failure of a significant proportion of patients cells to grow in vitro and the variable correlation of in vivo and in vitro sensitivity limits the overall utility of this tool in planning chemotherapy trials.

Table 3 T-11 ANLL, St. Jude Experience, 1980-86

	T-11 ANLL	Other ANLL
N	8	130
Male/female	6/2	80/50
Median WBC (X 10^9/L)	21.7 (range 5.8-171)	23.0 (range 1.5-990)
Age (yrs)	17 (12.5-18)	8.5 (0.1-18)
Morphology	Variable with bimorphic population	50% FAB M1-3 50% FAB M4-5
Positive Auer rods	5/8	52/130
Myeloid markers	+	+
T-11	+	–
E-rosettes	2/8 (1-5%)	N.A.
MPO	Weakly + (3-15% positivity)	>15% positivity
Response ANLL induction	4/8 CR	80% CR
Still in CCR	2/8	40%

CR = Complete remission.
CCR = Continuous complete remission.

IV. ACUTE MIXED-LINEAGE LEUKEMIA

Chapter 12 outlines in detail the biologic, immunologic and clinical aspects of lineage heterogeneity in the acute leukemias. Mirro et al. (1985a) reported patients with acute myeloid leukemia with mixed marrow morphology whose blasts strongly expressed the E-rosette-associated antigen of T-cell lineage. Since 1980, we have identified 8 children with ANLL whose blasts react strongly with OKT11 or 9.6 (CD-2) antibody, specific for the E-rosette-associated antigen (Tp50). Comparison of these cases (T-11 ANLL) with the remainder of newly diagnosed ANLL cases seen at our institution during this time period is shown in Table 3. As a group, T-11 ANLL patients were slightly older and more often were males. Morphologically, this leukemia does not fit a precise FAB classification. The majority of marrow cells are small blasts with scant cytoplasm lacking granules, most closely resembling lymphoblasts. Ten to twenty percent of the cells appear lymphoid and are larger with nucleoli and more abundant cytoplasm. By our diagnostic criteria, these cases are considered nonlymphoid leukemias since 5 of the 8 had readily apparent Auer rods, 7 expressed myeloperoxidase, and 1 demonstrated blast butyrate activity. All 8 of these T-11 ANLL cases expressed a battery of myeloid markers, with T-11 postivity ranging from 76-96%. Ability to form heat-stable E-rosettes was found in only 2 of these cases (1-5%

heat stable, 37°C rosettes). Clinically, these children had bulky cervical nodal disease. Response to antileukemic therapy as been variable (Mirro et al., 1985b). Although 4 patients achieved complete remission with ANLL directed therapy with daunomycin, cytosine arabinoside, 5-azacytidine, and etiposide, the remaining 4 failed the intensive induction scheme. These 4 ANLL-directed therapy failures responded to a prednisone, vincristine, and asparaginase regimen or so-called ALL-directed treatment. Only two patients survived with this entity, one after a bone marrow transplant, post ANLL-directed chemotherapy. Acute mixed-lineage leukemia is a significant subset of childhood myeloid leukemia for which the early addition of prednisone and vincristine should be considered.

V. CLINICAL IMPLICATIONS OF LEUKEMIC CELL HETEROGENEITY

It is clear that the acute leukemias are an extraordinarily diverse group of malignant diseases. The basis for this heterogeneity resides in the genetic changes responsible for the expression, maintenance, and progression of the malignant phenotype. Spontaneous mutations in clonogenic leukemic cells ultimately lead to the expression of a drug-resistant phenotype. The availability of powerful new techniques for examining the DNA of human cells has opened a new window on the molecular basis for leukemic phenotypes and the genetic instability inherent in such cells. This may lead to improved strategies of disease classification at diagnosis, to more accurately reflect the drug sensitivity of particular cases. Current evidence suggests that DNA or chromosomal rearrangements are the most critical factors determining the prognosis of acute leukemia. It is doubtful that modern leukemia therapy can cure 100% of patients. Recent data reported by Fearon 1986 indicate that even after apparent eradication of ANLL, a clone of hematopoietic preleukemic precursors capable of essentially normal differentiation can emerge and eventually cause relapse. The same scenario might be true in ALL. Thus, efforts to devise therapeutic alternatives seem justified. Perhaps simultaneous and sequential combinations of cytocidal chemotherapy and cytodifferentiation agents should be considered. Wider use of ablative therapy followed by bone marrow transplantation might also improve prognosis.

REFERENCES

Aur, R. J. A., Simone, J. V., Verzosa, M. S., Hustu, H. O., Barker, L. F., Pinkel, D. P., Rivera, G., Dahl, G. V., Wood, A., Stagner, S., and Mason, C. (1978). Childhood acute lymphocytic leukemia: Study VIII. *Cancer* 42:2123-2134.

Bennett, J. M. (1982). The French-American-British classification of the acute adult myeloid leukemia: Its clinical relevance. Chap. 4, In *Adult Leukemia*, C. D. Bloomfield (ed.). Nijhoff, Hague.

Bennett, J. M., Catovsky, D., Daniel, M. T., Flandrin, G., Galton, D. A. G., Gralnick, H. C., and Sultan, C. (FAB Co-operative Group) (1976). Proposals for the classification of the acute leukemias. *Br. J. Haematol.* 33:451-458.

Bennett, J. M., Begg, C. B., Sartiano, G. C., Tartaglia, A., Carbone, P. P. (1980). The chemotherapy of adult myeloid leukemias. *Proc. Am. Soc. Clin. Oncol.* 21:434.

Bennett, J. M., Catovsky, D., Daniel, M. T., Flandrin, G., Galton, D. A. G., Gralnick, H. R., and Sultan, C. (1981). The morphological classification of acute lymphoblastic leukemia: Concordance among observers and clinical correlations. *Br. J. Haematol.* 47:553-531.

Bennett, J. M., Catovsky, D., Daniel, M. T., Flandrin, G., Galton, D. A. G., Gralnick, H. R., and Sultan, C. (1985). Proposed revised criteria for the classification of acute myeloid leukemia. *Ann. Int. Med.* 103:620-625.

Berger, R., and Bernheim, A. (1982). Cytogenetic studies on Burkitt's lymphoma-leukemia. *Cancer Genet. Cytogenet.* 7:231-244.

Bernard, J., Weil, M., Bairon, M., Jacquillat, C., Flandrin, G., and Gemon, M.-F. (1973). Acute promyelocytic leukemia: results of treatment by daunorubicin. *Blood* 41:489-496.

Bernheim, A., Berger, R., and Lenoir, G. (1981). Cytogenetic studies on African Burkitt's lymphoma cell lines: t(8;14), t(2;8) and t(8;22) translocations. *Cancer Genet. Cytogenet.* 3:307-315.

Bloomfield, C. D., Goldman, A. I., Alimena, G., Berger, R., Borgstrom, G. H., Brandt, L., Catovsky, D., de la Chapelle, A., Dewald, G. W., Garson, O. M., Garwicz, S., Golomb, D. K., Hossfeld, D. K., Lawler, S. D., Mitelman, F., Nilsson, P., Pierre, R. V., Philip, P., Prigogina, E., Rowley, J. D., Sakurai, M., Sandberg, A. A., Secker Walker, L. M., Tricot, G., Van Den Berghe, H., Van Orshoven, A., Vuopio, P., and Whang-Pang, J. (1986). Chromosomal abnormalities identify high-risk and low-risk patients with acute lymphoblastic leukemia. *Blood* 67:415-420.

Borowitz, M. J., Dowell, B. L., Boyett, J. M., Falletta, J. M., Pullen, J., Crist, W. M., Humphrey, G. B., and Metzgar, R. S. (1985). Monoclonal antibody definition of T cell leukemia: A Pediatric Oncology Group study. *Blood* 65: 785-788.

Bowman, W. P., Melvin, S. L., Aur, R. J. A., and Mauer, A. M. (1981). A clinical perspective of cell markers in acute lymphocytic leukemia. *Cancer Res.* 41: 4704.

Bradstock, K. F., Papageorgiou, E. D., Janossy, G., Huffbrand, A. V., Willoughby, M. L., Roberts, P. D., and Bollum, F. J. (1980). Detection of leukemic lymphoblasts in CSF by immunofluorescence for terminal transferase. *Lancet* 1: 1144.

Brearley, R. L., Johnson, S. A. N., and Lister, T. A. (1979). Acute lymphoblastic leukaemia in adults: clinicopathologic correlations with the French-American-British (FAB) Co-operative group classification. *Eur. J. Cancer* 15:909-914.

Brodeur, G. M., Williams, D. L., Kalwinsky, D. K., Williams, J. K., and Dahl, G. V. (1983). Cytogenetic features of acute non-lymphoblastic leukemia in 73 children and adolescents. *Cancer Genet. Cytogenet.* 8:93-105.

Buick, R. N., Minden, M. D., and McCulloch, E. A. (1979). Self-renewal in culture of proliferative blast progenitor cells in acute myeloblastic leukemia. *Blood* 54:95-104.

Camitta, B. M., Pinkel, D., Thatcher, L. G., Casper, J., Kun, L. E., and Laver, S. (1980). Failure of early intensive chemotherapy to improve prognosis in childhood acute lymphocytic leukemia. *Med. Pediatr. Oncol.* 8:383-389.

Carroll, A. J., Crist, W. M., Parmly, R. T., Roper, M., Cooper, M. D., and Finley, W. H. (1984). Pre-B-cell leukemia associated with chromosome translocation 1;19. *Blood* 63:721-724.

Catovsky, D. (1975). T-cell origin of acid phosphate positive lymphoblasts. *Lancet* 2:327-328.

Catovsky, D., Galetto, J., Okos, A., Milani, G., and Galton, D. A. G. (1974). Cytochemical profile of B and T leukemia lymphocytes with special reference to acute lymphoblastic leukemia. *J. Clin. Pathol.* 27:767-771.

Chan, K. W., Steinherz, P. G., and Miller, D. R. (1981). Acute promyelocytic leukemia in children. *Med. Ped. Oncol.* 9:5-15.

Chessells, J. M., Hardisty, R. M., Rapson, N. T., and Greaves, M. F. (1977). Acute lymphoblastic leukemia in children: classification and prognosis. *Lancet* 2: 1307-1308.

Coccia, P., Miller, D. R., Kersey, J. H. (1980). Relationship of blast cells surface markers and morphology. FAB classification in childhood acute lymphocytic leukemia (ALL). *Proc. Am. Soc. Hematol.* 54:182a.

Coccia, P. F., Bleyer, W. A., Siegel, S. E., Lukens, J. N., Gross, S., Miller, D. R., Littman, P. F., Sather, H. N., and Hammond, G. D. (1983). Development and preliminary findings of CCSG protocols 161, 162, 163 for low, average and high-risk acute lymphoblastic leukemia in children. In *Leukemia Research: Advances in Cell Biology and Treatment*. S. B. Murphy and J. R. Gilbert (eds.). Elsevier, New York, pp. 241-250.

Coleman, M. S., Greenwood, M. F., Hutton, J. J., Bollum, F. J., Lampkin, B., and Holland, P. (1976). Serial observations on terminal deoxynucleotidyl transferase activity and lymphoblast surface markers in acute lymphoblastic leukemia. *Cancer Res.* 36:120-127.

Cordonnier, C., Vernant, J. P., Brun, B., Heilmann, M. G., Kuentz, M., Bierling, P., Farcet, J. P., Rodet, M., Duedari, N., Imbert, M., Jouault, H., Mannoni, P., Reyes, F., Dreyfus, B., and Rochant, H. (1985). Acute promyelocytic leukemia in 57 previously untreated patients. *Cancer* 55:18-25.

Costlow, M. E., Pui, C.-H., and Dahl, G. V. (1982). Glycocorticoid receptors in childhood acute lymphocytic leukemia. *Cancer Res.* 42:480.

Creutzig, V., Ritter, J., Riehm, H., Langermann, H.-J., Henze, G., Kabisch, H., Niethammer, D., Jürgens, H., Stollmann, B., Lasson, U., Kaufmann, U., Löffler, H., and Schellong, G. (1985). Improved treatment results in childhood acute myelogenous leukemia: a report of the German cooperative study AML-BFM-78. *Blood* 65:298-304.

Crist, W. M., Boyett, J., Roper, M., Pullen, J., Metzgar, R., Van Eys, J., Ragalo, A., Starling, K., Vietti, T., and Cooper, M. (1984). Pre-B-cell leukemia responds poorly to treatment: A Pediatric Oncology Group study. *Blood* 63: 407-414.

Crist, W. M., Grossi, C. E., Pullen, J., and Cooper, M. D. (1985). Immunologic markers in childhood acute lymphocytic leukemia. *Semin. Oncol.* 12:105-121.

Croce, C. M., Isobe, M., Palumbo, A., Puck, J., Ming, J., Tweardy, D., Evikson, J., Davis, M., and Rovera, G. (1985). Gene for α-chain of human T-cell receptor: Location on chromosome 14 regions involved in T-cell neoplasma. *Science* 227:1044-1047.

Dahl, G. V., Kalwinsky, D. K., Murphy, S., Look, A. T., Amadori, S., Kumar, M., Novak, R., George, S. L., Mason, C., Mauer, A. M., and Simone, J. V. (1982). Cytochemically based induction chemotherapy and splenectomy for childhood acute nonlymphocytic leukemia. *Blood* 60:856-863.

Dahl, G., Pui, C.-H., Kalwinsky, D., Ochs, J., Abromowitch, M., Mirro, J., Murphy, S., and Rivera, S. (1986). Teniposide (VM26) plus cytarabine (ara-C) improved outcome in extremely high-risk acute lymphocytic leukemia (ALL). *Proc. ASCO* 5:162.

Diaz, M. O., Le Beau, M. M., Pitha, P., and Rowley, J. D. (1986). Interferon and c-ets-1 genes in the translocation (9;11)(p22,q23) in human acute monocytic leukemia. *Science* 231:265-267.

Dow, L. W., Dahl, G. V., Kalwinsky, D. K., Mirro, J., Nash, M. B., and Robertson, P. K. (1986). Correlation of drug sensitivity in vitro with clinical regimens in childhood acute myeloid leukemia. *Blood* 68:400-405.

Dubé, I. D., Raimondi, S. C., Pi, D., and Kalovsek, D. K. (1986). A new translocation, t(10;14)(q24;q11), in T cell neoplasia. *Blood* 67:1181-1184.

Esber, E. C., Buell, D. N., and Leiken, S. L. (1976). Insulin binding of acute lymphocytic leukemia cells. *Blood* 48:33.

Fearon, E. R., Burke, P. J., Schiffer, C. A., Zehnbauer, B. A., and Vogelstein, B. (1986). Differentiation of leukemia cells to polymorphonuclear leukocytes in patients with acute nonlymphocytic leukemia. *N. Engl. J. Med.* 15-24.

Feldges, A. J., Aur, R. J. A., Verzosa, M. S., and Daniels, S. (1974). Periodic acid-Schiff reaction, a useful index of duration of complete remission in childhood acute lymphocytic leukemia. *Acta. Haematol.* 52:8-13.

Ferro, M. T., Roman, C. S., Guzman, M., Garcia-Larana, J., and Odriozola, J. (1985). Translocation (11;17)(q24;q21) as a variant of translocation (9;11) (p22,q24) in acute monoblastic leukemia. *Cancer Genet. Cytogenet.* 17:83-85.

Flandrin, G., and Daniel, M. T. (1973). Practical value of cytochemical studies for the classification of acute leukemias. *Recent Results in Cancer Res.* 43: 43-56.

Fourth International Workshop on Chromosomes and Leukemia. (1984). *Cancer Genet. Cytogenet.* 11:249-350.

George, S. L., Fernbach, D. J., Vietti, T. J., et al. (1974). Factors influencing survival in pediatric acute leukemia. *Cancer* 32:1542-1553.

Golomb, H. M., Rowley, J. D., and Vadiman, J. W. (1980). Microgranular acute monomyelocytic leukemia: a distinctive clinical, ultrastructural and cytogenetic entity. *Blood* 55:253-259.

Gordon, D. S., Hutton, J. J., Smalley, R. V., Meyer, Z. M., and Vogler, W. R. (1978). Terminal deoxynucleotidyl transferase (TdT) cytochemistry and membrane receptors in adult acute leukemia. *Blood* 52:1079-1088.

Greaves, M. F., Janossy, G., Peto, J., and Kay, H. (1981). Immunologically defined subclasses of acute lymphoblastic leukemia in children: Their relationship to presentation features and prognosis. Br. J. Haematol. 48:179-197.

Gustavsson, A., and Olofsson, J. (1984). Prediction of response to chemotherapy in acute leukemia by in vitro drug sensitivity testing on leukemic stem cells. *Cancer Res.* 44:4648-4652.

Hann, J. M., Evans, D. I. K., Palmer, M. K., Morris Jones, P. J., and Haworth, C. (1979). The prognostic significance of morphologic features in childhood acute lymphoblastic leukaemia. *Clin. Lab. Haematol.* 1:215-226.

Hect, F., Morgan, R., Gemmill, R. M., and Hect, B. K.-M. (1985). Translocations in T-cell leukemia and lymphoma. *N. Engl. J. Med.* (Letter) 313:758-759.

Hogge, D. E., Misawa, S., Parsa, N. Z., Pollak, A., and Testa, J. R. (1984). Abnormalities of chromosome 16 association with acute myelomonocytic leukemia and dysplastic bone marrow eosinophils. *J. Clin. Oncol.* 2:550-557.

Holmes, R., Keating, M. J., Cork, A., Broach, Y., Trujillo, J., Dalton, W. T., McCredie, K. B., and Freireich, E. J. (1985). A unique pattern of central nervous system leukemia in acute myelomonocytic leukemia associated with inversion (16)(p13,q22). *Blood* 65:1071-1078.

Huang, M.-J., Li, C.-Y., Nichols, W. L., Young, J.-H., and Katzmann, J. A. (1984). Acute leukemia with megakaryocytic differentiation: A study of twelve cases identified immunocytochemically. *Blood* 64:427-439.

Humphrey, G. B., Nesbit, M. S., and Brunning, R. D. (1974). Prognostic value of the periodic acid-Schiff (PAS) reaction in acute lymphoblastic leukemia. *Am. J. Clin. Pathol.* 61:393-397.

Janossy, G., Hoffbrand, A. V., Greaves, M. F., Ganesfraguru, K., Pain, C., Bradstock, K. F., Prentice, H. G., Kay, H. E. M., and Lister, T. A. (1980a). Terminal transferase enzyme assay and immunological membrane markers in diagnosis of leukemia, a multiparameter analyses of 300 cases. *Br. J. Haematol.* 44:221-234.

Kalwinsky, D. K., Weatherred, W. H., Dahl, G. V., Bowman, W. P., Melvin, S. L., Coleman, M. S., and Bollum, F. J. (1981). Clinical utility of initial terminal deoxynucleotidyl transferase determination in childhood acute leukemias. *Cancer Res.* 41:2877-2881.

Kalwinsky, D. K., Roberson, P., Dahl, G. V., Harber, J., Rivera, G. K., Bowman, W. P., Pui, C.-H., Ochs, J., Abromowitch, M., Costlow, M. E., Melvin, S. L., Stass, S., Williams, D., and Murphy, S. B. (1985). Clinical relevance of lymphoblastic biological features in children with acute lymphoblastic leukemia. *J. Clin. Oncol.* 3:477-484.

Kantarjian, H. M., Keating, M. J., McCredie, K. B., Beran, M., Walters, R., Dalton, W. T., Hittleman, W., and Freireich, E. J. (1985). A characteristic pattern of leukemic cell differentiation without cytoreduction during remission induction in acute promyelocytic leukemia. *J. Clin. Oncol.* 3:793-798.

Keleti, J., Révéz, T., and Schuler, D. (1978). Morphologic diagnosis in childhood leukemia. *Br. J. Haematol.* 40:501-502.

Kita, K., Nasu, K., Kamesaki, H., Doi, S., Tezuka, H., Tatsumi, E., Fukuhara, S., Nishikori, M., Uchino, H., and Shirakawa, S. (1985). Phenotypic analysis of acute lymphoblastic leukemia (ALL) cells which are classified as non-T and non-B and negative for common ALL antigen. *Blood* 66:47-52.

Klein, G. (1983). Specific chromosomal translocations and the genesis of B-cell derived tumors in mice and man. *Cell* 32:311-315.

Lampert, F., Henze, G., Langermann, H. J., Schellong, G., Gadner, H., and Riehm, H.-J. (1984). Acute lymphoblastic leukemia. *Recent results of cancer research.* 93:159-181.

Lanham, G. R., Bollum, F. J., Williams, D. L., and Stass, S. (1984). Simultaneous occurrence of terminal deoxynucleotidyl transferase and myeloperoxidase in individual leukemic blasts. *Blood* 64:318-320.

Lanham, G. R., Kalwinsky, D. K., Williams, D. L., Melvin, S. L., Harber, J. R., Motroni, T. H., and Stass, S. (1985). PAS stain in childhood ALL. Lack of independent prognostic value. *Amer. J. Clin. Path.* 83:494-497.

Larson, R. A., Le Beau, M. M., Vardiman, J. W., Testa, J. R., Golomb, H. M., and Rowley, J. D. (1983). The predictive value of initial cytogenetic studies in 148 adults with acute non-lymphocytic leukemia: a 12 year study 1973-82. *Cancer Genet. Cytogenet.* 10:219-236.

Laurie, H. C. (1968). Duration of remissions in lymphoblastic leukemia of childhood. 5-year survivals. *Br. Med. J.* 2:95-97.

Lester, T. J., Johnson, J. W., and Cuttner, J. (1985). Pulmonary leukostasis as the single worst prognostic factor in patients with acute myelocytic leukemia and hyperleukocytosis. *Am. J. Med.* 79:43-48.

Lihou, M. G., and Smith, P. J. (1985). Adriamycin and cytosine arabinoside contribute equally to prediction of response in acute myelocytic leukemia with improved confidence level. *Cancer Chemother. Pharmacol.* 14:116-119.

Lippman, M. E., Yarbo, G. S. K., and Leventhal, B. G. (1979). Glucocorticoid receptors in normal and leukemic human leukocytes. In *Glucocorticoid Action and Leukemia*, P. A. Bell and M. M. Borthwick (eds.). Alpha Omega, Cardiff, Wales, UK, p. 175.

Look, A. T. (1985). The emerging genetics of acute lymphoblastic leukemia: clinical and biological implications. *Semin. Oncol.* 12:92-104.

Look, A. T., Melvin, S. L., Williams, D. L., Brodeur, G. M., Dahl, G. V., Kalwinsky, D. K., Murphy, S. B., and Mauer, A. M. (1982). Aneuploidy and percentage of S-phase cells determined by flow cytometry correlate with cell phenotype in childhood acute leukemia. *Blood* 60:959-967.

Look, A. T., Melvin, S. L., Brown, K. L., Dockter, M. E., Roberson, D. R., and Murphy, S. B. (1984). Quantitative variation of the common acute lymphoblastic leukemia antigen (gp100) on leukemic marrow blasts. *J. Clin. Invest.* 73:1617-1628.

Look, A. T., Roberson, P. K., Williams, D. L., Rivera, G. K., Bowman, W. P., Pui, C.-H., Ochs, J., Abromowitch, M., Kalwinsky, D., Dahl, G. V., George,

S. L., and Murphy, S. B. (1985). Prognostic importance of blast cell DNA content in childhood acute lymphoblastic leukemia. *Blood* 64:1079-1086.

Magrath, I. T., and Ziegler, F. L. (1979). Bone marrow involvement in Burkitt's lymphoma and its relationship to acute B-cell leukemia. *Leuk. Res.* 4:33-59.

Marie, J.-P., Zittoun, R., Thevenin, D., Mathieu, M., and Viguie, F. (1983). In vitro culture of clonogenic leukemic cells in acute myeloid leukemias: growth pattern and drug sensitivity. *Br. J. Haematol.* 55:427-437.

Miller, D. R. (1975). Prognostic factors in childhood leukemia. *J. Pediatr.* 87: 672-676.

Miller, D. R., Leikin, S., Albo, V., Vitale, L., Sather, H., Coccia, P., Nesbit, M., Karon, M., and Hammond, D. (1980). Use of prognostic factors in improving the design and efficiency of clinical trials in childhood leukemia: Children's Cancer Study Group Report. *Cancer Treat. Rep.* 64:381-392.

Miller, D. R., Leikin, S., Albo, V., Sather, H., and Hammond, D. (1981). Prognostic importance of morphology (FAB classification) in childhood acute lymphoblastic leukemia (ALL). *Br. J. Haematol.* 48:199-206.

Miller, D. R., Leiken, S., Albo, V., Sather, H., Karon, M., and Hammond, D. (1983). Prognostic factors and therapy in acute lymphoblastic leukemia of childhood: CCG-141. *Cancer* 51:1041-1049.

Minden, M. D., Till, J. E., and McCulloch, E. A. (1978). Proliferative state of blast cell progenitors in acute myeloblastic leukemia (AML). *Blood* 52:592-600.

Mirro, J., Antoun, G. R., Zipf, T. F., Melvin, S., Stass, S. (1985a). The E-rosette associated antigen of T-cells can be identified on blasts from patients with acute myeloblastic leukemia. *Blood* 65:363-367.

Mirro, J., Zipf, T. F., Pui, C.-H., Kitchingman, G., Williams, D., Melvin, S., Murphy, S. B., and Stass, S. (1985b). Acute mixed lineage leukemia: Clinicopathologic correlation and prognostic significance. *Blood* 68:1115-1123.

Mirro, J., Kitchingman, J., Williams, D., Lauzon, G. J., Lin, C.-C., Calihan, T., and Zipf, T. F. (1986). Clinical and laboratory characteristics of acute leukemia with the 4;11 translocation. *Blood* 67:689-697.

Moore, M. A. S., Spitzer, G., Williams, N., Metcalf, D., and Buckley, J. (1974). Agar culture studies in 127 cases of untreated acute leukemia: the prognostic value of reclassification of leukemia according to in vitro growth characteristics. *Blood* 44:1-18.

Müller-Weihrich, S., Henze, G., Odenwald, E., and Rhiem, H. (1985). BFM trials for childhood non-Hodgkin's lymphoma. In *Malignant Lymphomas and Hodgkin's Disease: Experimental and Therapeutic Advances*. F. Cavalla, G. Bonnadonna, and M. Rozencweig (eds.). Martinus Nijhoff Publishers, Boston, Massachusetts, pp. 633-642.

Murphy, S. B., Bowman, W. P., Hustu, H. O., and Berard, C. W. (1985). Advanced stage (III/IV) Burkitt's lymphoma and B-cell ALL in children: Kinetic and pharmacologic rationale for treatment and recent results (1979-83). In *Burkitt's Lymphoma*, G. Lenoir, G. T. O'Connor, and C. L. M. Olweny (eds.). IARC Scientific Publications #60, Lyons, p. 405-418.

Murphy, S. B., Bowman, W. P., Abromowitch, M., Mirro, J., Ochs, J., Rivera, G., Pui, C.-H., Fairclough, D., and Berard, C. W. (1986). Results of treatment of advanced stage Burkitt's lymphoma and B-cell (SIg+) acute lymphoblastic leukemia with high-dose fractionated cyclophosphamide and coordinated high-dose methotrexate and cytarabine. *J. Clin. Oncol.* 4:1732-1739.

Nagasaka, M., Maeda, S., Maeda, H., Chen, H. L., Kita, K., Mabuchi, O., Misu, H., Matsuo, T., and Sugiyama, T. 91983). Four cases of t(4;11) acute leukemia and its myelomonocytic nature in infants. *Blood* 61:1174-1181.

Odom, L. F., and Gordon, E. M. (1984). Acute monoblastic leukemia in infancy and early childhood: successful treatment with an epipodophyllotoxin. *Blood* 64:875-882.

Palmer, M. K., Hann, I. M., Jones, P. M., and Evans, D. I. K. (1980). A score at diagnosis for predicting length of remission in childhood acute lymphoblastic leukemia. *Br. J. Cancer* 42:841-849.

Park, C. H., Wiernik, P. H., Morrison, F. S., Amare, J., VanSloten, K., and Maloney, T. R. (1983). Clinical correlation of leukemic clonogenic cell chemosensitivity assessed by in vitro continuous exposure to drugs. *Cancer Res.* 43: 2346-2349.

Pearson, M. G., Vardiman, J. W., Le Beau, M. M., Rowley, J. D., Schwartz, S., Kerman, S. L., Cohen, M. M., Fleischman, E. W., and Prigogina, E. L. (1985). Increased numbers of marrow basophils may be associated with a t(6;9) in ANLL. *Am. J. Hematol.* 18:393-403.

Preisler, H. D. (1982). An integrated approach to the study and treatment of acute myelocytic leukemia. In *Adult Leukemias*, Clara Bloomfield (ed.). Martinus Nijhoff, Boston, Massachusetts, Chapter 6.

Pui, C.-H., and Costlow, M. E. (1985a). Clinical and biological correlates of insulin binding by leukemic lymphoblasts. *Leuk. Res.* 9:843-849.

Pui, C.-H., Ochs, J., Kalwinsky, D. K., and Costlow, M. E. (1984). Impact of treatment efficacy on the prognostic value of glucocorticoid receptor levels in childhood acute lymphoblastic leukemia. *Leuk. Res.* 8:345-350.

Pui, C.-H., Dodge, R. K., Dahl, G. V., Rivera, G., Look, A. T., Kalwinsky, D., Bowman, W. P., Ochs, J., Abromowitch, M., Mirro, J., and Murphy, S. B. (1985b). Serum lactic dehydrogenase level as prognostic value in childhood acute lymphoblastic leukemia. *Blood* 66:778-782.

Pui, C.-H., Williams, D. L., Kalwinsky, D. K., Look, A. T., Melvin, S. L., Dodge, R. K., Rivera, G., Murphy, S. B., and Dahl, G. V. (1986a). Cytogenetic features and serum lactic dehydrogenase level predict a poor treatment outcome for children with pre-B-cell leukemia. *Blood* 67:247-254.

Pui, C.-H., Williams, D. L., Raimondi, S. C., Melvin, S. L., Behm, F. G., Look, A. T., Dahl, G. V., Rivera, G. K., Kalwinsky, D. K., Mirro, J., Dodge, R. K., and Murphy, S. B. (1986b). Unfavorable presenting clinical and laboratory features are associated with CALLA-negative non-T, non-B lymphoblastic leukemia in children. *Leuk. Res.* 10:1287-1292.

Pullen, D. J., Falletta, J. M., Crist, W. M., Vogler, L. B., Dowell, B., Humphrey, G. B., Blackstock, R., Van Eys, J., Cooper, M. D., Metzgar, R. S., and Meydrech, E. F. (1981). Southwest Oncology Group experience with immunological immunophenotyping in acute lymphocytic leukemia of childhood. *Cancer Res.* 41:4802-4809.

Pullen, D. J., Boyett, J. M., Crist, W. M., Falletta, J. M., Roper, M., Dowell, B., Van Eys, J., Jackson, J. F., Humphrey, G. B., Metzgar, R. S., and Cooper, M. D. (1984). Pediatric Oncology Group utilization of immunologic markers in the designation of acute lymphocytic leukemia (ALL) subgroups. Influence of treatment response. *Ann. N.Y. Acad. Sci.* 428:262.

Raimondi, S., Williams, D. L., Callihan, T., Peiper, S., Rivera, G. K., and Murphy, S. B. (1986). Nonrandom involvement of the 12p12 breakpoint in chromosome abnormalities of childhood acute lymphocytic leukemia. *Blood* 68: 69-75.

Raimondi, S., Pui, C.-H., Behm, F., and Williams, D. (1987). 7q32-q36 translocations in childhood T-cell leukemia: Cytogenetic evidence for involvement of the T-cell-receptor β-chain gene. *Blood* 69:131-134.

Reinherz, E. L., Acuto, O., Fabbi, M., Bensusson, A., Milanese, C., Royer, H. D., Meuer, S. C., and Schlossman, S. F. (1984). Clonogenic surface structure on human T lymphocytes: Functional and biochemical analysis of the antigen receptor complex. *Immunol. Rev.* 81:95-129.

Ribeiro, R., Abromowitch, M., Raimondi, S., and Williams, D. (1986). Clinical and biologic hallmarks of the Philadelphia (Ph) chromosome in childhood acute lymphoblastic leukemia (ALL). *Proc. AACR* 27:193 (abstract).

Riehm, H., Feickert, H.-J., and Lampert, F. (1986). Acute lymphoblastic leukemia. In *Cancer in Children: Clinical Management*, 2nd ed., H. J. Bloom (ed.). Heidelberg, Springer-Verlag, pp. 2-30.

Robinson, W. A., Kurnick, J. E., and Pike, B. L. (1971). Colony growth of human leukemia peripheral blood cells in vitro. *Blood* 38:500-508.

Rodenhuis, S., Smets, L. A., Slater, R. M., Behrendt, H., and Veerman, A. J. P. (1985). Distinguishing the Philadelphia chromosome of acute lymphoblastic leukemia from its counterpart in chronic myelogenous leukemia. *N. Engl. J. Med.* 313:51-52.

Rowley, J. D. (1984). Biological implications of consistent chromosomal rearrangements in leukemia and lymphoma. *Cancer Res.* 44:3159-3168.

Rowley, J. D. (1985). Report of the Children's Cancer Study Group. Editorial. *J. Clin. Oncol.* 3:1-2.

Sacchi, N., Watson, D. K., van Kessel, A. H. M. G., Hagemeijer, A., Kersey, J., Drabkin, H. D., Patterson, D., and Papas, T. S. (1986). Hu-*ets*-1 and hu-*ets* genes are transposed in acute leukemias with (4;11) and (8;21) translocations. *Science* 231:379-382.

Sakuii, M., and Sandberg, A. A. (1976). Correlation of karyotypes of clinical features of acute myeloblastic leukemia. *Cancer* 37:285-299.

Sallan, S. E., Weinstein, H. J., and Nathan, D. G. (1981). The childhood leukemias. *J. Pediatr.* 99:678-688.

Second International Workshop on Chromosomes and Leukemia. (1980). *Cancer Genet. Cytogenet.* 2:89-113.

Sen, L., and Borella, L. (1975). Clinical importance of lymphoblasts with T cell markers in childhood acute leukemia. *N. Engl. J. Med.* 292:828-832.

Shaw, M. T. (1978). The distinctive features of acute monocyte leukemia. *Am. J. Hematol.* 4:97-103.

Shaw, M. T., Humphrey, G. B., Lawrence, R., and Fischer, D. B. (1977). Lack of prognostic value of the periodic acid-Schiff reaction and blast cell size in childhood acute lymphocytic leukemia. *Am. J. Hematol.* 2:237-243.

Spitzer, G., Dicke, K. A., Gehan, E. A., Smith, T., McCredie, K. B., Barlogie, B., and Freireich, E. J. (1976). A simplified in vitro classification for prognosis in adult acute leukemias. The application of in vitro results in remission-predictive models. *Blood* 48:795-807.

Spitzer, G., Verma, D. S., Dicke, K. A., and McCredie, K. B. (1978). Culture studies in vitro in human leukemia. *Semin. Hematol.* 15:352-369.

Srivastava, B. I. S., Khan, S. A., and Henderson, E. S. (1976). High terminal deoxynucleotidyl transferase activity in acute myelogenous leukemia. *Cancer Res.* 36:3847-3850.

Stass, S. A., Pui, C.-H., Melvin, S., Rovigatti, U., Williams, D., Motroni, T., and Dahl, G. V. (1984). Sudan black B positive acute lymphoblastic leukaemia. *Br. J. Haematol.* 57:413-421.

Steinberg, P. G., Gaynon, P., Miller, D. R., Reaman, G., Bleyer, A., Finklestein, J., Evans, R. G., Meyers, P., Steinherz, L. J., Sather, H., and Hammond, D. (1986). Improved disease-free survival of children with acute lymphoblastic leukemia at high risk of early relapse with the New York regiman—A new intensive therapy protocol: A report from the Children's Cancer Study Group. *J. Clin. Oncol.* 4:744-752.

Stone, R. M., Maguire, M. E., Goldberg, M. A., Antin, J. H., Rosenthal, D. S., and Mayer, R. J. (1985). Acute promyelocytic leukemia (APL): Complete remission (CR) can occur without bone marrow aplasia. *Blood* 66:720 (abst).

Third International Workshop on Chromosomes in Leukemia. (1983). Chromosomal abnormalities and their clinical significance in acute lymphoblastic leukemia. *Cancer Res.* 43:868-873.

Tobelem, G., Jacquillat, C., Chastang, C., Auclerc, M. F., Lechevallier, T., Weil, M., Daniel, M. T., Flandrin, G., Harrousseau, J. L., Schaison, G., Boiron, M., and Bernard, J. (1980). Acute monoblastic leukemia: a clinical and biologic study of 74 cases. *Blood* 55:71-76.

Tricot, G., Broeckaert-Van Orshaven, A., Van Hoof, A., and Verwilghen, R. L. (1982). Suden black B positivity in acute lymphoblastic leukaemia. *Br. J. Haematol.* 51:615-621.

van Eys, J., Pullen, J., Head, D., Boyett, J., Crist, W., Falletta, J., Humphrey, G., Jackson, J., Riccardi, V., and Brock, B. (1986). The French-American-British (FAB) classification of leukemia. *Cancer* 57:1046-1051.

Vecchi, V., Rosito, P., Vivarelli, F., Mancini, A. F., Pession, A., Paolucci, G. (1980). *Br. J. Hematol.* 45:178-181.

Viana, M. B., Maurer, H. S., and Ferenc, C. (1980). Subclassification of acute lymphoblastic leukaemia in children: analysis of the reproductibility of morphologic criteria and prognostic implications. *Br. J. Haematol.* 44:383-388.

Vincent, P. C., Sutherland, R., Bardley, M., Lind, D., and Gunz, F. W. (1977). Marrow culture studies in adult acute leukemia at presentation and during remission. *Blood* 49:903-912.

Vogler, L. B., Crist, W. M., Brockman, D. E., Pearl, E. R., Lawton, A. R., and Cooper, M. D. (1978). Pre-B-cell leukemia: A new phenotype of childhood lymphoblastic leukemia. *N. Engl. J. Med.* 298:872-878.

Vowels, M. R., and Willoughby, M. L. N. (1973). Cyclic chemotherapy in acute lymphoblastic leukemia of childhood. 5-year survivals. *Arch. Dis. Child.* 48: 436-440.

Wagner, V. M., and Baehner, R. L. (1979). Correlations of the FAB morphologic criteria and prognosis in acute lymphocytic leukemia of childhood. *Am. J. Ped. Hem. Oncol.* 1:103-106.

Williams, D. L., Look, A. T., Melvin, S. L., Roberson, P. K., Dahl, G. V., Flake, T., and Stass, S. (1984). New chromosomal translocations correlate with specific immunophenotypes of childhood acute lymphoblastic leukemia. *Cell* 36:101-109.

Williams, D. L., Harber, J., Murphy, S. B., Look, A. T., Kalwinsky, D. K., Rivera, G., Melvin, S. L., Stass, S., and Dahl, G. V. (1986). Chromosomal translocations play a unique role in influencing prognosis in childhood acute lymphoblastic leukemia. *Blood* 68:205-212.

Winick, N., Steinherz, P. G., and Miller, D. R. (1985). Terminal deoxynucleotidyl transferase activity in childhood leukemia. *Cancer* 55:1943-1947.

Woods, W. G., Nesbit, N. E., Buckley, J., Lampkin, B. C., McCreadie, S., Kim, T. H., Piomelli, S., Kersey, J. H., Feig, S., Bernstein, I., and Hammond, D. (1985). Correlation of chromosome abnormalities with patient characteristics, histologic subtype and induction success in children with adult nonlymphoblastic leukemia. *J. Clin. Oncol.* 3:3-11.

Yunis, J. J., Bloomfield, C. D., and Ensrud, B. S. (1981). All patients with acute nonlymphocytic leukemia may have a chromosomal defect. *N. Engl. J. Med.* 305:135-139.

14

Leukemic Cell Characterization.

Clinical and Therapeutic Implications in Adult Acute Leukemia

MICHAEL J. KEATING *The University of Texas System Cancer Center, M. D. Anderson Hospital and Tumor Institute, Houston, Texas*

Great effort has been applied over many years to classify leukemia. The broad classifications into acute and chronic categories, and subsequently lymphoid, myeloid, and monocytic leukemia have been applied over at least 50 years. However, until 1960 most reports on the treatment of acute leukemia (AL) did not subclassify the results by even the broadest lymphoid and myeloid subclasses (1). A major reason for this omission was the lack of effective treatment for any form of AL at that time. Subcategorization into age groups was at least as meaningful as the morphologic subtype; responses, when they did occur, were more common in children (2).

Over the last quarter-century, major new therapies have been developed; patients of all age groups are able to achieve a remission with prospects of long-term survival. This has created a need for clinicians to identify the patients who benefit from present-day treatment for AL. As described in earlier chapters, a variety of tools are now available to characterize the leukemic cell. While these tools have brought us closer to an understanding of the biology and etiology of AL, they have, in addition, had a significant impact on identifying prognostic subgroups.

The most widely used initial classification of AL was into lymphoid (acute lymphoblastic leukemia, ALL) and myeloid (acute myelogenous leukemia, AML). The clinical significance of this classification, apart from the younger age of patients with ALL, was the different probability of response of these subtypes to some of the first therapeutically effective agents to be discovered. Vincristine, corticosteroids, and L-asparaginase are more effective in ALL than in AML. However, even within these morphologic subtypes, age is still an important factor; younger patients have a more favorable prognosis. Newer techniques such as use of surface markers and cytogenetic analysis have enabled investigators to further unravel the interrelationship of age, morphologic subtype, and response;

increasingly the age effect is being understood to be the result of a different incidence of subtypes of AL in different age categories (3,4).

Most clinical research protocols for treatment of AL are specifically designed for ALL or AML (also called acute nonlymphocytic leukemia, ANLL). With special stains, surface markers, and cytogenetic and electron microscopic studies, increasingly fewer patients cannot be classified as ALL or AML and are called *acute undifferentiated leukemia* (*AUL*). At the same time an increasing number of patients have been found to have simultaneous involvement of both lymphoid and myeloid cell lines (5). If separate populations of these cells exist which are lymphoid or myeloid, the term *biphenotypic leukemia* is used. However, dual-labeling studies have shown that individual cells can demonstrate both myeloid and lymphoid characteristics; some terms used for this phenomenon are *mixed lineage leukemia, lineage infidelity* and *lineage promiscuity* (6). For the purpose of this chapter, the clinical and therapeutic implications of cell characterization will be discussed for AML and ALL separately. Mixed-lineage leukemias will also be discussed.

I. ACUTE MYELOGENOUS LEUKEMIA (AML)

The need for the term *nonlymphocytic leukemia*, if it ever existed, has passed. Technologic advances have allowed the vast majority of cases of AL to be definitively assigned to the AML or ALL subcategories. For the last ten years, hematopathologists have been using the French-American-British (FAB) classification to classify AML into 6 subcategories, M1-M6 (7). In earlier chapters it was pointed out that M1 and M2 were cases of acute myeloblastic leukemia (AMbL) with

Table 1 Incidence and Response Rate According to FAB Subgroup in Selected Series

<table>
<tr><th></th><th colspan="2">Sultan</th><th colspan="2">Passe</th><th colspan="2">Bennett</th><th colspan="2">Mertelsman</th><th colspan="2">MDAH</th></tr>
<tr><th>FAB group</th><th>N</th><th>%CR</th><th>N</th><th>%CR</th><th>N</th><th>%CR</th><th>N</th><th>%CR</th><th>N</th><th>%CR</th></tr>
<tr><td>M1</td><td>27</td><td>59</td><td>10</td><td>50</td><td rowspan="2">113</td><td rowspan="2">49</td><td>18</td><td>50</td><td>79</td><td>58</td></tr>
<tr><td>M2</td><td>25</td><td>60</td><td>26</td><td>65</td><td>57</td><td>58</td><td>95</td><td>58</td></tr>
<tr><td>M3</td><td>19</td><td>63</td><td>10</td><td>30</td><td>30</td><td>50</td><td>31</td><td>65</td><td>31</td><td>65</td></tr>
<tr><td>M4</td><td>13</td><td>38</td><td>7</td><td>71</td><td>108</td><td>59</td><td>16</td><td>88</td><td>84</td><td>67</td></tr>
<tr><td>M5</td><td>14</td><td>36</td><td>22</td><td>50</td><td>22</td><td>32</td><td>65</td><td>49</td><td>28</td><td>79</td></tr>
<tr><td>M6</td><td>–</td><td>–</td><td>–</td><td>–</td><td>8</td><td>38</td><td>6</td><td>67</td><td>2</td><td>50</td></tr>
</table>

MDAH = M. D. Anderson Hospital.
CR = Complete remission.

varying degrees of differentiation, M3 was the equivalent of acute promyelocytic leukemia (APL), M4 of acute myelomonocytic leukemia (AMML), M5 of acute monocytic leukemia (AMoL), M6 of acute erythroleukemia (EL). The FAB classification of AML will now be discussed as regards its clinical significance.

A. FAB Classification

In the initial FAB proposal (7), 50% or greater myeloblasts were required for a diagnosis of AML; this number has subsequently been reduced to 30% (8). The patients who have less than 30% blasts in the bone marrow are considered to have a myelodysplastic syndrome. Substantial difficulties in concordance rates for the subcategories M1-M6 have been noted within single studies and the variation in the proportion of patients in the subcategories in different studies is also marked

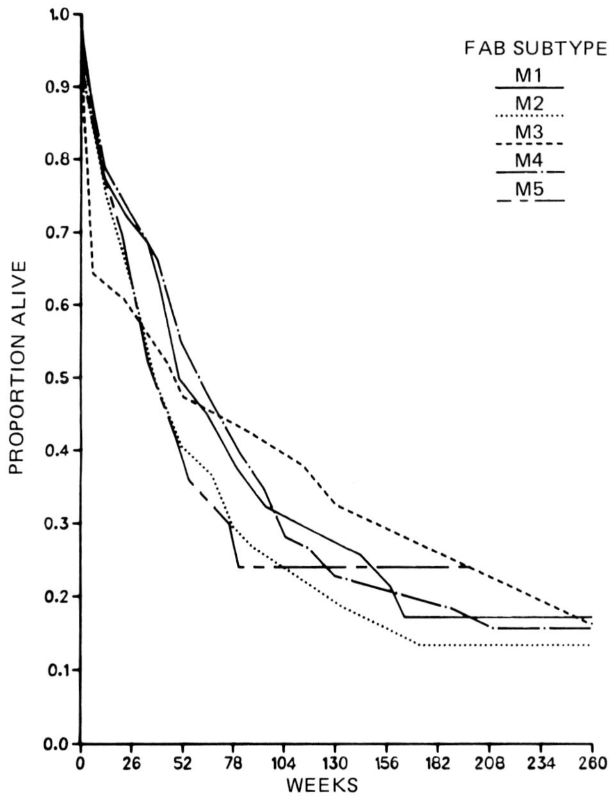

Figure 1 Survival of AML patients treated at the M. D. Anderson Hospital between 1975 and 1985, according to FAB subtypes.

(Table 1). The complete remission (CR) rates in the studies reported vary widely within each subcategory. In the M. D. Anderson Hospital (MDAH) series there was no significant difference in CR rate, CR duration, or survival between the various subsets although there is a suggestion of a higher porportion of long-term survivors in the M3 category (Figure 1) and shorter CR durations for the M5 patients (Figure 2).

Several reports have described the influence of Auer rods on survival and complete remission rate (Figure 3). Mertelsmann evaluated the interrelationship of Auer rod status with the FAB classification (42). The major impact of Auer rod status within the M2 subgroup was confirmed in the MDAH series. The majority of patients with a translocation between chromosomes number 8 and number 21 t(8;21) (q22;q22) are in the M2 category and this favorably influences survival. Other cytogenetic subgroups closely associated with the FAB classification are

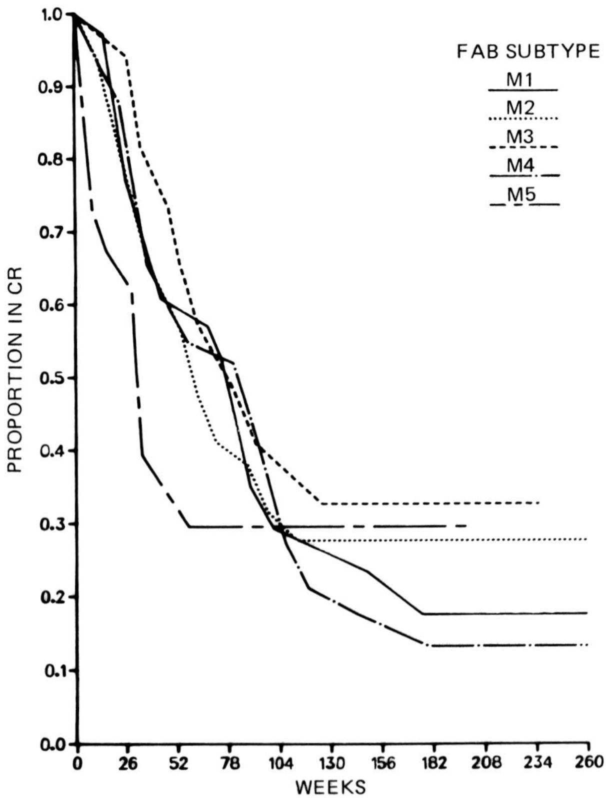

Figure 2 Remission duration of all AML patients treated at the M. D. Anderson Hospital between 1975 and 1985, according to FAB subtype.

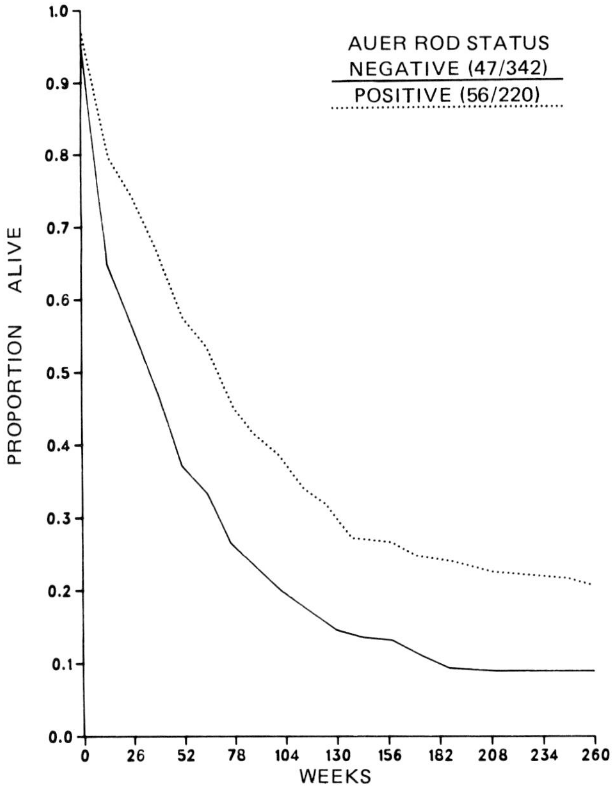

Figure 3 Survival of AML patients treated at the M. D. Anderson Hospital between 1975 and 1985, according to Auer rod status.

t(15;17)(q22;q21) in M3, inv(16)(p13;q22) in M4 with dysplastic eosinophils (M4e) and abnormalities involving the breakpoint q23 in chromosome number 11 with M5.

While the FAB classification has been useful in providing fixed, although arbitrary, guidelines for classification, the relatively poor reproducibility even among experienced hematopathologists limits its usefulness (9). The recent proposal for an M7 category for acute megakaryocytic leukemia (AMegaL) and further guidelines to separate erythroleukemia from myelodysplastic syndrome require clinical validation (10).

B. Cytogenetic Patterns

The introduction of banding techniques (Giemsa and quinacrine are most commonly used) allowed the accurate identification of all 22 pairs of chromosomes

Table 2 Correlation of FAB Subgroups with Cytogenetic Categories (MDAH)

		Percent in Each Subgroup					
Karyotype	N	M1	M2	M3	M4	M5	M6
Diploid	134	23	32	3	31	10	1
t(8;21)	18	11	84	0	6	0	0
t(15;17)	21	0	5	95	0	0	0
inv(16)	17	0	0	0	94	6	0
+8	19	21	21	—	26	32	0
-5,-7	34	41	41	—	15	0	3
Misc.	40	20	30	3	30	18	0
Total	283	24	30	10	26	9	1

and sex chromosomes. Numeric and structural abnormalities in AML have been demonstrated conclusively to be nonrandom; several cytogenetic abnormalities have been demonstrated to have unique clinico-cytogenetic syndromes. Specific translocations or inversions that are commonly found in AML are t(8;21), t(15;17), and inv16. Each is present in 5-10% of cases (11,12). Less common abnormalities are the presence of the Philadelphia chromosome, t(9;22)(q34;q11), and deletion or translocations involving 11q23 and t(6;9)(q23;q34).

The most common numeric changes include the addition of a number 8 chromosome (trisomy 8) or loss of all or part of chromosomes 5 and/or 7 (-5,-7; 5q-, 7q-). These abnormalities are common in secondary leukemia and myelodysplastic syndromes (13) and have been reportedly associated with occupational exposure to mutagens (14).

New techniques can produce elongated chromosomes, increasing the number of bands available for analysis; these have allowed for the detection of subtle changes in cases otherwise described as normal. Following such studies, Yunis and others suggested that nearly all patients with AML have a cytogenetic abnormality (15). The majority of the additional changes described using the extended-metaphase techniques have had subtle rearrangements or deletions and no new common karyotypic abnormalities with well-defined clinical or prognostic significance have been discovered so far.

t(8;21)(q22;q22)—usually M2 morphology. This specific abnormality was well described prior to the use of banding techniques as a complex abnormality (-C, +D, +E, -G) and an association with young age, presence of Auer rods on light microscopy, and nuclear blebs on electron microscopy and good prognosis was described (16). The incidence of this abnormality has been variously reported to be 5-7% in series of adults with AML (11,12) and it is possibly more common in children (17). One series has described an association with extramedullary deposits in 7 out of 30 patients (18). The response to treatment is usually good with a CR rate of approximately 90% usually reported, with a consequent favorable overall survival. In the MDAH series (1975-1986) the CR rate was 32/35 (91%) with a median survival of 18 months. The median CR duration was 16.5 months; 25% of all patients and 30% of the complete responding patients were long-term survivors (Figures 4 and 5).

A substantial proportion of patients with t(8;21) show a loss of an X or Y chromosome. Initial reports suggested that this was an adverse prognostic factor, but recent data does not support this conclusion. Similarly a group of patients who had a normal karyotype apart from loss of a Y chromosome did not demonstrate

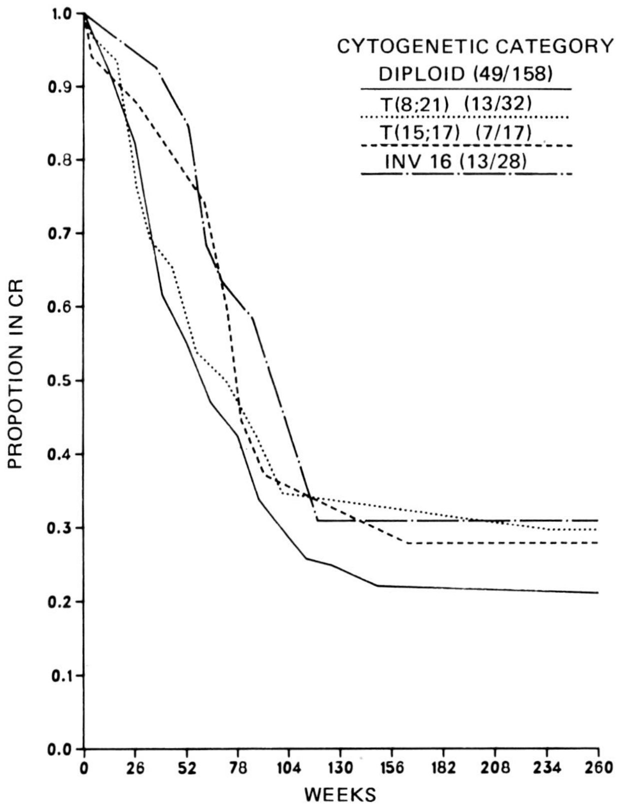

Figure 4 CR duration of diploid and favorable cytogenetic pattern in AML patients treated at the M. D. Anderson Hospital (1975-1985).

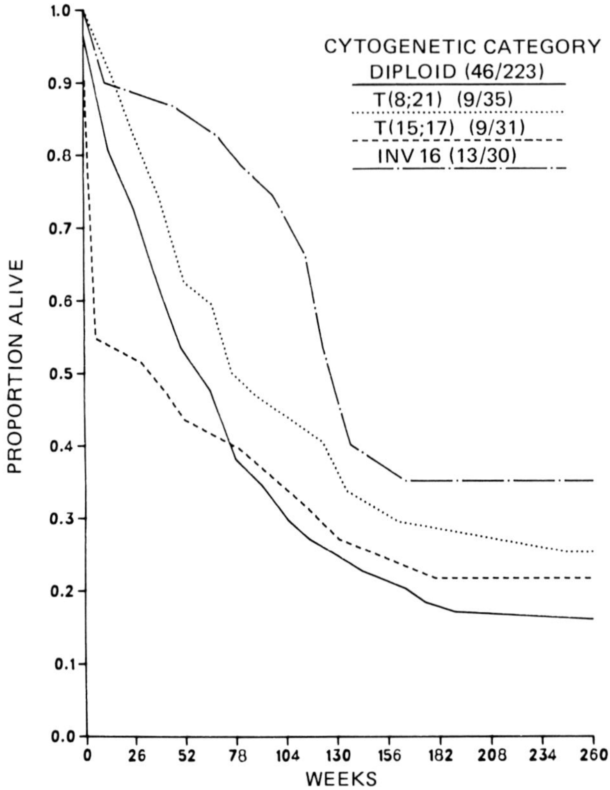

Figure 5 Survival of diploid and favorable cytogenetic patterns in AML patients treated at the M. D. Anderson Hospital (1975-1985).

any prognostic disadvantage when compared to patients with a diploid karyotype.

t(15;17)(q22;q21)–usually M3 morphology. Acute promyelocytic leukemia (APL) has been recognized to be a characteristic clinical syndrome since the 1970s, when the initial descriptions and promising therapeutic results were reported by Bernard (19). The association of a specific cytogenetic abnormality t(15;17) with APL has further clarified this clinical syndrome (20). In most series, more than 80% of patients with APL have the t(15;17) abnormality and patients with t(15;17) without the classical morphologic picture of APL have been shown to have characteristic microgranules in the cytoplasm on electron microscopy and are described as a microgranular variant of APL (21). The incidence of t(15;17) reported in the Fourth International Workshop on Chromosomes in

Leukemia (4th IWCL) was 65% (11); it was 73% in the MDAH series (22) and 100% in a recent series from Chicago (23).

Fatal intracranial and intrapulmonary hemorrhage is a major risk for patients with APL, most strikingly in the first two weeks after initiation of treatment (25-30%). The risk of bleeding is higher in patients with a low fibrinogen level, low platelet count, low hemoglobin, high circulating blast cell count, and advanced age (22). Heparin has been recommended for prevention of hemorrhage in APL but in many instances has not been successful.

The incidence of chemotherapy resistance is low in patients with t(15;17), yet the rate of cytoreduction is slow with a characteristic pattern of obtaining CR without a phase of marrow hypoplasia (24). Whether this pattern is due to leukemic cell differentiation is not known, but it is unlikely. While occasional reports in small patient series have given better results, the overall CR rate is probably 55-70% (22). Since Bernard's initial study, anthracyclines have been considered to be an essential ingredient of remission induction therapy, but recent results with amsacrine- (AMSA) containing regimens appears to be at least as effective (25).

Patients who obtain a CR have a high probability of staying in long-term remission. Two recent studies have reported that the use of 6-mercaptopurine and methotrexate in postremission therapy is associated with a greater likelihood of long-term remission (26,27).

inv(16)–M4 with eosinophilia. An increased number of eosinophils in the diagnostic bone marrow was noted to be a favorable prognostic factor for long-term survival in 1979 (28). Subsequently abnormalities in chromosome 16, whether a pericentric inversion or a deletion or a translocation, were found to be associated with dysplastic eosinophils of characteristic morphology (29,30). The blast cells were almost always of M4 morphology and the blasts and abnormal eosinophils have nuclear blebs on electron microscopy. The eosinophils differ morphologically from those in association with other karyotypes.

The clinical pattern of patients with inv16 is characteristic. The patient is usually young, with a high white blood cell count at diagnosis and a high incidence of hepatosplenomegaly. The CR rate is high (>90%) with long remission duration and a high incidence of long-term survivors. Surprisingly, there is a high probability of central nervous system leukemia (approximately 30%) with mass lesions being noted on CT scans of the brain (31). Other sites of extramedullary disease are not common but do occur. The CNS lesions are closely correlated with marrow relapse but can be effectively treated in some cases by high-dose cytosine arabinoside (ara-C) with or without cranial radiation (32). Upon relapse these patients have a good chance of obtaining second or third remissions.

t(9;22)(q34;q11)–Philadelphia-chromosome-positive AML. The Philadelphia (Ph^1) chromosome was initially thought to be found only in association with chronic myelogenous leukemia (CML) but is now known to be a common cytogenetic change in ALL. Less frequently, the Ph^1 is present at diagnosis in patients who present with AML without a preceding history suggestive of CML (33). Debate concinues as to whether these patients have CML with blast crisis emerging early and causing the initial clinical problem which brings the patient to the attention of the physician. Many series of patients reported in clinical trials omit these patients from analysis on the basis that they are CML patients in blast crisis.

The usual patient with Ph^1-positive AML is young and presents with a high white blood cell count and prominent hepatosplenomegaly, and has a high probability of failing to obtain a complete remission due to chemotherapy resistance (34,35). Surface marker studies suggest that the cells of several of these patients display both myeloid and lymphoid markers (35). Many of the patients have additional chromosome changes; an association with loss of chromosome 7 was reported in one series (34).

Abnormalities of chromosome 11q23 (abn11q23)–usually M5. Several different translocations have been described which share the feature of involving chromosome 11 with a breakpoint at q23; other cases are deletions of 11 at the same breakpoint. Most of these cases are classified as M4 or M5. One translocation t(4;11)(q21;q23) has been predominantly reported in ALL, but several of these cases appear to be biphenotypic, with monocytic differentiation being present (36). The incidence of abn11q23 in AML reported at the 4th International Workshop on Chromosomes in Leukemia (4th IWCL) was 4.2% (11); 70% were M5 and 17% were M4. Twelve percent of patients less than 20 years of age had abn11q23 versus only 3% of adults. Forty percent of all M5 cases had abn11q23; the abnormality was more marked in the monoblastic M5a cases than the more differentiated M5b cases. The CR rate was 8/15 (53%) with a median CR duration of only 5 months and a median survival of 9 months (11). In other series only 4/9 and 5/9 obtained CRs (37).

Abn11q23 appears to be clearly associated with monocytic differentiation in AML and has been associated with the Hu-ets-1 oncogene. The incidence appears to be low except in one series using high-resolution banding techniques, where 9/105 had abn11q23 (15). Overall prognosis appears to be poor.

Loss or deletion of chromosomes 5 or 7 (−5, −7; 5q−, 7q−). Loss of all or part of chromosomes 5 or 7 is common in AML (11,12), occurring in 11.8% of all cases of the 4th IWCL (11). Frequently, changes in other chromosomes occurred in conjunction with these abnormalities. Unlike the other abnormalities described above, the deletion in chromosomes 5 or 7 were not consistent and were noted at more than one breakpoint. These changes were more common in secondary leukemia than in de novo acute leukemia and were more common in patients who were older and had a preceding myelodysplastic syndrome. The response rate was low with a short CR duration and survival (Figures 6 and 7).

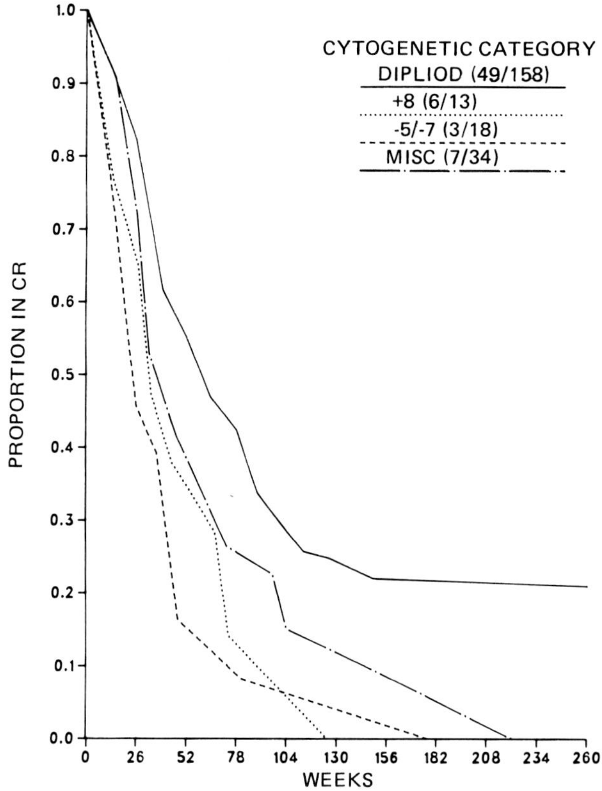

Figure 6 CR duration of diploid and unfavorable cytogenetic pattern in AML patients treated at the M. D. Anderson Hospital (1975-1985).

Trisomy 8. Addition of chromosome 8 is the most common change in hyperdiploid patients with AML, either as the sole abnormality or in conjunction with other changes (11,12). This abnormality shows many of the prognostic clinical features associated with abnormalities of chromosomes 5 and 7 and is also associated with secondary leukemia and myelodysplastic syndromes. The prognosis, although poor, is not as grave as patients with abnormalities in chromosomes 5 or 7.

Miscellaneous abnormalities. Several other karyotypic changes have been described in AML, but in insufficient numbers to be defined as to their prognostic roles, such as t(6;9)(p23;q34) (38), which is associated with marrow basophilia, trisomy 21, isochromosome 17q, etc. (11). With increasing accrual of data on such patients, the prognostic impact of these changes should be better defined.

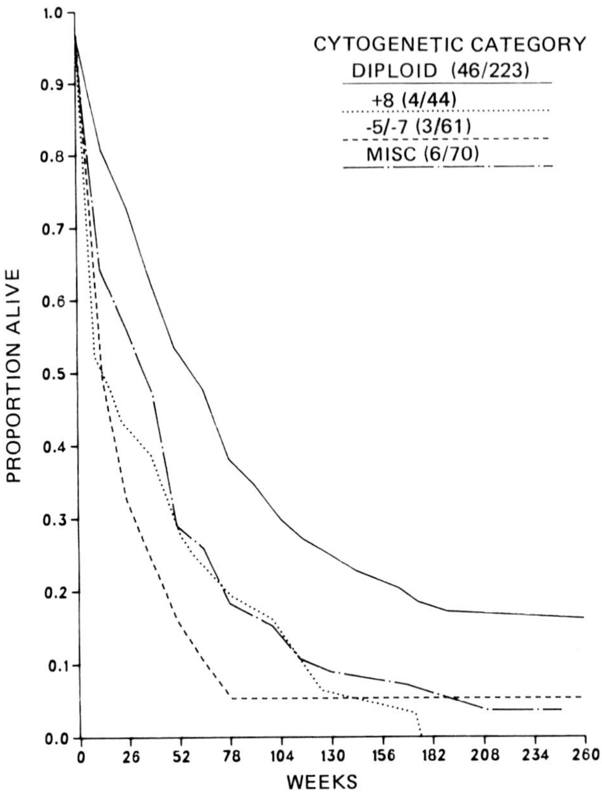

Figure 7 Survival of diploid and unfavorable cytogenetic patterns in AML patients treated at the M. D. Anderson Hospital (1975-1985).

C. Interrelationships of Cytogenetic Groups and Other Other Prognostic Characteristics

Several clinical characteristics have been correlated with survival and response to chemotherapy in AML. The most consistent of these have been age, history of an antecedent hematologic disorder (AHD) or myelodysplastic syndrome, previous malignancy or radiation or chemotherapy (secondary leukemia), temperature, organ function, performance status and extent of disease (11). The cytogenetic patterns are strongly associated with several of these factors, as shown in Table 3.

In both the 4th IWCL and the MDAH series, the cytogenetic findings were categorized in an hierarchial fashion (11,12). The MDAH classification initially identified the patients who are normal, and those with specific abnormalities such as t(8;21), t(9;22), t(15;17), inv(16), and abn11q23. Then patients were

Table 3 Correlation of Cytogenetic Groups with Prognostically Important Clinical Characteristics

		Proportion with clinical characteristics						
Characteristics	Value	inv(16)	t(8;21)	t(15;17)	Diploid	+8	−5/−7	Misc.
Age (yrs.)	> 50	.20	.27	.17	.55	.59	.67	.56
Sex	Male	.66	.57	.63	.55	.71	.61	.50
AHD	Yes	.23	.13	.07	.23	.46	.43	.24
Prior malignancy	Yes	.11	.03	.07	.11	.11	.30	.13
WBC (/cμmm)	>25,000	.29	.76	.20	.49	.34	.39	.46
Bilirubin (mg%)	⩾ 1	.09	.03	.37	.21	.34	.13	.21
Creatinine (mg%)	⩾ 1.4	.06	.02	.20	.17	.21	.21	.21
Liver	⩾ 5 cm	.14	.20	.17	.24	.39	.29	.26
Spleen	Palpable	.11	.33	.10	.21	.39	.23	.20
Auer rods	Yes	.97	.23	.80	.41	.16	.10	.26
Total No.		35	30	30	223	44	61	70

Table 4 Response Rate for Cytogenetic Subcategories During Different Time Periods

	N (%)		
Response rate	1975-79	1980-82	1983-85
Favorable			
t(8;21)	16/17 (94%)	9/10 (90%)	7/8 (88%)
inv(16)	10/11 (91%)	9/10 (90%)	9/9 (100%)
Intermediate			
Diploid	58/89 (65%)	65/86 (76%)	35/45 (78%)
45X,-Y	3/5 (60%)	3/4 (75%)	1/1 (100%)
t(15;17)	5/8 (63%)	5/12 (42%)	7/11 (64%)
Unfavorable			
+8	6/16 (38%)	5/15 (33%)	8/13 (62%)
-5/-7	7/24 (29%)	7/19 (37%)	4/17 (24%)
Miscellaneous	12/32 (38%)	11/22 (50%)	11/16 (69%)
Insufficient metaphases	17/35 (49%)	11/19 (58%)	5/9 (56%)

identified who had loss or deletion of chromosome 5 or 7; then addition of chromosome 8. The other patients were classified as "miscellaneous." Some patients have features of two categories such as inv(16) with an additional chromosome 8. In this case the patient was classified as inv(16) in the hierarchial classification. The complete remission (CR) rates, CR duration, and survival curves for all the cytogenetic subcategories are shown in Table 5 and Figures 4-7.

The cytogenetic classification has been shown to be consistent prospectively in the MDAH series and is a powerful tool to use in the design of new studies (Tables 4 and 5). It appears that the majority of long-term survivors are in the inv(16), t(15;17), t(8;21), and diploid groups; very few patients with other cytogenetic changes have a good chance of long-term survival with conventional chemotherapy (Figures 4-7).

One method of dealing with interrelationships has been to do multivariate regression analyses to determine which prognostic factors are most powerful and which are relatively independent of others (39). Using such techniques on the MDAH patient group from 1975-1983, the cytogenetic pattern was found to be the most powerful predictive factor for response to treatment, remission duration, and survival (Table 5). Similarly, the 4th IWCL found the cytogenetic pattern to have independent prognostic importance, after allowing for clinical variables (11).

Table 5 Ranking of Prognostic Variables for Probability of CR, Probability of Staying in CR for One Year, and Probability of Survival

Rank	Probability of CR	Possibility of > 1 yr CR duration	Probability of surviving
1	Cytogenetics	Cytogenetics	Cytogenetics
2	Bilirubin	Pre-Rx neutrophil count	Age
3	AHD	Courses to CR	AHD
4	Age	Albumin	Pre-Rx neutrophil count
5	Hemoglobin	Sex	Bilirubin
6	Temperature	Age	Albumin
7	Fibrinogen		
8	% Aneuploid cells		
9	Prior malignancy		

Data from studies at M. D. Anderson Hospital from 1975-1983.
AHD = Antecedent hematologic disorder
CR = Complete remission

D. Surface Marker Analysis

A large number of surface antigens can now be identified on the surface of normal and abnormal hemopoietic cells, as discussed in earlier chapters. These antigens are usually lineage-specific in normal cells and are present on the surface of myeloid or lymphoid cells. The antigens are expressed at different phases of hemopoietic differentiation. Several antigens appear to be expressed on cells of monocytic or granulocytic differentiation, while others are shared by both lines.

The FAB classification is an attempt to categorize the lineage of leukemic cells. Studies that attempt to compare surface antigen expression with FAB category are now being completed and immunophenotype is being used to supplement conventional diagnostic criteria. In a series of 100 consecutive patients with AL, immunophenotype made a major contribution to the final hematologic diagnosis in 19 cases (40). Obviously, this decision is of critical importance as most investigators treat AML and ALL with different regimens; this assignment is the major usefulness of surface antigen analysis at this time.

Interesting findings are available on surface antigen expression at various stages of differentiation; incidence figures for a variety of antigens in AML also are becoming available. Little has been published regarding the prognostic significance of AML, however. Griffin has reported on the preliminary findings of a study of

17 monoclonal antibodies in 196 patients with AML for the Cancer and Leukemia Group B (41). The antibodies used were anti Ia, MY4, MY7, MY8, MY9, MY10, Mo1, Mo2, MCS-1, PMN-81, AML-2-23, T101, T11, B1, J5, MY1, and B4. The frequency of positive reactions for the ALL antibodies T101, T11, B1, B4, and J5 was less than 5%. The frequency of positive reactions for the AML antibodies varied according to the FAB group; AML-2-23, PMN-81, Mo1 and Ia antigen expression were low in the FAB group M3; MY4 and MY8 were high in the FAB groups M4 and M5. While the FAB classification did not correlate with CR rate, MY4 and MY7 expression are adverse prognostic factors. One-third of patients had expression of neither MY4 nor MY7 and a CR rate of 82% was found in such patients. The immunophenotype and FAB classification did not correlate in half of the cases.

As the immunophenotype does not correlate with age, it is possible that it will provide independent prognostic information, which can be used in the design and analysis of clinical trials that could investigate the usefulness of different regimens in specific subsets of patients. Correlation with the common cytogenetic groups in AML should provide useful information.

E. Terminal Transferase (TdT)

Terminal deoxynucleotidyl transferase (TdT) is a polymerizing enzyme which catalyzes the addition of deoxyribonucleotide triphosphates to the 3'OH end of deoxynucleotide precursors without requiring a template. TdT is present in most cases of ALL; it is also present in 10-20% of cases of AML, although at a lower level (42,43). The CR rate has been reported to be lower in AML that has detectable TdT activity (TdT+) than TdT− cases in one study (21/40, 53% vs 69/99, 70%)(42). A poor prognosis (2 CRs of 11 evaluable patients) was noted by Bradstock et al. (43) in patients with detectable TdT activity. Contradictory data have been observed by Skoog et al., who found that the TdT+ AML patients had a higher CR rate and longer survival than TdT− patients (44). The Skoog study quantitated the level of TdT/microgram of DNA. The response rate for patients less than 60 years of age in the Skoog study was 10/12 (83%) for TdT+ patients and 7/18 (39%) for TdT− patients. At the MDAH (45) 19% of AML patients are TdT+ and the CR rate, CR duration, and survival are not significantly different for the two groups of patients: 96/153 (63%) CRs for TdT+ patients vs 19/35 (54%) for TdT− patients.

TdT activity in leukemic cells, while useful in separating ALL from AML, appears to be of uncertain usefulness as a prognostic characteristic. Whether the divergent results in various studies is due to differences in technique needs to be clarified.

F. Glucocorticoid Receptors

The response rate to glucocorticoids is lower in AML than in ALL for both children and adults. This clinical observation would suggest, in view of the correlation between estrogen receptors and response in breast cancer, that the number of glucocorticoid receptors present is lower in AML than in ALL. Recent studies, however, show that the number of receptors are the same in AML and ALL (46, 47). Reports of abnormal receptors in AML are probably due to sensitivity to proteolysis of the receptor-steroid complex, as in AML the level of activated complexes is low and the level of meroreceptors (proteolytic receptor fragments) is increased (48).

The glucocorticoid receptor level in AML was found to be equal to that of ALL in a group of 43 pediatric patients; it did not correlate with any clinical characteristics or with response to treatment, CR duration, or survival (46). Data from Skoog et al. in adults (44) are contradictory to this; Skoog found a higher CR rate and longer survival in patients with glucocorticoid receptors, especially if they were TdT+. These patients were not treated with glucocorticoids (44). Thus controversy persists as to the effect of TdT positivity and the level of glucocorticoid receptors on prognosis in AML.

G. Growth in Semisolid Media

Following the development of techniques for growing leukemic cells in agar, different laboratories sought to identify the clinical relevance of the growth characteristics. Initially, groups of cells greater than 40 in number were called *colonies* and smaller aggregates were called *clusters*. Normal bone marrow produced both colonies and clusters. The marrow of patients with AML grew few or no colonies and the number of clusters were either more or fewer than that of normals. The clusters were predominantly small (<20 cells) or large (20-40 cells). The initial report suggested that a pattern of small cluster growth was favorable (49). A later study (50) found good CR rates for patients with no growth or residual normal growth (4/6, 67%) or small cluster growth (26/35, 74%) and a poor CR rate in patients who grew large clusters (4/17, 23%). Separate studies emphasized the poor results in AML if more than 50 colonies or clusters were present after 14 days in culture (1/15, 7%) (51). A further report suggests a lower CR rate for patients with a large number of colonies or clusters and for clusters with more than 20 cells (52). These data suggest that if the leukemic cells are proliferative or clonogenic, the outcome of treatment is less likely to be successful.

More recently, McCulloch has applied the concept of secondary plating efficiency (PE2) to clinical studies. In the PE2 assay, cells from primary cultures of peripheral blood mononuclear cells in AML are pooled and replated. The number of colonies per 10^4 cells put into secondary cultures is then scored. The PE2 was the most powerful predictive test in a series of 45 patients, supporting the concept of a poor prognosis for highly clonogenic leukemic cells (53). A major problem in all these studies is the lack of standardization of the growth stimuli used and the variability of the arbitrary cut-points for colonies/clusters, etc. The true clinical impact of the culture techniques and their interactions with other clinical and biologic characteristics should be clarified when defined growth factors produced by recombinant DNA technology are applied.

H. Flow Cytometry in AML

Early studies of cytokinetics in AML used the cumbersome thymidine incorporation labeling index (LI), using autoradiography as a measure of the proportion of cells in S phase. Animal studies using highly clonogenic transplantable leukemia had demonstrated a positive association of cell kill with the proportion of cells undergoing DNA synthesis and as human acute leukemia was thought to be a highly proliferative tumor, drugs with preferential cytotoxic effect on cells in cycle were developed for clinical use. Studies of cell cycle in human AML have now established that AML is heterogenous and overall the leukemic blood cells have a lower labeling index (low S-phase percent) than do normal blast cells. The transit time and generation time of AML cells are prolonged and many cells appear to be in G_0 or prolonged G_1 phase.

Early studies suggest that a high percentage of cells in S phase correlated with a higher CR rate (54,55) but several studies are in conflict with these findings (56,57,58); at the present time no firm association with cytokinetic parameters and response has been found in AML. A significant weakness in most early studies has been the fact that bone marrow aspirates were used, which have variable degrees of dilution with peripheral blood, the cells of which have a lower S-phase percentage than blast cells from marrow biopsy specimens (58).

Two recent studies using flow cytometry have reported that while the percent of cells in $S + G_2 + M$ is not a significant prognostic factor for response in patients less than 50 years of age, a high percentage of cells in $S + G_2 + M$ is an adverse prognostic factor for older patients (59,60). This appeared to be most striking in older patients with cytogenetic abnormalities, and not for diploid patients (60). Additionally, cases with a high proportion of cells with a low protein content who were over the age of 50 years have a better survival (59). This finding presumably applies also to a low RNA content.

Flow cytometry does not give any information on generation time of leukemic cells. The high $S + G_2 + M$ in older patients may reflect a longer generation time. On the other hand, older patients have been reported to have several other differences from young patients, such as excessive growth in semisolid media and low surface antigenicity (61). Increasingly, the adverse effect of age on prognosis appears to be due to differences in the type of leukemia which can occur in the elderly.

I. Cell-Drug Interactions in AML

The major active drugs in AML are cytosine arabinoside (ara-C), the anthracyclines such as daunorubicin, adriamycin, rubidazone, and mAMSA. Several in vitro studies have been performed to attempt to predict the drugs' effects on outcome in clinical studies occurring at the same time. Most of these studies were performed on patients treated with a combination of drugs. The results have not demonstrated a strong correlation of in vitro and clinical outcome.

Some single-drug studies have provided interesting results, however. One study demonstrated a correlation between CR rate and the ratio of daunorubicin reductase in leukemic cells compared to that in red blood cells (62). Additionally, high retention of arabanosyl-cytosine ariphosphate (ara-CTP) in leukemic cells incubated in vitro was found to predict for long remission duration (63). Lack of inhibition of thymidine incorporation by leukemic cells after incubation with ara-C in vitro correlated with failure to respond to high dose ara-C (64), as did a low percent of cells in S phase (65).

In vivo studies have shown that a short half-life, low area under the curve (concentration X time), and low 12-hour level of ara-CTP in leukemic cells after a 2-hour infusion of 3 grams/m^2 predicts for failure to respond to high-dose ara-C (66). Another interesting clinical association is the significantly higher response rate to AMSA in AML patients whose cells have Auer rods present than for Auer-rod-negative patients (67). Cellular pharmacologic characteristics of leukemic cells in vivo should provide further keys to prognosis.

J. Age and Prognosis in AML

Previously, the adverse outcome with increasing age in AML has been attributed to poor tolerance of the myelosuppressive effects of therapy. While this is probably true, increasing evidence is accumulating that the leukemic cells in older patients have different karyotypes (12), and are more proliferative, and that having a high proportion of cells in $S + G_2 + M$ is an adverse factor (59,60). The impact of these findings in designing treatments specific to the type of leukemia regardless of age is uncertain. At the other end of the age spectrum, the only major characteristics predicting for a poor outcome in children with AML are loss of chromosome 7 or del(7q) (68) and monocytic morphology (69) particularly abn(11q23). The higher incidence in children of some clinical manifestations of AML suggest that other biologic differences exist, which escape identification with present techniques. Increasingly, evidence suggests that the cell type of leukemia, rather than the age of patient, is the key determinant of outcome.

III. ACUTE LYMPHOBLASTIC LEUKEMIA (ALL)

Most cases of ALL occur in childhood, although 20-25% of adults with AL have this diagnosis (70). The age cutoff for separation between the two groups is variable—from 14 to 20 years in different studies. As childhood and adult cases are treated and usually investigated by different groups, the studies of cellular characteristics are reported separately; the adult and childhood forms of the disease are therefore discussed separately in this chapter.

A. Childhood ALL

Age and the white blood cell count (WBC) were the major prognostic factors in ALL until techniques became available to identify the immunophenotype of the cells. Children between the ages 2 and 10 years have superior outcomes to those on either side of this range. A WBC greater than 25,000/mm^3 has consistently been a negative prognostic feature (71). Several studies were performed prior to immunophenotyping to evaluate the prognostic impact of special stains and morphology, but these have now been superseded by surface marker analysis.

Morphology

The FAB group developed a classification for ALL which separated cases into L1, L2, and L3 (see Chapter 2). L3 cases are very uncommon (approximately 1%) and have been shown to be cases of B-cell leukemia in most instances and to have a very poor prognosis; they are omitted from several studies. In most large series, the proportion of patients with L1 morphology was approximately 80-85%, and L2 was 15-20% (71,72,73). L2 morphology is more common than L1 in adults. In most series, the L1 patients have a superior survival to the L2 patients. After adjusting for age and WBC count, morphology was still significant in two series but not in the third (71,72,73).

Special Stains

The special stains most commonly evaluated as prognostic factors in ALL are the periodic acid-Schiff (PAS) reaction and TdT. PAS positivity does not appear to have prognostic significance. TdT is positive in most cases of ALL except for the B-cell phenotype. In non-B-cell ALL, it appears to have no prognostic significance.

Immunophenotype in Pediatric ALL

If cases are phneotyped using E-rosetting, a pan-T antibody, and tested for the presence of surface immunoglobulin (sIg) or cytoplasmic immunoglobulin (cIg) and for the common ALL antigen (CALLA), they can be classified to be T-cell, B-cell, pre-B, or early pre-B cell. Early pre-B cells are identified by evidence of immunoglobulin gene rearrangement in most cases that are not T-cell, B-cell or pre-B cell leukemia.

B-cell leukemia has a uniformly poor prognosis (75). Results to date indicate that early pre-B patients have the best results, followed by pre-B patients (76). The pre-B patients have a somewhat better early prognosis than those with T-cell ALL. The Pediatric Oncology Group (POG) showed that immunophenotype was an independent prognostic factor after accounting for age, WBC, and risk group (77). Both CNS relapse and bone marrow relapse occur more rapidly in the pre-B cell than in the "null" or early pre-B cell patients (77).

Pre-B cell ALL has been associated with a specific translocation t(1;19)(q23; q13) in a quarter of patients; these pre-B cell patients may have a worse prognosis than those without the abnormality (78,79). Pre-B ALL has clg present.

The term *null cell* has shifted in meaning as new tools for identifying cell lineage have developed. This creates difficulty in comparing previous studies to the present ones. The incidence of this group, who are negative for T- and B-cell markers and are CALLA-negative is approximately 5-10%; the outcome appears to be worse than for early pre-B cell CALLA-positive patients (80,81).

T-cell patients were initially identified by the ability to form rosettes with sheep erythrocytes (E+). A variety of antibodies are available which now identify T-cell-specific antigens. The antibodies also place the cells in the stage of T-cell differentiation—for example early, intermediate, late, or circulating T cell. T-cell leukemia was thought initially to be a very poor prognostic group. However, recently 40% of such patients have been found to stay in prolonged remission (82).

Other markers such as receptors for peanut agglutinin (83), Fc receptor (84) and the C_3 component of complement (85) have been less commonly studied. Although there are reports suggesting a poor outlook for patients whose cells are positive for these markers, their true significance has not been established.

Cytogenetic Pattern in Pediatric ALL

With improved techniques, the majority of children with ALL can now have an adequate cytogenetic analysis of their leukemic cells. Most of the karyotypes of children with ALL have been found to be abnormal (79). The number of known specific translocations and other changes in ALL is rapidly increasing, and their associations with specific immunophenotypes have been defined (78,79). The Third International Workshop on Chromosomes in Leukemia (3rd IWCL) (86) evaluated the prognostic impact of karyotype and found it to be an independent prognostic factor after allowing for age, WBC, FAB type, and immunophenotype. Children with a modal chromosome number greater than 50 had the longest CR duration; those having 47 to 50 chromosomes, 6q− and normal karyotypes were of intermediate CR duration; and those with hypodiploid or pseudodiploid chromosome numbers of translocations t(9;22), t(4;11), or t(8;14) had the shortest CR durations (79,86). The same groups, approximately, had significance for survival times.

The St. Jude's group studied 136 patients with an adequate karyotype analysis (87). Two-thirds of the patients in that study had an abnormal karyotype. Five categories were identified according to modal chromosome number: hyperdiploid >50; hyperdiploid 47-50; pseudodiploid; normal; and hypodiploid. The CR rate was significantly lower in the pseudodiploid group; the hyperdiploid >50 group had the highest CR rate. Survival analysis projected that only 5% of the hyperdiploid >50 patients were likely to fail prior to 30 months, compared with 40% for the hyperdiploid 47-50 or diploid groups, and 85% for the pseudodiploid group. Multivariate analysis showed that the cytogenetic pattern was the strongest prognostic variable and added significantly to the impact of WBC count.

The St. Jude's group has now identified an association of specific karyotypes with immunophenotype. They found 4/16 cases of E-rosette-positive patients had a karyotype t(11;14)(p13;q13); 7/23 patients with pre-B-cell ALL had a t(1;19)(79). The translocations t(2;8), t(8;14), and t(8;22) are known to be associated with B-cell leukemia (79).

The philadelphia chromosome (Ph^1), t(9;22), was found in 6% of cases of pediatric ALL vs 17% in adults by the 3rd IWCL (86). In all reports, this karyotype has a poor prognosis. In addition, the incidence of t(4;11) is approximately 5-6% in both adults and children and has a poor prognosis. This subset of patients, together with the Ph^1-positive patients are now being reported to be biphenotypic in many instances (88,89).

Cell Ploidy Using Flow Cytometry

Using propidium iodide or acridine orange as stains, the amount of DNA per leukemic cell can be compared to a normal diploid reference cell. While variations in stain affinity and other factors can theoretically interefere, the DNA content as measured by flow cytometry (FCM) is roughly proportional to the chromosome number, using cytogenetic analysis as the reference standard. This technique can rapidly screen large numbers of cells and can categorize patients into hypodiploid, diploid (which includes cytogenetically determined pseudodiploid patients), and near-haploid. Multiple leukemic stem cells can also be identified. The DNA index (the ratio of DNA of leukemic cells compared with diploid) has been separated by Look into DNA indices ≥ 1.16, 1.01-1.15, 1.0, and < 1.0. The relative proportion of pediatric ALL patients in these groups are 17%, 9%, 73%, and $< 1\%$ (90,91).

Most of the patients with a DNA index > 1.16 and of 1.01-1.15 are early pre-B patients. Most of the T-cell and pre-B cell patients have a DNA index of 1. Patients with a DNA index > 1.16 have the best prognosis.

Glucocorticoid Receptors

The good response of pediatric ALL to glucocorticoids has stimulated research into the correlation between glucocorticoid receptor (GR) cell number and response to treatment (92,93,94). The GR number is variable and certainly not an absolute predictor of response. However, in single- and multiple-agent studies, the resistant patients have a lower GR number than do CR patients. The GR number of B-cell ALL is very low, which correlates with the poor response to steroid therapy in this group (94). The GR levels are significantly associated with immunophenotype, they are higher in early pre-B ALL than in T-cell ALL; B-cell ALL has the lowest level (94). A significant correlation with CR and the early pre-B group has been found. More intensive treatment programs have been reported to overcome the adverse prognostic impact of a low GR number on CR rate, but have not overcome its effect on the length of the relapse-free interval

(92). Although a decrease in GR number is noted at relapse, the change does not appear sufficient to account for the marked decrease in steroid responsiveness at this time (93).

Cell Kinetics

The labeling index (LI) obtained using ^{3}H-thymidine autoradiography and the percent of cells in S phase using flow cytometry are closely correlated. In a study of 97 children with ALL, a low LI was associated with a high relapse rate, supporting earlier data (95,96). In the latter study, the LI provided prognostic information independent of the WBC count. The percent of cells in S phase (by FCM) was in the following order: B-cell ALL > T-cell ALL > non-B, non-T ALL. The percent of cells in S phase was higher for E-rosette-positive (E+) T-cell ALL than for E-rosette-negative (E−) T-cell patients (95). The percent of cells in S phase was higher for patients with a DNA index > 1 than for a DNA index = 1. However, patients with a DNA index > 1 are reported to have a good prognosis in other studies, which is contradictory to the univariate results with the percent of cells in S phase (95,96). This discordance with the demonstrated impact of LI on prognosis may be related to the observation that hyperdiploid patients with a higher LI have a long DNA synthesis time (97). Thus, the percent of cells in S phase found using FCM is an overestimate of the fractional birth rate of cells, which is lower than normal in ALL. The long DNA synthesis time may increase the susceptibility of the cells to S-phase-specific drugs.

Multivariate Analysis

The multiplicity of prognostic factors that are being identified in AL as newer techniques are applied to clinical samples has created a need to analyze the independence of the cellular characteristics from conventional clinical characteristics such as age and WBC. Multivariate regression analysis techniques are increasingly being applied (71,72,87,92,96) and certainly the chromosome pattern and immunophenotype have emerged as major new prognostic cellular characteristics. The independence of other factors such as GR number, labeling index, percent of cells in S phase, DNA index, etc. needs further clarification, with all techniques being applied to the same patient groups.

B. Adult ALL

The different prognosis for adult ALL compared with childhood ALL has been well documented and reviewed (98,99,100). Several differences in the cellular features of the disease in adults compared with that of children have been noted. The incidence of L1 morphology is lower in adults (30-40%) than in children. L2 morphology (50-60% in adults) and L3 morphology (5-10% in adults) are more common than in children (86,101,102). Even among adults who are CALLA+, the ratio of L1 to L2 is only 1:2. Three-quarters of children are CALLA+, vs only 50% in adults (103,104).

The surface marker phenotypes are less well defined in adult ALL, although in one series using monoclonal antibodies 64% were classified as B lineage (BA1+), 13% T lineage (T101 or OKT11 or 3A1+), 9% unclassified and 7% were positive for AML antigens (MCS2+) (105). The B lineage corresponds to early pre-B and pre-B immunophenotypes, although no studies for cytoplasmic immunoglobulin were performed. CALLA was present in 84% of B-lineage cases and 42% of the T-lineage cases. No definite prognostic information was noted in this study. In another series of 78 patients, the incidence of null cell (CALLA−, T antigen−, E-rosette−, sIg−) was 26%; CALLA+ 56%; pre-T 3% (T+, E-rosette−), T-cell 13%, and mixed lineage 3%. In that study, the T-cell and CALLA+ patients have a significantly longer CR duration than the null ALL group (106).

The incidence of adverse cytogenetic groups such as t(9;22), and abnormalities of 14q [t(8;14), 14q+] are threefold higher in adults with ALL than in children and the incidence of the favorable hyperdiploid group (modal number > 50) is three times less common (86).

The prognostic association with cellular characteristics is not well defined in adults with ALL. No major advantage for L1 over L2 morphology has been found; L3 morphology is considered to be an adverse factor (100). Whereas T-cell disease was formerly thought to be unfavorable, recent data do not support this; T-cell ALL and CALLA+ ALL had similar outcomes. An abnormal karyotype is an adverse factor for adults in ALL after considering age, immunophenotype and WBC.

The Memorial-Sloan Kettering Institute studies (MSKI) noted "no analyzable metaphases" on cytogenetic analysis to be a favorable sign; diploid patients to be intermediate; and t(9;22) and hypodiploid patients to be likely to have an unfavorable outcome (100). A high RNA index on flow cytometry was an adverse factor for CR duration in survival but not CR rate.

Much more data must be accumulated in adult ALL to draw conclusions about the prognostic significance of cellular characteristics. The age effect appears partly to be explained by a difference in incidence of different morphologic, cytogenetic, and immunophenotypic groups.

III. MULTIPLE PHENOTYPES AND MIXED LINEAGES IN ACUTE LEUKEMIA

Until recently, the cells of established leukemia cell lines and of patients with AL were thought to be restricted to either a myeloid or lymphoid lineage. With the availability of enzyme assays for TdT, surface antigen analysis using monoclonal antibodies, and techniques to study immunoglobulin and T-cell receptor rearrangement, more cases have been defined suggesting that both lineages are involved (107-111). If separate cell populations exist, one displaying myeloid and the other lymphoid markers, the term *biphenotypic leukemia* is used (6). *Lineage infidelity, lineage promiscuity* and *mixed lineage* are all terms which have been used to describe situations where there is evidence of single cells displaying involvement of both lineages (5,6,107-111).

When a patient displays involvement of one lineage at diagnosis and another at relapse, the term *lineage switch* has been used to describe it (6). Lineage infidelity can be intralineage (e.g., erythroid and myeloid) or interlineage (lymphoid and myeloid) (107).

Few objective data have been developed regarding the prognostic significance of these events. Smith and McCullough have reported a significantly lower CR rate for AML patients with lineage infidelity (5). Similarly, reports emphasize that two karyotypes, t(4;11) and t(9;22) which have a poor prognosis and are represented in both ALL and AML clinical series, often show evidence of mixed lineage (35,88,89). Certain abnormal karyotypes such as the t(8;21) and t(15;17) appear to be evident only in myeloid metaphases, whereas others involve both erythroid and myeloid cells (112). These two karyotypes are associated with a high cure fraction in AML.

Evidence is accumulating that these events, while not common (5-10%) are not rare and circumstantial evidence suggests that they do have a poorer outcome than restricted lineage cases. Further data must be accumulated before the true impact of mixed lineages etc. on natural and therapeutic history of patients is known.

IV. CONCLUSION

In recent years, improved technology has sharpened the clinician's ability to characterize the type(s) of cells involved in a particular patient. Clinical and prognostic associations have been defined in many instances and karyotype, immunophenotype, ploidy, etc. are emerging as major determinants of response to treatment and survival. Some treatment-specific associations have been noted. Multivariate analysis techniques are increasingly being employed to evaluate whether these characteristics have independent predictive value or are associated with well-known, simple clinical characteristics. Recent studies of treatment have been designed based on the scores obtained after considering prognostic variables, with different treatments being assigned to high- and low-risk groups. True individualization of treatment for patients awaits the detection of treatments specific for patients where cell display unique characteristics.

REFERENCES

1. Burchenal, J. H., Heyn, R., Sutow, W. W., Freireich, E. J., Whittington, R., and Louis, J. Investigations in acute leukemia. Presented at conference on Experimental Clinical Cancer Chemotherapy, Washington, D. C., November 11, 1959. JNCI.

2. Friereich, E. J., Gehan, E. A., sulman, D., Boggs, D. R., and Frei, III, E. (1961). The effect of chemotherapy on acute leukemia in the human. *J. Chron. Dis.* 14:593-608.
3. Rowley, J. D., Alimena, G., Garson, O. M., Hagemeijer, A., Mitelman, F., and Prigogina, E. L. (1982). A collaborative study of the morphologic type of acute nonlymphocytic leukemia with patient age and karyotype. *Blood* 59:1013-1022.
4. Woods, W. G., Nesbit, M. E., Buckley, J., Lampkin, B. C., McCreadie, S., Kim, T. H., Piomelli, S., Kersey, J. H., Feig, S., Bernstein, I., and Hammond, D. (1985). Correlation of chromosome abnormalities with patient characteristics, histologic subtype, and induction success in children with acute nonlymphocytic leukemia. *J. Clin. Oncol.* 3:3-11.
5. Smith, L. J., Curtis, J. E., Messner, H. A., Senn, J. S., Furthmayr, H., and McCulloch, E. A. (1983). Lineage infidelity in acute leukemia. *Blood* 61: 1138-1145.
6. Stass, S., and Mirro, J. (1985). Unexpected heterogeneity in acute leukemia: Mixed lineages and lineage switch. *Human Pathol.* 16:864-866.
7. Bennett, J. M., Catovsky, D., Daniel, M. T., et al. (1976). Proposals for the classification of the acute leukemias: French-American-British Cooperative Group. *Br. J. Haematol.* 33:451-458.
8. Bennett, J. M., Catovksy, D., Daniel, M. T., et al. (1982). Proposals for the classification of the myelodysplastic syndromes. *Br. J. Haematol.* 51:189-199.
9. Head, D. R., Savage, R. A., Cerezo, L., Craven, C. M., Bickers, J. N., Hartsock, R., Hosty, T. A., Saiki, J. H., Wilson, H. E., Morrison, F. S., Coltman, C. A., and Hutton, J. J. (1985). Reproducibility of the French-American-British Classification of acute leukemia: The Southwest Oncology Group experience. *Amer. J. Hematol.* 18:47-57.
10. Bennett, J. M., Catovsky, D., Daniel, M. T., Flandrin, G., Galton, D. A. G., Gralnick, H. R., and Sultan, C. (1985). Proposed revised criteria for the classification of acute myeloid leukemia: A report of the French-American-British Cooperative Group. *Ann. Intern. Med.* 103:620-625.
11. Fourth International Workshop on Chromosomes in Leukemia, 1982 (1984). Clinical significance of chromosomal abnormalities in acute nonlymphoblastic leukemia. *Cancer Genet. Cytogenet.* 11:332-350.
12. Keating, M. J., Cork, A., Broach, Y., Smith, T. L., Walters, R. S., McCredie, K. B., Trujillo, J., and Freireich, E. J. Toward a clinically relevant cytogenetic classification of acute myelogenous leukemia. *Leukemia Research*, in press.
13. Rowley, J. D., Golomb, H. M., Vardiman, J. W. (1981). Non-random chromosome abnormalities in acute leukemia and dysmyelopoietic syndromes in patients with previously treated malignant disease. *Blood* 58:759.
14. Mitelman, F., Brandt, L., Nilsson, P. G. (1978). Relation among occupational exposure to potential mutagenic/carcinogenic agents, clinical findings, and bone marrow chromosomes in acute nonlymphocytic leukemia. *Blood* 52:1229.

15. Yunis, J. J., Brunning, R. D., Howe, R. B., and Lobell, M. (1984). High-resolution chromosomes as an independent prognostic indicator in adult acute nonlymphocytic leukemia. *N. Eng. J. Med.* 311:812-818.
16. Trujillo, J. M., Cork, A., Ahearn, M. J., Youness, E. L., and McCredie, K. B. (1979). Hematologic and cytologic characterization of 8/21 translocation acute granulocytic leukemia. *Blood* 53:695-706.
17. Rowley, J. D. and Testa, J. R. (1983). Chromosome abnormalities in malignant hematologic diseases. *Adv. Cancer Res.* 36:103-148.
18. Swirsky, D. M., Li, Y. S., Matthews, J. G., Flemans, R. J., Rees, J. K. H., and Hayhoe, F. G. J. (1984). 8;21 translocation in acute granulocytic leukaemia: cytological, cytochemical and clinical features. *Brit. J. Hematol.* 56:199-213.
19. Bernard, J., Weil, J., and Jacquillant, C. (1977). Acute promyelocytic leukemia. In *Therapy of Acute Leukemias*, E. Mandelli (ed). Lombardo Editore, Rome, p. 456.
20. Rowley, J. D., Golomb, H. M., Vardiman, J., Fukuhara, S., Dougherty, C., and Potter, D. (1977). Further evidence for a non-random chromosomal abnormality in acute promyelocytic leukemia. *Int. J. Cancer* 20:869-872.
21. VanDerBerghe, H., Louwagie, A., Boeckaert-VanOrshover, A., et al. (1980). Chromosome abnormalities in acute promyelocytic leukemia. *Ann. Intern. Med.* 92:261.
22. Kantarjian, H. M., Keating, M. J., Walters, R. S., Estey, E. H., McCredie, K. B., Smith, T. L., Dalton, W. T., Cork, A., Trujillo, J. M., and Freireich, E. J. (1986). Acute promyelocytic leukemia–M.D. Anderson Hospital Experience. *Amer. J. Med.* 80:789-797.
23. Larson, R. A., Kondo, K., Vardiman, J, W., Butler, A. E., Golomb, H. M., and Rowley, J. D. (1984). Evidence for a 15;17 translocation in every patient with acute promyelocytic leukemia. *Amer. J. Med.* 76:827-841.
24. Kantarjian, H. M., Keating, M. J., McCredie, K. B., Beran, M., Walters, R., Dalton, Jr., W. T., Hittleman, W., and Freireich, E. J. (1985). A characteristic pattern of leukemic cell differentiation without cytoreduction during remission induction in acute promyelocytic leukemia. *J. Clin. Oncol.* 3:793-798.
25. Arlin, Z., Kempin, S., Mertelsmann, R., et al. (1984). Primary therapy of acute promyelocytic leukemia: Results of amsacrine- and daunorubicin-based therapy. *Blood* 63:211-212.
26. Kantarjian, H. M., Keating, M. J., Walters, R. S., Smith, T. L., McCredie, K. B., and Freireich, E. J. Role of maintenance chemotherapy in acute promyelocytic leukemia. *Cancer*, in press.
27. Marty, M., Ganem, G., Fischer, J., et al. (1984). Leucemie aigue promyelocytaire: etude retrospective de 119 malades traites par Daunorubicine. *Nouv. Rev. Fr. Hematol.* 26:371-378.
28. Keating, M. J., McCredie, K. B., Bodey, G. P., Smith, T. L., Gehan, E., and Freireich, E. J. (1982). Improved prospects for long-term survival in adults with acute myelogenous leukemia. *JAMA* 248:2481-2486.

29. Arthur, D. C., Bloomfield, C. D. (1983). Partial deletion of the long arm of chromosome 16 and bone marrow eosinophilia in acute nonlymphocytic leukemia: A new association. *Blood* 61:994-998.
30. Le Beau, M. M., Larson, R. A., Bitter, M. A., et al. (1983). Association of an inversion of chromosome 16 with abnormal marrow eosinophils in acute myelomonocytic leukemia. *N. Engl. J. Med.* 309:630-636.
31. Holmes, R., Keating, M. J., Cork, A., Broach, Y., Trujillo, J., Dalton, Jr., W. T., McCredie, K. B., and Freireich, E. J. (1985). A unique pattern of central nervous system leukemia in acute myelomonocytic leukemia associated with inv(16)(p13q22). *Blood* 65:1071-1078.
32. Glass, J. P., Van Tassel, P., Keating, M. J., Cork, A., Trujillo, J., and Holmes, R. Central nervous system complications of a newly recognized sub-type of leukemia: AMML pericentric inversion of chromosome #16. *J. Neurol.*, in press.
33. First International Workshop on Chromosomes in Leukemia, 1977. (1978). Chromosomes in acute non-lymphocytic leukemia. *Br. J. Haematol.* 39:311.
34. Maddox, A.-M., Keating, M. J., Trujillo, J., Cork, A., Youness, E., Ahearn, M. J., McCredie, K. B., and Freireich, E. J. (1983). Philadelphia-chromosome-positive adult acute leukemia with monosomy of chromosome number seven: A subgroup with poor response to therapy. *Leuk. Res.* 7:509-522.
35. Raza, A., Minowada, J., Barcos, M., Rakowski, I., and Preisler, H. D. (1984). Ph^1-positive acute leukemia. *Eur. J. Cancer. Clin. Oncol.* 20:1509-1516.
36. Stong, R. C., Korsmeyer, S. J., Parkin, J. L., Arthur, D. C., and Kersey, J. H. (1985). Human acute leukemia cell line with the t(4;11) chromosomal rearrangement exhibits B lineage and monocytic characteristics. *Blood* 65:21-31.
37. Berger, R., Bernheim, A., Sigaux, F., Daniel, M.-T., Valensi, F., and Flandrin, G. (1982). Acute monocytic leukemia chromosome studies. *Leuk. Res.* 6: 17-26.
38. Pearson, M. G., Vardiman, J. W., Le Beau, M. M., Rowley, J. D., Cohen, M. M., and Prigogina, E. L. (1983). A new cytogenetic subset of acute nonlymphocytic leukemia: t(6;9) associated with bone marrow basophilia. American Society for Hematology. *Blood* 62 (Supplement 1):180a.
39. Smith, T. L., Gehan, E. A., Keating, M. J., and Freireich, E. J. (1982). Prediction of remission in adult acute leukemia—development and testing of predictive models. *Cancer* 50:78-84.
40. Chan, L. C., Pegram, S. M., Greaves, M. F. (1985). Contribution of immunophenotype to the classification and differential diagnosis of acute leukemia. *Lancet* 8427:475-479.
41. Griffin, J. D. (1986). The application of monoclonal antibodies for the detection and classification of AML. In *Minimal Residual Disease in Acute Leukemia*, Martinus Nijhoff Publishers, Dordrecht, The Netherlands. pp. 58-67.
42. Mertelsmann, R., Moore, M. A. S., and Clarkson, B. (1982). Leukemia cell phenotype and prognosis: An analysis of 519 adults with acute leukemia. *Blood Cells* 8:561-583.

43. Bradstock, K. F., Hoffbrand, A. V., Ganeshaguru, K., Llewellin, P., Patterson, K., Wonke, B., Prentice, A. G., Bennett, M., Pizzolo, G., Bollum, F. J., and Janossy, G. (1981). Terminal deoxynucleotidyl transferase expression in acute non-lymphoid leukaemia: an analysis by immunofluorescence. *Brit. J. Haematol.* 47:133-143.
44. Skoog, L., Hagerstrom, T., Reizenstein, P., and Ost, A. (1986). Enzyme markers in acute myeloid leukemia. *Scand. J. Haemat.* 36:25.
45. Schachner, J., Kantarjian, H., Stass, S., Keating, M., and Freireich, E. J. Lack of prognostic significance of terminal transferase positivity in acute myelogenous leukemia. Submitted to *Blood*.
46. Pui, C.-H., Costlow, M. E., Kalwinsky, D. K., and Dahl, G. V. (1983). Glucocorticoid receptors in childhood acute non-lymphocytic leukemia. *Leuk. Res.* 7:11-16.
47. Bell, R., Lillquist, A., and McCaffrey, R. (1984). Glucocorticoid receptors in leukemia cells: an appraisal. *Leuk. Res.* 8:919-928.
48. Holbrook, N. H., Bloomfield, C. D., and Munck, A. (1983). Analysis of activated and nonactivated cytoplasmic glucocorticoid-receptor complexes from human leukemia cells by rapid DNA-DEAE mini-column chromatography. *Cancer Res.* 43:4478-4482.
49. Moore, M. A. S., Spitzer, G., Williams, N., and Buckley, T. (1974). Agar culture studies in 127 cases of untreated acute leukemia: The prognostic value of reclassification of leukemia, according to in vitro growth characteristics. *Blood* 44:1-18.
50. Spitzer, G., Dicke, K. A., Gehan, E. A., Smith, T., McCredie, K. B., Barlogie, B., and Freireich, E. J. (1976). A simplified in vitro classification for prognosis in adult acute leukemia: The application of in vitro results in remission-predictive models. *Blood* 48:795-807.
51. Kirshner, J. J., Goldberg, J., Nelson, D. A., and Gottlieb, A. J. (1982). Predictive value of the CFU-C assay in acute nonlymphocytic leukemia. *Amer. J. Med.* 72:715-619.
52. Preisler, H. D., Azarnia, N., and Marinello, M. (1984). Relationship of the growth of leukemic cells in vitro to the outcome of therapy for acute nonlymphocytic leukemia. *Cancer Res.* 44:1712-1717.
53. Curtis, J. E., Messner, H. A., Hasselback, R., Elhakim, T. M., and McCulloch, E. A. (1984). Contributions of host- and disease-related attributes to the outcome of patients with acute myelogenous leukemia. *J. Clin. Oncol.* 2: 253-259.
54. Hart, J. S., George, S. L., Frei, P., Bodey, G. P., Nickerson, R. C., and Freireich, E. J. (1977). Prognostic significance of pretreatment proliferative activity in adult acute leukemia. *Cancer* 39:1603.
55. Zittoun, R., Bouchard, M., Facquet-Danis, J., Precie-du-Sett, M., and Bousser, J. (1975). Prediction of the response to chemotherapy in acute leukemia. *Cancer* 35:507.
56. Amadori, S., Petti, M. C., Mastro Vicenzo, C., Testa, M. G., Antonelli, F., and Mandelli, F. (1980). Blast cell kinetics and prognosis in acute nonlymphocytic leukemia. *Leuk. Res.* 4:239.

57. Arlin, Z. A., Fried, J., and Clarkson, B. D. (1978). Therapeutic role of cell kinetics in acute leukemia. In *Clinics in Haematology 7.* Butler and Tanner, London, pp. 339-362.
58. Hiddeman, W., Buchner, T., Andreeff, M., Wormann, B., Melamed, M. R., and Clarkson, B. D. (1982). Cell kinetics in acute leukemia: A critical re-evaluation based on new data. *Cancer* 50:250.
59. Ffrench, M., Bryon, P. A., Fiere, D., Vuvan, H., Guyotat, D., Extra, J. M., and Viala, J. J. (1986). Cell-cycle prognostic value in adult acute myeloid leukemia. The choice of the best variables. *Leuk. Res.* 10:51-57.
60. Kantarjian, H. M., Barlogie, B., Keating, M. J., Hall, R. R., Smith, T. L., McCredie, K. B., and Freireich, E. J. (1985). Pretreatment cytokinetics in acute myelogenous leukemia–Age-related prognostic implications. *J. Clin. Invest.* 76:1-6.
61. Giannoulis, N., Ogier, C., Hast, R., Lindblom, B., Sjogren, A.-M., and Reizenstein, P. (1984). Difference between young and old patients in characteristics of leukemic cells: Older patients have cells growing excessively in vitro, with low antigenicity despite high HLA-DR antigens. *Amer. J. Hematol.* 16: 113-121.
62. Green, W., Huffman, D., Wiernik, P. H., et al. (1972). High-dose daunorubicin therapy for acute nonlymphocytic leukemia: Correlation of response and toxicity with pharmacokinetics and intracellular daunorubicin reductase activity. *Cancer* 30:1419-1427.
63. Rustum, Y. M., and Preisler, H. D. (1979). Correlation between leukemic cell retention of 1-β-D-arabinosylcytosine-5'-triphosphate and response to therapy. *Cancer. Res.* 39:42-49.
64. Preisler, H. D., Epstein, J., Raza, A., Azarnia, N., Browman, G., Booker, L., Goldberg, J., Gottlieb, A., Brennan, J., Grunwald, H., Rai, K., Vogler, R., Winton, L., Miller, K., and Larson, R. (1984). Inhibition of DNA synthesis by cytosine arabinoside: Relation to response of acute nonlymphocytic leukemia to remission induction therapy and to stage of the disease. *Eur. J. Cancer Clin. Oncol.* 20:1061-1068.
65. Preisler, H. D., Azarnia, N., Raza, A., Grunwald, H., Vogler, R., Browman, G., Goldberg, J., Chervenick, P., Miller, K., Brennan, J., Winton, L., Joyce, R., and Gottlieb, A. (1984). Relationship between the per cent of marrow cells in S phase and the outcome of remission-induction therapy for acute nonlymphocytic leukaemia. *Brit. J. Haematol.* 56:399-407.
66. Plunkett, W., Iacoboni, S., Estey, E., Danhauser, L., Liliemark, J. O., and Keating, M. J. (1985). Pharmacologically directed ara-C therapy for refractory leukemia. *Seminars. Oncol.* 12:20-30.
67. Estey, E. H., Keating, M. J., Smith, T. L., McCredie, K. B., Legha, S. S., Walters, R. S., Bodey, G. P., and Freireich, E. J. (1984). Prediction of complete remission in patients with refractory acute leukemia treated with AMSA. *J. Clin. Oncol.* 2:102-106.
68. Woods, W. G., Nesbit, M. E., Buckley, J., Lampkin, B. C., McCredie, S., Kim, T. H., Piomelli, S., Kersey, J. H., Feig, S., Bernstein, I., and Hammond, D. (1985). Correlation of chromosome abnormalities with patient character-

istics, histologic subtype, and induction success in children with acute nonlymphocytic leukemia. *J. Clin. Oncol.* 3:3-11.
69. Weinstein, H. J., Mayer, R. J., Rosenthal, D. S., Coral, F. S., Camitta, B. M., and Gelber, R. D. (1983). Chemotherapy for acute myelogenous leukemia in children and adults: VAPA update. *Blood* 62:315-319.
70. Keating, M. J., Smith, T. L., McCredie, K. B., Bodey, G. P., Hersh, E. M., Gutterman, J. U., Gehan, E., and Freireich, E. J. (1981). A four-year experience with anthracycline, cytosine arabinoside, vincristine and prednisone combination chemotherapy in 325 adults with acute leukemia. *Cancer* 47: 2779-2788.
71. Miller, D. R., Leikin, S., Albo, V., Sather, H., Karon, M., and Hammond, D. (1983). Prognostic factors and therapy in acute lymphoblastic leukemia of childhood: CCG-141. *Cancer* 51:1041-1049.
72. Kalwinsky, D. K., Roberson, P., Dahl, G., Harber, J., Rivera, G., Bowman, W. P., Pui, C.-H., Ochs, J., Abromowitch, M., Costlow, M. E., Melvin, S. L., Stass, S., Williams, D. L., and Murphy, S. B. (1985). Clinical relevance of lymphoblast biological features in children with acute lymphoblastic leukemia. *J. Clin. Oncol.* 3:477-484.
73. Crist, W., Pullen, J., Boyett, J., Falletta, J., van Eys, J., Borowitz, M., Jackson, J., Dowell, B., Frankel, L., Quddus, F., Ragab, A., and Vietti, T. (1986). Clinical and biologic features predict a poor prognosis in acute lymphoid leukemias in infants: A Pediatric Oncology Group study. *Blood* 67:135-140.
74. Miller, D. R., Leikin, S., Albo, V., et al. (1981). Prognostic importance of morphology (FAB classification) in childhood acute lymphoblastic leukemia (ALL). *Brit. J. Haematol.* 48:199-206.
75. Prokocimer, M., Matzner, Y., Ben-Bassat, H., et al. (1980). Burkitt's lymphoma presenting as acute leukemia (Burkitt's Lymphoma Cell Leukemia). *Cancer* 45:2884-2889.
76. Crist, W. M., Grossi, C. E., Pullen, D. J., and Cooper, M. D. (1985). Immunologic markers in childhood acute lymphocytic leukemia. *Seminars Oncol.* 12:105-121.
77. Crist, W. M., Boyett, J., Roper, M., et al. (1984). Pre B-cell leukemia responds poorly to treatment: A Pediatric Oncology Group study. *Blood* 63:407-414.
78. Carroll, A. J., Crist, W. M., Parmley, R. T., et al. (1984). Pre B-cell leukemia associated with chromosome translocation 1;19. *Blood* 63:721-724.
79. Williams, D. L., Look, A. T., Melvin, S. L., et al. (1984). New chromosomal translocations correlate with specific immunophenotypes of childhood acute lymphoblastic leukemia. *Cell* 36:101-109.
80. Morgan, E., and Hsu, C. C. S. (1980). Prognostic significance of the acute lymphoblastic leukemia (ALL) cell-associated antigen in children with null-cell ALL. *Amer. J. Ped. Hematol. Oncol.* 2:99-102.
81. Pullen, D. J., Boyett, J. M., Crist, W. M., et al. (1984). Pediatric Oncology Group utilization of immunologic markers in the designation of acute lymphocytic leukemia (ALL) sub-groups. Influence on treatment response. *Ann. N.Y. Acad. Sci.* 428:262.

82. Pullen, D. J., Sullivan, M. P., Falletta, J. M., et al. (1982). Modified LSA2-L2 treatment in 53 children with E-rosette-positive T-cell leukemia: results and prognostic factors. (A Pediatric Oncology Group study) *Blood* 60:1159-1168.
83. Levin, S., Russell, E. C., Blanchard, E., et al. (1980). Receptors for peanut agglutinin (*Arachus hypogea*) in childhood acute lymphoblastic leukemia: Possible clinical significance. *Blood* 55:37-39.
84. Esher, E. C., Movassaghi, N., and Leikin, S. L. (1978). Surface membrane determinants on childhood acute lymphocytic leukaemia cells: Immunoglobulin, Fc and C3 receptors. *Clin. Exp. Immunol.* 32:523-530.
85. Richie, E. R., Culbert, S. J., Sullivan, M. P., et al. (1978). Complement receptor-positive, sheep erythrocyte receptor-negative lymphoblasts in childhood acute lymphocytic leukemia. *Cancer Res.* 38:3616-3620.
86. Third International Workshop on Chromosomes in Leukemia, 1980. (1981). *Cancer Genet. Cytogenet.* 4:96-137.
87. Williams, D. L., Tsiatis, A., Brodeur, G. M., Look, A. T., Melvin, S. L., Bowman, W. P., Kalwinsky, D. K., Rivera, G., and Dahl, G. V. (1982). Prognostic importance of chromosome number in 136 untreated children with acute lymphoblastic leukemia. *Blood* 60:864-871.
88. Parkin, J., Abrahamson, C., McKenna, R., Heideman, R., Kersey, J., Brunning, R. (1981). t(4;11) acute leukemia: ultrastructural and immunological evidence for a myeloid progenitor cell proliferation. *Blood* 60:1321.
89. Nagasaka, M., Maeda, S., Maeda, H., Chen, H. L., Kita, K., Mabuchi, O., Misu, H., Matsuo, T., Sugiyama, T. (1983). Four cases of t(4;11) acute leukemia and its myelomonocytic nature in infants. *Blood* 61:1174.
90. Look, A. T., Melvin, S. L., Williams, D. L., Brodeur, G. M., Dahl, G. V., Kalwinsky, D. K., Murphy, S. B., and Mauer, A. M. (1982). Aneuploidy and percentage of S-phase cells determined by flow cytometry correlate with cell phenotype in childhood acute leukemia. *Blood* 60:959-967.
91. Look, A. T. (1985). The emerging genetics of acute lymphoblastic leukemia: Clinical and biologic implications. *Seminars Oncol.* 12:92-104.
92. Pui, C.-H., Ochs, J., Kalwinsky, D. K., and Costlow, M. E. (1984). Impact of treatment efficacy on the prognostic value of glucocorticoid receptor levels in childhood acute lymphoblastic leukemia. *Leuk. Res.* 8:345-350.
93. Pui, C.-H., Dahl, G. V., Rivera, G., Murphy, S. B., and Costlow, M. E. (1984). The relationship of blast cell glucocorticoid receptor levels to response to single-agent steroid trial and remission response in children with acute lymphoblastic leukemia. *Leuk. Res.* 8:579-585.
94. Quddus, F. F., Leventhal, B. G., Boyett, J. M., Pullen, D. J., Crist, W. M., and Borowitz, M. J. (1985). Glucocorticoid receptors in immunological subtypes of childhood acute lymphocytic leukemia cells: A Pediatric Oncology Group study. *Cancer Res.* 45:6482-6486.
95. Dow, L. W., Chang, L. J. A., Tsiatis, A. A., Melvin, S. L., and Bowman, W. P. (1982). Relationship of pretreatment lymphoblast proliferative activity and prognosis in 97 children with acute lymphoblastic leukemia. *Blood* 59:1197-1202.

96. Scarffe, J. H., Hann, I. M., Evans, D. I. K., Jones, P. M., Palmer, M. K., Lilleyman, J. S., and Crowther, D. (1980). Relationship between the pretreatment proliferative activity of marrow blast cells and prognosis of acute lymphoblastic leukaemia of childhood. *Brit. J. Cancer* 41:764-771.
97. Dormer, P., Ucci, G., Lau, B., Haas, R. J., and Janka, G. E. (1984). In vivo production of childhood acute lymphoblastic leukemia cells in relation to ploidy and immunological subtype. *Leuk. Res.* 8:587-595.
98. Hoelzer, D. (1984). Current status of ALL/AUL therapy in adults. *Recent Results in Cancer Res.* 93:182-203.
99. Jacobs, A. D., and Gale, R. P. (1984). Recent advances in the biology and treatment of acute lymphoblastic leukemia in adults. *New Eng. J. Med.* 311:1219-1231.
100. Clarkson, B., Ellis, S., Little, C., Gee, T., Arlin, Z., Mertelsmann, R., Andreeff, M., Kempin, S., Koziner, B., Chaganti, R., Jhanwar, S., McKenzie, S., Cirrincione, C., and Gaynor, J. (1985). Acute lymphoblastic leukemia in adults. *Seminars Oncol.* 12:160-179.
101. Bennett, J. M., Catovsky, D., Daniel, M. T., Flandrin, G., Galton, D. A. G., Gralnick, H. R., and Sultan, C. (1981). The morphological classification of acute lymphoblastic leukaemia: Concordance among observers and clinical correlations. *Brit. J. Haematol.* 47:553.
102. Brearly, R. L., Johnson, S. A. N., and Lister, T. A. (1975). Acute lymphoblastic leukemia in adults: Clinico-pathological correlations with the French-American-British (FAB) Co-operative Group classification. *Eur. J. Cancer* 15:905.
103. Greaves, M. F., and Lister, T. A. (1981). Prognostic importance of immunologic markers in adult acute lymphoblastic leukemia. *New Eng. J. Med.* 304:119-120.
104. Baccarani, M., Corbelli, G., Amadori, A., et al. (1982). Adolescent and adult acute lymphoblastic leukemia: prognostic features and outcome of therapy: a study of 293 patients. *Blood* 60:677-684.
105. Sobol, R. E., Royston, I., LeBien, T. W., Minowada, J., Anderson, K., Davey, F. R., Cuttner, J., Schiffer, C., Ellison, R. R., and Bloomfield, C. D. (1985). Adult acute lymphoblastic leukemia phenotypes defined by monoclonal antibodies. *Blood* 65:730-735.
106. Hoelzer, D., Thiel, E., Loffler, H., Bodenstein, H., Plaumann, L., Buchner, T., Urbanitz, D., Koch, P., Heimpel, H., Engelhardt, R., Muller, U., Wendt, F.-C., Sodomann, H., Ruhl, H., Herrmann, F., Kaboth, W., et al. (1984). Intensified therapy in acute lymphoblastic and acute undifferentiated leukemia in adults. *Blood* 64:38-47.
107. McCulloch, E. A. (1983). Stem cells in normal and leukemia hemopoiesis (Henry Stratton Lecture, 1982). *Blood* 62:1-13.
108. Greaves, M. F., Chan, L. C., Furley, A. J. W., Watt, S. M., and Molgaard, H. V. (1986). Lineage promiscuity in hemopoietic differentiation and leukemia. *Blood* 67:1-11.
109. Neame, P. B., Soamboonsrup, P., Browman, G., Barr, R. D., Saeed, N., Chan, B., Pai, M., Benger, A., Wilson, W. E. C., Walker, I. R., and McBride,

J. A. (1985). Simultaneous or sequential expression of lymphoid and myeloid phenotypes in acute leukemia. *Blood* 65:142-148.

110. Ferraris, A. M., Raskind, W. H., Bjornson, B. H., Jacobson, R. J., Singer, J. W., and Fialkow, P. J. (1985). Heterogeneity of B cell involvement in acute nonlymphocytic leukemia. *Blood* 66:342-344.
111. Rovigatti, U., Mirro, J., Kitchingman, G., Dahl, G., Ochs, J., Murphy, S., and Stass, S. (1984). Heavy chain immunoglobulin gene rearrangement in acute nonlymphocytic leukemia. *Blood* 63:1023-1027.
112. Berger, R., Bernheim, A., Daniel, M. T., Valensi, F., and Flandrin, G. (1983). Cytological types of mitoses and chromosome abnormalities in acute leukemia. *Leuk. Res.* 7:221-236.

Index

T

U

W

X